MEDICAL RADIOLOGY

Diagnostic Imaging

Editors:
A. L. Baert, Leuven
M. Knauth, Göttingen
K. Sartor, Heidelberg

E. J. Balthazar · A. J. Megibow · R. Pozzi Mucelli (Eds.)

Imaging of the Pancreas

Acute and Chronic Pancreatitis

With Contributions by

G. Armatura · M. A. Bali · E. J. Balthazar · P. A. Banks · D. Bar-Sagi · C. Bassi · C. Biasiutti
L. Boninsegna · C. Bruno · G. Butturini · C. Calciolari · P. Capelli · G. Carbognin
G. Cavallini · D. Cenzi · L. Cereser · D. Coser · M. Delhaye · D. L. Diehl · M. D'Onofrio
N. Faccioli · M. Falconi · G. Foti · F. Franzoso · L. Frulloni · R. Graziani · A. Guarise
E. M. Hecht · P. Kingman · G. Klöppel · R. S. Kwon · J. Mallen-St. Clair · G. Mansueto
C. Matos · A. J. Megibow · S. Minniti · G. Morana · K. J. Mortele · M. Neri · P. Pederzoli
R. Pozzi Mucelli · R. Sante Murano · N. Sartori · G. Schenal · P. Shamamian
A. Tognolini · G. Zamboni

Foreword by

A.L. Baert

With 335 Figures in 873 Separate Illustrations, 69 in Color and 47 Tables

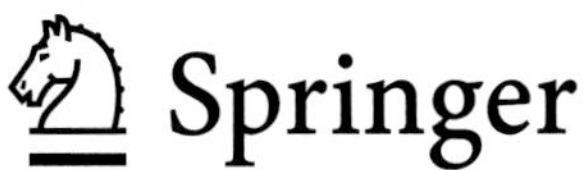
Springer

Emil J. Balthazar, MD
Professor, Department of Radiology
Bellevue Hospital
NYU-Langone Medical Center
Room 3W37
462 First Avenue
New York, NY 10016
USA

Roberto Pozzi Mucelli, MD
Professor, Department of Radiology
Policlinico "GB Rossi"
University of Verona
Piazzale LA Scuro 10
37134 Verona
Italy

Alec J. Megibow, MD, MPH, FACR
Professor, Department of Radiology
NYU-Langone Medical Center
550 First Avenue
New York, NY 10016
USA

Medical Radiology · Diagnostic Imaging and Radiation Oncology
Series Editors:
A. L. Baert · L. W. Brady · H.-P. Heilmann · M. Knauth · M. Molls · C. Nieder · K. Sartor

Continuation of Handbuch der medizinischen Radiologie
Encyclopedia of Medical Radiology

ISBN 978-3-540-00281-9 eISBN 978-3-540-68251-6

DOI 10.1007/978-3-540-68251-6

Medical Radiology · Diagnostic Imaging and Radiation Oncology ISSN 0942-5373

Library of Congress Control Number: 2006935427

Cover design and Layout: PublishingServices Teichmann, 69256 Mauer, Germany

Printed on acid-free paper

9 8 7 6 5 4 3 2 1 0

springer.com

Dedication for

Professor Carlo Procacci
(1950–2004)

Scholar, leader, friend.

Foreword

This second volume on modern multimodality pancreatic imaging deals with acute and chronic pancreatitis and pancreatic trauma. It comprehensively covers the diagnostic and interventional radiological techniques employed today in the management of patients with lesions related to one of these conditions.

As with the first volume, which deals with cystic and rare tumors of the pancreas, the various chapters are written by authors from both sides of the Atlantic, all internationally recognized experts in their particular field of interest. Their contributions, illustrated by high-quality images and figures, represent the state-of-the-art methods in pancreatic radiology.

I am particularly indebted to the editors, E. J. Balthazar, A. J. Megibow and R. Pozzi-Mucelli, for their great efforts in preparing this superb volume, which should be considered as the standard reference handbook on imaging of acute and chronic pancreatitis and pancreatic trauma for general and abdominal radiologists, gastroenterologists and abdominal surgeons. It will undoubtedly be of great help to guide them in the correct diagnostic and therapeutic decisions for their patients.

I am particularly grateful to R. Pozzi-Mucelli, who kindly accepted to take over the editor's task from our sadly deceased C. Procacci.

I am convinced that this outstanding work will meet with the same success as the first volume on cystic and rare tumors of the pancreas previously published in this series.

Leuven Albert L. Baert

Preface

Pancreatitis is a ubiquitous disease. Although it is more prevalent in developed countries, accounting for approximately 210,000 yearly hospital admissions in the US, the wide variety of causes accounts for it being seen in every country. Even though it is an old affliction, its clinical and pathologic manifestations were not recognized until late in the 19th and early 20th century. Seminal articles by CHIARI (1896), FITZ (1889) on acute pancreatitis and COMFORT 1946 on chronic pancreatitis defined the distinctive features of these related but separate clinical entities.

The radiologic evaluation of patients with these disorders paralleled the increasing clinical sophistication and, important to our current volume, the rapid technological advances as related to imaging. The modern era of pancreatic imaging began with the introduction of gray-scale ultrasound in the early 1970s and computed tomography (CT) in the mid 1970s. Pancreatic imaging progressed rapidly in the last two decades of the 20th century, specifically related to the appreciation of information provided by the proper use of iodinated intravenous contrast materials for both CT and magnetic resonance imaging (MRI). The development of multidetector-row CT (MDCT), advances in MRI beyond spin-echo techniques and of endoscopic ultrasound further improved and accelerated this trend. In addition to improving imaging diagnosis of pancreatitis and its complications, imaging techniques serve as a platform for increasingly innovative minimally invasive interventional therapies.

The present volume describes and illustrates the contributions, strengths and limitations of state-of-the-art imaging modalities used to diagnose and evaluate patients with pancreatitis and its abdominal complications. Additionally, we attempt to frame the imaging contributions in the context of what information is needed to make clinical decisions. The reader will notice several unavoidable overlapping opinions reflecting different points of view, distinct idiosyncratic experiences and various conflicting bibliographic references. This serves our purpose in providing a compendium of a variety of approaches to these complex patients. We are indebted to our eclectic experts, all recognized and experienced pancreatologists from Europe and the US, who contributed to this monograph.

This project has taken a significantly longer time to bring to publication than originally intended. While the editors bear the ultimate responsibility for timeliness of final publication, the effect of the untimely death of Professor Carlo Procacci of Verona cannot be minimized. The cruel irony that Professor Procacci was taken from us by pancreatic cancer is not lost. Professor Procacci conceived this project in 2000; he succumbed to his disease on January 1, 2004 at far too young an age. The appointment of Professor Roberto Pozzi-Mucelli at the Policlinico G. Rossi is guaranteed to sustain the contributions of this center to the world's knowledge of pancreatic disease.

A special note of thanks goes to our publisher, Springer-Verlag, to our editor, Ursula Davis, whose patience is truly remarkable, to the copy editors who worked hard to prepare the manuscripts and assure the illustrations are of the highest quality, and finally to Professor Albert Baert, who along with Professor Klaus Sartor are the "Diagnostic Imaging" series editors. Professor Baert's gentle and kindly encouragements along the way never failed to remind us of his belief in the potential value of this particular work.

New York — Emil J. Balthazar
New York — Alec J. Megibow
Verona — Roberto Pozzi Mucelli

Chiari H (1896) Ueber Selbstverdauung des menschlichen Pankreas. Zeitschrift fuer Heilkunde 17:69–96

Comfort MW, Gambill EE. Baggentoss AH (1945) Chronic relapsing pancreatitis: a study of twenty-nine cases without associated disease of the biliary or gastro-intestinal tract. Gastroenterology 4:239-85, 376–408

Fitz RH (1889) Acute pancreatitis: a consideration of pancreatic hemorrhage, hemorrhagic, suppurative, and gangrenous pancreatitis, and of disseminated fat necrosis. Boston Med Surg J 120:181–187

Contents

Acute Pancreatitis 1

1 Pathophysiology of Acute Pancreatitis
Peter Shamamian, Peter Klingman, John Mallen-St. Clair, and Dafna Bar-Sagi 3

2 Clinical Aspects of Acute Pancreatitis: Features, Prognosis and Use of Imaging Findings in Therapeutic Decision Making
Richard S. Kwon, Koenraad J. Mortele and Peter A. Banks 15

3 The Role of Ultrasound in Acute Pancreatitis
Costanza Bruno, Salvatore Minniti and Giacomo Schenal 33

4 The Role of Computed Tomography
Emil J. Balthazar 49

5 Magnetic Resonance Imaging of Acute Pancreatitis
Elizabeth M. Hecht 79

Pancreatic Trauma 105

6 Pancreatic Trauma
Alec J. Megibow 107

Chronic Pancreatitis 115

7 Pathophysiology of Chronic Pancreatitis
Giorgio Cavallini and Luca Frulloni 117

8 Clinical Aspects of Chronic Pancreatitis: Features and Prognosis
Luca Frulloni and Giorgio Cavallini 129

9 The Role of Ultrasound
Mirko D'Onofrio 139

10 The Role of Computed Tomography
Rossella Graziani, Daniela Cenci, Francesca Franzoso, Daniela Coser and Marinella Neri 149

11 The Role of MR Imaging
LORENZO CERESER, MARIA ANTONIETTA BALI, MYRIAM DELHAYE, and CELSO MATOS 183

12 The Role of Endoscopic Retrograde Cholangiopancreatography (ERCP)
MYRIAM DELHAYE 209

Complications of Acute and Chronic Pancreatitis 229

13 Pathology of Chronic Pancreatitis
GIUSEPPE ZAMBONI, PAOLA CAPELLI, and GÜNTER KLÖPPEL 231

14 Clinical Aspect of Complications: Features and Prognoses
CLAUDIO BASSI, GIOVANNI BUTTURINI, NORA SARTORI, MASSIMO FALCONI, and PAOLO PEDERZOLI 261

15 Imaging of Pancreatic Pseudocyst
GIOVANNI CARBOGNIN, CARLO BIASIUTTI, CHIARA CALCIOLARI. GIOVANNI FOTI, and ROBERTO POZZI MUCELLI 269

16 Imaging of Biliary and Vascular Complications
GIANCARLO MANSUETO, DANIELA CENCI, GIULIA ARMATURA, RICARDO SANTE MURANO, and ALESSIA TOGNOLINI 295

17 Imaging of Local Extension and Fistulas
GIOVANNI CARBOGNIN, CHIARA CALCIOLARI, and GIOVANNI FOTI 311

18 Chronic Pancreatitis vs Pancreatic Tumors
ALESSANDRO GUARISE, NICCOLO' FACCIOLI, GIOVANNI MORANA, and ALEC J. MEGIBOW 329

19 The Role of Endoscopy in Acute and Chronic Pancreatitis
DAVID L. DIEHL 371

20 Surgical and Interventional Perspective in Chronic Pancreatitis
MASSIMO FALCONI, LETIZIA BONINSEGNA, NORA SARTORI, CLAUDIO BASSI, and PAOLO PEDERZOLI 383

Subject Index 391

List of Contributors 399

Acute Pancreatitis

Pathophysiology of Acute Pancreatitis

1

Peter Shamamian, Peter Kingman, John Mallen-St. Clair, and Dafna Bar-Sagi

CONTENTS

1.1 **Introduction** *3*

1.2 **Etiology** *3*
1.2.1 Mechanical Etiology *4*
1.2.1.1 Biliary Calculi *4*
1.2.1.2 Pancreatic Obstruction from Neoplasm and Ascariasis *4*
1.2.1.3 Congenital Anomalies – Pancreas Divisum *5*
1.2.1.4 Trauma *5*
1.2.2 Metabolic Etiology *5*
1.2.2.1 Alcohol *5*
1.2.2.2 Hypertriglyceridemia *6*
1.2.2.3 Hypercalcemia *6*
1.2.2.4 Post Cardiac Surgery *7*
1.2.3 Miscellaneous Etiologies *7*

1.3 **Biochemical Pathogenesis of Acute Pancreatitis** *7*
1.3.1 Enzyme Co-localization and Mediators of Inflammation *7*
1.3.2 Mediators of Inflammation in Acute Pancreatitis *9*
1.3.3 Systemic Manifestations of Inflammation in Acute Pancreatitis *11*

References *12*

P. Shamamian, MD
Department of Surgery, Medical University of South Carolina, Charleston, South Carolina 29425, USA
P. Kingman, MD
Department of Surgery, Memorial Sloan-Kettering Cancer Center, New York, NY 10021, USA
J. Mallen-St. Clair, BA, MSc
D. Bar-Sagi, PhD
Department of Biochemistry, NYU-Langone Medical Center, 550 First Avenue, New York NY 10016, USA

1.1 Introduction

Acute pancreatitis is a common clinical entity that follows a variable course ranging from mild abdominal pain to multisystem organ failure and death. There are numerous known causes of acute pancreatitis, all of which are thought to precipitate the disease by causing acinar cell injury. Although acinar injury may be a common trigger for pancreatitis, the mechanisms linking causal entities to induction of cellular injury remain unclear. Similar to the variability of clinical presentation, the pattern of pancreatic pathology following injury can manifest in many ways including: simple edema, necrosis, pseudocysts, and abscesses.

1.2 Etiology

Acute pancreatitis can be triggered by a mechanical, metabolic, vascular, or infectious event (Table 1.1). Although the molecular mechanisms responsible for the induction of pancreatitis for each of these causes remain elusive, leading theories have been gaining evidence and will be discussed subsequently. Gallstone disease and chronic ethanol abuse account for greater than 80% of cases of acute pancreatitis; however, the incidence of pancreatitis in patients with these conditions is low (5%–10%) suggesting that additional co-factors are necessary to precipitate pancreatitis. Idiopathic causes are common and apply to patients with confirmed pancreatitis in which a causative agent cannot be identified. Regardless of the etiology, the clinical manifestations of acute pancreatitis are remarkably similar, suggesting that the pathogenesis involves a common pathway.

Table 1.1. Etiologies of clinical acute pancreatitis. [Modified from CAPPELL (2008); GREENBERGER and TOSKES (2008)]

Common etiologies
- Biliary calculi and sludge (Sect. 1.2.1.1)
- Alcoholism (Sect. 1.2.2.1)
- Hypertriglyceridemia (Sect. 1.2.2.2)
- Endoscopic retrograde cholangiopancreatography
- Traumatic Pancreatitis

Drug-induced (Sect. 1.2.3)
- Azathioprine
- 6-MP
- Sulfonamides
- Estrogens
- Tetracycline
- Anti-epileptic
- Anti Retroviral
- Furosemide

Hypercalcemia with or without hyperparathyroidism (Sect. 1.2.2.3)
Posterior penetrating duodenal ulcer
Scorpion venom
Uncommon etiologies
- Ischemia/vasculitis (hypoperfusion)
- Pancreatic cancer (histologic evidence is present in many cases)
- Pancreas divisum

Genetic/hereditary (Sect. 1.2.3)
Cystic fibrosis
Infections (Sect. 1.2.3)
- Ascariasis
- Mumps
- Coxsackievirus
- Herpetic/CMV (HIV patients)

1.2.1 Mechanical Etiology

The common inciting event in pancreatitis with a mechanical etiology is pancreatic duct obstruction. Gallstones, tumors, pancreas divisum, ascariasis, and trauma can all result in obstructive pancreatitis. Pancreatic ductal epithelial cells function to convey digestive enzymes in an inactive zymogen state from acinar cells to the duodenum where the enzymes are cleaved to an active form by enterokinase. Cells that line the pancreatic ducts secrete water, bicarbonate, and mucus to minimize activation of the transported enzymes. Fat and protein in the duodenum induce cholecystokinin (CCK) secretion from small intestine mucosal endocrine cells, which in turn leads to the release of inactive digestive enzymes from the acinar cells. When the pancreatic duct is obstructed, acinar cells continue secreting digestive enzymes against a closed system. It is thought that ultimately, intrinsic protective mechanisms to prevent zymogen activation are overwhelmed, resulting in the premature activation of the digestive enzymes, which in turn leads to acinar cell injury and pancreatitis. (GRADY et al. 1992; SAKORAFAS and TSIOTOU 2000; LIGHTNER and KIRKWOOD 2001).

1.2.1.1 Biliary Calculi

It is generally accepted that gallstone-induced pancreatitis results from a gallstone migrating through the ampulla of Vater. Several mechanisms have been proposed to explain how the migrating stone can cause inflammation of the pancreas. The most likely explanation for the pathogenesis of gallstone pancreatitis is that as stone passes through the ampulla it either directly occludes the pancreatic duct by impaction or indirectly leads to pancreatic duct hypertension by creating inflammation and edema of the ampulla as the stone passes (MOODY et al. 1990). Other theories that have been put forth suggest that bile reflux into the pancreatic duct activates pancreatic enzymes and leads to pancreatic inflammation. The once popular common channel hypothesis suggested that a stone impacts in the ampulla causing bile to reflux through the common channel that exists between the distal ends of the pancreatic and common bile ducts (CBD) has been called into question because normally there is higher resting pressure in the pancreatic duct compared to the CBD. Additionally, pancreatic zymogens are activated by bile only after at least 8–12 h of incubation time. There are also reports that 20% of the general population has separate common bile duct and pancreatic duct openings (ARENDT et al. 1999).

A study examining potential unidentified causes of idiopathic acute pancreatitis found that 73% of these patients had biliary sludge or microlithiasis. The authors hypothesized that over 75% of idiopathic attacks of acute pancreatitis are, in fact, caused by microscopic gallstones that were not detected using standard radiological techniques (ROS et al. 1991). Treating these patients with cholecystectomy has proven to decrease the rate of recurrence of acute pancreatitis, suggesting that the rates of gallstone pancreatitis may be globally underestimated.

1.2.1.2 Pancreatic Obstruction from Neoplasm and Ascariasis

Pancreatic neoplasms cause approximately 3% of acute pancreatitis cases with a wide range of severity. The etiology of neoplasm-associated pancreatitis is thought to result from an obstructed or stenotic pancreatic duct that leads to an increase in pressure distal to the obstruction. Evidence suggests that any pancreatic lesions, benign, malignant, solid or cystic can be a potential cause of pancreatitis. Thus, neoplastic lesions of the pancreas must be considered in all idiopathic cases, it is important to note the potential requirement for repeat imaging after the acute inflammation has resolved as surrounding inflammation makes CT diagnosis of a carcinoma more difficult (Grendell 1990).

It should be stressed that any insult which causes obstruction of the pancreatic duct can induce acute pancreatitis. For example, ascariasis, the most common helminth worldwide, is the second most common cause of acute pancreatitis in India. The worms move into the ampulla and block drainage from both the pancreatic and CBD. It is rare to find pancreatic duct invasion by ascariasis, due to the narrow duct lumen. Presence of ascariasis can be diagnosed by ultrasound demonstrating tubular structures in the ducts and ERCP can aid in the diagnosis and extraction of invading worms (Khuroo et al. 1992).

1.2.1.3 Congenital Anomalies – Pancreas Divisum

ERCP and autopsy studies demonstrate pancreas divisum in up to 10% of the population. Pancreas divisum occurs when non-fusion of the dorsal and ventral ducts results in a dominant dorsal duct that collects the majority of pancreatic secretions and drains through a patent minor papilla. The smaller ventral duct collects secretions from the inferior portion of the head of the pancreas and the uncinate process and drains via the ampulla of Vater. Several clinical studies support the conclusion that pancreas divisum predisposes some patients to acute pancreatitis, but the majority of patients with pancreas divisum have no symptoms throughout their lifetime, in fact it is estimated that only 5% of patients with pancreas divisum develop acute pancreatitis. One hypothesis about the etiology of pancreatitis resulting from pancreas divisum is that in the setting of a stenotic lesser papilla successful pancreatic drainage does not occur, resulting in a relative pancreatic duct obstruction. Some reports suggest that stenting the duct of Santorini can decrease the frequency of attacks of pancreatitis in these individuals (Sakorafas and Tsiotou 2000). In the absence of severe pancreatitis no therapeutic maneuvers are indicated for pancreatic divisum. If the pancreatitis is severe or there are multiple attacks, then the minor papilla may need to be stented, surgical drainage may be required, or sphincterotomy may be indicated (Grendell 1990).

1.2.1.4 Trauma

Trauma to the pancreas results from iatrogenic and external traumatic causes. Post-procedural pancreatitis can be caused by direct manipulation of the pancreas or the pancreatic duct. ERCP has a 3%–4% pancreatitis rate. If the patient has a minor papilla and an accessory pancreatic duct, these rates decrease. Of the complications that occur after ERCP 59% are mild complications, 32% are moderate, 7% are severe, and 2% are fatal. Post-ERCP pancreatitis is thought to occur when more contrast is injected than the duct can hold. Furthermore, there is animal evidence that the iodinated contrast materials, as used in imaging studies, can contribute to the severity of acute pancreatitis (Trap et al. 1999; Pezzilli et al. 2002). Factors that increase the risk of post-ERCP pancreatitis are: prior history of pancreatitis, operator inexperience, elevated injection pressures, multiple injections into the pancreatic duct, and depth of cannulation into the pancreatic duct. External pancreatic trauma, often undetected at the time of injury, can result in ductal strictures that manifest years later with chronic obstructive pancreatitis.

1.2.2 Metabolic Etiology

The common metabolic etiologies that can cause pancreatitis include excess ethanol use, hyperlipidemia, hypercalcemia, and medications.

1.2.2.1 Alcohol

There is no universally accepted hypothesis explaining the etiology of alcoholic pancreatitis. Symptoms usually develop between 2 and 10 years after initiation of heavy drinking, but acute pancreatitis can develop in some patients following brief exposure. Patients that develop alcohol-induced acute pancreatitis average a daily consumption of 100–150 g of alcohol. It has been established that the type of alcoholic beverage does not affect the risk of developing pancreatitis or the presentation of the disease

(Wilson et al. 1985). Despite the clear connection between alcohol consumption and pancreatitis, only 10%–15% of heavy alcohol users develop the disease, suggesting additional co-factors are required to trigger an attack of pancreatitis. One theory of the etiology of alcohol-induced pancreatitis is that oxidative metabolism of ethanol by alcohol dehydrogenase in the pancreas yields acetaldehyde that is toxic to acinar cells. Acetaldehyde toxicity may be direct or stem from the production of reactive oxygen species generated during metabolism that results in oxidative stress in the pancreas (Majumdar et al. 1986; Nordback et al. 1991; Altomare et al. 1996). Alternative byproducts of non-oxidative ethanol metabolism, particularly fatty acid ethyl esters (FAEE) also have deleterious effects on the pancreas. Indeed, FAEE causes pancreatic edema, acinar vacuolization and trypsinogen activation when infused in rats (Criddle et al. 2004; Criddle et al. 2006). Recent reports have suggested that alcohol may increase the inflammatory response to an episode of pancreatitis by augmenting NF-κB translocation following activation of protein kinase C (Satoh et al. 2006). Although the precise mechanism of alcohol-induced pancreatitis is still under debate, current evidence supports a model in which metabolic byproducts of ethanol metabolism either cause direct injury to pancreatic acinar cells or sensitize these cells to injury by other toxic agents.

1.2.2.2 Hypertriglyceridemia

Elevated triglycerides (>1000 mg/dl) is a well established cause of acute pancreatitis. Patients with familial type V hyperlipoproteinemia develop hypertriglyceridemia and have an increased risk of pancreatitis. Other situations that can lead to dramatic elevations in triglyceride levels occur in pregnancy, oral contraceptive use (particularly in the setting of obesity, diabetes, or pre-existing hyperlipidemia), and vitamin A treatment. Women are particularly vulnerable to developing hypertriglyceridemia-induced pancreatitis in the third trimester of pregnancy when triglyceride levels typically increase three-fold. This is clinically relevant as there is a 10%–20% mortality rate for the fetus during an attack of acute pancreatitis in the third trimester (Ramin and Ramsey 2001).

The mechanism of hypertriglyceridemia-induced pancreatitis remains under investigation. Under normal conditions, triglycerides are hydrolyzed to free fatty acids by lipase expressed on endothelial cells. These free fatty acids are normally safely conveyed to the liver by lipoproteins and albumin. One model to explain the pathogenesis of triglyceride-induced pancreatitis is that in the context of elevated triglycerides, available albumin is saturated, and pancreatic capillaries are exposed to highly cytotoxic concentrations of circulating free fatty acids that can cause vascular endothelial damage, ischemic injury and inflammation (Sakorafas and Tsiotou 2000). Genetically engineered mice that mimic hyperlipidemic conditions in humans support this model and will be useful to further elucidate the mechanisms underlying hyperlipidemia-induced pancreatitis (Wang et al. 2008).

Diagnosing hyperlipidemic pancreatitis is a challenge because patients with abdominal pain and hypertriglyceridemia often do not have elevated amylase or lipase levels, as elevated circulating lipids block the chemical determination of amylase resulting in false negative test results. Urinary amylase testing is still accurate in these patients. The treatment is to decrease TG level to <500 mg/dl. Oral pancreatic enzymes are used to decrease pancreatic stimulation and decrease abdominal pain until triglyceride levels are stabilized. The diet should then consist of polyunsaturated fat, starch and fiber (instead of sucrose) (Toskes 1990).

1.2.2.3 Hypercalcemia

The association between acute pancreatitis and hypercalcemia has long been recognized. The most common underlying cause of hypercalcemia is hyperparathyroidism; however, only 1.5% of these patients develop acute pancreatitis, suggesting that other factors are required to develop pancreatitis in the context of hypercalcemia (Bess et al. 1980). Hypercalcemia associated with malignancy has also been shown to increase the risk of acute pancreatitis (Goldberg and Herschmann 1976). One mechanism that has been proposed for calcium-induced pancreatitis is that high levels of circulating calcium result in elevated intra-cellular calcium. Research has demonstrated that elevated cytosolic calcium can facilitate premature activation of zymogen granules within the acinar cell and cause injury or death to the cell injury. More detailed information regarding the role of calcium in the induction of pancreatitis will be discussed in Sect. 1.3.

1.2.2.4
Post Cardiac Surgery

Pancreatitis is a relatively common complication of cardiac surgery. Elevations in pancreatic amylase are detected in 27% of patients following cardiac surgery; however, CT and autopsy studies suggest that the incidence is only 0.12%–5%. Acute pancreatitis following cardiac surgery is thought to be the result of ischemia caused by reductions in pancreatic blood flow during bypass and the use of pressors during surgery. Risk factors for post-operative acute pancreatitis include: the use of peri-operative calcium chloride, valve surgery, and renal insufficiency. It has also been proposed that pancreatitis following cardiac surgery may be caused by the showering of atheromatous emboli that obstructs pancreas blood flow and causes ischemia (Fernandez-del Castillo et al. 1991).

1.2.3
Miscellaneous Etiologies

Numerous medications are thought to cause pancreatitis, but the etiology remains unclear. There are multiple reports that steroids, diuretics, calcium, warfarin, cimetidine, sulfonamides, tetracyclines, clonidine, and methyldopa can cause pancreatitis. In a study of 45 German hospitals over 1 year 22/1613 patients with pancreatitis had drug-induced pancreatitis from azathioprine, sulfasalazine, ddI, estrogen, and furosemide (Lankisch et al. 1995), suggesting that medication-induced pancreatitis is a rare but significant clinical entity.

Hereditary pancreatitis is a rare inherited disease. Patients with hereditary pancreatitis usually have multiple bouts of acute pancreatitis, often starting in childhood, but presenting as late as 50 years old (Pandol et al. 2007). There is an autosomal dominant pattern, with 80% penetrance. The genetic basis of hereditary pancreatitis is a mutation in cationic trypsinogen that eliminates an autoregulatory tryptic cleavage site (Whitcomb et al. 1996). Absence of this autoregulatory cleavage site is thought to result in inappropriately elevated levels of trypsin activity within the pancreas, ultimately leading to autodigestion of the gland (Bruno 2001). The primacy of trypsin in hereditary pancreatitis has been further supported by additional recently discovered genetic causes of hereditary pancreatitis. Inactivating mutations in a serine protease inhibitor (Spink 1) that inhibits trypsin activity have been identified in a cohort of individuals with idiopathic hereditary pancreatitis (Witt et al. 2000). Finally, mutations in chymotrypsin C, an enzyme that cleaves and inactivates trypsin have also been discovered in individuals with chronic pancreatitis (Masson et al. 2008). These genetic studies suggest that mutations that increase the activity of trypsin, or decrease the effectiveness of an inhibitor of trypsin increase the risk of developing pancreatitis.

There are many infectious agents that can cause pancreatitis, including mumps, coxsackie B, Rubella, EBV, CMV, and hepatitis A and B. Two-thirds of pancreatitis cases in patients with HIV result from opportunistic infections of the pancreas. CMV is the most common causative agent; others include cryptococcus, cryptosporidium, and mycobacterium avium. Many antiretroviral medications also may cause pancreatitis, so it is important to distinguish infectious from iatrogenic causes in HIV patients (Cappell and Hassan 1993).

1.3
Biochemical Pathogenesis of Acute Pancreatitis

1.3.1
Enzyme Co-localization and Mediators of Inflammation

Clinical acute pancreatitis results from varying degrees of cellular autodigestion triggered by a wide variety of agents or events that can injure the pancreatic acinar cell; the acinar cells are actually injured by the digestive enzymes they produce (van Acker et al. 2006). A leading theory suggests that the mechanism of acinar injury is premature intracellular activation of digestive enzymes (particularly trypsin to trypsinogen) within pancreatic acini. In the healthy acinar cell, digestive enzymes are present in an *inactive* state as either pro-enzymes or zymogen granules. When stimulated by CCK, acinar cells release zymogen granules into the pancreatic ductal system where they are conveyed (in a *still* inactive state) into the duodenal lumen. Pancreatic digestive enzymes are activated in duodenum when exposed to a low pH and are processed to an active form by enterokinase. In acute pancreatitis, it is hypothesized that acinar cell injury results in inactive zymogens inappropriately co-localized with lysosomal hydrolases (such as cathepsin B) within acinar cell cytoplasmic vacuoles. These lysosomal proteases can cleave the digestive enzymes to a mature form resulting in premature trypsinogen activation within the acinar cell and cause cell injury or death (Van Acker et al. 2007) (Fig. 1.1). Further evidence to support the role of cathepsin B in promoting premature trypsin activation came from studies that demonstrated that inhibition of cathepsin B by chemical or genetic means decreases trypsin activity and reduces the severity of acute pancreatitis in mice (Van Acker et al. 2007; Halangk et al. 2000). The mechanism through which these cytoplasmic vacuoles form and result in inappropriate co-localization is unclear. One compelling theory suggests that the cytoplasmic vacuoles are autophagic in origin. This study demonstrated that autophagic vacuoles form during the induction of acute pancreatitis. Furthermore, these vacuoles form around lysosomes and secretory vesicles and provide the site of inappropriate trypsinogen activation. Interfering with the process of autophagy during the course of pancreatitis lead to a complete protection from the pathophysiological hallmarks of acute pancreatitis in this model (Hashimoto et al. 2008).

In addition to causing cellular injury, trypsin has been shown to directly stimulate cytokine production both in acinar cells and in intra-pancreatic or circulating macrophages (Hirota et al. 2006; Lundberg et al. 2000). As previously discussed, genetic evidence supports the relevance of trypsin activation in pancreatitis, as individuals with mutations that increase trypsin activity or decrease the effectiveness of a factor that inhibits trypsin activity can result in hereditary pancreatitis characterized by multiple episodes of acute pancreatitis (Teich and Mossner 2008). If premature trypsinogen activation and inappropriate protease activity are the culprit in acute pancreatitis than one would expect that inhibition of these proteases would have a beneficial effect on the course of acute pancreatitis and, in fact, protease inhibitors have been found to reduce the severity of pancreatitis in animal models and post ERCP in humans (Zyromski and Murr 2003; Whitcomb 2000).

An alternative hypothesis suggests that inappropriate secretion of digestive enzymes across the ba-

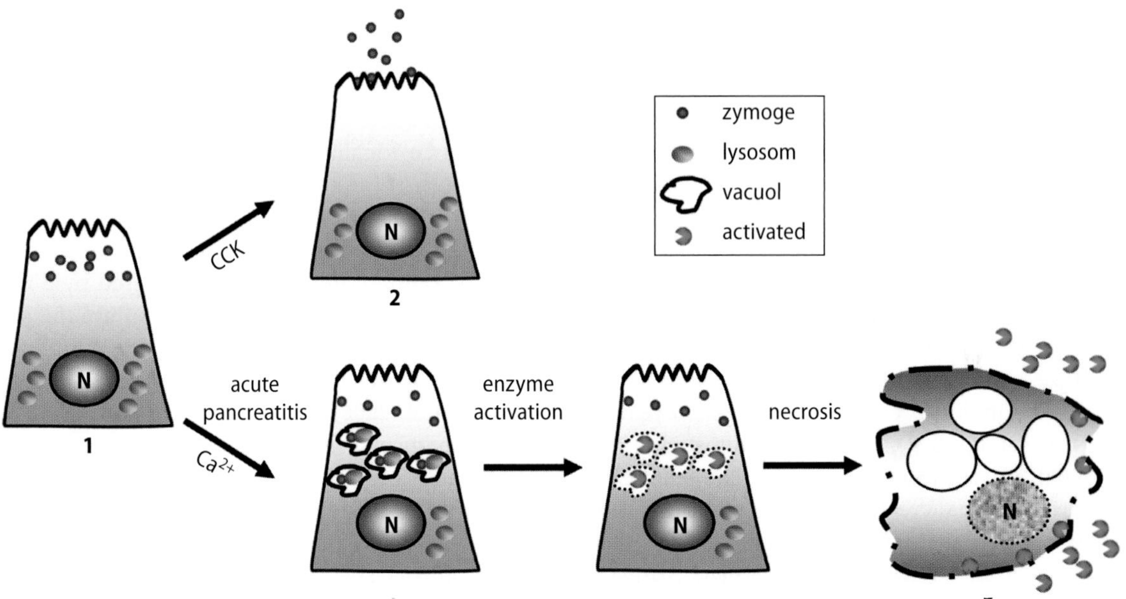

Fig 1.1. Co-localization hypothesis: In the normal pancreas, acinar cell zymogen granules are localized to the apical region, lysosomes to the basolateral region (*1*). In response to cholecystokinin (CCK) stimulation, zymogens are secreted into the ductal system where they are conveyed to the duodenum and activated (*2*). Any insult that triggers an attack of acute pancreatitis causes sustained calcium fluxes, vacuole formation, and mis-sorting of zymogens and lysosomes (*3*). Vacuoles and mis-sorted lysosomes can result in inappropriate co-localization of lysosomal hydrolases, most notably cathepsin B, which can activate digestive enzymes within the cell (*4*). Inappropriate activation of digestive enzymes results in an autodigestive process that can progress to necrotic cell death, loss of membrane integrity, and release of active enzymes into surrounding tissue (*5*)

solateral membrane of the acini into the interstitial spaces can trigger acute pancreatitis. Alterations in ductal cell permeability that allow proteases to leak through the ductal epithelium into the interstitium have also been invoked as a potential mechanism for autodigestive tissue injury in acute pancreatitis. There is less experimental evidence to support these two hypotheses. Regardless of the mechanism, it is clear that acinar injury is a critical precipitating event in the pathogenesis of acute pancreatitis and that autodigestion of the pancreas is a consequence of this injury.

A key question that remains unanswered in regards to the pathophysiology of acute pancreatitis is: what are the key cellular and molecular events that trigger co-localization, premature zymogen activation, and acinar cell necrosis? Experimental evidence suggests that calcium is one of the critical regulators of these processes. In the normal acinar cell, secretion of digestive enzymes is directly linked to CCK-mediated calcium fluxes. In a physiological setting these calcium fluxes are well controlled and follow a defined spatiotemporal pattern. A leading hypothesis suggests that precipitants of acute pancreatitis cause sustained cytosolic elevations of calcium that trigger premature activation of zymogens and subsequent necrosis (Criddle et al. 2007). All animal models of acute pancreatitis, including hyperstimulation (Raraty et al. 2000), duct ligation (Mooren et al. 2003), bile acid infusion (Kim et al. 2002), and injection of FAEE, demonstrate sustained elevations of calcium. Therapeutic attempts to reduce calcium levels using chelating agents or calcium channel blockers have been shown to block premature activation of trypsin and acinar necrosis in these models (Raraty et al. 2000), supporting a critical role for sustained calcium levels in the etiology of acute pancreatitis. Determining the molecular pathway that links elevated cytosolic calcium levels to co-localization and premature zymogen activation will be instrumental to our understanding of the pathogenesis of acute pancreatitis.

1.3.2 Mediators of Inflammation in Acute Pancreatitis

Following the initial injury phase of acute pancreatitis, a sequential inflammatory response is triggered, the severity of which can ultimately determine the outcome of the disease. Resident macrophages and acinar cells themselves trigger an intense cytokine response that ultimately leads to an influx of neutrophils and macrophages into the pancreas (Fig. 1.2).

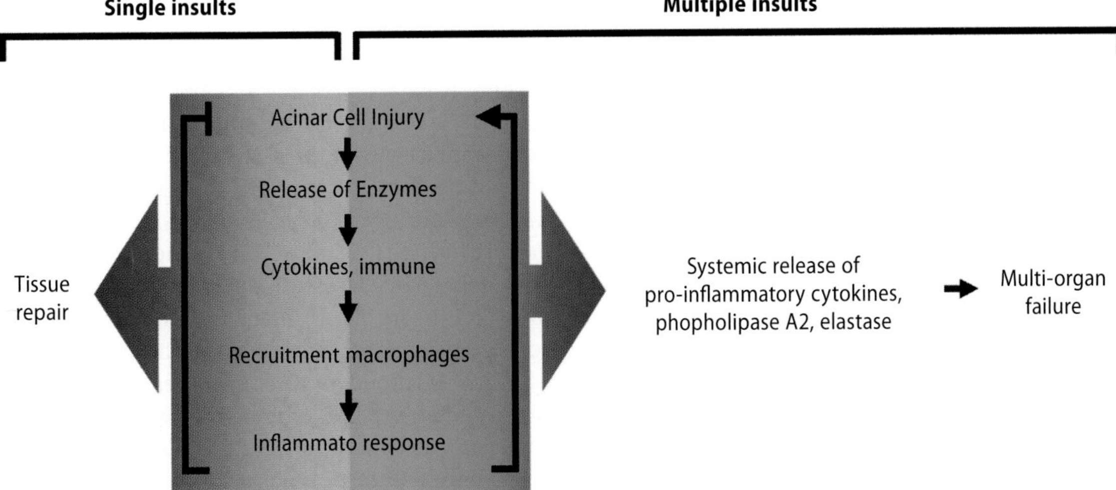

Fig. 1.2. Temporal progression of acute pancreatitis: Acinar cell injury and death is the common connection between the different types of acute pancreatitis. This injury results in the release of activated digestive enzymes from the dying cells, which triggers the secretion of cytokines from resident macrophages and acinar cells. Neutrophils and macrophages respond to these cytokines and are recruited into the pancreas. In the majority of patients the inflammation is resolved without adverse consequences (*blue arrow*). In some patients the inflammatory response results in further acinar injury, perpetuating a cycle that can ultimately result in the systemic release of pro-inflammatory cytokines, phospholipase A2, and elastase. These factors can target multiple organs including the lung, kidney, and heart and cause microvascular collapse, multi-organ failure and death (*green arrow*)

Activated neutrophils can lead to further acinar injury and zymogen activation by increasing levels of reactive oxygen species and neutrophil proteases, thus increasing the level of pancreatic damage following injury. Evidence to support the deleterious role of neutrophils has come from studies demonstrating beneficial effects on the course of animal models of pancreatitis following neutrophil depletion. Within hours of the initial insult, mononuclear cells invade the pancreas and produce multiple inflammatory mediators. There is a persistent amplification of the inflammatory response with hyperactivated inflammatory mediators such as complement, nitric oxide, free radicals, cytokines, platelet activating factor (PAF), IL-1β, MIF, IL-6, and tumor necrosis factor-α (TNF-α). In animal models, IL-1β, TNF-α, and PAF are produced within 30 min of initiation of pancreatitis (Pereda et al. 2004). Although the initial mediators derive from acinar cells and cells that have invaded the pancreas (monocytes and PMN), eventually organs such as the lungs, liver, and spleen produce additional inflammatory mediators. To summarize, acute pancreatitis causes necrosis with subsequent neutrophil influx; this is followed by infiltration of activated macrophages that release a "second wave" of cytokines that further stimulate neutrophils potentially causing organ damage. This phenomenon has been referred to as the "second attack" (Ogawa 1998).

The extent of the inflammatory phase of an episode of acute pancreatitis is dependent on the level of acinar cell damage. The effect of the inflammatory response on distant tissues results from cytokines and active proteases that are released into the circulation from the inflamed pancreas. Systemic release of cytokines can prime inflammatory responses in distant organs and proteases cause activation of elastase and phospholipase, enzymes that ultimately digest cellular membranes in distant organs. The lung is particularly susceptible to this form of cellular injury and acute respiratory distress and multiorgan failure may occur.

Induction and nuclear translocation of the transcription factors nuclear factor κB (NF-κB) and activator protein 1 (AP-1) in acinar cells and resident macrophages in the early stages of pancreatitis are thought to mediate the transcription of pro-inflammatory cytokines and chemokines that participate in recruitment of neutrophils. The cytokines IL-1β, TNF-α, IL-6, IL-8, and PAF are all thought to play a critical role in the inflammatory phase of acute pancreatitis. Other mediators implicated in disease pathogenesis in experimental models include complement, bradykinin, nitric oxide, reactive oxygen intermediates, substance P, and higher polyamines (Granger and Remick 2005). In particular, the complement and the kallikrein-kinin system become activated during the course of acute pancreatitis and cause increased vascular permeability and neutrophil accumulation.

In general, it has been thought that cytokines alone do not precipitate pancreatitis, but that they can exacerbate the course of pancreatitis by promoting cell death (Zyromski and Murr 2003); however, recent experiments have suggested that in certain contexts, cytokines can directly trigger pancreatic necrosis. Infusion of IL-12 and IL-18 in obese leptin-deficient mice have been found to precipitate massive acute pancreatitis, suggesting a potential link between the increased risk of severe acute pancreatitis and obesity (Sennello et al. 2008). These results suggest that certain risk factors can "prime" the pancreas for cytokine-mediated cellular injury.

Although there is currently some debate about whether cytokines directly or indirectly cause pancreatic injury, it is clear that cytokines can act on multiple target cells. Cytokines have the property of amplifying their own production and that of other cytokines, which can result in extremely unfortunate consequences for the host as high levels of cytokines can ultimately cause death. For example, it is known that IL-1β can cause hypotension, DIC, shock, and death. IL-6 can also cause fever. Elevated serum levels are predictive of the severity of pancreatitis, leading to the notion that IL-6 levels could be measured within the first 24 h of the clinical episode of pancreatitis to assess the need for intensive care monitoring. IL-8 levels also coincide with disease severity. IL-8 causes leukocyte degranulation and release of elastase and other enzymes. IL-1β and TNF-α are the primary inflammatory mediators of severe pancreatitis and they both induce IL-6 and IL-8. It should be noted that these cytokines are not uniformly present but are frequently elevated in serum of patients with severe disease and correlate with a poor prognosis. IL-10 is produced late during the course of acute pancreatitis and has an anti-inflammatory effect that inhibits the activity of TNF-α and IL-1β. Because of the anti-inflammatory actions of IL-10, some view this cytokine as a potential treatment to dampen cytokine production in severe acute pancreatitis (Norman 1998), and pretreatment with IL-10 has been shown to decrease the severity of pancreatitis in animal models.

Further evidence for the roles of IL-1β and TNF-α in propagating the systemic inflammatory response is demonstrated by the decrease in mortality of genetically engineered mice lacking these cytokines when subjected to models of severe acute pancreatitis (Parsons et al. 1992; Kingsnorth 1997). The importance of systemic cytokines levels in regulating severity of pancreatitis has also been validated in clinical studies demonstrating that TNF-α, TNF-α receptors, IL-6, and CRP levels are significantly higher in the first 2 days following admission in patients with acute pancreatitis that ultimately develop organ failure (de Beaux et al. 1996).

In addition to the importance of classic pro-inflammatory cytokines in acute pancreatitis numerous other inflammatory factors are involved in the pathogenesis of the disease. One such mediator is PAF, a vasodilator and leukocyte activator, and its concentrations are closely related to IL-1β and TNF-α levels. Inhibition of PAF causes a decrease in IL-1β and TNF-α. PAF is synthesized and secreted when phospholipase A2 is activated. It is an autocrine, paracrine, and endocrine mediator depending on the concentrations that are activated and released. It stimulates enzyme release from normal pancreatic tissue. When serum levels of PAF are elevated, it has similar effects to endotoxin, increasing vascular permeability in the kidneys, heart, lungs, and GI tract. In animal studies, injection of PAF into the pancreatic blood supply causes acute pancreatitis. It is implicated in both the pathogenesis of the local inflammatory response and the systemic features of the disease, probably by increasing vascular permeability and through its chemotactic properties attracting inflammatory cells to the pancreas. Activated cytokines such as PAF cause increased expression of adhesion molecules on endothelium, activation of white blood cells, and acute phase reactant production (Kingsnorth et al. 1995). Further proof of the importance of PAF to the pathologic cascade of pancreatitis is the reduction in severity of acute pancreatitis in experimental models given PAF antagonists (Kingsnorth 1997).

1.3.3 Systemic Manifestations of Inflammation in Acute Pancreatitis

The inflammatory response to acinar injury can result in multiple systemic complications including fever, acute respiratory distress syndrome (ARDS), renal failure, and myocardial depression. Fever is thought to be a direct impact of pro-inflammatory cytokines acting on the hypothalamus. Acute renal failure is thought to occur secondary to volume depletion and hypotension from increased capillary permeability. Shock and myocardial depression are thought to result from elevation of vasoactive peptides. ARDS is thought to result from microvascular thrombosis as well as phospholipase A2-mediated cleavage of lecithin, a key component of surfactant.

In addition to inflammatory mediators that are locally produced and released from the pancreas, pancreatitis can also affect the permeability of both the gut and lung. Increased intestinal permeability in pancreatitis is thought to occur secondary to hypovolemic ischemia and can cause bacterial translocation through the gut and the systemic release of endotoxin. Bacterial translocation is associated with adverse consequences and can be lethal, resulting in the infection of the pancreas or peri-pancreatic tissue. Endotoxin release can further activate the innate immune system and increase the permeability of vascular beds exacerbating hypovolemia. Clinical evidence supports an association between endotoxin levels in the peripheral circulation and severity of acute pancreatitis. Experimental evidence suggests that there is a dysfunction of the gut barrier following induction of acute pancreatitis characterized by epithelial atrophy and decreased numbers of mucosal immune cells. In the early stages of acute pancreatitis, gut pH is decreased as a result of decreased blood flow and mucosal ischemia, in later stages malnutrition can cause further mucosal epithelial atrophy. It should be noted that although serum endotoxin is detected in 90% patients that ultimately die from acute pancreatitis, it is not a prognostic indicator for mortality. Because of the adverse consequences of gut permeability in acute pancreatitis, considerable efforts have been focused on maintaining the barrier function of the intestine. There is some evidence that enteral feeding can reduce bacterial translocation and may have a beneficial impact on the course of the disease.

Lung injury is the most comprehensively studied systemic complication of acute pancreatitis and it serves as a model to elucidate the systemic inflammatory response (De Campos et al. 2007). Lung injury with pancreatitis ranges from hypoxia, pulmonary edema, and atelectasis, to ARDS. Pulmonary injury following acute pancreatitis is thought to result from increased vascular permeability leading ultimately to edema formation. PAF may regulate this process as experimental evidence has demonstrated that PAF antagonists can decrease the fluid accumulation in the lungs and capillary permeability in the pancreas itself. PAF antagonists may decrease lung injury by blocking PAF within the pancreas where it reduces acinar injury, and decreases coagulation and complement activation (Galloway and Kingsnorth 1996; Sakorafas and Tsiotou 2000).

In addition to the role of systemic inflammatory cytokines in eliciting lung damage, inflammatory cell infiltration into the lung may be directly responsible for pancreatitis-induced lung injury. The amount of lung neutrophils are increased within 4 h after the induction of pancreatitis, and depletion of neutrophils has been shown to ameliorate pancreatitis-induced lung pathology in animal models, suggesting that neutrophils are the main mediators of pulmonary endothelial injury. A current model suggests that granulocytic-mediated lung injury is exacerbated in the context of inflammatory mediators released from the pancreas and that the neutrophils from acute pancreatitis patients can produce more severe tissue damage than those from healthy donors (Paulino et al. 2007).

References

Altomare E, Grattagliano I et al. (1996) Acute ethanol administration induces oxidative changes in rat pancreatic tissue. Gut 38:742–746

Arendt T, Nizze H et al. (1999) Biliary pancreatic reflux-induced acute pancreatitis – myth or possibility? Eur J Gastroenterol Hepatol 11:329–335

Bess MA, Edis AJ et al. (1980) Hyperparathyroidism and pancreatitis. Chance or a causal association? Jama 243:246–247

Bruno MJ (2001) Current insights into the pathogenesis of acute and chronic pancreatitis. Scand J Gastroenterol Suppl (234):103–108

Cappell MS (2008) Acute pancreatitis: etiology, clinical presentation, diagnosis, and therapy. Med Clin North Am 92:889–923, ix–x

Cappell MS, Hassan T (1993) Pancreatic disease in AIDS – a review. J Clin Gastroenterol 17:254–263

Criddle DN, Raraty MG et al. (2004) Ethanol toxicity in pancreatic acinar cells: mediation by nonoxidative fatty acid metabolites. Proc Natl Acad Sci U S A 101:10738–10743

Criddle DN, Murphy J et al. (2006). Fatty acid ethyl esters cause pancreatic calcium toxicity via inositol trisphosphate receptors and loss of ATP synthesis. Gastroenterology 130:781–793

Criddle DN, McLaughlin E et al. (2007) The pancreas misled: signals to pancreatitis. Pancreatology 7:436–446

de Beaux AC, Goldie AS et al. (1996) Serum concentrations of inflammatory mediators related to organ failure in patients with acute pancreatitis. Br J Surg 83:349–353

De Campos T, Deree J et al. (2007) From acute pancreatitis to end-organ injury: mechanisms of acute lung injury. Surg Infect (Larchmt) 8:107–120

Fernandez-del Castillo C, Harringer W et al. (1991) Risk factors for pancreatic cellular injury after cardiopulmonary bypass. N Engl J Med 325:382–387

Galloway SW, Kingsnorth AN (1996) Lung injury in the microembolic model of acute pancreatitis and amelioration by lexipafant (BB-882), a platelet-activating factor antagonist. Pancreas 13:140–146

Goldberg LD, Herschmann EM (1976) Letter: hypercalcemia and pancreatitis. Jama 236:1352

Grady T, Saluja AK et al. (1992) In vivo and in vitro effects of the azidothymidine analog dideoxyinosine on the exocrine pancreas of the rat. J Pharmacol Exp Ther 262:445–449

Granger J, Remick D (2005) Acute pancreatitis: models, markers, and mediators. Shock 24[Suppl 1]:45–51

Greenberger NJ, Toskes PP (2008) Acute and chronic pancreatitis. In: Fauci AS, Braunwald E, Kasper DL, Hauser SL, Longo DL, Jameson JL, Loscalzo J (eds) Harrison's principles of internal medicine, 17th edn. McGraw-Hill Professional, New York

Grendell JH (1990) Idiopathic acute pancreatitis. Gastroenterol Clin North Am 19:843–848

Halang, W, Lerch MM et al. (2000) Role of cathepsin B in intracellular trypsinogen activation and the onset of acute pancreatitis. J Clin Invest 106:773–781

Hashimoto D, Ohmuraya M, et al. (2008) Involvement of autophagy in trypsinogen activation within the pancreatic acinar cells. J Cell Biol 181:1065–1072

Hirota M, Ohmuraya M et al. (2006) The role of trypsin, trypsin inhibitor, and trypsin receptor in the onset and aggravation of pancreatitis. J Gastroenterol 41:832–836

Khuroo MS, Zargar SA et al. (1992) Ascaris-induced acute pancreatitis. Br J Surg 79:1335–1338

Kim JY, Kim KH et al. (2002) Transporter-mediated bile acid uptake causes Ca2+-dependent cell death in rat pancreatic acinar cells. Gastroenterology 122:1941–1953

Kingsnorth A (1997) Role of cytokines and their inhibitors in acute pancreatitis. Gut 40:1–4

Kingsnorth AN, Galloway SW et al. (1995) Randomized, double-blind phase II trial of Lexipafant, a platelet-activating factor antagonist, in human acute pancreatitis. Br J Surg 82:1414–1420

Lankisch PG, Droge M et al. (1995) Drug induced acute pancreatitis: incidence and severity. Gut 37:565–567

Lightner AM, Kirkwood KS (2001) Pathophysiology of gallstone pancreatitis. Front Biosci 6: E66–76

Lundberg AH, Eubanks JW 3rd et al. (2000) Trypsin stimulates production of cytokines from peritoneal macrophages in vitro and in vivo. Pancreas 21:41–51

Majumdar AP, Vesenka GD et al. (1986) Morphological and biochemical changes of the pancreas in rats treated with acetaldehyde. Am J Physiol 250(5 Pt 1):G598–606

Masson E, Chen JM et al. (2008) Association of rare chymotrypsinogen C (CTRC) gene variations in patients with idiopathic chronic pancreatitis. Hum Genet 123:83–91

Moody FG, Calabuig R et al. (1990) Stenosis of the sphincter of Oddi. Surg Clin North Am 70:1341–1354

Mooren F, Hlouschek V et al. (2003) Early changes in pancreatic acinar cell calcium signaling after pancreatic duct obstruction. J Biol Chem 278:9361–9369

Nordback IH, MacGowan S et al. (1991) The role of acetaldehyde in the pathogenesis of acute alcoholic pancreatitis. Ann Surg 214:671–678

Norman J (1998) The role of cytokines in the pathogenesis of acute pancreatitis. Am J Surg 175:76–83

Ogawa M (1998) Acute pancreatitis and cytokines: "second attack" by septic complication leads to organ failure. Pancreas 16:312–315

Pandol SJ, AK Saluja et al. (2007) Acute pancreatitis: bench to the bedside. Gastroenterology 133:1056

Parsons PE, Moore FA et al. (1992) Studies on the role of tumor necrosis factor in adult respiratory distress syndrome. Am Rev Respir Dis 146:694–700

Paulino EC, de Souza LJ et al. (2007) Neutrophils from acute pancreatitis patients cause more severe in vitro endothelial damage compared with neutrophils from healthy donors and are differently regulated by endothelins. Pancreas 35:37–41

Pereda J, Sabater L et al. (2004) Effect of simultaneous inhibition of TNF-alpha production and xanthine oxidase in experimental acute pancreatitis: the role of mitogen activated protein kinases. Ann Surg 240:108-116

Pezzilli R, Romboli E et al. (2002) Mechanisms involved in the onset of post-ERCP pancreatitis. Jop 3:162–168

Ramin KD, Ramsey PS (2001) Disease of the gallbladder and pancreas in pregnancy. Obstet Gynecol Clin North Am 28:571–580

Raraty M, Ward J et al. (2000) Calcium-dependent enzyme activation and vacuole formation in the apical granular region of pancreatic acinar cells. Proc Natl Acad Sci U S A 97:13126–13131

Ros E, Navarro S et al. (1991) Occult microlithiasis in 'idiopathic' acute pancreatitis: prevention of relapses by cholecystectomy or ursodeoxycholic acid therapy. Gastroenterology 101:1701–1709

Sakorafas GH, Tsiotou AG (2000) Etiology and pathogenesis of acute pancreatitis: current concepts. J Clin Gastroenterol 30:343–356

Satoh A, Gukovskaya AS et al. (2006) Ethanol sensitizes NF-kappaB activation in pancreatic acinar cells through effects on protein kinase C-epsilon. Am J Physiol Gastrointest Liver Physiol 291:G432–438

Sennello JA, Fayad R et al. (2008) Interleukin-18, together with interleukin-12, induces severe acute pancreatitis in obese but not in nonobese leptin-deficient mice. Proc Natl Acad Sci U S A 105:8085–8090

Teich N, Mossner J (2008) Hereditary chronic pancreatitis. Best Pract Res Clin Gastroenterol 22:115–130

Toskes PP (1990) Hyperlipidemic pancreatitis. Gastroenterol Clin North Am 19:783–791

Trap R, Adamsen S et al. (1999) Severe and fatal complications after diagnostic and therapeutic ERCP: a prospective series of claims to insurance covering public hospitals. Endoscopy 31:125–130

van Acker GJ, Perides G et al. (2006) Co-localization hypothesis: a mechanism for the intrapancreatic activation of digestive enzymes during the early phases of acute pancreatitis. World J Gastroenterol 12:1985–1990

Van Acker GJ, Weiss E et al. (2007) Cause-effect relationships between zymogen activation and other early events in secretagogue-induced acute pancreatitis. Am J Physiol Gastrointest Liver Physiol 292:G1738–1746

Wang Y, Sternfeld L et al. (2008) Enhanced susceptibility to pancreatitis in severe hypertriglyceridemic lipoprotein lipase deficient mice and agonist-like function of pancreatic lipase in pancreatic cells. Gut 31:31

Whitcomb DC (2000) Genetic predispositions to acute and chronic pancreatitis. Med Clin North Am 84:531–547, vii

Whitcomb DC, Gorry MC et al. (1996) Hereditary pancreatitis is caused by a mutation in the cationic trypsinogen gene. Nat Genet 14:141–145

Wilson JS, Bernstein L et al. (1985) Diet and drinking habits in relation to the development of alcoholic pancreatitis. Gut 26:882–887

Witt H, Luck W et al. (2000) Mutations in the gene encoding the serine protease inhibitor, Kazal type 1 are associated with chronic pancreatitis. Nat Genet 25:213–216

Zyromski N, Murr MM (2003) Evolving concepts in the pathophysiology of acute pancreatitis. Surgery 133:235–237

Clinical Aspects of Acute Pancreatitis: Features, Prognosis and Use of Imaging Findings in Therapeutic Decision Making

2

Richard S. Kwon, Koenraad J. Mortele, and Peter A. Banks

CONTENTS

2.1 **Features of Acute Pancreatitis** *15*

2.2 **Prognosis and Severity** *16*
2.2.1 Clinical Assessment of Severity *17*
2.2.2 Laboratory Assessment of Severity *17*
2.2.3 Radiologic Assessment of Severity *19*

2.3 **Timing and Use of Imaging in Therapeutic Decision Making** *19*
2.3.1 At Time of Diagnosis *19*
2.3.1.1 Identification of Gallstones *19*
2.3.1.2 Confirmation of Acute Pancreatitis *20*
2.3.1.3 Assessment of Severity *20*
2.3.2 During the First Week and Thereafter *21*
2.3.2.1 Interstitial Pancreatitis *21*
2.3.2.2 Necrotizing Pancreatitis *22*
2.3.2.3 Infected Pancreatic Necrosis *24*
2.3.2.4 Sterile Pancreatic Necrosis *27*
2.3.2.5 Organized Necrosis *27*
2.3.3 Venous Thrombosis and Solid Organ Involvement *28*
2.3.4 Acute Hemorrhage *29*

2.4 **Summary** *30*

References *30*

R. S. Kwon, MD; P. A. Banks, MD
Center for Pancreatic Disease, Division of Gastroenterology, Brigham and Women's Hospital, Harvard Medical School, Boston, MA 02115, USA
K. J. Mortele, MD
Center for Pancreatic Disease, Department of Radiology, Division of Abdominal Imaging and Intervention, Brigham and Women's Hospital, Harvard Medical School, Boston, MA 02115, USA

Acute pancreatitis is a challenging illness characterized by abdominal pain and elevated pancreatic enzymes. In the majority of cases, acute pancreatitis is mild and resolves with conservative therapy. In 10%–20% of cases, the disease is severe and may lead to significant morbidity and mortality, usually due to multi-system organ failure or complications from infected necrosis. The challenge for clinicians is to determine quickly and accurately which patients are most likely to develop severe disease and require intensive care. In this chapter, we will briefly discuss the clinical features of acute pancreatitis, methods of assessing severity and use of imaging in patient care.

2.1 Features of Acute Pancreatitis

The main symptom of acute pancreatitis is abdominal pain which is invariably in the epigastric area but frequently diffuse in the upper abdomen. Pain associated with pancreatitis is constant with very little fluctuation. In approximately half the cases, the pain radiates to the back. The onset of pain is acute, reaching maximal levels within 30–60 min. The level of pain is strong enough to require medical evaluation and at times may be excruciating. In the majority of patients, abdominal pain is associated with nausea and vomiting.

The differential diagnosis of acute pancreatitis includes perforated peptic ulcer, cholecystitis or biliary colic, intestinal obstruction or infarction, appendicitis, inferior wall myocardial infarction, and ectopic pregnancy or ovarian torsion in women. Because many of these are medical or surgical emergencies, the correct diagnosis must be made promptly.

Low-grade fever is common. High fever may indicate cholangitis in the appropriate clinical setting. Jaundice supports the diagnosis of biliary pancreatitis. The patient may be tachypneic due to abdominal pain or diaphragmatic irritation from pancreatic exudate. Pulmonary examination may reveal signs of pleural effusion, which are usually on the left and occasionally bilateral. Cardiac examination usually shows tachycardia. Abdominal examination is characterized by epigastric or diffuse upper abdominal tenderness and minimal distension in mild cases of pancreatitis. In severe cases, the patient's abdomen may be very tender and show peritoneal signs, including rigidity and rebound tenderness. Bowel sounds are usually hypoactive due to ileus. Ecchymoses in the flanks (Grey-Turner's sign) or near the umbilicus (Cullen's sign) are rare physical findings that result from local spread of pancreatic exudate. These findings are present in only 3% of pancreatitis (Dickson and Imrie 1984). Very rare physical findings include subcutaneous fat necrosis (panniculitis) and ophthamological abnormalities including arcus lipoides, band keratopathy or retinal thrombosis, known as Purtscher's retinopathy.

The gold standard for diagnosing acute pancreatitis is a serum amylase that is elevated ≥3 times above normal (Chase et al. 1996; Steinberg et al. 1985). In a detailed analysis of prospective trials, the sensitivity and specificity of an increased amylase was 83% and 90%, respectively (Dominguez-Munoz 1999). Serum levels increase within 2 h of the onset of pain but can normalize within 3–5 days (Zieve 1996).

This test has several limitations. Serum amylase levels may be normal in acute pancreatitis if associated with hypertriglyceridemia (because of an inhibitor) (Claiven et al. 1998; Warshaw et al. 1975), if there is delayed determination of serum amylase (because it may have normalized), or if the patient has chronic pancreatitis (because baseline amylase production is already low) (Claiven et al. 1989). Also, there are numerous non-pancreatic sources of amylase, including ovaries, salivary glands, and Fallopian tubes. Hyperamylasemia in the absence of pancreatitis can also occur with intrabdominal diseases including intestinal ischemia, perforation or obstruction. It can occur in renal failure, head trauma and lung cancer.

Lipase is another pancreatic enzyme used for diagnosing acute pancreatitis. When increased three times above normal, lipase is considered a more accurate test than amylase (Chase et al. 1996). Its sensitivity and specificity are 95% and 96%, respectively, in part because there are fewer non-pancreatic sources of lipase (Dominguez-Munoz 1999). Its half-life is longer than that of amylase and, as a consequence, lipase levels remain elevated in serum longer than amylase (Tichtin et al. 1965; Tietz and Shuey 1993). Of note, the levels of either enzyme have no bearing on etiology or severity.

Serum pancreatic isoenzymes and a urinary amylase-creatinine clearance ratio have been investigated as more accurate methods to diagnose acute pancreatitis but are no more useful than serum amylase or lipase. In recent studies, urinary trypsinogen-2 measurement has shown encouraging preliminary results but is not yet commercially available (Kemppainen et al. 1997; Hedstrom et al. 2001).

2.2 Prognosis and Severity

In 1992, a multidisciplinary symposium in Atlanta proposed a clinically based classification for acute pancreatitis (Table 2.1). Mild acute pancreatitis was defined as pancreatitis with minimal or no organ dysfunction and an uneventful recovery. Severe acute pancreatitis was defined as pancreatitis with severe pathology (including pancreatic necrosis, pseudocysts, or fluid collections) and/or organ failure (renal or pulmonary insufficiency, hypotension or gastrointestinal bleeding). Pancreatic necrosis

Table 2.1. Atlanta criteria for mild and severe pancreatitis

Mild acute pancreatitis:	defined as pancreatitis with minimal organ dysfunction and an uneventful recovery.
Severe acute pancreatitis:	defined as pancreatitis associated with organ failure and/or local complications, such as necrosis, abscess, or pseudocyst; ≥3 Ranson's criteria, ≥8 APACHE II score
Organ failure:	defined as
	1. Shock: systolic blood pressure <90 mm Hg
	2. Pulmonary insufficiency: PaO_2 ≤60 mm Hg
	3. Renal failure: serum creatinine >2 mg/dL after rehydration
	4. Gastrointestinal bleeding: >500 mL/24 h

Adapted from Bradley (1993)

and multi-system organ failure are the two most important determining factors of severity.

The establishment of severity is important because it correlates with prognosis. In cases of mild pancreatitis, mortality is approximately 1%–2%. Mortality is as high as 50% in necrotizing pancreatitis associated with multi-organ failure (PEREZ et al. 2002).

The challenge for the clinician is to identify within a few hours of admission those who will progress to multi-system organ failure and to provide appropriate care, including fluid resuscitation, respiratory support, and intensive care if needed. To date, there is no ideal way to assess severity of acute pancreatitis at admission.

2.2.1 Clinical Assessment of Severity

Bedside clinical assessment, even by experts in the field, has been largely inaccurate in determining severity and predicting prognosis. MCMAHON et al. (1980) reported that only 39% of severe cases of pancreatitis were accurately predicted at presentation. However, there are several risk factors of severity at admission that can be identified at the bedside.

Age and obesity have been linked to higher severity and mortality. In one study, the mortality of patients with necrotizing pancreatitis over 70 years of age was reported to be 26.5% vs 7.8% in those under 70 years (UOMO et al. 1998). Obesity, as defined by body mass index (BMI = weight/height^2[kg/m^2]) > 30, has been shown to be a risk factor for organ failure (FUNNELL et al. 1993; PORTER and BANKS 1991) and mortality (MARTINEZ et al. 1999). A recent study reported that android fat distribution and higher waist circumference, in particular, are associated with a greater risk for developing severe acute pancreatitis (MERY et al. 2002). Obesity has a sensitivity of 63% and a specificity of 95% for predicting disease severity (FUNNELL et al. 1993). It is speculated that increased fat deposits in the peripancreatic and retroperitoneal spaces in obese patients may increase the risk of peripancreatic fat necrosis and infection (FUNNELL et al. 1993).

Information regarding past history of pancreatitis can be helpful. The first or second episodes of pancreatitis are more likely to result in severe disease than a later episode (RANSON 1997; PEREZ et al. 2002). A reasonable explanation is that the amount of viable pancreatic tissue diminishes with each episode. Also, a short interval between the onset of symptoms and medical evaluation (< 18 h) correlates with severity (BROWN et al. 2000). Presumably severe disease causes more excruciating abdominal pain that forces the patient to seek medical attention early.

Certain findings on physical exam can warn of severe disease. While present in only 1%–3% patients with pancreatitis, the presence of the Grey-Turner's sign or the Cullen's sign is associated with a higher mortality (DICKSON and IMRIE 1984).

2.2.2 Laboratory Assessment of Severity

Hemoconcentration has received recent attention as an early marker of severity and organ failure (BAILLARGEON et al. 1998; BROWN et al. 2000; LANKISCH et al. 2001a). In a retrospective study of 64 patients, Baillargeon et al. found that a hematocrit ≥47% or a failure of hematocrit to decrease in 24 h were the best factors for necrotizing pancreatitis (BAILLARGEON et al. 1998). In a later prospective study from the same institution, Brown et al. found that a hematocrit > 44% was the best predictor of necrotizing pancreatitis and organ failure (BROWN et al. 2000). A study from Germany found that a hematocrit above the gender-specific mean of normal hematocrit range correlated with pancreatic necrosis on CT but not with organ failure (LANKISCH et al. 2001a). All three studies found similarly high negative predictive values (88%–96%), indicating that in the absence of hemoconcentration, necrotizing pancreatitis rarely occurs.

Individual markers have been used to assess severity, including elevated creatinine (> 2 mg/dL) (TALAMINI et al. 1999) or hyperglycemia (> 250 mg) (BLUM et al. 2001). However, multivariable scoring systems, most notably Ranson's criteria and the APACHE II score, are the usual standards to determine severity. These tabulate markers of both systemic inflammation and organ failure.

RANSON et al. (1974) developed a scoring system to predict severity in alcoholic pancreatitis based upon 11 objective criteria (Table 2.2). Five are determined at admission and the remaining six during the next 48 h. With ≤2 positive signs, mortality was < 1% whereas with ≥6 signs, mortality was 100% (RANSON 1982). One major shortcoming of this system is that intermediate scores of 3–5 do not accurately predict the incidence of necrosis or organ

Table 2.2. Ranson's early prognostic signs

At admission or diagnosis
Age > 55 years
WBC > 16,000/mm^3
LDH > 350 IU/L
AST > 250 IU/L
Glucose > 200 mg/dL
Within 48 h
Hematocrit fall > 10%
BUN elevation > 5 mg/dL
Serum calcium < 8 mg/dL
PaO_2 < 60 mm Hg
Base deficit > 4 mEq/L
Fluid sequestration > 6 L

WBC = white blood count, LDH = lactic dehydrogenase, AST = aspartate aminotransferase, BUN= blood urea nitrogen, PaO_2 = arterial pressure of oxygen

Adapted from Ranson et al. (1974)

failure. Another is that 48 h are required to complete data collection, by which time the prognostic information may be too late to help the patient.

The Glasgow criteria were developed to simplify Ranson's criteria (Imrie et al. 1978) but still require 48 h for complete data collection. The Glasgow criteria and later modifications are generally no more accurate than Ranson's criteria.

The Acute Physiology and Chronic Health Evaluation (APACHE II) system uses 12 variables representing seven major organ systems. The advantage of the system is its ability to assess severity on admission, though it is more accurate after 48 h. An APACHE II score > 9 at 48 hs is as accurate as Ranson's criteria (Larvin and McMahon 1989; Wilson et al. 1990). The APACHE II scores can be recalculated daily and can monitor response to therapy. A major drawback to this scoring system is the need to measure many variables. The Atlanta conference defined an APACHE II score >7 at admission as severe disease but this cutoff may be too low. In a modification, obesity has been added to the list of variables (APACHE-O), which has a positive predictive value of severity of 74% when the score is >9 (Martinez et al. 1999). APACHE III decreased the number of variables but has not afforded any greater advantage (Chatzicostas et al. 2002) and may be less accurate at the early stages.

Markers of pancreatic inflammation are also available for use. C-reactive protein (CRP) is an acute phase reactant, which is a good predictor of necrosis (Uhl et al. 1991; Gross et al. 1990; de Beaux et al. 1996; Leser et al. 1991; Pezzilli et al. 1995; Viedma et al. 1994). The sensitivity and specificity are 77.5% and 75%, respectively when greater than 140 mg/dL (Puolakkainen et al. 1987). A level of > 150 mg/L is now accepted as cutoff for severe disease (Dervenis et al. 1999). The advantage of this test is its low cost and wide availability. Its main drawback is the slow increase in serum to peak levels such that the test is most useful after 36–48 h.

Increased urinary trypsinogen activation peptide (TAP), an activation peptide released during pancreatitis, is also useful as a marker for severity if measured within 48 h of the onset of symptoms (Gudgeon et al. 1990; Neoptolemos et al. 2000; Tenner et al. 1997; Heath et al. 1995). However, this test is not commercially available. Urinary levels of the activation peptide from procarboxypeptidase B (CAPAP), which is also released by during pancreatitis, may prove to be a more useful assay in the future (Appelros et al. 1998, 2001).

Trypsinogen is a pancreatic proenzyme thought to play a central role in the pathophysiology of pancreatitis. One isoenzyme, trypsinogen-2 (anionic trypsinogen), is elevated in both serum and urine in acute pancreatitis (Kempainnen et al. 1997). In one study, a cut-off serum level of 1,000 μg/L differentiated complicated from uncomplicated necrotizing pancreatitis with a sensitivity of 91% and a specificity of 71% (Saino et al. 1996). Urinary levels of trypsinogen-2 lack sensitivity to distinguish mild from severe disease (Lempinen et al. 2003, 2001; Kyplanpaa et al. 2000). These test are not yet commercially available.

Other markers of pancreatic injury that are being investigated include trypsin complexes (Hedstrom et al. 1996), phospholipase A2 (Wereszycynska-Seimiatkowska et al. 1998), pancreatitis-associated protein (Kemppainen et al. 1996), methemalbumin (Lankisch et al. 1989), and pancreatic ribonuclease (Warshaw et al. 1975). Markers of inflammation (Warshaw and Lee 1979) that are currently investigational include interleukin(IL)-6 (Pezzilli et al. 1999; Chen et al. 1999), IL-8 (Chen et al. 1999), polymorphonuclear elastase (Wereszycynska-Seimiatkowska et al. 1998), tumor necrosis factor (Chen et al. 1999), and serum amyloid A (Pezzillli et al. 2000).

2.2.3 Radiologic Assessment of Severity

At the time of admission, a pleural effusion demonstrated on chest radiograph indicates a higher risk for severe disease. HELLER et al. (1997) reported that 84% of patients with severe pancreatitis (as defined by Atlanta criteria) had a pleural effusion on chest radiograph as compared to 8.6% of patients with mild disease. TALAMINI et al. (1999) reported that a pleural effusion on chest radiograph, coupled with an increased serum creatinine (>2 mg/dL), was associated with an increased risk of necrotizing pancreatitis and mortality.

With the original Balthazar grading system (Table 2.3), Grades D and E were associated with a higher morbidity and mortality. The CT severity index (CTSI) is the current system by which severity is usually determined (Table 2.3) (BALTHAZAR et al. 1990) and improves upon the original classification by including the amount of necrosis as identified following intravenous contrast administration. CTSI scores of 0–3 are associated with 8% morbidity and 3% mortality, but scores of 7–10 are associated with 92% morbidity and 17% mortality. SIMCHUK et al. (2000) found similar findings and reported that a CTSI more than 5 also correlated with length of hospital stay and need for surgical necrosectomy. A disadvantage is that the scoring is susceptible to interobserver variability.

Table 2.3. CT severity index

Grade	CT finding	Score
A.	Normal pancreas	0
B.	Pancreatic enlargement	1
C.	Pancreatic inflammation and/or peripancreatic fat changes	2
D.	Single peripancreatic fluid# collection	3
E.	Two or more fluid collections# and/or retroperitoneal air	4
% necrosis		**Score**
0		0
< 30		2
30–50		4
> 50		6

CT severity index score = Grade score + % necrosis score#
Adapted from BALTHAZAR et al. (1985, 1990)

2.3 Timing and Use of Imaging in Therapeutic Decision Making

Imaging provides critical information for clinicians in the management of acute pancreatitis. This information includes confirmation of the diagnosis, visualization of the cause of pancreatitis, stratification of severity of pancreatitis, and identification of complications (BANKS 1997). Imaging also provides vital information when therapeutic intervention is required and can be used as a guide to perform interventions.

2.3.1 At Time of Diagnosis

At the time of diagnosis, the primary roles of imaging are to determine whether the cause of pancreatitis (e.g. gallstones or pancreas divisum) can be determined, confirm the diagnosis of acute pancreatitis and exclude other condition such as mesenteric infarction or perforated duodenal ulcer, and provide preliminary information as to the severity of acute pancreatitis.

2.3.1.1 Identification of Gallstones

At the time of admission, it is important to identify the cause of acute pancreatitis. A careful history and physical examination, and evaluation of laboratory tests and imaging are all helpful. In gallstone pancreatitis, abdominal ultrasound is the best initial test to identify biliary sludge and cholelithiasis, but is not as accurate in identifying stones in the common bile duct (ELMAS 2001). Other imaging studies that can accurately identify choledocholithiasis but are not usually performed at admission are magnetic resonance cholangiopancreatography (MRCP), endoscopic ultrasound (EUS), and endoscopic retrograde cholangiopancreatography (ERCP) (Fig. 2.1).

If imaging studies reveal the presence of choledocholithiasis or if there is a strong clinical suspicion based on characteristic abnormalities of liver function tests and/or dilatation of the common bile duct, the clinician must decide whether urgent (<48 h) ERCP should be performed for the purpose of identifying and then removing common bile duct stones. There are two major clinical concerns when gallstones lodge in the common bile duct. The first is ascending cholangitis. The second is that an obstructing common bile duct stone may lead to additional pancreatic damage and thereby increase morbidity and mortality. There have been four studies that have addressed these concerns (Neoptolemos et al. 1998; Fan et al. 1993; Folsch et al. 1997; Nowak et al. 1995). There is general agreement that in mild pancreatitis urgent ERCP with removal of gallstones from the common bile duct does not alter the clinical course and, therefore, is not indicated. However, the role of ERCP in severe pancreatitis remains controversial. In one study, ERCP with removal of common bile duct stones was helpful in preventing biliary sepsis but not in influencing the natural history of the acute pancreatitis (Fan et al. 1993). Other studies have yielded conflicting results as to the impact of urgent ERCP with removal of common bile duct stones in severe acute pancreatitis. There has not been agreement that urgent ERCP decreases morbidity and mortality in severe acute pancreatitis. At the present time, urgent ERCP is considered a reasonable option for patients who are either strongly suspected of cholangitis or who are exhibiting evidence of organ failure. The optimal timing of urgent ERCP appears to be within 48 hours of onset of symptoms. Urgent ERCP in severe pancreatitis should be performed only by those with considerable experience in therapeutic endoscopy.

2.3.1.2 Confirmation of Acute Pancreatitis

At admission, CT scan is indicated if there is doubt on the part of the clinician as to whether severe abdominal pain is due to pancreatitis or some other serious intra-abdominal condition. The Balthazar-Ranson scoring system (A–E) is sufficient to confirm that the patient has pancreatitis if the score is ≥B.

Abdominal ultrasound performed at the time of admission may also support the diagnosis of pancreatitis; however, visualization of the pancreas is often hindered by overlying bowel gas. Findings consistent with pancreatitis include diffuse glandular enlargement, hypoechoic texture of the pancreas indicating interstitial edema, focal areas of hemorrhage within the pancreas, acute retroperitoneal fluid accumulation, and free intraperitoneal fluid (Jeffrey 1989).

2.3.1.3 Assessment of Severity

The Balthazar-Ranson scoring system provides useful information in assessing the severity of acute pancreatitis. In general, patients with one or more fluid collections (that is, Balthazar-Ranson score of D or E) have a more prolonged course of pain and are more likely to have organ failure and necrotizing pancreatitis than those with a score of A, B, or C (Ranson et al. 1985).

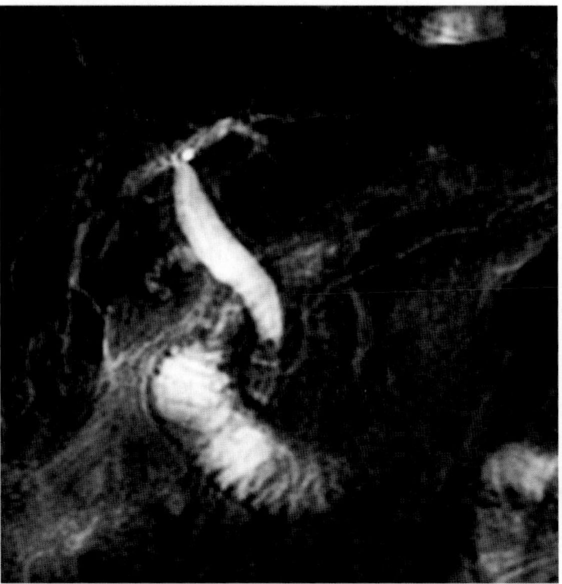

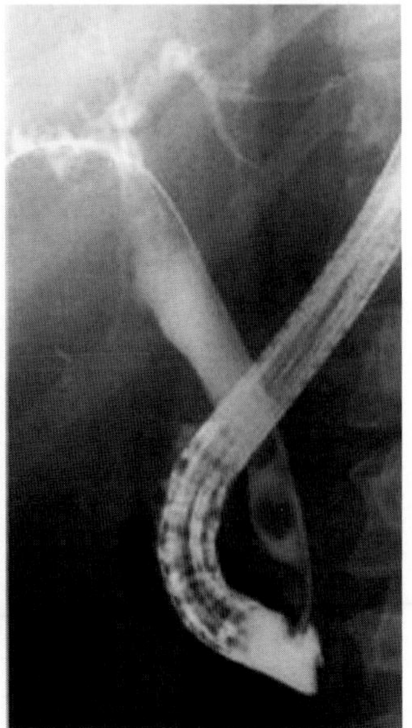

Fig. 2.1. a Projective MR cholangiographic image shows a mildly dilated common bile duct and the presence of two filling defects consistent with common bile duct stones. **b** ERCP image obtained in the same patient confirms the presence of two common bile duct stones

The radiologic modality of choice to determine whether the patient has interstitial or necrotizing pancreatitis is contrast-enhanced thin section multidetector-row CT (Fig. 2.2). Although a contrast-enhanced CT scan is frequently performed at the time of admission for the purposes of making this distinction, it remains unproven whether this knowledge can impact clinical care in the first few days. Standard of care during the first several days includes aggressive fluid resuscitation, bowel rest, analgesia, and vigilant assessment for the development of organ failure. Indeed, the opinion has been expressed that CT scan is not essential in the first 48–72 h of hospitalization (Lankisch et al. 2001b). It should also be noted that pancreatic necrosis is more accurately identified 48–72 h after the onset of disease (Balthazar 2002).

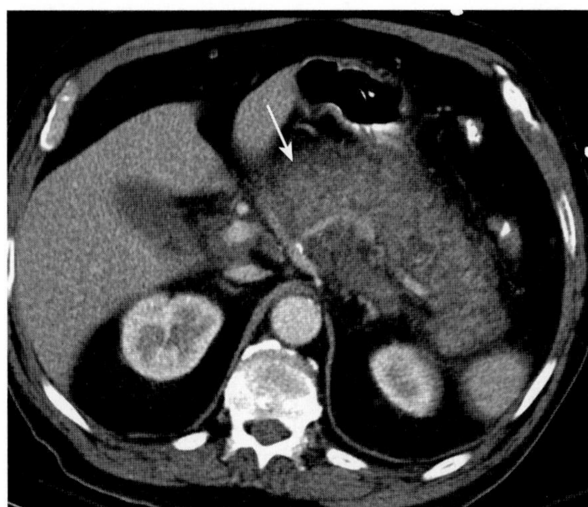
a

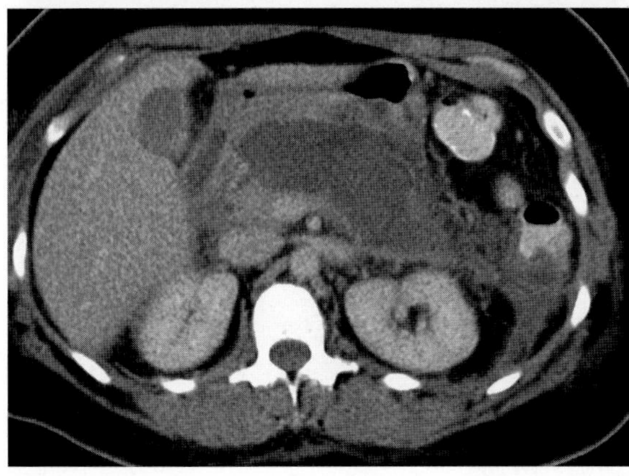
b

Fig. 2.2. a Axial contrast-enhanced CT image shows an enlarged and edematous pancreas without evidence of necrosis. Note, there is mild peripancreatic fat stranding (*arrow*) in the anterior pararenal space. **b** Axial contrast-enhanced CT image in another patient shows subtotal necrosis of the pancreatic gland

2.3.2
During the First Week and Thereafter

As many as 80%–90% of patients with acute pancreatitis have interstitial pancreatitis. Most recover within a few days and are discharged within 4–7 days. Less than 10% experience organ failure, which is usually transient. The overall mortality in interstitial pancreatitis is less than 3% and is usually caused by intractable organ failure in patients with comorbid disease.

Among the 10%–20% of patients with necrotizing pancreatitis, one half experiences organ failure which frequently is prolonged. Mortality in necrotizing pancreatitis in the absence of organ failure is probably 0%–3%. The mortality of single organ failure is less than 10%. The mortality associated with multi-system organ failure is approximately 40%–50%.

Patients who do not recover rapidly within the first several days require a contrast-enhanced CT scan to determine whether they have interstitial or necrotizing pancreatitis. Signs and/or symptoms of failure to recover or respond to appropriate therapy include persistent abdominal pain requiring narcotic medication, persistent leukocytosis or fever, or persistence or development of organ failure.

Magnetic resonance imaging (MRI), and in particular, magnetic resonance cholangiopancreatography (MRCP) has been increasingly utilized in the care of patients with acute pancreatitis. MR imaging can detect pancreatic necrosis (Saifuddin et al. 1993) and determine severity as accurately as CT scan (Lescesne et al. 1999; Arvanitakis et al. 2004), and is superior in delineating pancreatic duct anatomy and detecting choledocholithiasis (Fig. 2.3). In addition, potential contrast-mediated nephrotoxicity is minimized by the use of gadolinium chelates. Nonetheless, despite these benefits, CT scan can be obtained in a much more timely and cost-effective manner than MR imaging in most hospitals and, therefore, remains the preferable radiologic test.

2.3.2.1
Interstitial Pancreatitis

If CT scan reveals evidence of interstitial pancreatitis, the expectation of the clinician is that there will be gradual improvement with continued supportive therapy. Abdominal pain usually resolves within 3–5 days, and analgesic medication can be gradually withdrawn. Leukocytosis, fever and any evidence of organ failure also usually resolve within this time frame. However, if abdominal pain, fever or leukocytosis persists, and particularly if organ failure does not resolve, repeat imaging is advisable to determine the cause of persistent toxicity. There are several possible causes. First, the patient may have pancreatic necrosis rather than interstitial pancreatitis (Fig. 2.4a,b). Second, the patient may have interstitial pancreatitis with persistence of large fluid collections in the anterior pararenal space, lesser sac, or elsewhere. These fluid collections usually resolve over the next several weeks. If they do, systemic toxicity usually then resolves. However, if fluid collections persist and are associated with ongoing systemic toxicity (such as fever or leukocytosis) there is a possibility that the extrapancreatic fluid collections have become secondarily infected. While this does not occur very often in the absence of necrotizing pancreatitis, image-guided percutaneous aspiration with Gram stain and culture is advisable to exclude infection. If Gram stain and culture reveal the presence of infection, percutaneous catheter drainage can be utilized to manage the infected peripancreatic fluid collection.

Another possible cause of unresolved toxicity associated with persistence of fluid collections is a pancreatic ductal disruption. This entity can be suggested by a CT scan that shows an intrapancreatic collection of fluid at the neck as well as increasing peripancreatic fluid collections and confirmed by ERCP (Fig. 2.4c). The treatment of choice for a ductal disruption is the endoscopic insertion of a stent within the pancreatic duct that bridges the disruption (Telford et al. 2002). The stent is usually left in place for approximately 3 weeks, and is then removed if endoscopic injection of contrast into the pancreatic duct shows that the disruption has healed.

A third possibility for persistent toxicity after 4–6 weeks is the development of a pancreatic pseudocyst (Fig. 2.5). If a pseudocyst develops and remains asymptomatic, present thinking is that there is no need for intervention. However, if the pseudocyst causes abdominal pain, signs of biliary or gastric obstruction, or becomes secondarily infected, it should be drained. Choices include CT- or ultrasound-guided percutaneous catheter drainage, surgical drainage via cystgastrostomy or cystjejunostomy, or endoscopic drainage if feasible through the stomach or duodenum.

2.3.2.2 Necrotizing Pancreatitis

If, in the context of persisting toxicity such as fever and leukocytosis and/or unresolved organ failure, CT shows the presence of pancreatic necrosis, the hospital stay is likely to be prolonged, perhaps for as long as 2–6 months. The major concerns for the clinician are development or persistence of organ failure (including azotemia, hypoxemia, or shock) and the development of secondary pancreatic infection (infected pancreatic necrosis, see below).

Interestingly, the extent of necrosis does not necessarily correlate with toxicity. Although some pa-

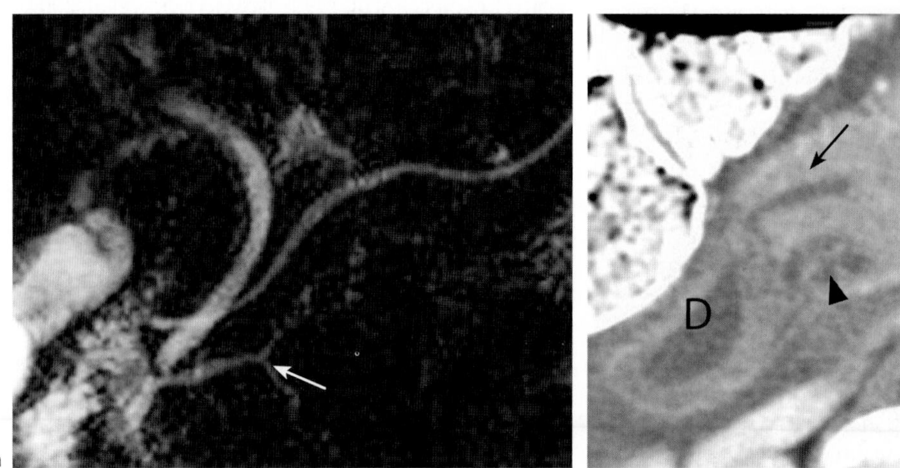

Fig. 2.3. a Projective MRCP image shows drainage of the main pancreatic duct through the duct of Santorini consistent with pancreas divisum. Note ventral duct remnant (*arrow*). **b** Axial contrast-enhanced CT image shows a dilated duct of Santorini (*arrow*) and diffuse peripancreatic fluid in this patient with interstitial pancreatitis caused by pancreas divisum. A small cystic lesion (*arrowhead*) was incidentally discovered in the posterior aspect of the pancreatic head. (*D* = duodenum)

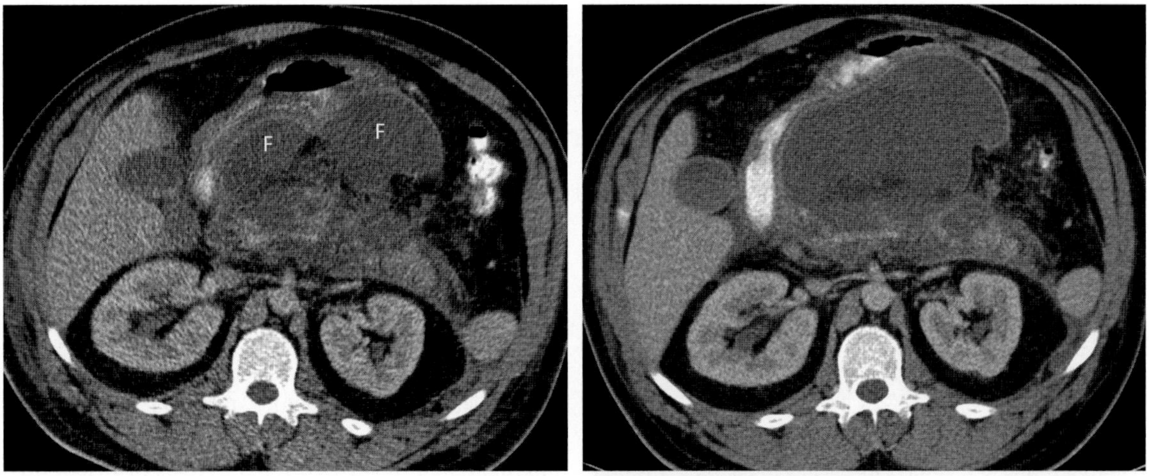

Fig. 2.4. a Axial contrast-enhanced CT image shows areas of necrosis (*F*=fluid). **b** Axial contrast-enhanced CT image obtained 4 weeks later shows organized necrosis in the pancreas and lesser sac. The necrosis was drained percutaneously. **c** ERCP image obtained after incomplete resolution shows main pancreatic duct disruption (*arrow*) and spillage of contrast in the retroperitoneum and lesser sac surrounding the drainage catheter

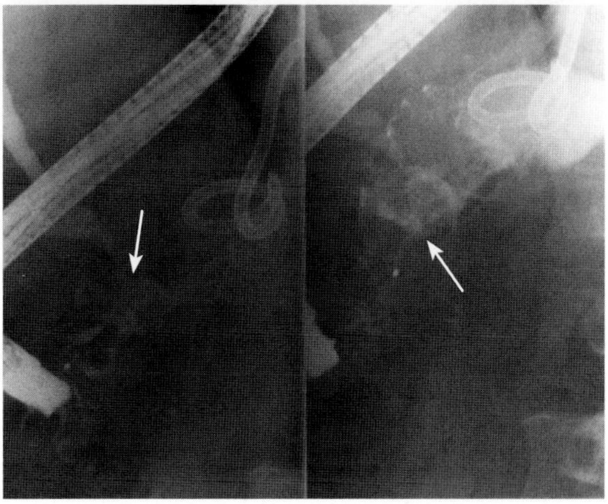

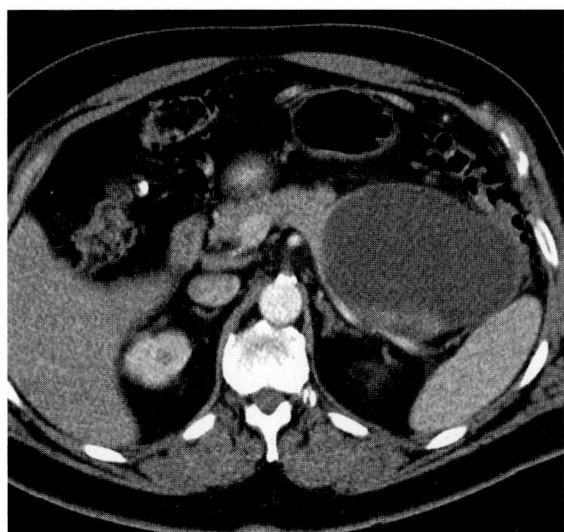

Fig. 2.5. Axial contrast-enhanced CT image shows a well-defined pseudocyst in the pancreatic tail 6 weeks after necrotizing pancreatitis

tients with extended pancreatic necrosis have considerable toxicity including multi-system organ failure, others, surprisingly, have no manifestations of toxicity (Fig. 2.6). Some patients with less than 30% of necrosis have considerable toxicity, while others do not. Balthazar's initial data and that of others had supported the concept that extensive necrosis correlates with higher morbidity and mortality, including organ failure, infected necrosis, and death, but these correlations have recently come into question. Perez et al. (2002) found that morbidity and mortality in necrotizing pancreatitis correlated better with multiorgan failure than extent of necrosis. In particular, patients with extensive pancreatic necrosis were not more likely to have pancreatic infection or multi-system organ failure than those with lesser amounts of necrosis (Perez et al. 2002). De Sanctis et al. (1997) reported no significant correlation with the extent of necrosis and outcome. It would appear that the finding of extensive necrosis on CT scan

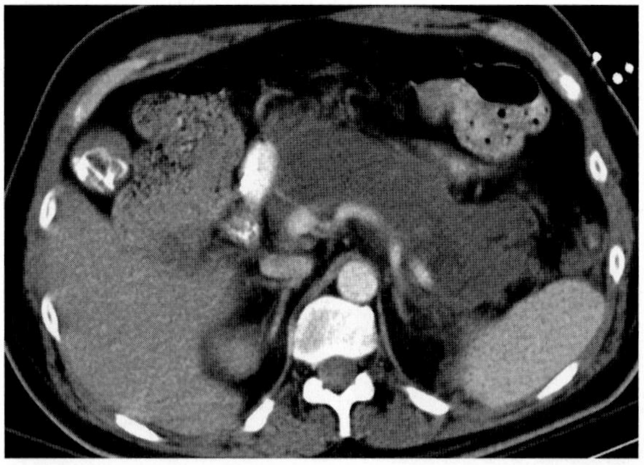

Fig. 2.6. Axial contrast-enhanced CT image in a patient who required intubation and pressor support during the course of his pancreatitis shows near-total necrosis of the pancreatic gland. The patient recovered fully without the need for surgical or radiologic intervention

does not necessarily mean that the patient is or will become seriously ill. In necrotizing pancreatitis, extensive or not, the main concerns for the clinician are the multi-system organ failure (which usually occurs within the first 7 days), and pancreatic infection (which usually occurs after the 7th day). In most series, one half of the deaths from acute pancreatitis take place within the first 7–14 days as a direct result of multi-system organ failure, and the remainder after 14 days, usually as a consequence of pancreatic infection (Mutinga et al. 2000).

Patients who exhibit evidence of organ failure require treatment in an intensive care unit. Treatment for progressive organ failure may require intubation with assisted ventilation, renal dialysis, and pharmacological support of blood pressure. There are additional treatment options that should be considered. First, clinicians should reevaluate for the possibility of biliary sepsis caused by a common bile duct stone. Rather than from the pancreatitis itself, progressive organ failure could be a result of biliary sepsis. If this is suspected, ERCP or MRCP should be considered. Secondly, patients require prolonged bowel rest and nutritional support, either with the use of total parenteral nutrition (TPN) or enteral feeding via a nasal jejunal feeding tube. Third, the clinician could consider the use of broad spectrum antibiotics to prevent pancreatic infection (Golub et al. 1998; Uhl et al. 2002). The role of prophylactic antibiotics has recently been called into question because of concerns for fungal superinfection (Grewe et al. 1999; Isenmann et al. 2002), which can increase morbidity and possibly mortality, and also because of concerns that antibiotics may be ineffective to prevent pancreatic infection (Isenmann et al. 2004).

In general, CT scans are repeated every 7–10 days to follow the evolution of necrotizing pancreatitis and to look for complications. Patients with necrotizing pancreatitis who do not exhibit systemic toxicity or whose systemic toxicity resolves within a few days do not require pancreatic interventions. Patients who improve clinically over 7–10 days then cautiously receive oral nourishment and are discharged after a hospitalization that may vary from 3–4 weeks. However, some patients continue to show clinical instability with persistent tachycardia, persistent fever and leukocytosis or organ failure. When this occurs, image-guided percutaneous aspiration is required to exclude the possibility of infected pancreatic necrosis (see below).

2.3.2.3 Infected Pancreatic Necrosis

While CT scan is very accurate in determining necrosis, it cannot distinguish between infected and sterile necrosis in the absence of retroperitoneal air bubbles (Fig. 2.7). In general, more than half of pancreatic infections are documented between the 7th and 21st day of hospitalization, and the remainder thereafter. Fungal infections in particular may take place after 4–6 weeks, especially among patients who have been on potent broad-spectrum antibiotic therapy. Percutaneous CT-guided fine needle aspiration (FNA) has been shown to be a safe and accurate method to determine the presence of infected necrosis (Banks et al. 1995; Gerzof et al. 1984, 1987). Aspirated pancreatic fluid should be submitted immediately for Gram stain and bacterial and fungal culture to ensure greatest accuracy. Infected pancreatic necrosis has traditionally been managed with urgent surgical necrosectomy and appropriate antibiotic coverage, and remains the treatment of choice (Uhl et al. 2002). However, when patients are too ill to undergo surgical treatment, our experience and the experience of others provide evidence that percutaneous catheter drainage may be successful in reducing toxicity associated with infection and stabilizing the patient's condition (Figs. 2.8 and 2.9). Surgical debridement can then be more safely performed if catheter drainage is unable to eliminate all infected material (Freeny et al. 1998). Successful catheter drainage requires daily conscientious management by interventional radiologists, including frequent flushing and up-sizing of the catheters. Other options to eliminate infected necrotic material include endoscopic necrosectomy (Baron et al. 2002) (Fig. 2.10) and percutaneous endoscopic necrosectomy (Carter et al. 2000). Additional experience with these two techniques will be required to evaluate these options more fully. At the present time, there have been no prospective studies which have compared the various techniques to eliminate infected pancreatic necrosis.

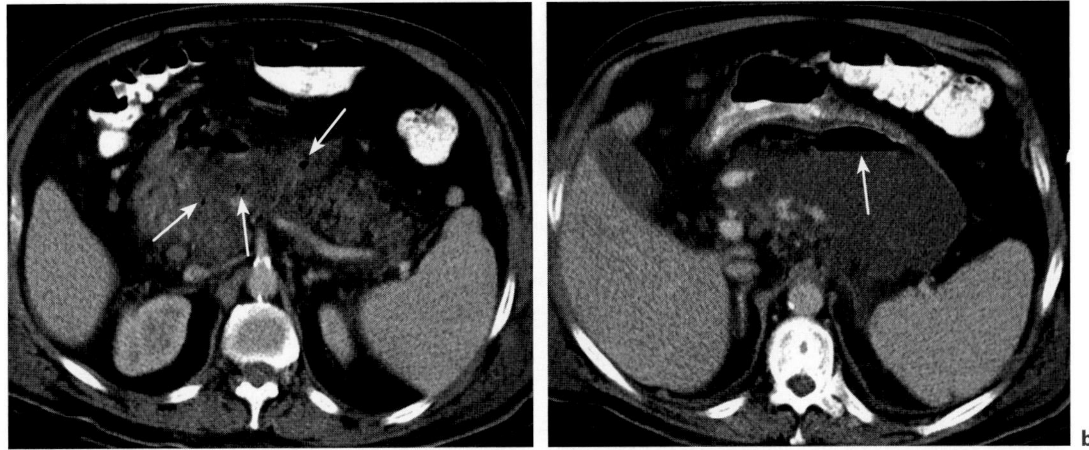

Fig. 2.7. a Axial contrast-enhanced CT image in a patient with sepsis shows subtotal necrosis of the pancreatic gland and the presence of air bubbles (*arrows*), suggestive of infected necrosis. **b** Axial contrast-enhanced CT image in the same patient at a higher level shows the presence of an air-fluid level (*arrow*) in the lesser sac

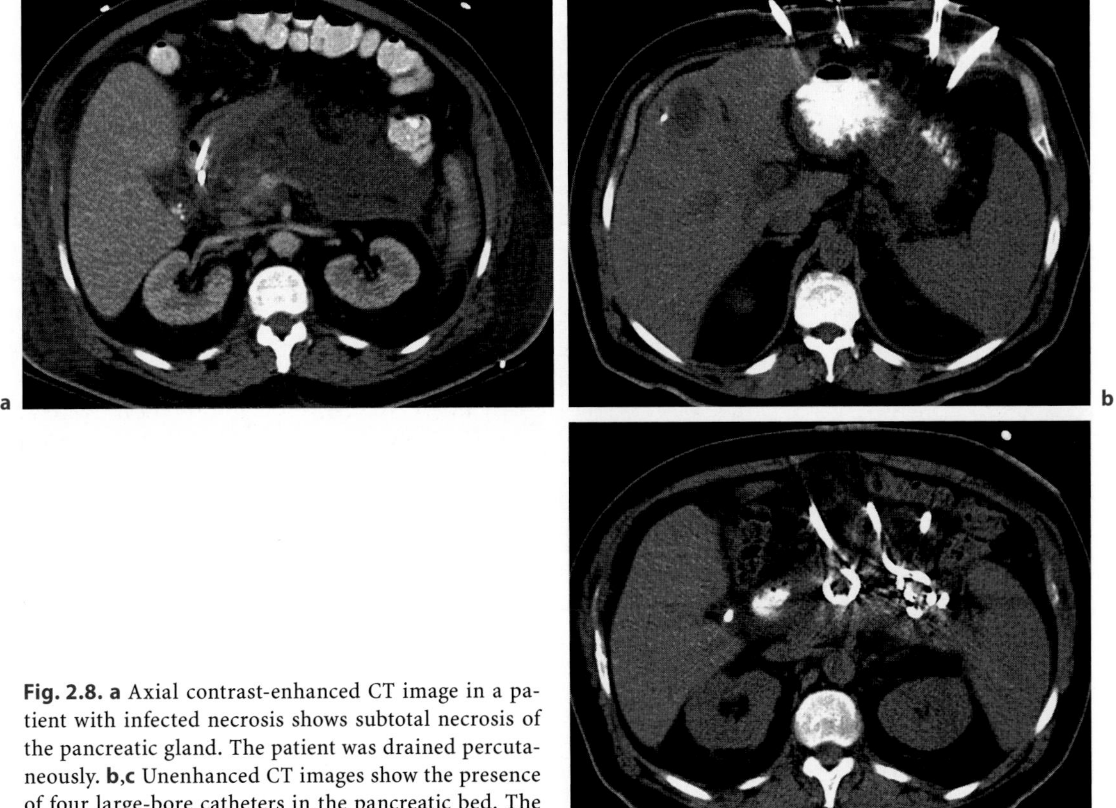

Fig. 2.8. a Axial contrast-enhanced CT image in a patient with infected necrosis shows subtotal necrosis of the pancreatic gland. The patient was drained percutaneously. **b,c** Unenhanced CT images show the presence of four large-bore catheters in the pancreatic bed. The patient recovered without the need for surgery

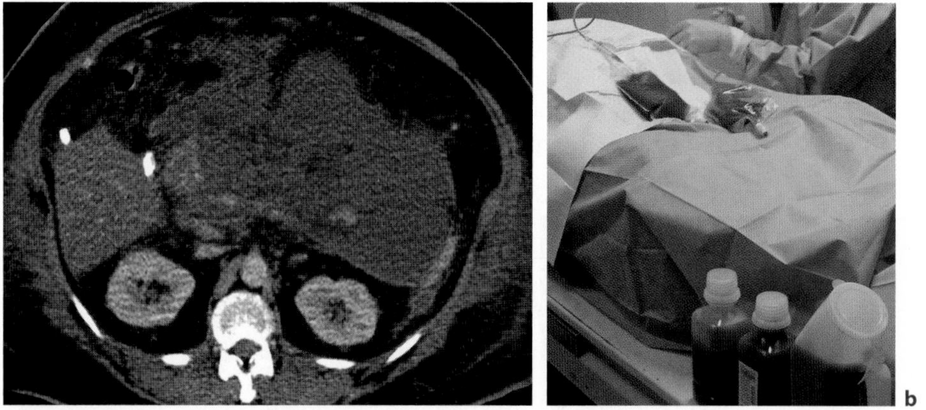

Fig. 2.9. **a** Axial contrast-enhanced CT image shows subtotal necrosis of the pancreatic gland and extensive fluid accumulation in the retroperitoneum and lesser sac. Because of hyperbilirubinemia and gastric outlet obstruction patient underwent CT guided-aspiration and drainage. **b** Photograph obtained during the procedure shows bottles filled with brownish pancreatic exudates. Gram-stain and culture showed no organisms

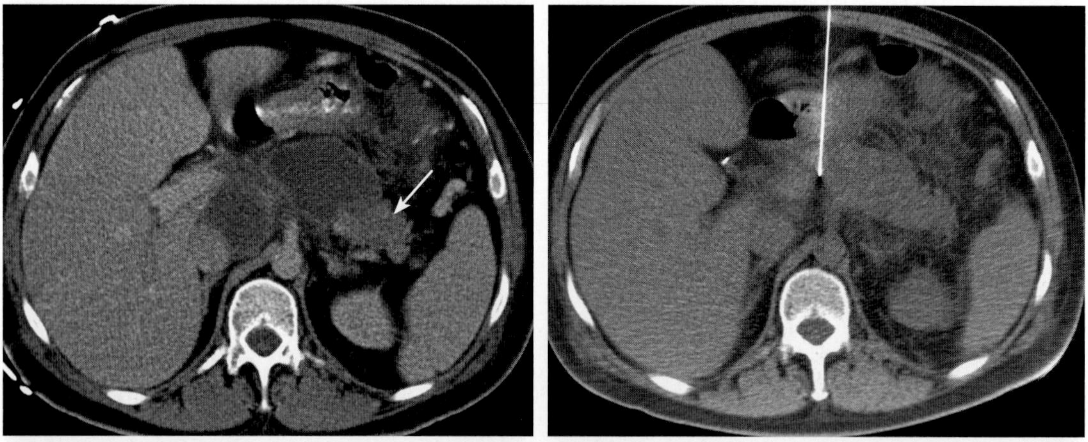

Fig. 2.10. **a** Axial contrast-enhanced CT image shows subtotal necrosis of the pancreatic gland with viable remnant pancreatic tail (*arrow*). **b** CT-guided needle aspiration revealed infected pancreatic necrosis. **c** Endoscopic image shows endoscopic transgastric debridement of the necrosis. **d** Post-debridement unenhanced CT image shows presence of two double pigtail catheters connecting the stomach with the pancreatic bed

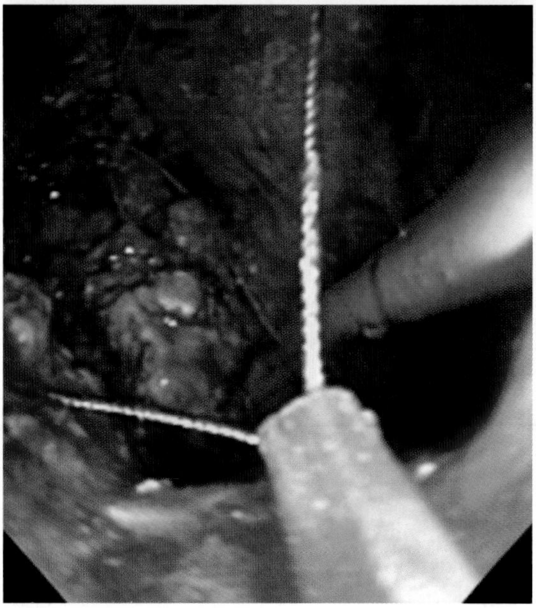

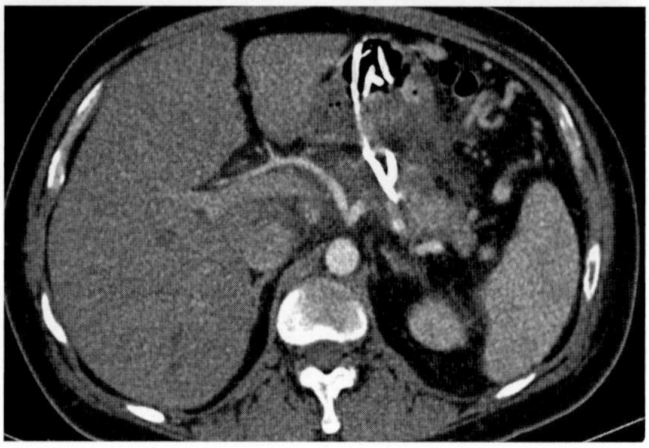

2.3.2.4
Sterile Pancreatic Necrosis

Patients who have undergone percutaneous aspiration because of persistent toxicity are considered to have sterile necrosis if the aspirate is sterile. Some patients recover rapidly and require no additional intervention. Others who continue to exhibit clinical toxicity should continue to receive aggressive medical support in an intensive care unit. Historically, these patients with unresolved toxicity would have undergone urgent surgical debridement (RATTNER et al. 1992), but within the last 15 years these patients have been increasingly managed successfully non-surgically (BUCHLER et al. 2000; BRADLEY and ALLEN 1991). This change in approach reflects an overall impression that early surgery may contribute to mortality and that persistent medical therapy may yield a better result. To date, there are no randomized clinical trials that have compared early surgical debridement with continuation of medical management to treat severe sterile necrosis.

Patients with ongoing toxicity being managed in the intensive care unit should undergo image-guided aspiration every 7–10 days in order to ensure that the necrosis remains sterile. If infection is found, surgical debridement or aggressive percutaneous catheter drainage is usually then required. Most patients who continue to have negative aspirates show clinical improvement after 3–6 weeks.

In some centers, rather than performing aspiration every 7–10 days, a catheter is left in place and irrigated in accordance with radiologic protocol in an attempt to provide a radiologic necrosectomy. In theory, the removal of sterile necrotic material may reduce systemic toxicity. While colonization may be expected with an indwelling catheter, experienced radiologists believe that a serious infection is not likely to occur if the catheter is managed properly. To date, there are no clinical studies that have compared the results of therapy utilizing weekly percutaneous aspiration to rule out infection versus prolonged catheter drainage of sterile necrosis.

Some patients with ongoing toxicity but with negative aspirates do not show clinical improvement after 3–6 weeks. One possible explanation is that there is a pancreatic ductal disruption (or possibly even several ductal disruptions) with continued extravasation of noxious pancreatic juice into areas of peripancreatic necrosis. An ERCP is not generally recommended to stent across a disruption in the setting of sterile necrosis for several reasons. First, there may be a ductal obstruction such that the disruption cannot be visualized. Second, if there is no obstruction, the contrast will extravasate through the disruption and possibly infect the necrotic area. Third, the area of necrosis is often very extensive such that the upstream portion of the duct cannot be visualized or accessed by a stent. Finally, even if a bridging stent can be placed, it may act as a foreign body and convert sterile necrosis into infected necrosis. Thus, medical management should be continued in the setting of sterile necrosis.

2.3.2.5
Organized Necrosis

After approximately 3–6 weeks or longer, there is general subsidence of the inflammatory component associated with sterile necrosis with some organization of the pancreatic necrosis in a somewhat ovoid configuration, which has traditionally been called a pseudocyst and more recently has been termed organized necrosis. The value of the term organized necrosis is to remind the physician that the low attenuation structure on CT scan contains necrotic pancreatic and peripancreatic tissue and not simply fluid and that any attempt at intervention that does not eliminate the necrotic debris is likely to encourage infection. The evolution of necrotizing pancreatitis into organized necrosis can be well seen on serial CT scans.

During this transformation to organized necrosis, most patients improve clinically with subsidence of abdominal pain, fever, leukocytosis, and resolution of organ failure. In these circumstances, the patient should be fed cautiously. In the setting of sterile necrosis, if there is no abdominal pain or other symptoms, there is no intervention required and the patient can be weaned off of TPN and discharged.

Some patients are unable to tolerate oral intake because of exacerbation of pain or have intractable nausea and vomiting if the organized necrosis causes either gastric outlet or duodenal obstruction. The cause of these symptoms is usually increased pressure within the organized necrosis caused by continued extravasation of pancreatic fluid from the residual viable tail of the pancreas (sometimes called a "remnant tail") (Fig. 2.11). There is invariably a concomitant pancreatic duct disruption which serves as the entry for pancreatic juice into the organized necrosis.

The physician has several options when abdominal pain occurs in association with organized necro-

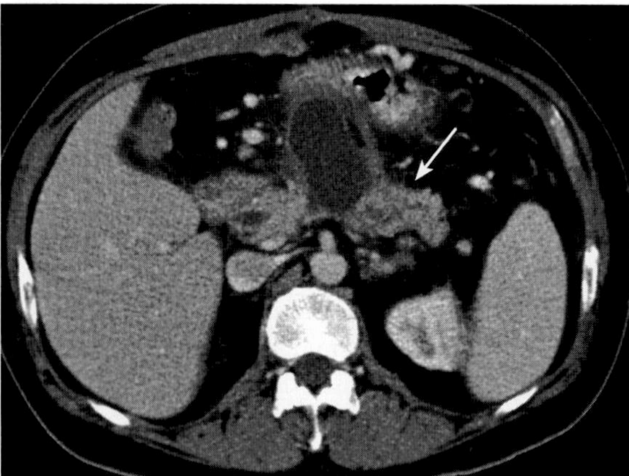

Fig. 2.11. Axial contrast-enhanced CT image obtained in a patient with known sterile pancreatic necrosis shows presence of a remnant pancreatic tail (*arrow*) and fluid reaccumulation

sis. The first is continuation of TPN, but this rarely is helpful. The second would be an ERCP with an insertion of a stent into the area of organized necrosis. This may cause secondary infection of the organized necrosis and is not likely to allow the egress of the semisolid necrotic material. The third and best choice is debridement of the organized necrosis. Debridement can be done in three ways. The first is surgical cystjejunostomy or cystgastrostomy (Fig. 2.12). The surgeon takes care to finger debride residual necrotic material while evacuating the fluid component of organized necrosis. A second choice is endoscopic debridement if the organized necrosis is impacted against the stomach or duodenum. In this technique, an opening is created endoscopically through the posterior wall of the stomach or duodenum into the area of organized necrosis and an endoscopic snare is used to retrieve loose necrotic debris from within the cavity. Additional egress of necrotic debris and fluid is achieved by irrigation and the insertion of double pig tail catheters between the cavity and the stomach (or duodenum) (Fig. 2.10c,d). The catheters can then be removed 3–4 weeks later. A third choice is percutaneous catheter drainage with vigorous irrigation of the necrotic debris. A possible drawback of the radiologic approach would be the difficulty in irrigating the semisolid pancreatic debris such that the residual debris may predispose to infection. Another disadvantage of this approach is that pancreatic juice from the remnant tail usually continues to drain through the catheter thereby creating an external fistula.

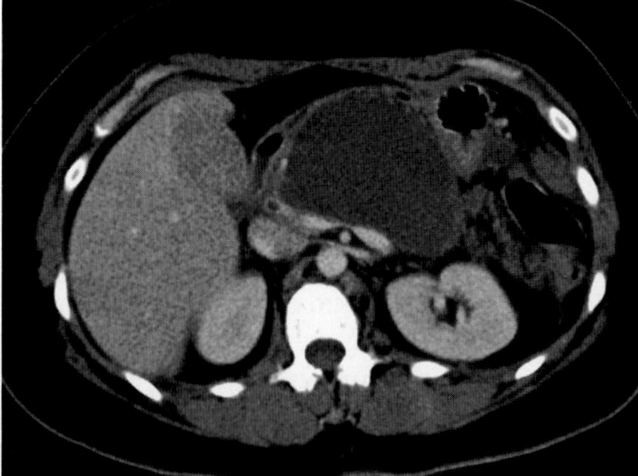

a

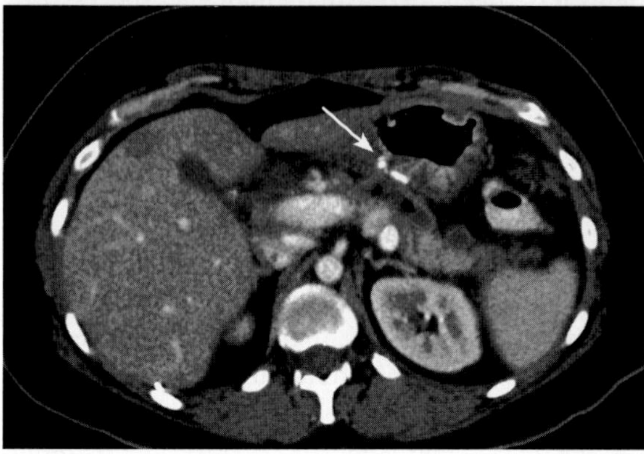

b

Fig. 2.12. **a** Axial contrast-enhanced CT image obtained 6 weeks after necrotizing pancreatitis shows the presence of organized necrosis in the lesser sac. **b** Axial contrast-enhanced CT image obtained after surgical debridement with cystgastrostomy (*arrow*) shows sutures at the level of the anastomosis between the stomach and retroperitoneum. Residual fluid and air bubbles are seen in the lesser sac

2.3.3 Venous Thrombosis and Solid Organ Involvement

Clinicians also rely on CT scan to identify local complications, such as venous thrombosis or surrounding organ involvement. Venous thrombosis secondary to peripancreatic inflammation or mass effect is rare and usually occurs in the splenic, superior mesenteric and portal vein (Fig. 2.13a). Rarely, a splenic vein thrombosis causes bleeding from gastric varices and require splenectomy.

The surrounding solid organs, including spleen, kidney, and liver (in order of frequency) may have a subcapsular fluid collection or even infarction. Solid organ involvement may ultimately require surgical intervention (Mortele et al. 2003).

2.3.4 Acute Hemorrhage

Acute bleeding is a rare event that can occur at any time in the course of acute pancreatitis. If bleeding occurs, clinicians use endoscopy to evaluate and treat gastrointestinal sources of bleeding, and CT scan to rule out retroperitoneal hemorrhage, pseudoaneurysms, or varices secondary to venous thrombosis (Fig. 2.13b).

Pseudoaneurysms result from autodigestion of arterial walls, usually the splenic artery, by pancreatic enzymes and may cause significant hemorrhage. Pseudoaneurysms usually occur late in the disease course (weeks to months) and may require radiologic embolization (Fig. 2.14). Splenic venous thrombosis (and rarely, portal vein thrombosis) can cause gastrointestinal bleeding from gastric varices (e.g. segmental portal hypertension).

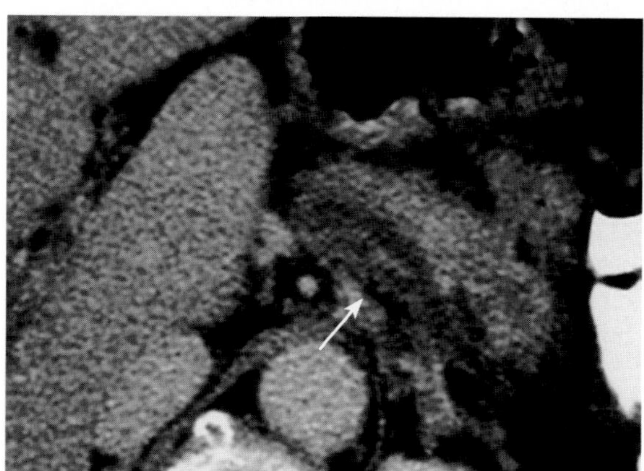

a

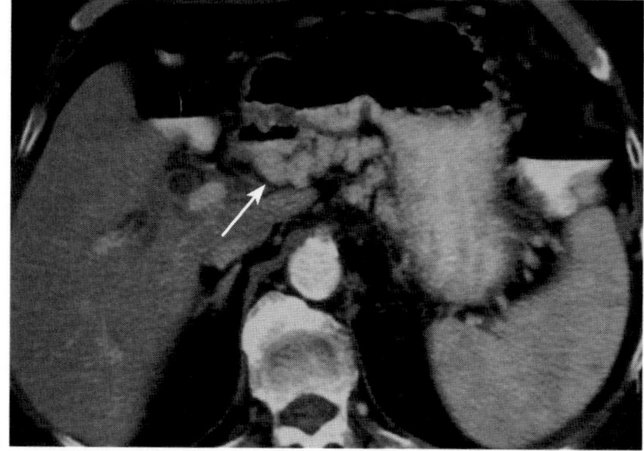

b

Fig. 2.13. a Axial contrast-enhanced CT image shows the hypoattenuating appearance of the splenic vein (*arrow*) consistent with acute splenic vein thrombosis. **b** Axial contrast-enhanced CT image in another patient with a splenic vein thrombosis shows varices (*arrow*) along the lesser curvature of the stomach consistent with segmental portal hypertension

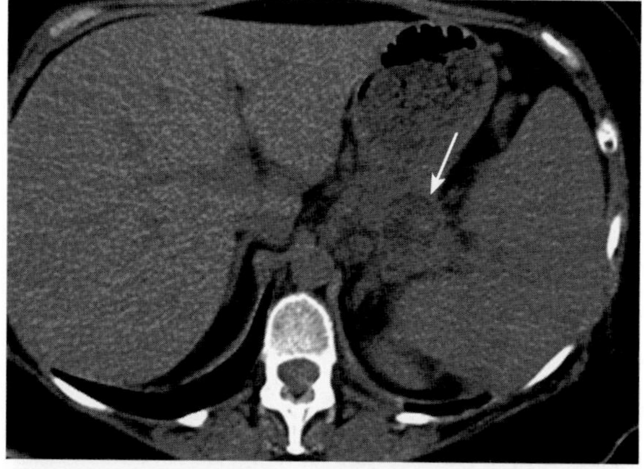

a

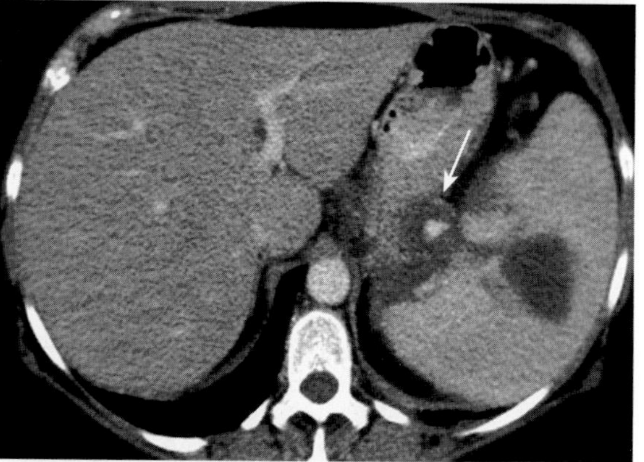

b

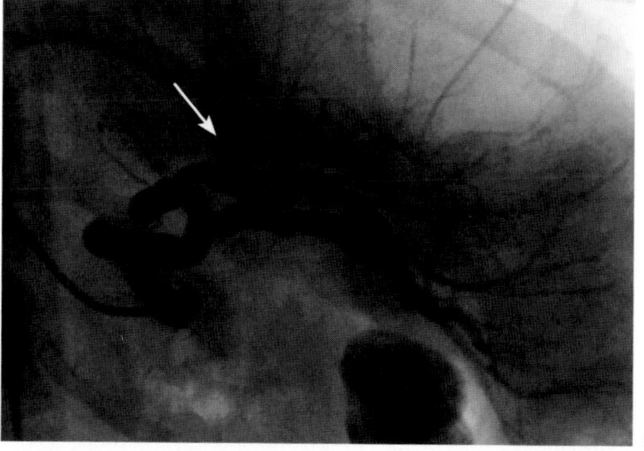

c

Fig. 2.14. a Axial unenhanced CT image obtained one year after acute pancreatitis shows a small hypoattenuating collection (*arrow*) in the splenic hilum. **b** Axial contrast-enhanced CT image in the same patient shows significant enhancement of the hypoattenuating structure (*arrow*) consistent with a pseudoaneurysm. **c** Digital subtraction angiogram shows the saccular pseudoaneurysm (*arrow*) originating from a segmental splenic artery branch

2.4 Summary

Imaging is an indispensable tool in the care of patients with pancreatitis. On admission, ultrasound can identify cholelithiasis, and CT scan helps confirm diagnosis and assess severity. During the course of acute pancreatitis, repeat CT scans identify interval changes and local complications. In necrotizing pancreatitis, image-guided aspiration distinguishes between infected and sterile necrosis. In the appropriate clinical setting, interventional radiologic techniques can be used to debride necrosis, to drain pancreatic fluid collections, and to embolize pseudoaneurysms.

References

Appelros S, Thim L, Borgstrom A (1998) Activation peptide of carboxypeptidase B in serum and urine in acute pancreatitis. Gut 42:97–102

Appelros S, Petersson U, Toh S et al (2001) Activation peptide of carboxypeptidase B and anionic trypsinogen as early predictors of the severity of acute pancreatitis. Br J Surg 88:216–221

Arvanitakis M, Delhaye M, De Maertelaere V et al (2004) Computed tomography and magnetic resonance imaging in the assessment of acute pancreatitis. Gastroenterology 126:715–723

Baillargeon JD, Orav J, Ramagopal V et al (1998) Hemoconcentration as an early risk factor for necrotizing pancreatitis. Am J Gastroenterol 93:2130–2134

Balthazar EJ (2002) Complications of acute pancreatitis: clinical and CT evaluation." Radiol Clin North Am 40(6): 1211–1127

Balthazar EJ, Ranson JHC, Naidich D et al (1985) Acute pancreatitis: prognostic value of CT. Radiology 156:767–772

Balthazar EJ, Robinson DL, Megibow AJ et al (1990) Acute pancreatitis: value of CT in establishing prognosis. Radiology 174:331–336

Banks PA (1997) Practice guidelines in acute pancreatitis. Am J Gastroenterol 92:377–386

Banks PA, Gerzof SG, Langevin RE et al (1995) CT-guided aspiration of suspected pancreatic infection: bacteriology and clinical outcome. Int J Pancreatol 18:265–270

Baron TH, Harewood GC, Morgan DE et al (2002) Outcome differences after endoscopic drainage of pancreatic necrosis, acute pancreatic pseudocysts, and chronic pancreatic pseudocysts. Gastrointest Endosc 56:7–17

Blum T, Maisonneuve P, Lowenfels AB et al (2001) Fatal outcome in acute pancreatitis: its occurrence and early prediction. Pancreatology 1:237–241

Bradley EL III, Allen K (1991) A prospective longitudinal study of observation versus surgical intervention in the management of necrotizing pancreatitis. Am J Surg 161:19–24

Bradley EL 3rd (1993) A clinically based classification system for acute pancreatitis. Summary of the International Symposium on Acute Pancreatitis, Atlanta, Ga, September 11 trough 13, 1992. Arch Surg 128(5):586–590

Brown A, Orav J, Banks PA (2000) Hemoconcentration is an early marker for organ failure and necrotizing pancreatitis. Pancreas 20:367–372

Buchler MW, Gloor B, Muller CA et al (2000) Acute necrotizing pancreatitis: treatment strategy according to the status of infection. Ann Surg 232:619–626

Carter CR, McKay CJ, Imrie CW (2000) Percutaneous necrosectomy and sinus tract endoscopy in the management of infected pancreatic necrosis: an initial experience. Ann Surg 232:175–180

Chase CW, Barker DE, Russell WL et al (1996) Serum amylase and lipase in the evaluation of acute abdominal pain. Ann Surg 62:1028–1033

Chatzicostas C, Roussomoustakaki M, Vlachonikolis IG et al (2002) Comparison of Ranson, APACHE II and APACHE III scoring systems in acute pancreatitis. Pancreas 25:331–335

Chen CC, Wang SS, Lee FY et al (1999) Proinflammatory cytokines in early assessment of the prognosis of acute pancreatitis. Am J Gastroenterol 94:213–218

Claiven PA, Meyer, RJ, Meyer P et al (1989) Acute pancreatitis and normoamylasemia. Not an uncommon combination. Ann Surg 210:614–620

Claiven PA, Hauser H, Meyer P et al (1998) Value of contrast-enhanced computerized tomography in the early diagnosis and prognosis of acute pancreatitis. Am J Surg 155:457–466

De Beaux AC, Goldie AS, Ross JA et al (1996) Serum concentrations of inflammatory mediators related to organ failure in patients with acute pancreatitis. Br J Surg 83:349–353

De Sanctis JT, Lee MJ, Gazelle GS et al (1997) Prognostic indicators in acute pancreatitis: CT v Apache II. Clin Radiol 52:842–848

Dervenis C, Johnson CD, Bassi C (1999) Diagnosis, objective assessment of severity, and management of acute pancreatitis. Santorini Consensus conference. Int J Pancreatol 25:193–210

Dickson AP, Imrie CW (1984) The incidence and prognosis of body wall ecchymosis in acute pancreatitis. Surg Gynaecol Obstet 159:323–347

Dominguez-Munoz JE (1999) Diagnosis of acute pancreatitis: any news or still amylase? In: Buchler M, Uhl E, Friess H, Malfertheiner P (eds) Acute pancreatitis: novel concepts in biology and therapy. Blackwell Science, London

Elmas N (2001) The role of diagnostic radiology in pancreatitis. Eur J Radiol 38:120–132

Fan ST, Lai EC, Mok FP et al (1993) Early treatment of acute biliary pancreatitis by endoscopic papillotomy. N Engl J Med 328:228–232

Folsch UR, Nitsche R, Ludtke R et al (1997) German Study Group on Acute Biliary Pancreatitis: early ERCP and papillotomy compared with conservative treatment for acute biliary pancreatitis. N Engl J Med 336:237–242

Freeny PC, Hauptmann E, Althaus SJ et al (1998) Percutaneous CT-guided catheter drainage of infected acute necrotizing pancreatitis: techniques and results. AJR Am J Roentgenol 170:969–975

Funnell IC, Bornman PC, Weakley SP et al (1993) Obesity: an important prognostic factor in acute pancreatitis. Br J Surgery 80:484–486

Gerzof SG, Johnson WC, Robbins AH et al (1984) Percutaneous drainage of infected pancreatic pseudocysts. Arch Surg 119:888–893

Gerzof SG, Banks PA, Robbins AH et al (1987) Early diagnosis of pancreatic infection by computed tomography-guided aspiration. Gastroenterology 93:1315–1320

Golub R, Siddiqi F, Pohl D (1998) Role of antibiotics in acute pancreatitis: A meta-analysis. J Gastrointest Surg 2:496–503

Grewe M, Tsiotos GG, Luque de-Leon E et al (1999) Fungal infection in acute necrotizing pancreatitis. J Am Coll Surg 188:408–414

Gross V, Scholmerich J, Leser H-G et al (1990) Granulocyte elastase in assessment of severity of acute pancreatitis. Comparison with acute-phase protein C-reactive protein, α1-antitrypsin, and protease inhibitor a2-macroglobulin. Dig Dis Sci 35:97–105

Gudgeon AM, Heath DI, Hurley P et al (1990) Trypsinogen activation peptides assay in the early prediction of severity of acute pancreatitis. Lancet 335:4–8

Heath DI, Cruickshank A, Gudgeon AM et al (1995) The relationship between pancreatic enzyme release and activation and the acute-phase protein response in patients with acute pancreatitis. Pancreas 10:347–353

Hedstrom J, Sainio V, Kemppainen E et al (1996) Serum complex of trypsin 2 and alpha 1 antitrypsin as diagnostic and prognostic marker of acute pancreatitis: clinical study in consecutive patients. BMJ 313:333–337

Hedstrom J, Kemppainen, Andersen J et al (2001) A comparison of serum trypsinogen-2 and trypsin2-a1-antitrypsin complex with lipase and amylase in the diagnosis and assessment of severity in the early phase of acute pancreatitis. Am J Gastroenterol 96:424–430

Heller SJ, Noordhoek E, Tenner SM et al (1997) Pleural effusion as a predictor of severity in acute pancreatitis. Pancreas 15:222–225

Imrie CW, Benjamin IS, Ferguson JE et al (1978) A single-center double-blind trial of trasylol therapy in primary acute pancreatitis. Br J Surg 65:337–341

Isenmann R, Schwarz M, Rau B et al (2002) Characteristics of infection with Candida species in patients with necrotizing pancreatitis. World J Surg 2002 26:372–376

Isenmann R, Runzi M, Kron M et al (2004) Prophylactic antibiotic treatment in patients with predicted severe acute pancreatitis: a placebo-controlled, double-blind trial. Gastroenterology 126:997–1004

Jeffrey RB (1989) Sonography in acute pancreatitis. Rad Clin N Am 27:5–17

Kemppainen E, Sand J, Puolakkainen P et al (1996) Pancreatitis associated protein as an early marker of acute pancreatitis. Gut 39:675–678

Kemppainen EA, Hedstrom JL, Puolakkainen PA et al (1997) Measurement of urinary trypsinogen-2 as a screening test for acute pancreatitis. N Engl J Med 336:1788–1793

Kyplanpaa ML, Kemppainen E, Puolakkainen P et al (2000) Reliable screening for acute pancreatitis with rapid urine trypsinogen-2 test strip. Br J Surgery 87:49–52

Lankisch PG, Schirren CA, Otto J (1989) Methemalbumin in acute pancreatitis: an evaluation of its prognostic value and comparison with multiple prognostic parameters. Am J Gastroenterol 84:1391–1395

Lankisch PG, Mahlke R, Blum T et al (2001a) Hemoconcentration: an early marker of severe and/or necrotizing pancreatitis? A critical appraisal. Am J Gastroenterol 96(7):2081–2085

Lankisch PG, Struckmann K, Assmus C et al (2001b) Do we need a computed tomography examination all patients with acute pancreatitis within 72 h after admission to hospital for the detection of pancreatic necrosis? Scan J Gastroenterol 36:432–436

Larvin M, McMahon MJ (1989) APACHE-II score for assessment and monitoring of acute pancreatitis. Lancet 2:201–205

Lempinen M, Kylanpaa-Back ML, Stenman UH et al (2001) Predicting the severity of acute pancreatitis by rapid measurement of trypsinogen-2 in urine. Clin Chem 47:2103–2107

Lempinen M, Stenman UH, Finne P et al (2003) Trypsinogen-2 and trypsinogen activation peptide (TAP) in urine of patients with acute pancreatitis. J Surg Res 111:267–273

Lescesne R, Tourel P, Bret PM et al (1999) Acute pancreatitis: interobserver agreement and correlation of CT and MR cholangiopancreatography with outcome. Radiology 211:727–735

Leser HG, Gross V et al. (1991) Elevation of serum interleukin-6 concentration precedes acute-phase response and reflects severity in acute pancreatitis. Gastroenterology 101(3): 782–785

Martinez J, Sanchez-Paya J, Palazon JM et al (1999) Obesity: a prognostic factor of severity in acute pancreatitis. Pancreas 19:15–20

McMahon MJ, Playforth MJ, Pickford IR (1980) A comparative study of methods for the prediction of severity of attacks of acute pancreatitis. Br J Surg 69:29–32

Mery CM, Rubio V, Duarte-Rojo A et al (2002) Android fat distribution as predictor of severity in acute pancreatitis. Pancreatology 2:543–549

Mortele KJ, Banks PA, Silverman SG (2003) State-of-the-art imaging of acute pancreatitis. JBR-BTR 86:193–208

Mutinga M, Rosenbluth A, Tenner SM et al (2000) Does mortality occur early or late in acute pancreatitis? Int J Pancreatol 28:91–95

Neoptolemos JP, Carr-Locke DL, London NJ et al (1988) Controlled trial of urgent endoscopic retrograde cholangiopancreatography and endoscopic sphincterotomy versus conservative treatment for acute pancreatitis due to gallstones. Lancet 2:979–983

Neoptolemos JP, Kemppainen EA, Mayer JM et al (2000) Early prediction of severity in acute pancreatitis by urinary trypsinogen activation peptide: a multicentre study. Lancet 355:1955–1960

Nowak A, Nowakowska-Dulawa E, Marek T et al (1995) Final results of the prospective, randomized, controlled study on endoscopic sphincterotomy versus conventional management in acute biliary pancreatitis (abstr). Gastroenteroloy 108:A380

Perez A, Whang EE, Brooks DC et al (2002) Is severity of necrotizing pancreatitis increased in extended necrosis and infected necrosis? Pancreas 25:229–233

Pezzilli R, Billi P, Miniero R et al (1995) Serum interleukin-6, interleukin-8, and beta 2-microglobulin in early assessment of severity of acute pancreatitis. Comparison with serum C-reactive protein. Dig Dis Sci 40:2341–2348

Pezzilli R, Morselli-Labate AM, Miniero R (1999) Simultaneous serum assays of lipase and interleukin-6 for early diagnosis and prognosis of acute pancreatitis. Clin Chem 45:1762–1767

Pezzilli R, Melzi d'Eril GV, Morselli-Labate AM et al (2000) Serum amyloid A, procalcitonin, and C-reactive protein in early assessment of severity of acute pancreatitis. Dig Dis Sci 45:1072–1078

Porter KA, Banks PA (1991) Obesity as a predictor of severity in acute pancreatitis. Int J Pancreatol 10:247–252

Puolakkainen P, Valtonen V, Paananen A et al (1987) C-reactive protein (CRP) and serum phospholipase a1 in the assessment of the severity of acute pancreatitis. Gut 28:764–771

Ranson JHC (1982) Etiologic and prognostic factors in human acute pancreatitis: a review. Am J Gastroenterol 77:633–638

Ranson JH (1997) Diagnostic standards for acute pancreatitis. World J Surg 21:136–142

Ranson JH, Balthazar E et al. (1985). Computed tomography and the prediction of pancreatic abscess in acute pancreatitis. Ann Surg 201(5):656–665

Ranson JHC, Rifikind KM, Roses DF et al (1974) Prognostics signs and the role of operative management in acute pancreatitis. Surg Gynaecol Obstet 139:69–81

Rattner DW, Legermate DA, Lee MJ et al (1992) Early surgical debridement of symptomatic pancreatic necrosis is beneficial irrespective of infection. Am J Surgery 163:105–109

Saifuddin A, Ward J, Ridgway J et al (1993) Comparison of MR and CT scanning in severe acute pancreatitis: initial experiences. Clinical Radiology 48:111–116

Sainio V, Puolakkainen P, Kemppainen E et al (1996) Serum trypsinogen-2 in the prediction of outcome in acute necrotizing pancreatitis. Scan J Gastroenterol 31:818–824

Simchuk EJ, Traverso LW, Nukui Y et al (2000) Computed tomography severity index is a predictor of outcomes for severe pancreatitis Am J Surg 179:352–355

Steinberg W, Goldstein SS, Davis ND et al (1985) Diagnostic assays in acute pancreatitis: a study of sensitivity and specificity. Ann Int Med 102:576–580

Talamini G, Uomo G, Pezzilli R et al (1999) Serum creatinine and chest radiographs in the early assessment of acute pancreatitis. Am J Surg 177:7–14

Telford JJ, Farrell JJ, Saltzman JR et al (2002) Pancreatic stent placement for duct disruption. Gastrointest Endosc 56:18–24

Tenner S, Fernandez-del Castillo C, Warshaw A et al (1997) Urinary trypsinogen activation peptide (TAP) predicts severity in patients with acute pancreatitis. Int J Pancreatology 21:105–110

Tichtin HE, Trujillo NP, Evans NF et al (1965) Diagnostic value of a new serum lipase method. Gastroenterology 48:12–19

Tietz NW, Shuey DF (1993) Lipase in serum – the elusive enzyme: an overview. Clinical Chemistry 39:746–756

Uhl W, Buchler M, Malfertheiner P et al (1991) PMN-elastase in comparison with CRP, antiproteases, and LDH as indicators of necrosis in human acute pancreatitis. Pancreas 6:253–259

Uhl W, Warshaw A, Imrie C et al (2002) IAP guidelines for the surgical management of acute pancreatitis. Pancreatology 2:565–573

Uomo G, Talamini G, Rabitti PG et al (1998) Influence of advanced age and related comorbidity on the course and outcome of acute pancreatitis. Ital J Gastroenterol Hepatol 30:616–621

Viedma JA, Perez-Mateo M, Agullo J et al (1994) Inflammatory response in the early prediction of severity in human acute pancreatitis. Gut 35:822–827

Warshaw AL, Lee KH (1979) Serum ribonuclease elevation and pancreatic necrosis in acute pancreatitis. Surgery 86:227–234

Warshaw AL, Bellini CA, Lesser PB (1975) Inhibition of serum and urine amylase activity in pancreatitis with hyperlipidemia. Ann Surg 182:72–75

Wereszczynska-Siemiatkowska, Dabrowski A, Jedynak M et al (1998) Oxidative stress as an early prognostic factor in acute pancreatitis (AP): its correlation with serum phospholipase A2 (PLA2) and plasma polymorphonuclear elastase (PMN-E) in different-severity forms of human AP. Pancreas 17:163–168

Wilson C, Heath DI, Imrie CW (1990) Prediction of outcome in acute pancreatitis: a comparative study of APACHE II, clinical assessment and multiple factor scoring systems. Br J Surg 77:1260–1264

Zieve L (1996) Clinical value of determinations of various pancreatic enzymes in serum. Gastroenterology 46:62–71

The Role of Ultrasound in Acute Pancreatitis

3

Costanza Bruno, Salvatore Minniti, and Giacomo Schenal

CONTENTS

3.1 **Introduction** *33*

3.2 **Diagnosis** *33*
3.2.1 Size of the Pancreas *34*
3.2.2 Echotexture of the Pancreas *34*
3.2.3 Focal Changes *35*

3.3 **Extra-glandular Changes** *35*
3.3.1 Fluid Collections *35*
3.3.2 Pancreatic Ascites *37*

3.4 **Etiologic Diagnosis** *37*
3.4.1 Gallstones *38*
3.4.2 Biliary Ducts Stones *38*
3.4.3 Idiopathic Pancreatitis *38*

3.5 **Clinical Evaluation** *40*
3.5.1 Severity Grading *40*
3.5.2 Resolution of Acute Pancreatitis *40*

3.6 **Complications** *40*
3.6.1 Glandular Infections *40*
3.6.2 Pseudocysts *41*
3.6.3 Vascular Complications *43*

3.7 **Conclusions** *43*

References *43*

C. Bruno, MD; S. Minniti, MD
Department of Radiology, Policlinico "GB Rossi", University of Verona, Piazzale LA Scuro 10, 37134 Verona, Italy
G. Schenal, MD
Department of Radiology, Ospedale Borgo Trento, Piazzale Stefani 1, 37126 Verona, Italy

3.1 Introduction

Ultrasound (US) is frequently used as an initial diagnostic study for patients suffering from acute abdominal pain (Merkle and Goerich 2002; Panzironi et al. 1997). It can both diagnose acute pancreatitis (AP) and exclude many other causes of abdominal pain (Bennett and Hann 2001; Lecesne and Drouillard 1999). Both increasing operator experience and technological advances in equipment (such as tissue harmonics), the pancreas can now be evaluated by US in over 90% of cases (Atri and Finnegan 1998; Bennett and Hann 2001; Jeffrey 1989; Karlson et al. 1999; Minniti et al. 2003). In AP, ultrasonographic evaluation is hampered in 25%–30% of patients due to overlapping gastrointestinal gas (Manfredi et al. 2001).

In addition to excessive intestinal gas, ultrasound has limited capabilities in evaluating the presence and extent of necrosis, in detecting the full extent of pancreatic related fluid collections and in identifying gastrointestinal tract complications (Manfredi et al. 2001). Despite these limitations there is sufficient literature to support the use of US to follow-up (assuming access is not hindered by excessive surgical drains) and for guiding needle aspiration or percutaneous drainage procedures (Gerzof et al. 1987; Malecka-Panas et al. 1998; Merkle and Goerich 2002; Panzironi et al. 1997; Rau et al. 1998; Van Sonnenberg et al. 1989).

3.2 Diagnosis

The accuracy of diagnostic ultrasound in AP depends on the evolution of the disease and its severity.

It is likely that the examination would be inconclusive in the early phases and in the mild forms of AP (Atri and Finnegan 1998; Bennett and Hann 2001; Freeny 1989; Jeffrey 1989; Lawson 1983; Lecesne and Drouillard 1999; Merkle and Goerich 2002).

3.2.1 Size of the Pancreas

Because of interstitial edema induced by the inflammatory process, the pancreas increases in size diffusely (Fig. 3.1) (Atri and Finnegan 1998; Bennett and Hann 2001; Jeffrey 1989; Lecesne and Drouillard 1999). Sometimes, however, the enlargement is segmental (Fig. 3.2) and affects the head of the pancreas (Blery et al. 1987). A modest size increase of the pancreas is better appreciated on a longitudinal scan along and adjacent to the superior mesenteric vein.

Caution is necessary when assessing the increase in size of the pancreas with US, especially when the size of the gland cannot be compared with a previous baseline examination. (Merkle and Goerich 2002). In fact, the normal variations in the size range are wide. The normal antero-posterior diameter of the pancreas varies from between 21 and 28 mm at the head, 12 and 22 mm at the body and 8 and 24 mm at the tail (De Graaff et al. 1978; Haber et al. 1976; Kolmannskog et al. 1982, 1983). The pancreas tends to atrophy with age (Manfredi et al. 2001). Thus ultrasound is more reliable in follow-up than on the initial evaluation of the actual size of the pancreas (Manfredi et al. 2001; Merkle and Goerich 2002).

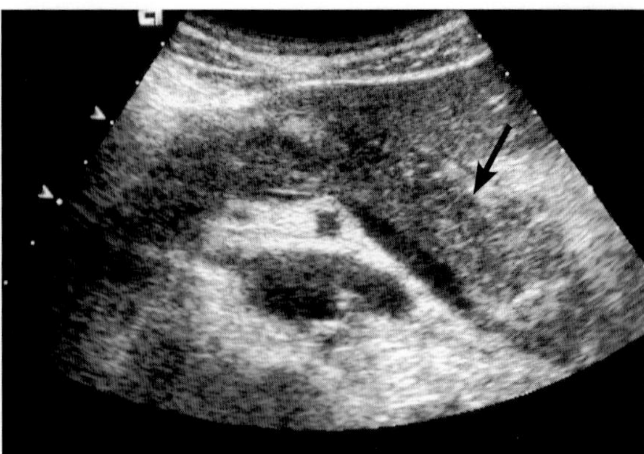

a

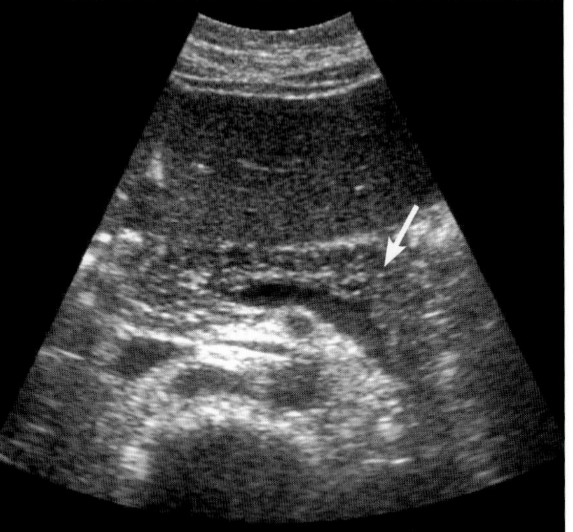

b

Fig. 3.1a,b. Acute edematous pancreatitis: transverse scans showing enlarged hypoechoic pancreas (*arrows*)

3.2.2 Echotexture of the Pancreas

The decreased echogenicity of the pancreatic parenchyma in patients with AP is related to the presence of amount of interstitial edema (Fig. 3.3) (Bennett and Hann 2001; Manfredi et al. 2001; Merkle and Goerich 2002). The change in echotexture is best seen 2–5 days after clinical onset (Freise 1987).

As with size, the decreased echogenicity may be difficult to appreciate on a single study. If the pancreas was inherently hyperechoic because of fatty infiltration seen in advanced age, or if the acute inflammation is superimposed on pre-ex-

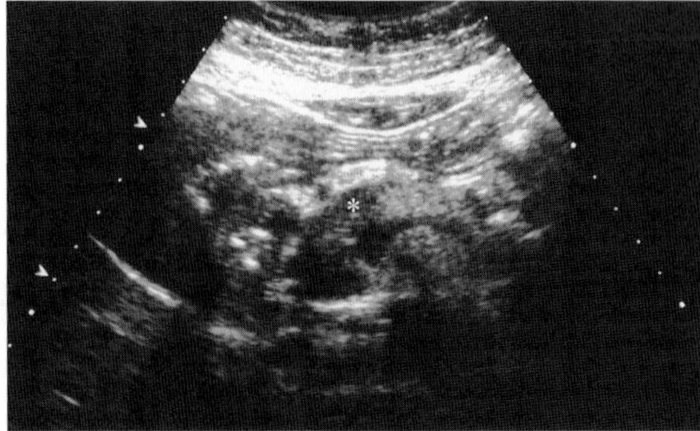

Fig. 3.2. Acute edematous pancreatitis: transverse scan demonstrates an enlarged hypoechoic head (*asterisk*) secondary to inflammatory changes

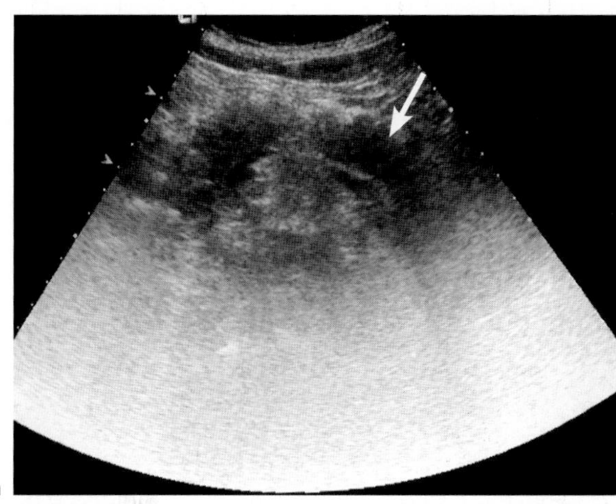

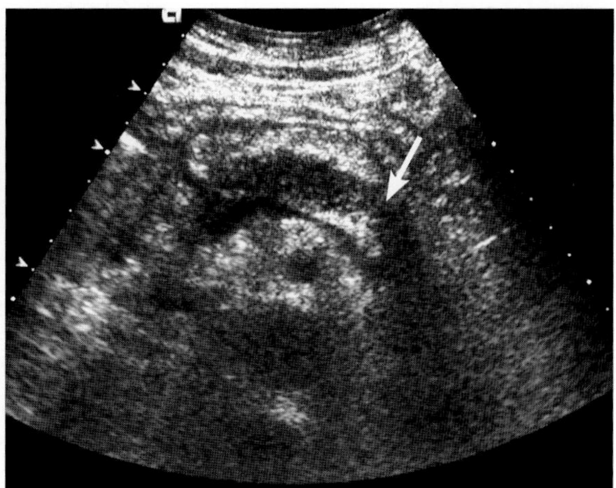

Fig. 3.3a,b. AP related changes in parenchymal echogenicity: transverse scan. As a consequence of edema pancreas becomes hypoechoic and inhomogeneous (*arrows*)

isting chronic pancreatitis, the resultant echogenicity can appear normal (Manfredi et al. 2001). Comparing the echogenicity of the pancreas and the liver can also be misleading as the latter undergoes fatty infiltration in AP patients who are alcoholics and/or dyslipidemics (Atri and Finnegan 1998). The contours of the pancreas are usually irregular and poorly defined due to the inflammation of the peri-pancreatic fat (Bennett and Hann 2001).

It is possible, although uncommon, for the main pancreatic duct to be dilated in AP, especially if it is obstructed by a focal inflammatory or neoplastic stricture (Atri and Finnegan 1998; Bennett and Hann 2001). This finding can be apparent in both the acute episode and during the healing phases (Malfertheiner and Buechler 1987). Ductal dilatation, according to some authors, is common with AP in children and is a more reliable diagnostic feature than glandular shape and size. It is also useful during a follow-up since it apparently correlates with the increase serum lipase level (Chao et al. 2000).

3.2.3 Focal Changes

Several findings involving different portions of the pancreas can occur in AP:

- AP can affect a portion of the pancreas, resulting in focal enlargement and decreased echogenicity in the affected region. This occurs most frequently in the head of the gland (Fig. 3.4) (Bennett and Hann 2001; Merkle and Goerich 2002). In rare cases, focal AP can be due to a nearby inflammatory condition, for example a penetrating duodenal ulcer (Atri and Finnegan 1998).
- It is also possible to see focal changes in the echotexture of the pancreas, usually presenting with hazy contours, due to fluid collections, necrotic foci or hyperechoic hemorrhages (Fig. 3.5) (Atri and Finnegan 1998; Bennett and Hann 2001; Lecesne and Drouillard 1999; Merkle and Goerich 2002).

The finding of a well-defined hypoechoic area in the pancreas raises the suspicion of neoplasm particularly if the patient has no acute symptoms and a normal serum amylase (Neff et al. 1984). This finding should be followed and correlated with further imaging; either MDCT, dedicated pancreatic MRI or endoscopic ultrasound (US) needle aspiration should be performed if the abnormality persists (Fig. 3.6); however, a result that does not show tumor does not exclude the possibilty and close clinical follow-up is essential. Differential diagnosis of a focal abnormality in the pancreas includes: pancreas divisum, focal lipomatosis, idiopathic fibrosclerosis, hypoechoic ventral pancreas, diverticulum of the duodenum. The sonographer should carefully attempt to exclude the presence of metastatic lesions, adjacent normal parenchyma, dilatation of the common bile duct or main pancreatic duct, normal peri-pancreatic vessels (Loren et al. 1999).

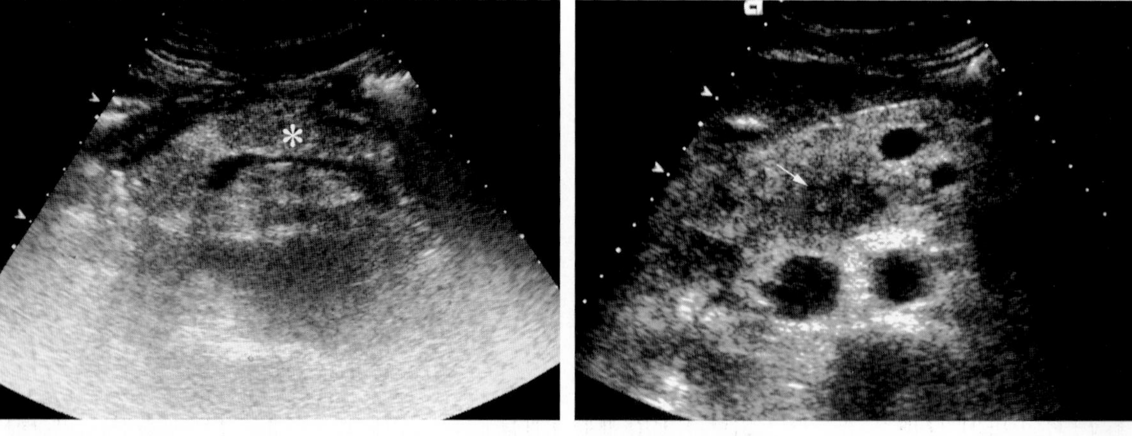

Fig. 3.4a,b. Focal involvement in AP, transverse and sagittal scans: there may be focal inflammatory changes in the body (*asterisk*) or in the head (*arrow*)

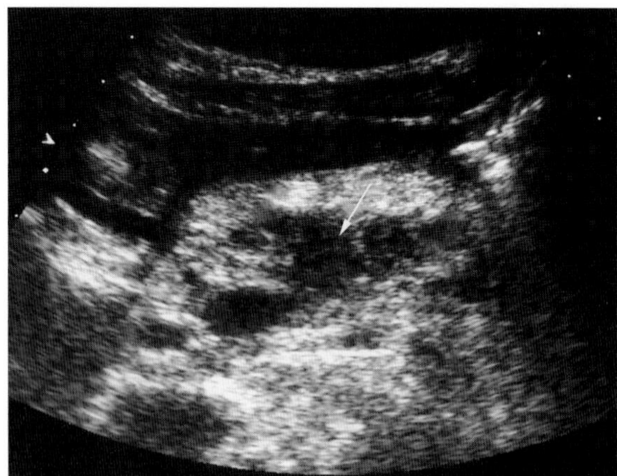

Fig. 3.5. Acute necrotizing pancreatitis, transverse scan: necrotic foci are an evolution of edema and can cause other focal changes (*arrow*)

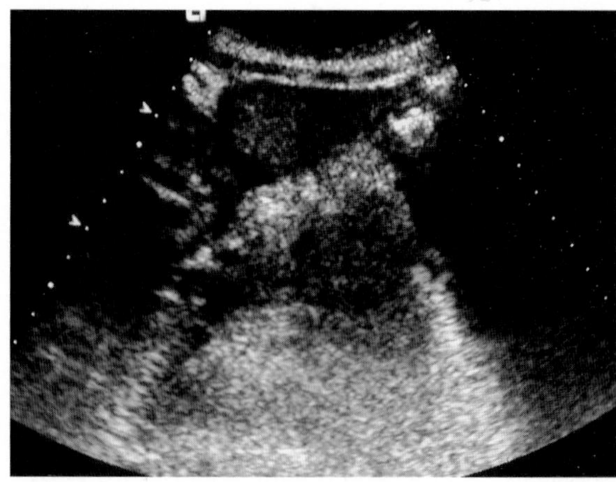

Fig. 3.6. Acute edematous pancreatitis, sagittal scans: differentiation of focal pancreatitis from neoplasm may be difficult because both conditions create a focal hypoechoic mass on sonograms

3.3 Extra-glandular Changes

3.3.1 Fluid Collections

Ultrasound is excellent for detecting the presence of fluid collections. However, MDCT or MRI are superior in evaluating the extent of these collections. Peripancreatic collections may be simple fluid with a hypoechoic appearance or more complex as they become filled with debris and/or necrotic tissue (Jeffrey et al. 1986; Atri and Finnegan 1998; Lecesne and Drouillard 1999; Bennett and Hann 2001; Manfredi et al. 2001; Merkle and Goerich 2002).

The following regions should be carfully interrogated for the presence of fluid collections in patients with AP:

- The lesser sac – they are easily recognized (Fig. 3.7). The caudate medial border of the caudate lobe should be visualized to assess the presence of fluid in the upper recesses of the lesser sac. EUS has significantly higher sensitivity in detection of peripancraetic fluid collections

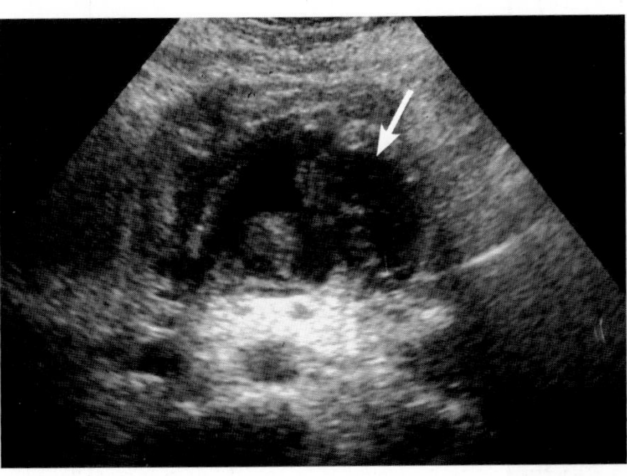
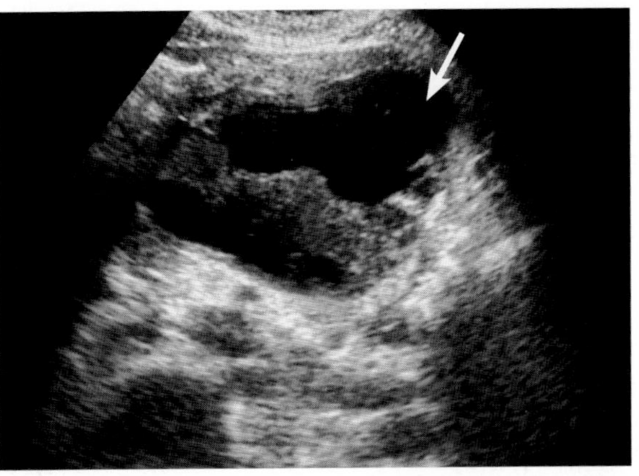

Fig. 3.7a,b. Acute pancreatitis, lesser sac fluid, transverse scans: fluid can be easily found in the lower lesser sac. Lower lesser sac fluid located between the pancreas and the stomach is the easiest to be localized with ultrasound and it often shows debris (*arrows*)

(Lecesne and Drouillard 1999; Sugiyama and Atomi 1998).

- Perirenal spaces, left more frequently than right (Fig. 3.8).
- Pararenal spaces (Fig. 3.9) (Chen et al. 1995).
- In mild cases, only a thin band of fluid surrounding the pancreas may be the only finding of fluid (Fig 3.10) (Atri and Finnegan 1998; Jeffrey et al. 1986).
- It is difficult to detect any thickening of Gerota fascia with ultrasound, although this is easily visualized with CT imaging (Lecesne and Drouillard 1999).

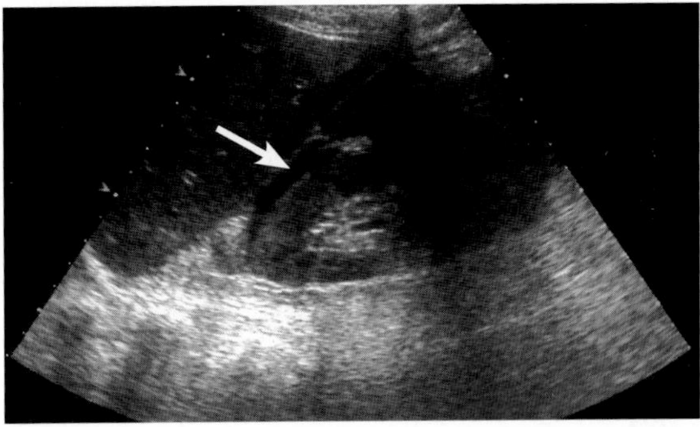

Fig. 3.8. Acute pancreatitis, perirenal fluid: sagittal scan, fluid in the perirenal right space surrounding superior pole of the right kidney (*arrow*)

3.3.2 Pancreatic Ascites

Pancreatic ascites is caused by the slow leakage of pancreatic secretions (Fig. 3.11) resulting from a disruption of the duct of Wirsung, from a fistula or a ruptured pseudocyst (Atri and Finnegan 1998). The appearance of ascites associated to a sudden reduction in size of a pseudocyst raises the suspicion of a fistula between the main pancreatic duct the cyst and the peritoneal cavity (Procacci et al. 2002). The appearance of pancreatic ascites is identical with benign ascites from any other cause. The diagnosis is established by recognizing the presence of ascites, and establishing high amylase levels within the effusion.

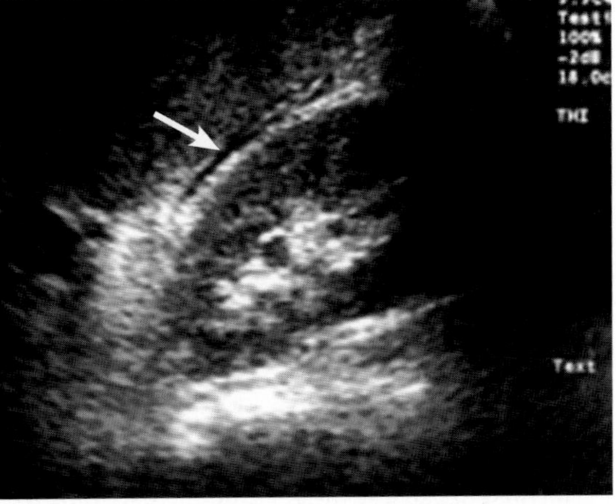

Fig. 3.9. Acute pancreatitis, perirenal fluid and fat changes: echogenic perirenal fat (*arrow*) is separating fluid from superior pole of the kidney

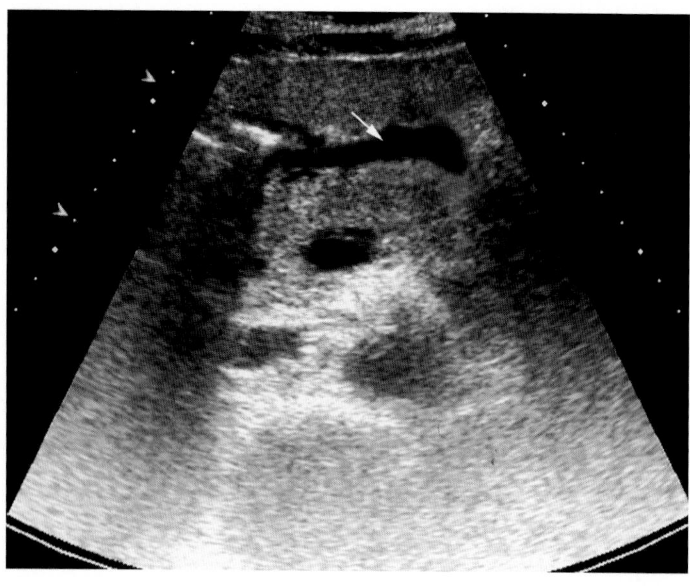

Fig. 3.10. Minimal fluid in AP, transverse scan: small amount of fluid surrounding pancreas (*arrow*)

Retroperitoneal fluid can extend into the mediastinum and accumulate in the pleural cavity (Belfar et al. 1987).

3.4 Etiologic Diagnosis

US examination can determine the cause of AP in patients with biliary calculi (Atri and Finnegan 1998; Bennett and Hann 2001; Gandolfi et al. 2003; Harvey and Miller 1999; Merkle and Goerich 2002; Pezzilli et al. 1999).

The ability to demonstrate biliary stones at any level (intra-hepatic, gallbladder, common duct) using ultrasound has improved with the introduction of second harmonic imaging (Shapiro et al. 1998).

3.4.1 Gallstones

It is standard of care that in ANY patient presenting with acute pancreatitis, a US examination must be performed to exclude biliary calculi. The finding of gallstones in patients with AP is of significant diagnostic value. In all, 4% of patients with gallstone disease will result in AP (Glasgow et al. 2000).

Ultrasound the gold standard modality to diagnose gallstones (Fig. 3.12) (Jeffrey et al. 1996). It is far more reliable than CT, having a higher than 95% sensitivity, specificity and accuracy (Cooperberg and Burhenne 1980; Goodman et al. 1985; Hessler et al. 1989; Laing et al. 1981). Because US is limited in its ability to detect choledocholithiasis, MRI is becoming more frequently used in the evaluation of patients with AP; however, it is expensive and not readily available.

3.4.2 Biliary Ducts Stones

For the diagnosis of dilatation of the biliary tree, ultrasound has 99% sensitivity (Cooperberg et al. 1980) and 93% accuracy, but it is not as reliable at defining the site (accuracy 60% – 92%) and, the cause of the obstruction (accuracy 39% – 71%) (Baron et al. 1982; Laing et al. 1986).

The diagnosis of choledocholithiasis requires visualization of an echogenic spot surrounded by bile with a posterior shadow (Fig. 3.13) – ultrasound has a reported 47% – 85% sensitivity, 89% – 91% specificity and 92% positive predictive value. Typical pitfalls in this diagnosis are the presence of stones in undilated ducts, the absence of shadowing and the stone's location in the distal common bile duct, which in about 8% of patients is not visible due to the overlapping intestinal gas (Baron et al. 1982;

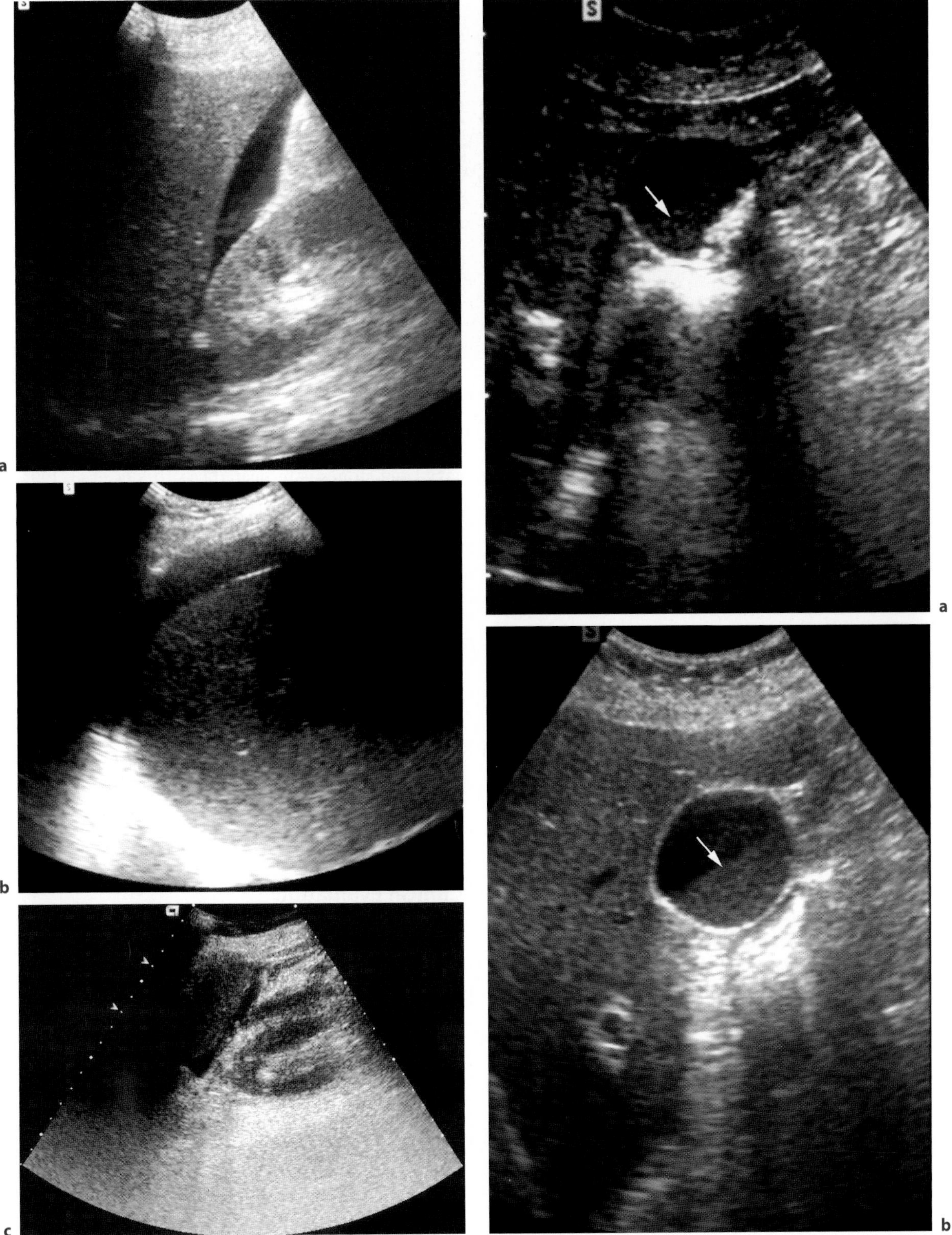

Fig. 3.11a–c. Pancreatic ascites. Sagittal US (**a**,**c**) and transverse scans (**b**), pancreatic ascites can be found in the Morrison's pouch (**a**) and in the right (**b**) and left (**c**) subphrenic spaces

Fig. 3.12a,b. Cholelithiasis: sagittal scans. US can detect stones with acoustic shadows (*arrow*, **a**) and biliary sludge slightly echogenic without acoustic shadows (*arrow*, **b**)

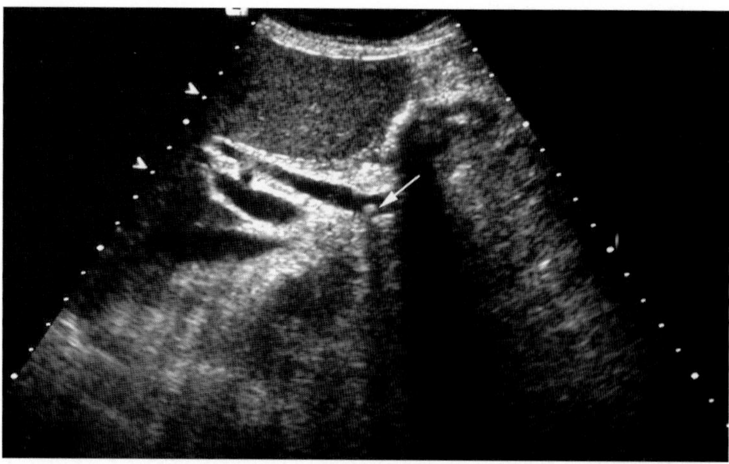

Fig. 3.13. Choledocholithiasis: sagittal scan showing small echogenic focus with acoustic shadows in the common bile duct (*arrow*)

Cooperberg et al. 1980). The correlation between ultrasonography and ERCP for diagnosing the presence of stones or sludge in the biliary tracts is only 60% (Pezzilli et al. 1999).

Current literature recommends that confirmation of choledocholithiasis in AP is unnecessary in the acute phase unless the patient develops fever. In those cases, therapeutic ERCP with sphincterotomy and stone removal is indicated (Folsch et al. 1997; Harvey and Miller 1999; Merkle and Goerich 2002). The literature regarding different imaging modalities to detect common duct stones did not agree until a few years ago. Some authors reported a high sensitivity (90%) for spiral CT (Neitlich et al. 1997; Harvey and Miller 1999; Bennett and Hann 2001), while others were of the opinion that the best examination was endoscopic ultrasound (Sugiyama and Atomi 1998), because of the poor sensitivity of abdominal US and spiral CT (47%). The introduction of the MR cholangiopancreatography (MRCP) has dramatically improved the noninvasive diagnosis of common duct stones.

3.4.3 Idiopathic Pancreatitis

Between 20% and 30% of cases of AP remain "idiopathic" (Frossard et al. 2000). Some of these cases are due to the presence of tiny unrecognizable stones or sludge wedged in the papilla of Vater. If biliary microlithiasis is suspected, EUS, which has a positive predictive value of 98% for the diagnosis of biliary tract stones is indicated (Amouyal et al. 1994, Buscail et al. 1995; Chak et al. 1999; Frossard et al. 2000; Lecesne and Drouillard 1999; Liu et al. 2000; Norton and Alderson 2000; Prat et al. 2001; Shaffer 2001; Snady 2001; Sugiyama and Atomi 1998). In patients in whom endoscopic ultrasound has demonstrated the presence of stones in the biliary tracts, an endoscopic sphincterotomy can then be performed at the same session (Prat et al. 2001).

3.5 Clinical Evaluation

3.5.1 Severity Grading

Ultrasound cannot reliably detect necrosis in patients with AP (Atri and Finnegan 1998; Bennett and Hann 2001).

It has been stated that the presence of necrosis can be suspected when considerable heterogeneity in the pancreatic echotexture is found, appearing late after the onset of the acute attack (Cotton et al. 1980). According to other authors, however, ultrasound is claimed to be reliable in distinguishing between edematous and necrotizing forms of AP (Fig. 3.14) (Panzironi et al. 1997). The diagnosis is more reliably made with endoscopic ultrasound, which apparently has 100% sensitivity discriminating mild

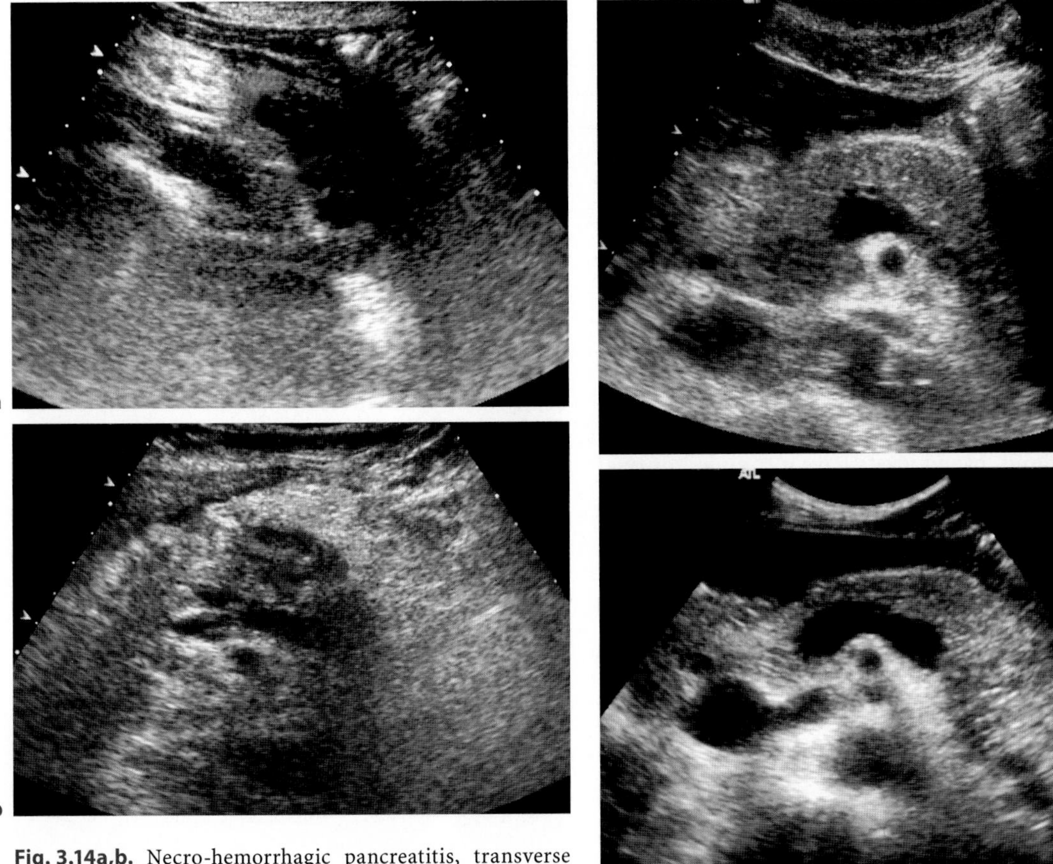

Fig. 3.14a,b. Necro-hemorrhagic pancreatitis, transverse scans: pancreatic necrosis can be detected as inhomogeneous hypoechoic areas different in extension (**a**,**b**)

Fig. 3.15a,b. US documentation of resolution of AP. Image (**a**) compatible with edematous AP. There is return to normal coincident with clinical resolution (**b**)

from severe forms of AP (LECESNE and DROUILLARD 1999; SUGIYAMA and ATOMI 1998).

Some authors have noted that, during the early phases of the disease, cases of AP that may develop necrosis are characterized by an increase in the velocity of the flow in the hepatic artery and a decrease in the pulsatility index of the superior mesenteric artery (SAKAGAMI et al. 2002).

3.5.2 Resolution of Acute Pancreatitis

Ultrasound is a reliable follow-up imaging method of the resolution of the acute inflammatory process (Fig. 3.15) that usually characterizes mild forms of AP.

3.6 Complications

3.6.1 Glandular Infections

There are three complications in AP that are susceptible to infection: infected necrosis, infected pseudocysts and abscess. Their imaging findings are nonspecific and, in the case of necrosis and pseudocyst, may be indistinguishable from sterile forms (MORGAN et al. 1997). When infection is clinically suspected, needle aspiration and culture of all fluid collections is necessary. Needle aspiration can be effectively performed under ultrasonographic guidance with reported sensitivity of 88% and specificity of 90% for diagnosis (ATRI and FINNEGAN 1998; RAU et al. 1998). Ultrasound can also be used for guiding percutaneous drainage. In the absence of gas within the collection, it may be impossible to distinguish an infected collection from a sterile one (Fig. 3.16). Infected pseudocyst or fluid collections may be treated by percutaneous drainage, but effective control of infected necrosis requires open surgical debridement (Morgan et al. 1997; Procacci et al. 2002). In the absence of gas, it cannot.

3.6.2 Pseudocysts

At ultrasound, pseudocysts have a rounded or oval shape with smooth well-defined contours and intraluminal fluid contents (Fig. 3.17) (Sarti 1980; Atri and Finnegan 1998). In the early stage of formation, they may display internal echoes generated by residual necrotic material, which tends to disappear over time (Laing et al. 1979; Lee et al. 1988). Pseudocysts are unilocular but sometimes have thin septa, which divide them into several cavities (Laing et al. 1979). The walls rarely calcify (Atri and Finnegan 1998). The ultrasonographic features of pseudocysts can be better evaluated with endoscopic ultrasound (Byrne et al. 2002).

Drainage is considered if the pseudocyst persists for a long time (more than 6 weeks), if the cyst is > 5 cm and if it causes symptoms or complications (Atri and Finnegan 1998). Drainage can be performed under ultrasonographic or echo-endoscopic guidance (Breslin and Wallace 2002; Byrne et al. 2002). Ultrasound, either traditional or endo-

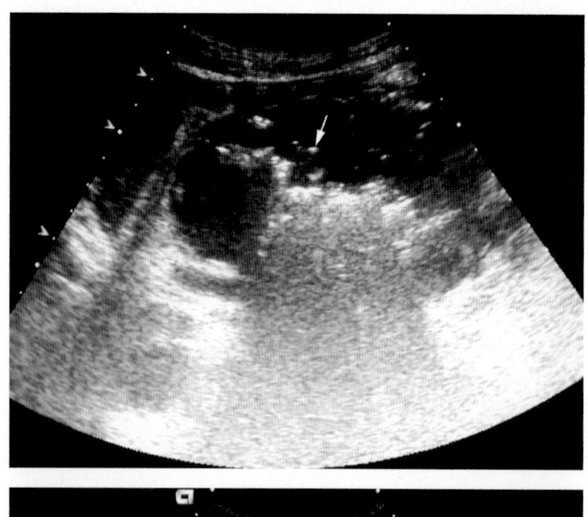

a

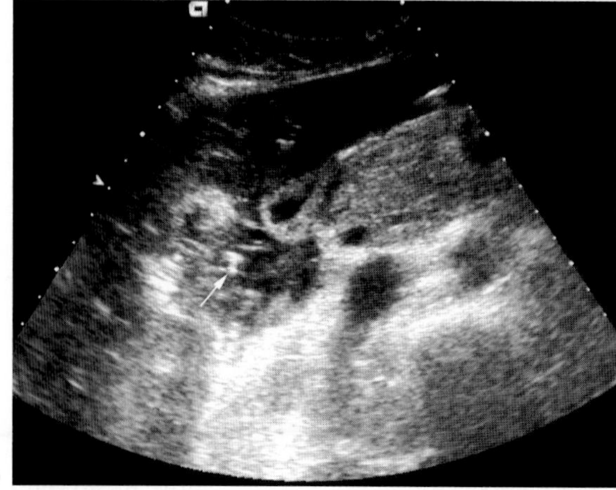

b

Fig. 3.16a,b. Necro-hemorrhagic pancreatitis, transverse scans: US can evaluate the evolution of fluid collections showing eventual complications. Infected fluid collections often show debris (*arrow*, **a**) or bright echoes from gas bubbles (*arrow*, **b**)

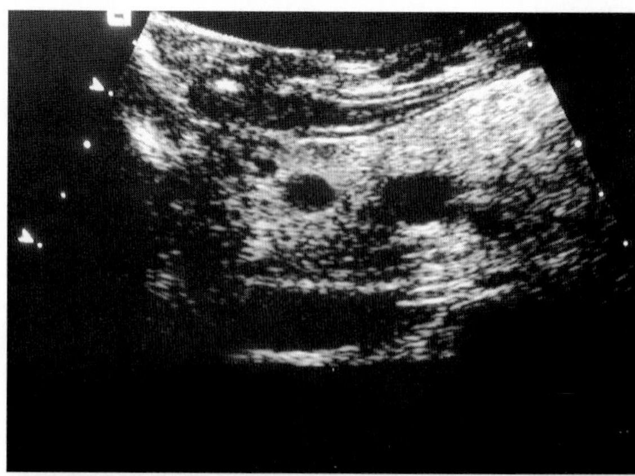

a

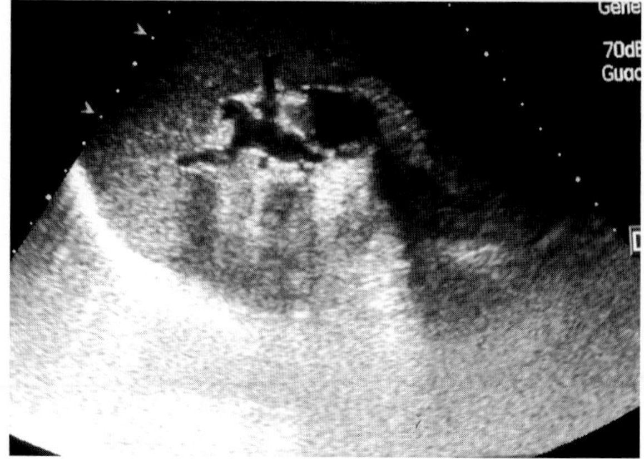

b

Fig. 3.17a,b. Simple pseudocysts: sagittal scans through pancreatic head (**a**) and tail (**b**). They are fluid collections with well defined nonepithelized wall with anechoic structure showing acoustic enhancement

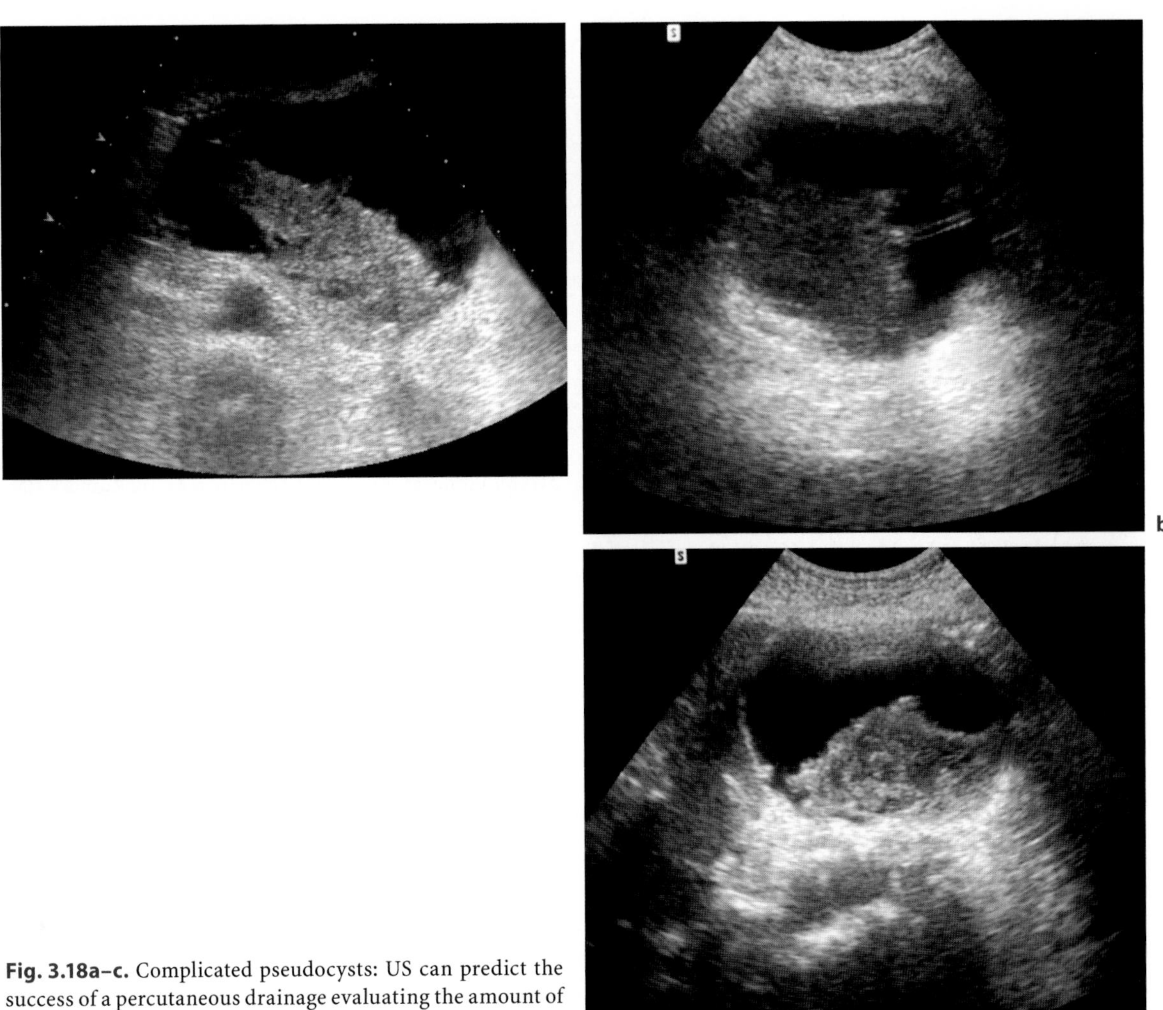

Fig. 3.18a–c. Complicated pseudocysts: US can predict the success of a percutaneous drainage evaluating the amount of debris in the lesion (**a**), can be used to guide the procedure (**b**) and to monitor the result (**c**)

scopic can also evaluate the resolution of a pseudocyst following a drainage procedure (BRESLIN and WALLACE 2002; BYRNE et al. 2002; MERKLE and GOERICH 2002).

Complications from pseudocysts are amenable to US diagnosis (Fig. 3.18). These complications include:

- Extesnive cephalad or caudal migration as they dissect across fascial planes (MAIER et al. 1986; LYE et al. 1987).
- Direct extension into the parenchyma of adjacent solid organs (liver, spleen, kidney).
- Gastrointestinal or billiary obstructuin (VICK et al. 1981; RHEINGOLD et al. 1978).
- Spleno-portal vein thrombosis (FALKOFF et al. 1986).
- Erosion into adjacent arteries causing the formation of pseudoaneurysms.
- Gastrointestinal bleeding either from arterial erosion or portal hypertension (GRACE and JORDAN 1976; STANLEY et al. 1976).
- Sterile or infected peritonitis.
- Superinfection.

Presence of infection does not correlate with size of cyst or thickness of cyst wall. Endocavity gas bubbles are seen in infected pseudocysts but occasionally they may be the consequence of a cyst-enteric fistula (LEE et al. 1988; BENNETT and HANN 2001).

3.6.3
Vascular Complications

Vascular complications can be caused directly by AP or by pseudocysts. The addition of Doppler interrogation improves diagnosis (Atri and Finnegan 1998; Bennett and Hann 2001; Merkle and Goerich 2002; Dorffel et al. 2000; Bennett and Hann 2001).

The most frequent vascular complication of AP is the formation of a pseudoaneurysm. In order of frequency, the arteries most commonly involved are splenic, gastro-duodenal, pancreatico-duodenal, left gastric and hepatic arteries. Pseudoaneurysms develop in 3.5%–10% of AP cases, they rarely rupture but when they do, the mortality rate is around 50% (MacMahon 1994). A ruptured pseudoaneurysm can bleed in a pseudocyst, in the pancreatic parenchyma, in the peritoneal cavity or in the gastro-intestinal tract. US with Doppler is an excellent examination for suspected pseudoaneurysms (Ishida et al. 1999; Lecesne and Drouillard 1999).

In all patients with AP the US examination must include the Doppler examination of all intra- or peri-pancreatic fluid collections in order to distinguish pseudocysts from pseudoaneurysms (Maus 1993; Waslen et al. 1998). A non-symptomatic pseudoaneurysm can occasionally be suspected if the B-mode ultrasound reveals, at a short interval, any size increase or variation in the echogenicity of the fluid collection (Kahn et al. 1994; Procacci et al. 2002).

The Doppler examination shows a whirling flow with an uneven variable velocity (Kahn et al. 1994). These variations depend on the size of the pseudoaneurysm and on the presence of clots (Waslen et al. 1998). If the pseudoaneurysm is totally thrombosed, the diagnosis can be difficult (Kahn et al. 1994; Waslen et al. 1998).

3.7
Conclusions

In patients with acute pancreatitis the use of ultrasonographic abdominal examination contributes to the diagnosis, evaluation and management. Conventional abdominal and endoscopic sonographic studies are mainly used to detect gallbladder and common duct stones, to follow up the presence and size of fluid collections and pseudocysts and to guide interventional procedures in patients with complications such as needle aspirations and drainage of fluid collections and pseudocysts.

References

Amouyal P, Amouyal G, Levy P, Tuzet S, Palazzo L, Vilgrain V, Cayet B, Belghiti J, Fekete F, Bernades P (1994) Diagnosis of choledocolithiasis by endoscopic ultrasonography. Gastroenterology 42:225–231

Atri M, Finnegan PW (1998) The pancreas. In: Rumack CM, Wilson SR, Charboneau JW (eds) Diagnostic ultrasound, 2nd edn. Mosby, St. Louis, pp 241–256

Balthazar EJ, Freeny PC, Van Sonnenberg E (1994) Imaging and intervention in acute pancreatitis. Radiology 193:297–306

Baron RL, Stanley RJ, Lee JKT, Koehler RE, Melson GL, Balfe DM, Weyman PJ (1982) A prospective comparison of the evaluation of biliary obstruction using computed tomography and ultrasonography. Radiology 145:91–98

Belfar HL, Radecki PD, Friedman AC, Caroline DF (1987) Pancreatitis presenting as pleural effusions: computed tomography demonstration of pleural extension of pancreatic exudate. Comput Tomogr 11:184–186

Bennett GL, Hann LE (2001) Pancreatic ultrasonography. Surg Clin North Am 81:259–281

Blery M, Hautefeuille P, Jacquenod P (1987) Pancreatites aigues. Apport de l'échographie et de la tomodensitométrie. Feuillets de Radiologie 27:259–271

Breslin N, Wallace MB (2002) Diagnosis and fine needle aspiration of pancreatic pseudocysts: the role of endoscopic ultrasound. Gastrointest Endosc Clin North Am 12:781–790

Buscail L, Escorrou J, Moreau J, Delvaux M, Louvel D, Lapeyre F, Tregant P, Frexinos J (1995) Endoscopic ultrasonography in chronic pancreatitis: a comparative prospective study with conventional ultrasonography, computed tomography and ERCP. Pancreas 10:251–257

Byrne MF, Mitchell RM, Baillie J (2002) Pancreatic pseudocysts. Curr Treat Options Gastroenterol 5:331–338

Chak A, Hawes RH, Cooper GS, Hoffman B, Catalano MF, Wong RC, Herbener TE, Sivak MV Jr (1999) Prospective assessment of the utility of EUS in the evaluation of gallstone pancreatitis. Gastrointest Endosc 49:599–604

Chao H, Lin S, Kong M, Luo C (2000) Sonographic evaluation of the pancreatic duct in normal children and in children with pancreatitis. J Ultrasound Med 19:757–763

Chen JJ, Changchien CS, Kuo CH (1995) Causes of increasing width of right anterior extrarenal space seen in ultrasonographic examinations. J Clin Ultrasound 23:287–292

Cooperberg PL, Burhenne HJ (1980) Real-time ultrasonography: diagnostic technique of choice in calculous gallbladder disease. N Engl J Med 302:1277–1279

Cooperberg PL, Li D, Wong P, Cohen MM, Burhenne HJ (1980) Accuracy of common hepatic duct size in the evaluation of extrahepatic biliary obstruction. Radiology 135:141–144
Cotton PB, Lees WR, Vallon AG, Cottone M, Croker JR, Chapman M (1980) Gray-scale ultrasonography and endoscopic pancreatography in pancreatic diagnosis. Radiology 134:453–459
Cronan JJ (1986) US diagnosis of choledocholithiasis: a reappraisal. Radiology 161:133–134
Cronan JJ, Mueller PR, Simeone JF, O'Connell RS, Van Sonnenberg E, Wittenberg J, Ferrucci JT Jr (1983) Prospective diagnosis of choledocholithiasis. Radiology 146:467–469
De Graaff CS, Taylor KJ, Simonds BD, Rosenfield AJ (1978) Gray-scale echography of the pancreas. Re-evaluation of normal size. Radiology 129:157–161
Dorffel T, Wruck T, Ruckert RI, Romaniuk P, Dorffel Q, Wermke W (2000) Vascular complications in acute pancreatitis assessed by color duplex ultrasonography. Pancreas 21:126–133
Falkoff GE, Taylor KJW, Morse SS (1986) Hepatic artery pseudoaneurysm: diagnosis with real-time and pulsed Doppler ultrasound. Radiology 58:55–56
Flunker S, Aube C, Anglade E, Vuillemin E, Bourree Y, Burtin P, Caron-Poitreau C (2001) Value of tissue harmonic imaging in biliary lithiasis. Gastroenterol Clin Biol 25:589–594
Folsch UR, Nitsche R, Ludtke R, Hilgers RA, Creutzfeldt W (1997) Early ERCP and papillotomy compared with conservative treatment for acute biliary pancreatitis. The German Study Group on Acute Biliary Pancreatitis. N Engl J Med 336:237–242
Freeny PC (1989) Classification of pancreatitis. Radiol Clin North Am 27:1–3
Freise J (1987) Evaluation of sonography in the diagnosis of acute pancreatitis. In: Beger HG, Buechler M (eds) Acute pancreatitis. Springer, Berlin Heidelberg New York, pp 118–138
Frossard JL, Sosa-Valencia L, Amouyal G, Marty O, Hadengue A, Amouyal P (2000) Usefulness of endoscopic ultrasonography in patients with "idiopathic" acute pancreatitis. Am J Med 109:196–200
Fugazzola C, Procacci C, Caudana R, Bergamo IA (1984) The role of computed tomography in acute pancreatitis. In: Banks PA, Porro GB (eds) Acute pancreatitis. Advances in pathogenesis, diagnosis and treatment. Masson, Milano, pp 79–86
Gandolfi L, Torresan F, Solmi L, Puccetti A (2003) The role of ultrasound in biliary and pancreatic disease. Eur J Ultrasound 16:141–159
Gerzof SG, Banks PA, Robbins AH, Johnson WC, Spechler SJ, Wetzner SM, Snider JM, Langevin RE, Jay ME (1987) Early diagnosis of pancreatic infection by computed tomography-guided aspiration. Gastroenterology 93:1315–1320
Glasgow RE, Cho M, Hutter MM, Mulvihill SJ (2000) The spectrum and cost of complicated gallstone disease in California. Arch Surg 135:1021–1027
Goodman AJ, Neoptolemos JP, Carr-Locke DL, Finlay DB, Fossard DP (1985) Detection of gall stones after acute pancreatitis. Gut 26:125–132
Grace RR, Jordan PH (1976) Unresolved problems of pancreatic pseudocysts. Ann Surg 184:16–21
Gross BH, Harter LP, Gore RM, Callen PW, Filly RA, Shapiro HA, Goldberg HI (1983) Ultrasonic evaluation of common bile duct stones: prospective comparison with endoscopic retrograde cholangiopancreatography. Radiology 146:471–474
Haber K, Freimanis AK, Asher WM (1976) Demonstration and dimensional analysis of the normal pancreas with gray-scale echography. Am J Roentgenol 126:624–628
Harvey RT, Miller WT (1999) Acute biliary disease: initial CT and follow-up US versus initial US and follow-up CT. Radiology 213:831–836
Hessler PC, Hill DS, Deforie FM, Rocco AF (1989) High accuracy sonographic recognition of gallstones. Am J Roentgenol 136:517–520
Ishida H, Konno K, Komatsuda T, Sato M, Naganuma H, Hamashima Y, Ishida J (1999) Gastrointestinal bleeding due to ruptured pseudoaneurysm in patients with pancreatitis. Abdom Imaging 24:418–421
Jeffrey RB (1989) Sonography in acute pancreatitis. Radiol Clin North Am 27:5–17
Jeffrey RB, Laing FC, Wing VW (1986) Extrapancreatic spread of acute pancreatitis: new observations with real-time ultrasound. Radiology 159:707–711
Kahn LA, Kamen C, McNamara MP (1994) Variable color Doppler appearance of pseudoaneurysm in pancreatitis. AJR Am J Roentgenol 162:187–188
Kane RA (1988) The biliary system. In: Kurtz A, Goldberg BB (eds) Gastrointestinal ultrasonography. Churchill Livingstone, New York, pp 75–138
Karlson BM, Ekbom A, Lindgren PG, Kallskog V, Rastad J (1999) Abdominal US for diagnosis of pancreatic tumor: prospective cohort analysis. Radiology 213:107–111
Kolmannskog F, Swensen T, Vatn MH, Larsen S (1982) Computed tomography and ultrasound of the normal pancreas. Acta Radiol Diagn (Stockh) 23:443–451
Kolmannskog F, Larsen S, Swensen T, Larssen T (1983) Reproducibility and observer variation at computed tomography and ultrasound of the normal pancreas. Acta Radiol Diagn (Stockh) 24:21–25
Laing FC, Jeffrey RB (1983) Choledocholithiasis and cystic duct obstruction: difficult ultrasonographic diagnosis. Radiology 146:475–479
Laing FC, Gooding GW, Brown T, Leopold GR (1979) Atypical pseudocysts of the pancreas: an ultrasonographic evaluation. J Clin Ultrasound 7:27–33
Laing FC, Federle MP, Jeffrey RB (1981) Ultrasonographic evaluation of patients with acute right upper quadrant pain. Radiology 140:449–455
Laing FC, Jeffrey RB, Wing VW (1984) Improved visualization of choledocholithiasis by sonography. AJR Am J Roentgenol 143:949–952
Laing FC, Jeffrey RB, Wing VW, Nyberg D (1986) Biliary dilatation: defining the level and cause by real-time US. Radiology 160:39–42
Lawson TL (1983) Acute pancreatitis and its complications. Computed tomography and sonography. Radiol Clin North Am 21:495–513
Lecesne R, Drouillard J (1999) Acute pancreatitis. In: Baert AL, Delorme G, Van Hoe L (eds) Radiology of the pan-

creas, 2nd edn. Springer, Berlin Heidelberg New York, pp 123–143

Lee CM, Chang-Chien CS, Lin DY, Yang CY, Sheen IS, Chen WJ (1988) Real-time ultrasonography of pancreatic pseudocysts: comparison of infected and uninfected pseudocysts. J Clin Ultrasound 16:393–397

Lee MJ, Choi TK, Lai ECS (1986) Endoscopic retrograde cholangiopancreatography after acute pancreatitis. Surg Gynecol Obst 163:354–358

Liu CL, Lo CM, Chan JK, Poon RT, Fan ST (2000) EUS for detection of occult cholelithiasis in patients with idiopathic pancreatitis. Gastrointest Endosc 51:28–32

London NJM, Neoptolemos JP, Lavelle J, Bailey I, James D (1989) Serial computed tomography scanning in acute pancreatitis: a prospective study. Gut 30:397–403

Loren I, Lasson A, Fork T, Genell S, Nilsson A, Nilsson P, Nirhov N (1999) New sonographic imaging observations in focal pancreatitis. Eur Radiol 9:862–867

Lye DJ, Stark RH, Cullen GM, Wepfer JF (1987) Ruptured pancreatic pseudocysts: extension into the thigh. AJR Am J Roentgenol 49:937–938

MacMahon MJ (1994) Acute pancreatitis. In: Misiewicz JJ, Pounder RE, Venables CW (eds) Diseases of the gut and pancreas. Blackwell, London, pp 3427–3440

Maier W, Roscher R, Malfertheiner P, Schmidt E, Buechler M (1986) Pancreatic pseudocyst of the mediastinum: evaluation by computed tomography. Eur J Radiol 6:70–72

Malecka-Panas E, Juszynski A, Chrzastek J, Nowacka B, Jarkowska J, Studniarek M (1998) Pancreatic fluid collections: diagnostic and therapeutic implications of percutaneous drainage guided by ultrasound. Hepatogastroenterology 45:873–878

Malfertheiner P, Buechler M (1987) Clinical symptoms and diagnostic requirements in acute pancreatitis. In: Beger HG, Buechler M (eds) Acute pancreatitis. Springer, Berlin Heidelberg New York, pp 104–124

Manfredi R, Brizi MG, Canade A, Vecchioli A, Marano P (2001) Imaging of acute pancreatitis. Rays 26:135–142

Maus TM (1993) Pseudoaneurysm hemorrhage as a complication of pancreatitis. Mayo Clin Proc 68:895–896

Merkle EM, Goerich J (2002) Imaging of acute pancreatitis. Eur Radiol 12:1979–1992

Minniti S, Bruno C, Biasiutti C, Tonel D, Falzone A, Falconi M, Procacci C (2003) Sonography versus helical CT in identification and staging of pancreatic ductal adenocarcinoma. J Clin Ultrasound 31:175–182

Morgan DE, Baron TH, Smith JK, Robbin ML, Kenney PJ (1997) Pancreatic fluid collections prior to intervention: evaluation with MR imaging compared with CT and US. Radiology 203:773–778

Neff CC, Simeone JF, Wittenberg J, Mueller PR, Ferrucci JT Jr (1984) Inflammatory pancreatic masses: problems in differentiating focal pancreatitis from carcinoma. Radiology 150:35–40

Neitlich JD, Topazian M, Smith RC, Gupta A, Burrell MI, Rosenfield AT (1997) Detection of choledocholithiasis: comparison of unenhanced helical CT and endoscopic retrograde cholangiopancreatography. Radiology 203:753–757

Neoptolemos JP, Hall AW, Finlay DF, Berry JM, Carr-Locke DL, Fossard DP (1984) The urgent diagnosis of gallstones in acute pancreatitis: a prospective study of three methods. Br J Surg 71:230–233

Norton SA, Alderson D (2000) Endoscopic ultrasonography in the evaluation of idiopathic acute pancreatitis. Br J Surg 87:1650–1655

Panzironi G, Franceschini L, Angelini P, Ascarelli A, De Siena G (1997) Role of ultrasonography in the study of patients with acute pancreatitis. G Chir 18:47–50

Pezzilli R, Billi P, Barakat B, D'Imperio N, Miglio F (1999) Ultrasonographic evaluation of the common bile duct in biliary acute pancreatitis patients: comparison with endoscopic retrograde cholangiopancreatography. J Ultrasound Med 18:391–394

Prat F, Edery J, Meduri B, Chiche R, Ayoun C, Bodart M, Grange D, Loison F, Nedelec P, Sbai-Idrissi MS, Valverde A, Vergeau B (2001) Early EUS of the bile duct before endoscopic sphincterotomy for acute biliary pancreatitis. Gastrointest Endosc 54:724–729

Procacci C, Mansueto G, D'Onofrio M, Gasparini A, Ferrara RM, Falconi M (2002) Non-traumatic abdominal emergencies: imaging and intervention in acute pancreatic conditions. Eur Radiol 12:2407–2434

Rau B, Pralle U, Mayer GM, Beger HG (1998) Role of ultrasonographically guided fine-needle aspiration cytology in the diagnosis of infected pancreatic necrosis. Br J Surg 85:179–184

Rheingold OJ, Wilbar JA, Barkin JS (1978) Gastric outlet obstruction due to pancreatic pseudocyst: a report of two cases. Am J Gastroenterol 69:92–96

Rothlin M (2000) Does every patient with pancreatic disease need ultrasound examination? Swiss Surg 6:211–215

Sakagami J, Kataoka K, Sogame Y, Usui N, Mitsuyoshi M (2002) Ultrasonographic splanchnic arterial flow measurement in severe acute pancreatitis. Pancreas 24:357–364

Sankaran S, Walt A (1976) Pancreatic ascites: recognition and management. Arch Surg 3:430–434

Sarti DA (1980) Ultrasonography of the pancreas. In: Sart DA, Sample WF (eds) Diagnostic ultrasound, text and cases. M. Nijoff, The Hague, pp 168–225

Shaffer EA (2001) Gallbladder sludge: what is its clinical significance? Curr Gastroenterol Rep 3:166–173

Shapiro RS, Wagreich J, Parsons RB, Stancato-Pasik A, Yeh HC, Lao R (1998) Tissue harmonic imaging sonography: evaluation of image quality compared with conventional sonography. AJR Am J Roentgenol 171:1203–1206

Snady H (2001) Endoscopic ultrasonography in benign pancreatic disease. Surg Clin North Am 81:329–344

Stanley JL, Frey CF, Miller TA, Lindenauer SM, Child CG III (1976) Major arterial hemorrhage: a complication of pancreatic pseudocyst and chronic pancreatitis. Arch Surg 111:435–440

Sugiyama M, Atomi Y (1998) Acute biliary pancreatitis: the roles of endoscopic ultrasonography and endoscopic retrograde cholangiopancreatography. Surgery 124:14–21

Van Sonnenberg E, Wittich GR, Casola G, Brannigan TC, Karnel F, Stabile BE, Varney RR, Christensen RR (1989) Percutaneous drainage of infected and nonifected pancreatic pseudocysts: experience in 101 cases. Radiology 170:757–762

Vick CW, Simeone JF, Ferrucci JT Jr, Wittenberg J, Mueller PR (1981) Pancreatitis-associated fluid collection involving the spleen: sonographic and computed tomographic appearance. Gastrointest Radiol 6:247–250

Vujic I (1989) Vascular complications of pancreatitis. Radiol Clin North Am 27:81–91

Wang SS, Lin XZ, Tsai YT, Lee SD, Pan HB, Chou YH, Su CH, Lee CH, Shiesh SC, Lin CY (1988) Clinical significance of ultrasonography, computed tomography and biochemical tests in the rapid diagnosis of gallstone-related pancreatitis: a prospective study. Pancreas 3:153–158

Waslen T, Wallace K, Burbridge B, Kwauk S (1998) Pseudoaneurysm secondary to pancreatitis presenting as GI bleeding. Abdom Imaging 23:318–321

The Role of Computed Tomography

4

Emil J. Balthazar

CONTENTS

4.1 **Introduction** *49*
4.2 **Pathophysiology** *50*
4.3 **Clinical Significance of Pancreatic Necrosis** *52*
4.4 **Classification of Pancreatitis** *52*
4.5 **Diagnosis of Acute Pancreatitis** *53*
4.5.1 Clinical and Laboratory Features *53*
4.6 **CT Diagnosis** *54*
4.6.1 Technical Considerations *54*
4.6.2 Normal Pancreas *54*
4.6.3 Diagnostic CT Features of Acute Pancreatitis *55*
4.6.4 Limitations in the CT Diagnosis *58*
4.6.5 Less Common CT Presentations *58*
4.6.5.1 Segmental Pancreatitis *58*
4.6.5.2 Groove Pancreatitis *58*
4.6.5.3 Autoimune Pancreatitis *60*
4.6.5.4 Acute Exacerbation of Chronic Pancreatitis *60*
4.7 **Staging of Acute Pancreatitis** *61*
4.7.1 Clinical and Laboratory Evaluation *61*
4.7.2 Numerical Systems *62*
4.8 **CT Staging** *63*
4.8.1 CT Severity Index *65*
4.8.2 Limitations and Pitfalls of CT Staging *65*
4.9 **Complications of Acute Pancreatitis** *66*
4.9.1 Intermediate Complications *68*
4.9.1.1 Infected Pancreatic Necrosis *68*
4.9.1.2 Pancreatic Abscess *68*
4.9.1.3 Pancreatic Pseudocysts *69*
4.9.2 Other Complications *70*
4.10 **Late Complications** *71*
4.10.1 Vascular and Hemorrhagic Complications *71*
4.10.2 Pancreatic Ascites *73*
4.11 **Summary** *74*
References *74*

E. J. Balthazar, MD
Professor, Department of Radiology, Bellevue Hospital, NYU-Langone Medical Center, 462 First Avenue, New York, NY 10016, USA

4.1 Introduction

For over one hundred years since its original description by Fitz (1889), acute pancreatitis has remained a ubiquitous and somewhat perplexing disease. The clinical entity called pancreatitis can be better defined as a "syndrome" distinguished by the sudden onset of a nonspecific acute inflammatory reaction of the pancreas and by its secondary morphologic and physiologic consequences. It is further characterized by an unusually diverse etiology, by protean clinical manifestations, by an unforeseen clinical course and outcome and by a relatively high morbidity and mortality (Beger et al. 1997; Malfertheiner and Dominguez-Munoz 1993; Renner et al. 1985; Banks 1994). Its clinical importance, potential health hazards and medical financial implications stem from its frequent occurrence, particularly in the more developed countries and affluent economic environments. A prevalence of about 30 patients with acute pancreatitis per 100,000 inhabitants per year has been reported, with over 100,000 hospitalizations a year in the USA (National Hospital Discharge Survey 1989; National Center for Health Statistics 1987). Moreover, despite a recent decreasing trend in mortality, the overall incidence of lethal attacks in patients with acute pancreatitis are known to occur in 2%–10% of cases (Beger et al. 1997; Banks 1994; Dervenis et al. 1999).

Although alcohol intake and cholelithiasis are by far the most common known etiologic factors (60%–80% of reported cases), 66 other entities that potentially may induce pancreatitis have been recognized in comprehensive reviews (Ranson 1982; Steinberg and Tenner 1994). This long list of causative agents is impressive not only by its sheer number but by the diversity of pathologic processes and pathways (metabolic, mechanical, drugs, vascular, infections, hereditary), all able to induce a similar inflammatory reaction in the affected pancreas (Table 4.1). Furthermore, there is no reliable relationship established between any specific etiologic factor and the clinical manifestations, severity of disease and eventual outcome (Ranson 1982; Berk 1995; Lankisch et al. 1996; Uhl et al. 1996).

Because of the great diversity of etiologic agents, it is safe to assume that the initial biochemical events that occur at the cellular level within the pancreas, are triggered by diverse mechanisms and remain the subject of intense speculation and extensive ongoing investigations (Singh and Simsek 1990; Opie 1901; Weber and Adler 2001; Uhl et al. 1991; Wilson et al. 1989; Gross et al. 1993). At this time there is still a poor understanding of the initial cellular and enzymatic alterations involved, and a lack of a unified pathophysiologic concept.

In the past, limitations in the clinical diagnosis and evaluation of patients suspected of harboring acute pancreatitis have prompted the use of conventional radiographic procedures such as plain abdominal films and barium fluoroscopic studies. These procedures however, have been found to be helpful only occasionally, being nonspecific and revealing liabilities and serious shortcomings in this cohort of patients (Davis et al. 1980; Millward et al. 1983; Stein et al. 1959; Price 1956; Safrit and Rice 1989; Berenson et al. 1971; Balthazar and Henderson 1973; Poppel 1968). As late as 1984, in a leading article published in the New England Journal of Medicine, Moosa stated that "there is no foolproof way of diagnosing acute pancreatitis except by direct inspection of the gland at laparotomy" (Moossa 1984). The introduction of computed tomography (CT) and particularly the contrast enhanced helical or multidetector high resolution imaging, has altered this view. CT has greatly enhanced our ability to evaluate patients suspected of having acute pancreatitis and has, by enlarged, rendered diagnostic laparotomies superfluous. CT has become the standard imaging test and the imaging procedure of choice in the evaluation of patients suspected of having acute pancreatitis.

The role of CT examination in patients suspected of acute pancreatitis is twofold. First, to confirm the clinical diagnosis, stage the severity of an acute attack and detect local pancreatic, retroperiteneal and abdominal complications. Second, to discover or rule out alternative intraperitoneal pathologic conditions that may mimic the clinical presentation and laboratory abnormalities seen in patients with acute pancreatitis.

4.2 Pathophysiology

Depending on the population studied, alcohol abuse and cholelithiasis are the two most common etiologies of acute pancreatitis (Ranson 1982; Steinberg and Tenner 1994). Other causes, less frequently encountered in clinical practice, are hyperlipidemia, endoscopic retrograde cholangio-pancreatography (ERCP), abdominal or cardiac surgery, different drugs and infections, and pancreatitis associated with acquired immunodeficiency syndrome (AIDS), (Table 4.1) (Ranson 1982; Parenti et al. 1996; Steer 1989; Pelucio et al. 1995; Seidlin et al. 1992; Cotton 1977; Cohen et al. 1996; Feiner 1976; White et al.

Table 4.1. Etiologic factors in acute pancreatitis. Modified from Ranson JHC. Am J Gastroenterl 1982; 77:633–638

Metabolic	Mechanical	Vascular	Infection
Alcohol	Choletithiasis	Postoperative (cardiopulmonary bypass)	Mumps
Hyperlipidemia	Postoperative (gastric, biliary)	Periateritis nodosa	Coxsackie virus
Drugs	Post-traumatic	Atheroembolism	AIDS
Scorpion venom	Retrograde pancreatography	Systemic lupus erythemotosus	
Genetic	Pancreatic duct obstruction		
Autoimmune	Pancreatic tumor		
	Ascaris infestation		
	Duodenal obstruction		

1970; Cappell and Hassan 1993). In approximately 10%–15% of patients the etiology will remain unknown and these individuals will be considered to have idiopathic pancreatitis. In most of these patients occult microlithiasis or biliary sludge are probably the leading predisposing factors (Ranson 1982; Lee et al. 1992).

The common denominator that mediates the clinical onset of the disease, is the premature activation of pancreatic enzymes and their extravasation in the pancreatic gland and peripancreatic tissues. The mechanism by which pancreatic enzymes are activated outside the intestinal tract remains obscure. Intraparenchimal and extrapancreatic extravasation of these activated enzymes leads to autodigestion and explains the pathologic changes seen in patients with acute pancreatitis. Depending on the degree of premature activation and the amount of extravasation, a variety of pathologic abnormalities from mild edema and reactive inflammatory response to severe tissue injury, damage of the pancreatic capillary network, hemorrhage and necrosis will ensue. These phenomena explain the development of perilobular and/or panlobular necrosis affecting the acinar cells, islet cells, pancreatic ductal system and interstitial fatty tissue (Kloppel 1994). Furthermore, extravasation of pancreatic lipase results in the development of ratroperitoneal fat necrosis, a serious development by itself.

Alcoholic pancreatitis occurs predominantly in men who consume large quantities of alcohol usually for a long period of time. It is presumed that alcohol is toxic to the pancreas, changes the permeability of the pancreatic ducts and may cause precipitation of protein plugs in the secondary and main pancreatic ducts (Singh and Simsek 1990). Furthermore, chronic alcohol intake may cause edema of the papilla of Vater, papillary dysfunction, spasm of the sphincter of Oddi and pancreatic hypersecretion which probably plays a role in increasing pancreatic duct pressure (Ranson 1982; Singh and Simsek 1990).

Passage of calculi from the gallbladder into the common bile duct impacted at the papilla of Vater and obstruction of the main pancreatic duct is accepted as the triggering mechanism for the unfolding of an acute attack of pancreatitis. It is assumed that continuous pancreatic secretion into an obstructed ductal system leads to ductal hypertension and probably ductal disruption, with intravasation and extravasation of pancreatic enzymes (Ranson 1982; Opie 1901; Balthazar 2003). Cholecystolithiasis (gallbladder stones) estimated to occur in about 25 million adults in the USA, is associated with choledocholithiasis (common bile duct stones) in approximately 15% of the patients (Balthazar 2003). Most of these patients, however, while developing other symptoms and jaundice, do not have pancreatitis. To explain this discrepancy, the common channel theory of Opie suggests that in some individuals who have a common biliary-pancreatic channel, the impacted stone located distal to the convergence of the two ducts, obstructs both systems and facilitates bile to reflux into the pancreatic ductal system, inducing pancreatitis (Opie 1901). In clinical practice, the detection of gallbladder calculi in patients with acute pancreatitis is considered diagnostic of biliary pancreatitis. That is despite the fact that the evidence of common duct stones or impacted stones is only presumptive, and that common duct stones may not be present or may have already passed at the time of the diagnosis. Indeed, in patients diagnosed of biliary pancreatitis with gallstones, persistent ampullary or common duct stones are found at surgery in only 7%–18% of patients (Ranson 1982; Balthazar 2003).

Clinical and experimental investigations have estimated that at the beginning of an acute attack of pancreatitis and, related to the degree of pancreatic injury, several toxic, biologically active compounds are produced and liberated in the blood stream and ascitic fluid (Weber and Adler 2001; Uhl et al. 1991; Wilson et al. 1989; Gross et al. 1993). Increased levels of serum and/or urinary trypsinogen- activated peptide, phospholipase A2, and polymorphonuclear cell elastase have been detected in patients with severe pancreatitis (Weber and Adler 2001; Uhl et al. 1991; Wilson et al. 1989; Gross et al. 1993; Tenner et al. 1997). Moreover, a variety of other inflammatory mediators called cytokines are manufactured and have been isolated in the ascitic fluid (Gross et al. 1993; Denham and Norman 1999).

Cytokines are a group of low-molecular-weight protein that are physiologically active in very small concentrations and have a diverse range of pharmacologic activities. Once produced and excreted by different cells they induce the production of other inflammatory mediators such as interleukin (IL)-1 and tumor necrosis factor (TNF) not only in the pancreas but in the lungs, liver and spleen as well. Some cytokins (IL-1, TNF) considered mediators of disease progression tend to start and amplify the rapid progression of a several postinflammatory cascades, inducing severe systemic and distal organ dysfunction (GROSS et al. 1993; DENHAM and NORMAN 1999). Additionally, the diffusion of TNF in the pancreatic parenchima is toxic to the acinar cells and contributes to the severity of parenchimal pancreatic injury. It has been suggested that in addition to the autodigestion and ischemic theories previously proposed, TNF may be a contributing factor to the development of necrosis and severity of pancreatic injury (GROSS et al. 1993; DENHAM and NORMAN 1999).

Pathologic examination of patients with severe pancreatitis shows extensive necrotizing vasculitis with thrombosis and occlusions of the small arterial and venous pancreatic vessels, areas of hemorrhage, and devitalized pancreatic parenchima (KLOPPEL 1994). Similar findings are present in variable degrees in the extrapancreatic retroperitoneal fatty tissue. Necrosis occurs early, within the first 24–48 h and, with few exceptions, remains stable during an acute episode of pancreatitis (BEGER et al. 1997; UHL et al. 1991). Zones of ischimia followed by nonviable pancreatic tissue develop, which may be diffuse or patchy, superficial or deep and which may affect any part of the pancreatic gland.

4.3 Clinical Significance of Pancreatic Necrosis

The clinical relevance of the presence and the detection of pancreatic necrosis cannot be overemphasized. Reported mortality rates of less than 1% in patients with interstitial pancreatitis show a dramatic increase to 10%–23% in patients with necrotizing pancreatitis (BEGER et al. 1997; MALFERTHEINER and DOMINGUEZ-MUNOZ 1993; BANKS 1994; DERVENIS et al. 1999; BERK 1995; BANKS 1997). Virtually all life-threatening complications occur in patients with necrotizing pancreatitis. Secondary bacterial contamination is present in 40%–70% of patients with pancreatic necrosis and it constitutes a major risk of death (RENNER et al. 1985). A mortality rate of 67% was found to be present in patients with extended (> 50%) necrosis of the pancreatic gland in one series (BEGER et al. 1997). Multiorgan failure is more common and more severe in patients with necrotizing pancreatitis and more than 80% of deaths occur in patients with pancreatic necrosis (BEGER et al. 1997). In the past decade, attempts to improve medical care and decrease morbidity and mortality have focussed on clinical, laboratory or radiologic means of detecting necrosis and thus separating patients with mild, from those with severe forms of disease. Patients with pancreatic necrosis are closely monitored in the intensive care unit, their systemic and organ disturbances are corrected and, follow-up CT examinations are routinely performed in this setting.

4.4 Classification of Pancreatitis

Based on a better understanding of pathophysiology and of the relevance of pancreatic necrosis, acute pancreatitis has been classified, by the 1992 Atlanta, Ga, International Symposium on Acute Pancreatitis, into mild acute pancreatitis and severe acute pancreatitis (BANKS 1993). Intermediate forms of disease with different clinical and morphologic manifestations certainly occur, but the presence of necrosis seems to be the distinguishing feature at the pathologic level. This new classification defines the severity of disease in practical, clinical relevant terms. It is essentially based on the presence and extent of multiorgan failure (clinical and laboratory parameters) and on the morphology of the pancreatic gland as depicted at CT imaging performed with intravenously administrated contrast material.

Mild pancreatitis previously called edematous or interstitial pancreatitis occurs in about 70%–80% of patients. It is a self-limiting disease with absent or minimal organ failure, without complications, and with an uneventful recovery. Severe acute pancreatitis on the other hand, previously called hemorrhagic or necrotizing pancreatitis, occurs in the minority of patients with acute pancreatitis (20%–30%), and is defined by pancreatic necrosis, its pathologic hallmark. Severe pancreatitis has a protracted clinical course, shows evidence of distal organ dysfunction, a high incidence of abdominal complications, and a high mortality rate (BEGER et al. 1997; MALFERTHEINER and DOMINGUEZ-MUNOZ 1993; BERK 1995; BANKS 1997). Clinical and laboratory parameters as well as the CT examinations have shown certain advantages and a number of limitations in detecting acute pancreatitis and in staging the severity of the initial clinical attack.

4.5 Diagnosis of Acute Pancreatitis

4.5.1 Clinical and Laboratory Features

The clinical diagnosis of acute pancreatitis is based on the association of symptoms, mainly abdominal pain, nausea and vomiting with an increase in the concentration of serum amylase and/or lipase levels. There is usually a sudden onset of epigastric pain of variable intensity which may radiate to the back or both flanks. The pain may be partially relieved by sitting or lying in a fetal position and may have been triggered by the ingestion of a heavy meal or a drinking binge (Ranson 1982). In mild forms of pancreatitis the physical examination is unremarkable, whereas in more severe disease there may be abdominal distension, epigastric fullness and upper abdominal tenderness. More specific signs of flank ecchymosis (Gray-Turner's sign) or periumbilical ecchymosis (Cullen's sign) are helpful but are present in only about 1% of patients (Dickson and Imrie 1984). The presence of tachycardia, tachypnea, orthostatic hypotension, cyanosis, leukocytosis and hemoconcentration heralds the development of severe pancreatitis. Most of the presenting symptoms and clinical signs are confusing, leading to a differential diagnosis which includes other acute abdominal conditions e.g. perforated peptic ulcer, biliary disease, cholecystitis, bowel obstruction and mesenteric vascular occlusions with bowel infarction (Banks 1997). The diagnosis therefore relies heavily on the twofold or threefold increase in the serum amylase concentration or an elevated serum lipase level.

The association of clinical symptoms with an elevation in the serum concentration of pancreatic amylase has been reported in about 80% of patients with acute pancreatitis (Agarwal et al. 1990; Clavien et al. 1989; Spechler et al. 1983). While measurement of serum amylase is the most common diagnostic test used in acute pancreatitis, its real sensitivity cannot be accurately estimated because the test has become the diagnostic criterion for detecting the disease. Important pitfalls in diagnosis are evident in clinical practice mainly related to the limited sensitivity and lack of specificity of the serum amylase concentration. Elevated amylase levels are sometimes present in the previously mentioned acute abdominal conditions leading to false positive diagnostic errors. Normal serum amylase concentrations, on the other hand, may be found in patients with CT or surgical proven pancreatitis leading to false negative diagnostic errors. Reported data in the literature regarding the relevance of elevated serum amylase level in acute pancreatitis, varies greatly, because of patients selection process, etiology of pancreatitis and time of the examination after the onset of an acute attack. Serum amylase levels tend to return rapidly (48–72 h) to normal levels while elevated lipase levels tend to decrease more slowly (Agarwal et al. 1990; Clavien et al. 1989; Spechler et al. 1983; Ranson 1997).

In a large review of patients with acute abdominal disorders, 20% had elevated serum amylase level; 75% of patients with hyperamylasemia had acute pancreatitis while 25% had other abdominal conditions (Ranson 1997). In a comparative study of patients with pancreatitis vs other acute abdominal conditions, the initial serum amylase was elevated in 95% of patients with acute pancreatitis and in only 5% of those with other acute abdominal disorders (Ranson 1997). It is important to consider however that biliary colic/cholecystitis is 20 times more common than acute pancreatitis and perforated ulcer 3 times more common. Moreover in a study of 318 subjects with CT evidence of acute pancreatitis, 19% of patients had a normal serum amylase on admission while another survey demonstrated that up to one-third of the patients with alcoholic pancreatitis had a normal amylase at presentation (Clavien et al. 1989; Spechler et al. 1983). Analysis of several published series have shown that serum lipase estimation has only a slightly superior sensitivity and specificity and a slightly greater overall accuracy than serum amylase. The benefits are enhanced when there is a delay in the initial blood sampling (Agarwal et al. 1990; Ranson 1997).

It is difficult to estimate the sensitivity of the clinical diagnosis in patients with acute pancreatitis. In patients with mild pancreatitis with transitory nonspecific symptoms or in patients with acute abdominal symptoms and normal amylase concentration the diagnosis is probably often missed. We know, however, that even with severe pancreatitis the diagnosis was not made in 30%–40% of patients until the time of autopsy (Corfield et al 1985). Lack of characteristic clinical findings or a specific laboratory test had established CT imaging as a non-invasive and widely accessible complimentary diagnostic test, routinely used today to confirm the clinical suspicion of acute pancreatitis.

4.6 CT Diagnosis

CT scanning can adequately visualize the pancreas and the adjacent retroperitoneal structures in almost all individuals. High resolution images are rapidly obtained, and show a remarkable capacity to evaluate the morphology of the pancreatic gland and detect early peripancreatic inflammatory changes and extrapancreatic fluid collections (Balthazar 1989).

4.6.1 Technical Considerations

Optimal images of the pancreas requires helical (spiral) CT or multidetector row CT (MDCT) combined with a rapid administration of intravenous contrast material. The goal is to eliminate respiratory artifacts and increase the conspicuity of the pancreatic gland by reliably augmenting its attenuation values. Oral contrast agents are habitually given as well as one cup of water just before the start of acquisition. We routinely administer a rapid 3–4 mL/s intravenous bolus injection of 150 mL of 60% nonionic contrast material after the digital scout film is obtained.

With helical scanning, axial images 5-mm collimation, pitch 1.5 over the upper abdomen, and 7-mm collimation, pitch 2 for the rest of the abdomen can be obtained.

Acquisition starts from the top of the diaphragm at approximately 60 s after beginning of intravenous contrast administration.

With the MDCT scanner, a two-phase acquisition technique can be employed. The first arterial dominant phase starts obtaining images at 40 s over the pancreatic gland, from the top of the vertebral body T12 to the superior edge of the vertebral body L4. We use a collimation of 2.5 mm, with a table speed of 3.75 mm. The second, portal dominant phase starts at about 70 s and acquires axial images of 5-mm collimation, with a table speed of 15 mm, from the dome of the diaphragm through the pubic symphysis. Once images are generated they can be viewed as planer two-dimensional axial images or they can be reconstructed into any plane at a commercially available workstation. Images can be examined on printed films, workstations or PACS systems. For dual-phase pancreatic imaging, with data sets containing hundreds of images, the use of film has become impractical. Similar high resolution images can be acquired by changing some of these technical parameters, as long as the pancreas is imaged at the peak of vascular enhancement (late arterial, early portal phase) and narrow collimation axial images are obtained.

4.6.2 Normal Pancreas

The pancreatic gland has an oblique orientation in the upper abdomen with the tail located adjacent to splenic hilum and the head located more inferiorly in the duodenal sweep. Several adjacent axial images are required to visualize the entire gland. The normal pancreas appears as a sharply defined, homogeneously enhancing structure, having a smooth contour or a slightly corrugated acinar configuration (Fig. 4.1). The size of the gland shows individual variations with smaller atrophic glands seen in elderly individuals. The head of the pancreas measures about 3–4 cm, body 2–3 cm, and tail, about 1–2 cm in the anteroposterior diameter with a gradual transition between segments (Balthazar 1989). The inferior aspect of the head of the pancreas, called the uncinate process, located just anterior and superior to the horizontal, third duodenal segment, has a triangular configuration with its apex extending towards the midabdomen (Fig. 4.1). The body of the pancreas is reliably located just anterior to the splenic artery and vein, relationship which helps identify the pancreas on more limited quality studies or in cachectic individuals devoided of retroperitoneal fat. Dorsal pancreas (body and tail) may be rarely congenitally absent and the tail of the pancreas may be occasionally slightly enlarged, having a bulbous appearance. A normal pancreatic duct measuring no more than 1–2 mm in diameter, is often depicted with narrow collimation, high resolution scanning.

Baseline attenuation values of the normal pancreas on CT images acquired without intravenous contrast administration are 40–50 HU. Lower baseline measurements should be expected in patients with pancreatic fatty infiltration. A homogeneous enhancement of the entire pancreatic gland to 100–150 HU occurs during the administration of intravenous contrast (Fig. 4.1). These measurements may show slight individual density variations, usually of no more than 10–20 HU, between different

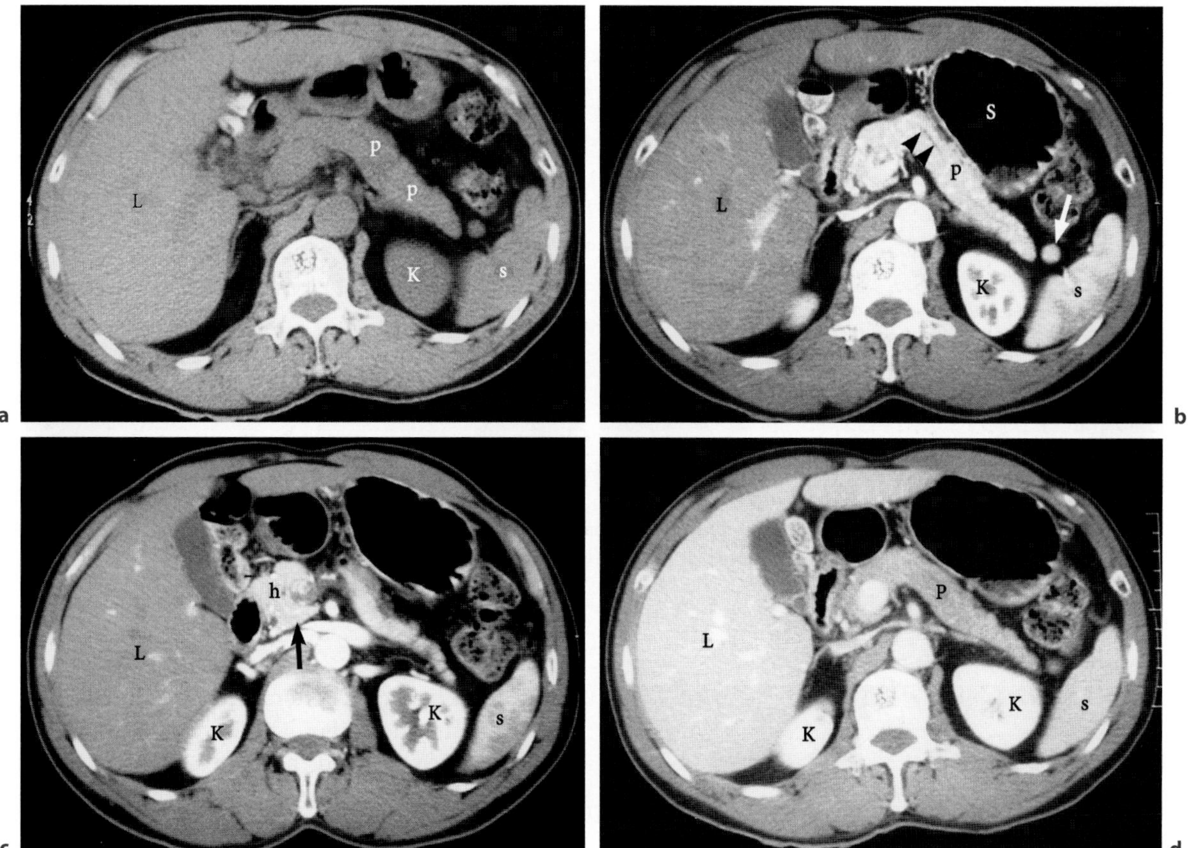

Fig. 4.1a–d. Normal pancreas, three phase multidetector CT examination. **a** Preliminary noncontrast phase. Pancreas is well visualized (*p*) with a basic attenuation value of 50 HU similar to the spleen and liver. *P*: pancreas, *s*: spleen, *L*: liver, *K*: kidney. **b,c** Arterial phase. There is homogeneous enhancement of the pancreas (160 HU) and visualization of a normal pancreatic duct (*arrowheads*). Head of pancreas (*h*) and uncinate process (*black arrow*) are well seen. A small accessory spleen is present adjacent to tail of pancreas and the spleen (*white arrow*). *s*: spleen, *S*: stomach, *L*: liver, *K*: kidney. **d** Portal phase shows homogeneous enhancement (100 HU) of the pancreas (*P*), and normal peripancreatic structures. *P*: pancreas, *s*: spleen, *L*: liver, *K*: kidney

segments of pancreatic gland. Small bulges or mild contour abnormalities should be considered variants to normal, as long as the gland maintains a homogenous attenuation and a uniform morphologic texture.

4.6.3 Diagnostic CT Features of Acute Pancreatitis

The CT findings in acute pancreatitis reflect the presence and extent of the pancreatic and retroperitoneal developing inflammatory process. The appearance is similar irrespective of etiology with the exception of traumatic pancreatitis in which pancreatic lacerations and high density hemorrhagic collections may be detected. Acute pancreatitis is in majority of cases, a diffuse disease involving the entire pancreatic gland (Balthazar 1989, 1994; Balthazar et al. 1990). In milder clinical forms there is a slight to moderate increase in the size of the gland and discrete peripancreatic inflammatory changes (Fig. 4.2). Pancreatic parenchyma becomes slightly heterogeneous and the degree of enhancement is variable depending on the extent of hyperemia and/or edema induced by the inflammatory process. Since the pancreas does not have a well-developed fibrous capsule, extravasation of pancreatic enzymes outside of the gland occurs early. Subtle peripancreatic abnormalities seen at the beginning of an acute attack of pancreatitis are, a slight increase in the density of peripancreatic fatty tissue

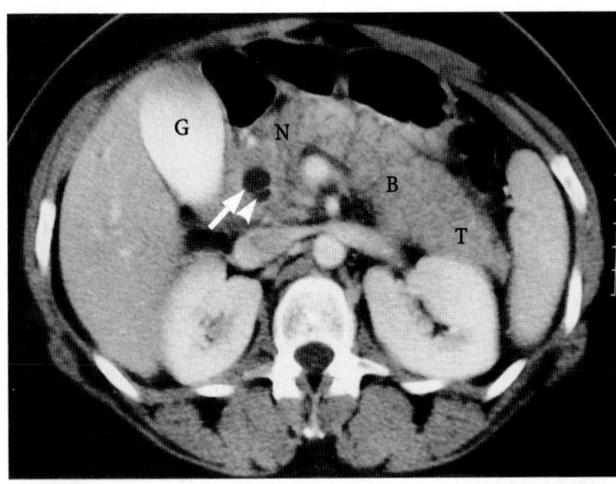

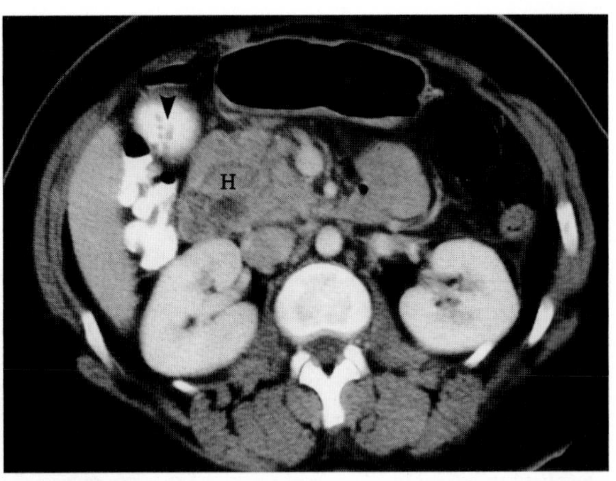

Fig. 4.2a,b. Acute pancreatitis in 34-year-old woman status post ERCP examination. **a** Tail (*T*), body (*B*) and neck (*N*) of the pancreas are enlarged and homogeneously enhancing. Common duct is dilated (*white arrow*) and large cystic duct (*arrowhead*) is seen. Gallbladder is filled with contrast material (*G*). **b** Head of pancreas (*H*) is enlarged and slightly heterogeneous. A few small stones are detected in contrast filled gallbladder (*black arrowhead*). Stage B pancreatitis, no necrosis, CT severity index 1

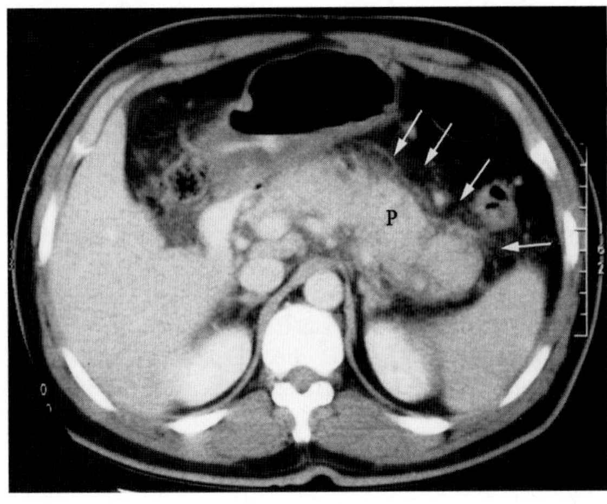

Fig. 4.3. Alcoholic pancreatitis in 36-year-old man. CT shows a diffusely enlarged pancreas (*P*) and streaky densities in the peripancreatic fat (*arrows*) consistent with peripancreatic inflammation. Stage C pancreatitis, no necrosis, CT severity index 2

with a dirty, hazy or lacelike appearance (Fig. 4.3). Small ill defined fluid collections begin to develop and often mild thickening of the adjacent fascial planes become apparent. In some cases, the contours of the pancreatic gland becomes shaggy, extraglandular inflammatory reaction is evident, however the gland appears intrinsically normal in size, contour and attenuation values.

In the more severe forms of acute pancreatitis the amount of peripancreatic inflammatory exudate, which for a lack of a better term we call fluid collections, is increased (Fig. 4.4). These collections are initially poorly defined, heterogeneous in attenuation (20–40 HU) and represent a combination of retroperitoneal fat necrosis, extravasated pancreatic secretions, inflammatory exudate and hemorrhage. The usual locations of the extravasated fluid are the anterior pararenal space, more common and more severe on the left side, and the lesser peritoneal sac (Fig. 4.4) (Balthazar 1989, 1994); . When massive, fluid collections tend to dissect fascial planes and extend inferiorly along the pararenal spaces, continue over the psoas muscles and enter the pelvis. Less commonly, the exudates may invade the mesentery, mesocolon, perirenal space and the peritoneal cavity. Free intraperitoneal fluid with high amylase levels (pancreatic ascites) is detected by CT in about 7% of cases of acute pancreatitis (Balthazar et al. 1985) and is seen mainly in patients with more severe forms of disease.

Acute fluid collections occur in approximately 40%–50% of patients with pancreatitis, early in the course of disease (Fig. 4.4) (Balthazar et al. 1990; Balthazar 1994). They develop in the retroperitoneum, and lesser peritoneal sac mainly outside of the pancreas, although small fluid collections may also be detected in the gland. In more then 50% of cases the fluid resolves without complications while in the rest, they linger, tend to partially encapsulate, develop into pseudocysts or get infected and become pancreatic abscesses (Balthazar et al. 1985, 1990;

BALTHAZAR 1994; HILL et al. 1982). They can also dissect mesenteric and fascial planes and /or involve solid organs such as spleen, left kidney, liver or the wall of the adjacent segments of the gastrointestinal tract, mainly transverse colon and splenic flexure.

Areas of nonenhancing pancreas, representing zones of ischemia and/or necrosis is considered the CT hallmark of severe acute pancreatitis (Fig. 4.5). In these patients, either the entire pancreas or only part of the gland fails to enhance during the intravenous contrast examination. A quantitative evaluation of extent of necrosis can be made by grossly dividing necrosis into mild, less than one third of the volume of the gland, moderate, up to 50% and sever, over 50% of the pancreas (Fig. 4.6). Surgical correlation studies have documented that CT has shown an overall sensitivity of 77%–85% in detecting pancreatic necrosis, with 100% sensitivity for diagnosing extended necrosis and 50% sensitivity for depicting smaller patchy necrotic areas (BEGER et al. 1986). The CT findings seen in acute pancreatitis should be considered reliable and characteristic with very few false positives and with a reported specificity approaching 100% (MAIER 1987).

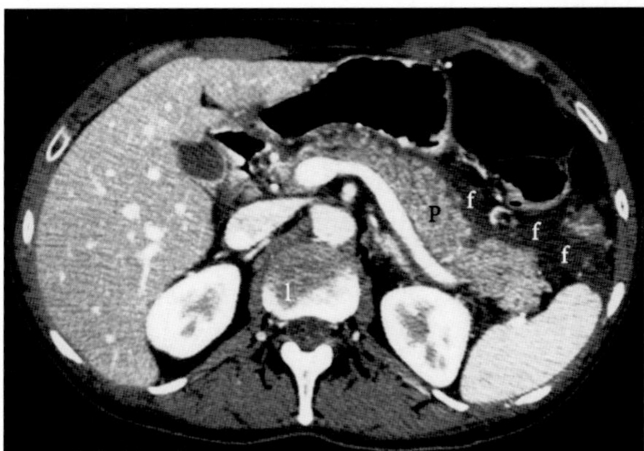

a

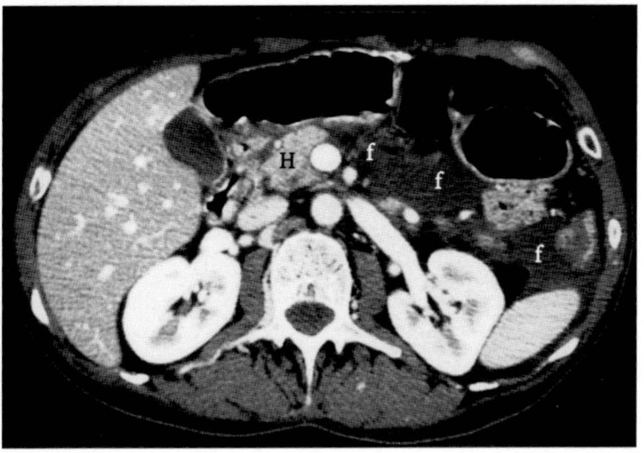

b

Fig. 4.4a,b. Acute pancreatitis in 51-year-old man. **a** Arterial phase CT reveals diffuse enlargement of the pancreas with homogeneous attenuation values of only 92 HU due to parenchymal edema. The normal texture of the gland is preserved (*P*). Fluid is noted adjacent to body and tail of pancreas (*f*). **b** A more caudal image shows similar enhancement of the head of pancreas (*H*) and fluid accumulation (*f*) in the left anterior pararenal space. Stage D pancreatitis, no necrosis, CT severity index 3

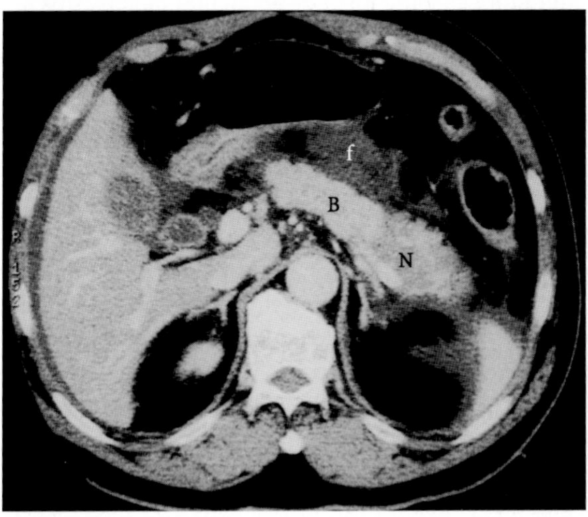

a

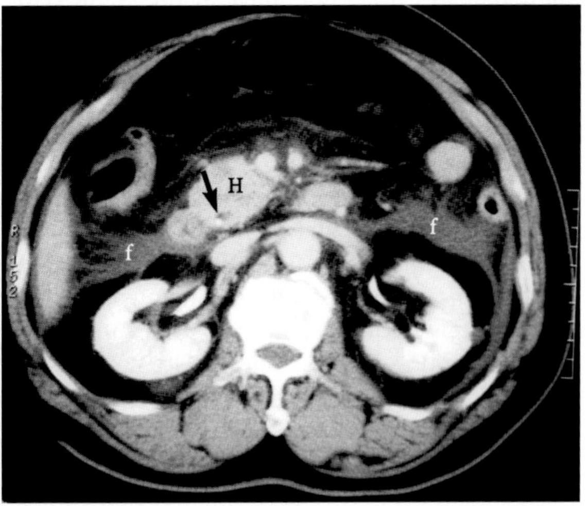

b

Fig. 4.5a,b. Gallstone acute pancreatitis in 64-year-old man. **a** Decreased attenuation in the tail of the pancreas compared to the body (*B*) is consistent with focal area of pancreatic necrosis (*N*). Fluid (*f*) is detected around the body and tail of the pancreas. **b** Head of the pancreas (*H*) is enlarged and small calcified stone is present in the distal common duct (*arrow*). There is fluid collecting in the right and left anterior pararenal space (*f*). Stage E pancreatitis, focal necrosis, CT severity index 6

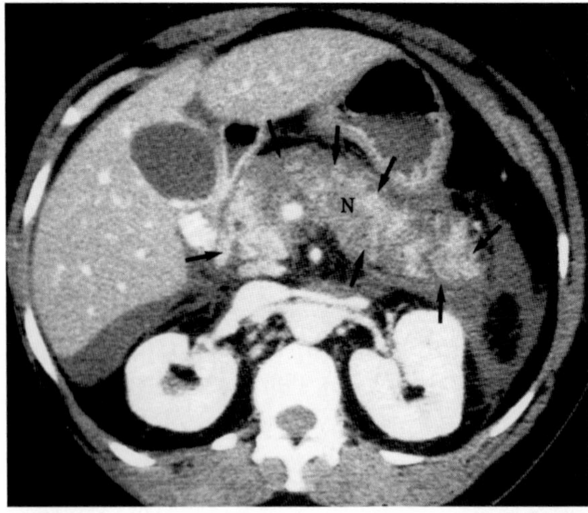

Fig. 4.6. Acute pancreatitis in 47-year-old woman. Pancreas (*arrows*) is enlarged with multiple enhancing islands of pancreatic parenchyma, interspaced with large areas of decreased attenuation consistent with necrosis (*N*). There is fluid in left and right anterior pararenal space. Grade E pancreatitis, moderate (up to 50%) necrosis, CT severity index 8

4.6.4 Limitations in the CT Diagnosis

Poor quality studies, motion artifacts, absent introabdominal fat and lack of intravenous contrast administration are some of the most common limitations of the CT diagnosis of acute pancreatitis. Without vascular and parenchymal enhancement the diagnosis can still be made in the majority of cases. Some of the more subtle parenchymal and peripancreatic abnormalities however, become harder to depict, decreasing the sensitivity of CT to diagnose pancreatitis.

The incidence of a normal pancreatic gland seen on CT in patients with acute pancreatitis is difficult to establish. Surgical and pathologic proof is lacking and the clinical diagnosis is based on nonspecific symptoms and a rise in the serum amylase level. Based on these criteria, a normal pancreatic gland may be visualized in as many as 14%–28% of patients, depending on the severity of disease and type of population examined (Balthazar et al. 1985; Beger et al. 1986). There is general agreement that, given a good quality CT performed during a bolus of intravenous contrast administration, all patients with moderate or severe pancreatitis will exhibit salient CT abnormalities. A normal pancreas on CT occurs only in the very mild forms of pancreatitis.

In the context of these potential pitfalls and heavily dependent on the severity of disease in the groups of individuals tested, CT sensitivity in acute pancreatitis was reported to be 77% (Maier 1987) and 92% (Clavien et al. 1988) respectively. These figures should be expected to improve, following the recent technical advances achieved in abdominal and pancreatic CT imaging.

4.6.5 Less Common CT Presentations

4.6.5.1 Segmental Pancreatitis

Pancreatic inflammatory changes can occasionally affect only part of the gland. The segment involved in most cases is the head of the pancreas and only rarely the pancreatic tail (Fig. 4.7). This presentation is more commonly seen in patients with biliary pancreatitis, it develops mostly after repeated episodes of pancreatitis and it is associated with milder clinical forms. It was reported in up to 18% of patients with pancreatitis and it involves only a part of the gland either exclusively or predominantly (Balthazar et al. 1985).

4.6.5.2 Groove Pancreatitis

Groove pancreatitis can be defined as a more severe and more chronic form of segmental pancreatitis affecting the head of the pancreas (Fujita et al. 1997; Stolte et al. 1982; Becker and Mischke 1991). Pancreatic head becomes enlarged and heterogeneous, and fluid with secondary inflammatory changes accumulates in the groove between the head of the pancreas and duodenal sweep (Fig. 4.8). This development leads, overtime, to intrinsic inflammatory reaction and fibrosis involving the duodenal wall and common bile duct which defines the clinical aspects of the syndrome. Duodenal stenosis and/or bile duct strictures have been reported in about 50% of these patients (Fujita et al. 1997). Abdominal pain, vomiting and obstructive jaundice are the common manifestations, and the syndrome appears to be associated with alcoholism in most patients (Fujita et al. 1997; Stolte et al. 1982; Becker and Mischke 1991). Carcinoma of the head of the pancreas if difficult to rule out and in many patients incidental Whipple resections are performed (Fujita et al. 1997).

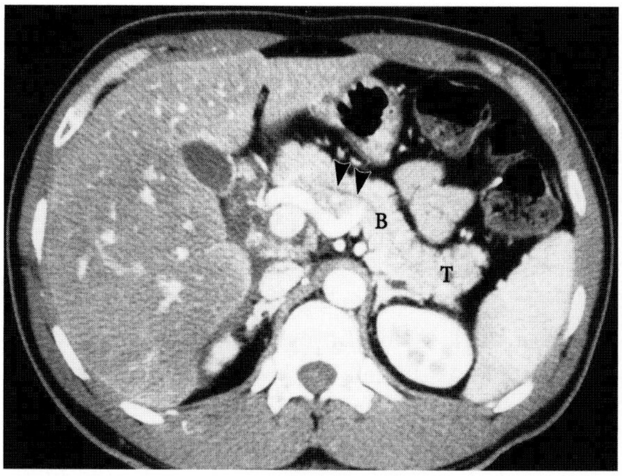

Fig. 4.7a–c. Focal acute pancreatitis in 28-year-old man with a previous episode of alcoholic pancreatitis. **a** Tail (*T*) and Body (*B*) of the pancreas are unremarkable. A normal pancreatic duct is visualized (*arrowheads*). **b** Head of the pancreas is enlarged and slightly heterogeneous (*H*). There is fluid collecting only around the head of the pancreas (*arrows*). **c** Duodenum (*d*) is enveloped by retroperitoneal fluid (*arrows*) located mainly to the right of midline

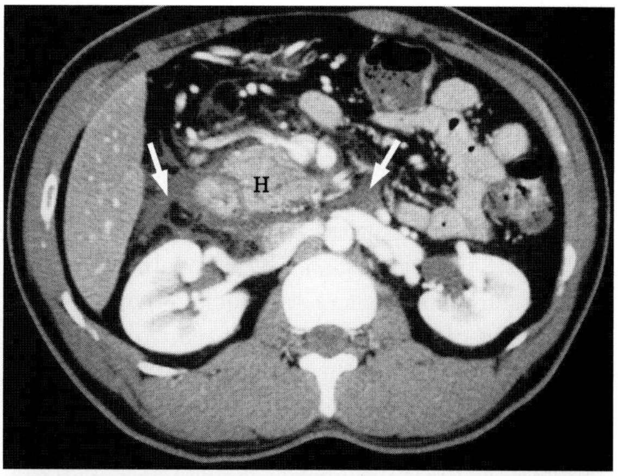

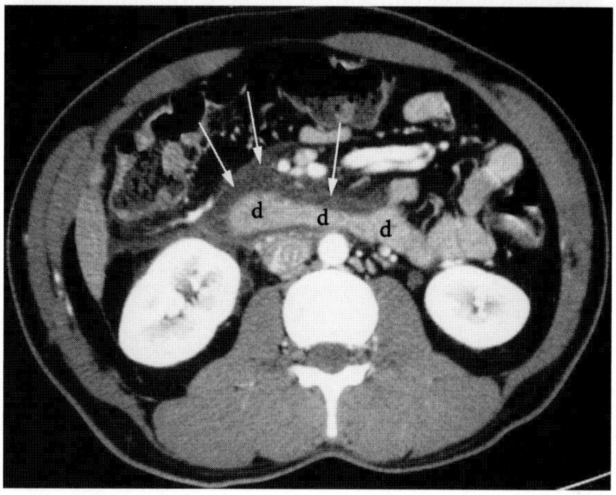

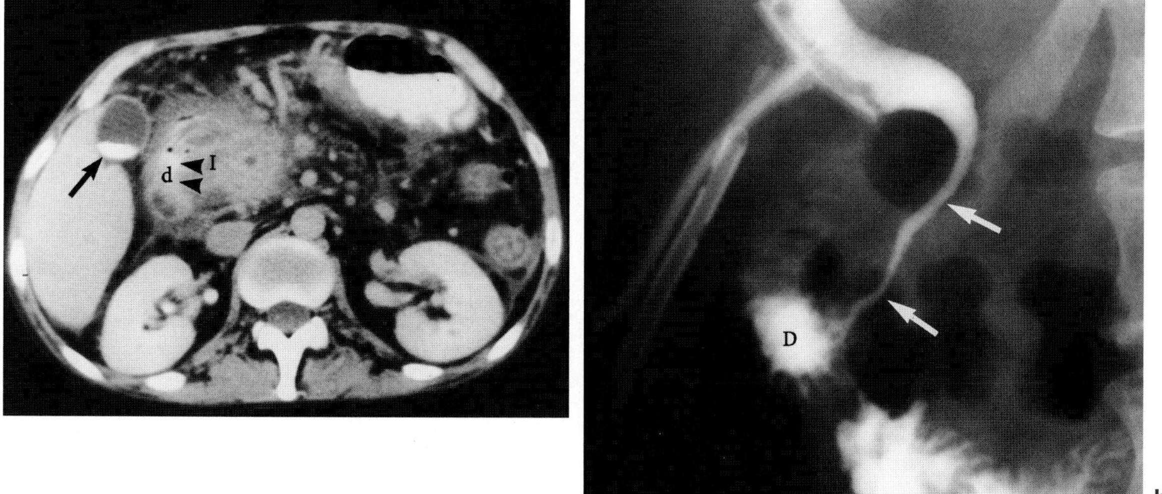

Fig. 4.8a,b. Groove pancreatitis in 32-year-old man following repeated episodes of acute pancreatitis presenting with jaundice. **a** Head of pancreas is enlarged and there is fluid and inflammation (*I*) around the second duodenal segment (*d*). Gallstones are present in the gallbladder (*arrow*). **b** T-tube cholangiogram following cholecystectomy shows long segment of narrowing of the distal common duct (*arrows*). *D*: duodenum

4.6.5.3
Autoimune Pancreatitis

Sarles et al. (1961) described an unusual form of pancreatitis associated with autoimune disease and characterized by hypergamaglobulinemia, eosinophilia and the presence of antinuclear antibodies (ANA) (Sarles et al. 1961; Saito et al. 2002). The histopathologic findings of autoimune pancreatitis include lymphocytes and plasma call infiltration of the pancreas, and fibrosis, with damage of the pancreatic islets and acini. Morphologic changes detectable by CT are diffuse or segmental enlargement with a slightly decreased homogeneous enhancement of the pancreas. Patients have little or no pain, may have obstruction of the common duct with jaundice and they may develop regional lymphadenopathy (Fig. 4.9). These findings are suspicious for a pancreatic neoplasm particularly lymphoma. When the correct diagnosis is suspected, hematologic work up and fine needle aspiration biopsy can confirm it. Excellent response to steroid therapy with resolution of the clinical and CT morphologic findings has been reported (Saito et al. 2002).

4.6.5.4
Acute Exacerbation of Chronic Pancreatitis

Patients with chronic pancreatitis may occasionally present with acute symptoms and an elevated serum amylase level. Clinical presentation is often mild to moderate and stigmata of chronic pancreatitis is detected on CT examination. There is usually evidence of parenchymal atrophy, dilatation of the pancreatic duct (finding absent in acute pancreatitis), intraductal calcifications and mild peripancreatic inflammatory reaction and/or small fluid collections. Associated pseudocepts or pancreatic abscesses may be present. The intrinsic pancreatic morphologic changes are permanent while the acute CT changes and clinical symptoms usually resolve with conservative therapy.

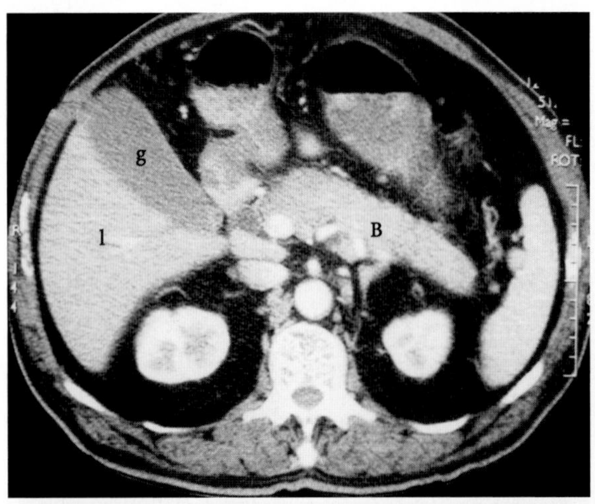

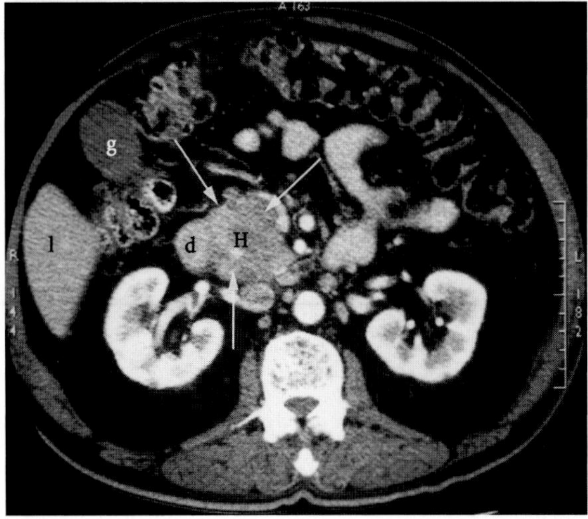

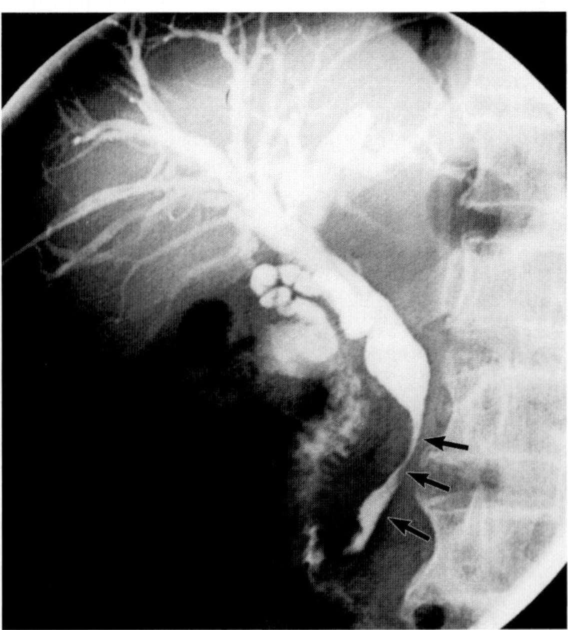

Fig. 4.9a–c. Autoimune pancreatitis in 73-year-old man presenting with jaundice. **a** Body of pancreas (*B*) is normal. *g*: gallbladder, *l*: liver. **b** Head of the pancreas (*H*) is enlarged and has a slightly lower attenuation compared with the rest of the pancreas (*arrows*). There are no peripancreatic fluid collections. *d*: duodenum, *g*: gallbladder, *l*: liver. **c** Percutoneous cholangiogram reveals external compression and narrowing of the distal common duct (*arrows*) consistent with mass in the head of pancreas. Biopsies of the head of pancreas and regional nodes revealed lymphocytic infiltration and follow-up examination 3 months later showed resolution of the clinical and CT findings

4.7 Staging of Acute Pancreatitis

Treatment of patients with acute pancreatitis depends on the early assessment of severity of disease. The initial evaluation should be based on objective parameters and should be able to detect and quantify the severity of an acute attack of pancreatitis. In the last 10 years it has become evident that the 2%–10% overall mortality of acute pancreatitis is directly related with the presence and the extent of pancreatic necrosis (MALFERTHEINER and DOMINGUEZ-MUNOZ 1993; BANKS 1994; DERVENIS et al. 1999; BERK 1995; BANKS 1997; Maier 1987). Thus the early detection of patients with severe pancreatitis is mainly based on the depiction of pancreatic necrosis (necrotizing pancreatitis) and is being used as a grave prognostic indicator of the outcome in these patients. An ideal staging system should be able to identify necrosis early, be reliable based on objective parameters, be performed rapidly, and be easily available and affordable (DERVENIS et al. 1999). Clinical and CT parameters used to assess and quantify the severity of an acute attack of pancreatitis have been used and discussed in the literature.

4.7.1 Clinical and Laboratory Evaluation

Several clinical symptoms including hypotension, tachycardia, fever, respiratory distress or cyanosis are occasionally seen in a severe attack, but are not specific. They may appear late after an acute attack and individually are not reliable predictive indicators (DERVENIS et al. 1999; Banks 1993; AGARWAL and PITCHUMONI 1991). Flank ecchymosis (Grey Turner's sign) or periumbilical ecchymosis (Cullen's sign) are rarely seen, appear late in the course of disease and are more specific (DICKSON and IMRIE 1984). It has been reported that a severe attack of pancreatitis can be detected based on clinical evaluation alone, in only 34%–39% of patients at the time of clinical onset (McMAHON et al. 1980; WILSON et al. 1990). At the beginning, at the admission to the hospital, reliable clinical signs are often lucking; when signs develop, they are difficult to interpret and lack objective quantification.

Abnormal values of certain routine laboratory test are often present in patients with severe pancreatitis. A low serum calcium level (<7.5 mg/dL), an elevated serum glucose level (>250 ml/dL), and high serum creatinine level (>2 mg/dL), are disturbing prognostic signs that correlate with an increased risk of death (BEGER et al. 1997; MALFERTHEINER and DOMINGUEZ-MUNOZ 1993; BANKS 1994; DERVENIS et al. 1999; BERK 1995). Moreover in Bank's series (BANKS et al. 1983), the development of one or several signs of distal organ failure (Table 4.2) was associated with a 50% mortality rate. However, none of these single parameters are sufficiently sensitive or specific to reliable identify patients with necrotizing pancreatitis.

A variety of biologically active substances – called vasoactive peptides, cytokines and inflammatory mediators – are produced and liberated in the bloodstream and ascitic fluid in patients with pancreatitis (WEBER and ADLER 2001; UHL et al. 1991; WILSON et al. 1989; GROSS et al. 1993; TENNER et al. 1997). It has been postulated that identification and measurements of some of these toxic compounds may correlate with the development and severity of an acute attack of pancreatitis.

Methemalbumine and pancreatic ribonuclease are considered specific markers for the presence of hemorrhagic or necrotizing pancreatitis. Pancreatic necrosis can be diagnosed or strongly suspected when an elevated serum level of tumor necrosis factor is detected (LANKISCH et al. 1989; WARSHAW and LEE 1979; KEMMER et al. 1991; EXLEY et al. 1992; PAAJAINEN et al. 1995). A number of cytokines including, interleukin 6 and phospholipase A2 have been shown able to detect and quantify the severity of an acute attack of pancreatitis (DE BEAUX et al. 1996; NEVALAINEN 1980; BUCHLER et al. 1989; BIRD et al. 1989). An accuracy of about 80% in detecting pancreatic necrosis has been reported with phospholipase A2 determinations (NEVALAINEN 1980; BUCHLER et al. 1989; BIRD et al. 1989). In addition, plasma concentration of polymorphonuclear elastase has been reported to possess a positive predictive value of over 90% in predicting a severe episode of pancreatitis (DOMINGUEZ-MUNOZ et al. 1991). Premature activation of trypsinogen, which

Table 4.2. Acute pancreatitis: signs of organ failure

Shock, systolic BP <90 mm Hg
Pulmonary insufficiency, PaO_2 <60 mm Hg
Renal failure, creatinine >2 mg/dL
Gastroitestinal bleeding >500 mL/24h

occurs mainly in patients with severe pancreatitis can be depicted by measuring trypsinogen activation peptide in the urine (Tenner et al. 1997).

Despite remarkable progress, the clinical utility of most of these laboratory indices remains to be further tested in clinical trials. They had not yet gained widespread clinical acceptance in most hospitals. A clinically useful correlation with the development of pancreatic necrosis and its extent at the onset of an acute attack of pancreatitis, remains to be proven.

4.7.2 Numerical Systems

Since individual clinical signs or single laboratory parameters do not reliably identify severity of disease or predict outcome, numerical detection systems have been devised to better evaluate the potential risk of death in patients with acute pancreatitis. All clinically available systems are based on counting the number and degree of systemic abnormalities (organ failure, metabolic alterations) - called grave signs, prognostic indices or risk factors - and correlating the results with mortality and morbidity rates. It should be remembered however, that the detected alterations reflect systemic dysfunction; they do not reflect the severity of intraabdominal disease and they certainly have no diagnostic value, being seen in a variety of other acute abdominal conditions.

Historically, the first numerical system, proposed by Ranson et al. (1974), is still the most popular in the USA. It is based on 11 objective signs: 5 determined at the onset, and 6 within the first 48 h (Table 4.3). With a higher number of risk factors, there is a corresponding worsening of the outcome and a gradual increase in the morbidity and mortality. In the original survey, there was less than 1% mortality with fewer than three grave signs, 16% in patients with three or four signs, 40% in patients with five or six signs, and 100% in patients with more than six grave signs. The system is a good indicator of disease severity particularly useful at the two ends of the numerical scale. Pancreatitis is mild with two or fewer grave signs, whereas pancreatitis is severe when more than six grave signs are present. Inaccuracies in correlation with morbidity and mortality are however present in cases presenting with three to five signs, which is a common clinical occurrence (Banks 1994, 1997).

Table 4.3. Ranson's criteria of severity in acute pancreatitis

At admission
• Age > 55 years
• White blood cell count > 16,000/mm^3
• Glucose > 200 mg/dL
• Serum Lactic dehydrogenase (SLDH) > 350 IU/L
• Aspartate aminotransferase > 250 IU/L
During initial 48 h
• Hematocrit fall of > 10 vol. %
• Serum urea nitrogen rise of > 5 mg/dL
• Ca++ < 8 mg/dL
• PaO_2 < 60 mg Hg
• Base deficit > 4 mEq/L
• Fluid sequestration > 6 L

Several other grading systems, each using slightly different parameters, have since been proposed, with a prognostic efficiency similar to that of Ranson system. The best known are the Glasgow original or modified system, the Simplified Acute Physiology (SAP) score and the simplified prognostic criteria (Agarwal and Pitchumoni 1986; Imre et al. 1978). Imrie's modification of the Ranson system uses eight prognostic criteria; it omits hematocrit level, base deficit, age and fluid sequestration but includes albumin level of less than 32 g/L as an important criterion of severity (Imre et al. 1978).

A slightly more reliable prognostic numerical method called the Acute Physiology and Chronic Health Evaluation (APACHE II) that can be used at the onset of an acute attack as well as in monitoring patients progression has been reported (Knaus et al. 1985; Larvin and McMahon 1989). The system is however more complex based on 12 physiologic measurements, and more difficult to perform (Table 4.4). An APACHE II cutoff score of more than 8 grave signs is consistent with the development of severe pancreatitis (Knaus et al. 1985; Larvin and McMahon 1989). The accuracy of the APACHE II method for identifying patients with severe pancreatitis on admission to the hospital has been about 75%. The test is used as a prognostic indicator to help select patients for intensive care treatment. After 48 h, Apachy II scores are similar to the previously mentioned other numerical system. The general accu-

Table 4.4. APACHE. II grading system. Points assigned for each variable are summed, given the acute physiology score (APS). The higher the score the greater likelihood for morbidity and mortality.

Severity of Disease Classification system
Rectal temperature
Mean arterial pressure
Heart rate
Respiratory rate
Arterial pO_2
Arterial pH
Serum sodium
Serum potassium
Serum creatinine
Hematocrit
White blood cell count
Glascow coma score

racy of these numerical systems is about 70%–80% with an overall sensitivity ranging from 57% to 85% and with a specificity of 68% to 85% (Dervenis et al. 1999; Agarwal and Pitchumoni 1991; Agarwal and Pitchumoni 1986; Blamey et al. 1984).

4.8 CT Staging

The ability of intravenous contrast enhanced CT imaging to directly assess the morphology of pancreatic gland and of the adjacent retroperitaneal structures has greatly improved the diagnosis and staging of acute pancreatitis. Clinical parameters previously discussed evaluate systemic abnormalities, but are not able to discern the presence and extend of pancreatic injury and /or peripancreatic fluid collections. Modern CT imaging has become a fast, noninvasive and reliable examination, available in most hospitals, and able to diagnose and quantify pancreatic necrosis. Thus, CT has become a required and essential component of our new classification system (Balthazar et al. 1985, 1990; Balthazar 1994).

Previous investigations have tried to gauge the potential use of CT imaging in assessing the severity of an acute attack of pancreatitis (Mendez et al. 1980; Nordestgaaard et al. 1986). In our 1985 paper (Balthazar et al. 1985) we have divided the CT features of acute pancreatitis into five separate grades (Table 4.5) and correlated the CT features with the development of local complications and death. We observed that most morbidity and all lethal attacks occurred in our D and E grades patients presenting with peripancreatic fluid collections (Figs. 4.4–4.6). Patients with grade D or E had a mortality rate of 14% and a morbidity rate of 54%, as compared with no mortality and a morbidity rate of only 4% in patients with grade A, B or C (Fig. 4.10). Similar general observations were later published by other clinical researches (Clavien et al. 1988; London et al. 1989). Moreover we have noticed that the developing fluid collections resolved spontaneously in about half of our patients while in other half they partially or completely encapsulated, developing into abscesses or pseudocysts (Balthazar et al. 1985).

The advantages of our initial grading system rely on the ability to select a sub group of patients (with grade D or E), at high risk of death and with a potentially higher morbidity rate. This CT grading is easy to perform, does not necessarily require intravenous contrast administration or it can be performed with slower intravenous rates of injection, and with slower CT scanners and 5–7 mm collimation. Its drawbacks relate to its limited capacity to better foretell mortality and morbidity rates in patients with D or E grades, since 54% of patients with peripancreatic fluid collection did not developed complications, in our original survey (Balthazar et al. 1985). Furthermore, images obtained with slow rates of intravenous contrast perfusion, or without intravenous contrast, cannot reliably depict pancreatic necrosis at the onset of an acute attack, lowering its sensitivity as a prognostic indicator of severity of pancreatitis.

More recent developments, starting with the introduction of incremental dynamic bolus technique and followed by rapid CT scanning, faster intravenous injection rates and narrow collimation, have dramatically improved CT staging of acute pancrea-

Table 4.5. CT grading in acute pancreatitis

Grade	
A	Normal pancreas
B	Pancreatic enlargement
C	Inflammation pancreas and peripancreatic fat
D	Single small peripancreatic fluid collection
E	Large fluid collections or retroperitoneal air

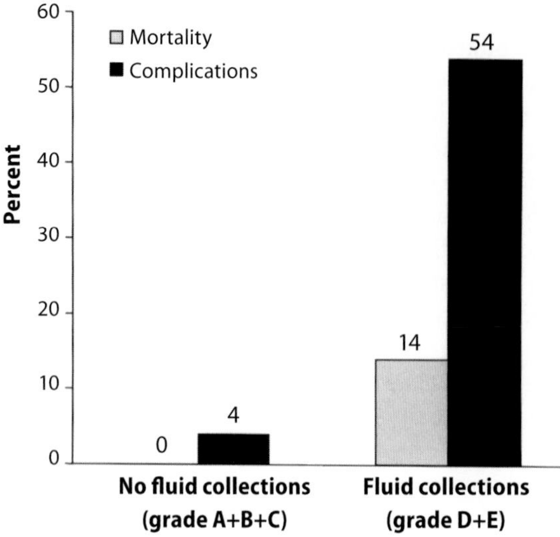

Fig. 4.10. CT grading vs morbidity and mortality

titis (Freeny 1993). Previous investigations have recognized a casual relationship between lack of pancreatic parenchymal enhancement and the development of pancreatic necrosis (Beger et al. 1986; Kivisaari et al. 1983). In patients with interstitial mild pancreatitis, the capillary network in intact, vasodilatation is often present and the entire gland is expected to show a significant increase in its attenuation values of at least 50–60 HU above its basic values (Figs. 4.2, 4.3). When the arterial flow is impeded or the capillary network is damaged, there is a striking decrease or a total lack of parenchymal enhancement, signifying the presence of ichemia and often the development of necrosis (Balthazar 2002) (Figs. 4.5, 4.6). This process can be diffuse or patchy, it can be superficial or deep and it can affect any segment of the pancreas. It can be grossly quantified into severe, affecting most of the gland, or segmental involving up to 50% or less then 30% of the pancreas (Figs. 4.5, 4.6). Once necrosis develops, usually within 48–72 h from the clinical onset of acute pancreatitis, the normal glandular CT texture changes, it liquefies and it becomes better defined when compared with the adjacent still viable enhancing pancreatic tissue (Fig. 4.11). Criteria for the CT diagnosis of pancreatic necrosis have been proposed, as focal or diffuse zones of nonenhanced pancreatic parenchyma detected on examination performed with intravenous bolus administration of contrast material (Banks 1993).

An excellent correlation between CT findings in acute pancreatitis, length of hospitalization, development of local complications and death was documented in our 1990 published series (Balthazar et al. 1990). While patients without necrosis (as previously defined) had no mortality and only a 6% complication rate (Figs. 4.2, 4.3), patients with CT evidence of necrosis exhibited a 23% mortality and a 82% morbidity (Fig. 4.12). The extent of necrosis was found, in addition, to have prognostic significance. Mortality and morbidity in patients with extensive necrosis far exceeded those observed in patients with small, patchy areas of necrosis (Figs. 4.5, 4.6 and 4.10). There were no statistical meaningful differences in prognosis, once the necrotic zones were larger than 40%–50% of the volume of the gland. The combined morbidity in patients with over than 30% necrosis was 94%, and the mortality was 29% (Figs. 4.6, 4.10).

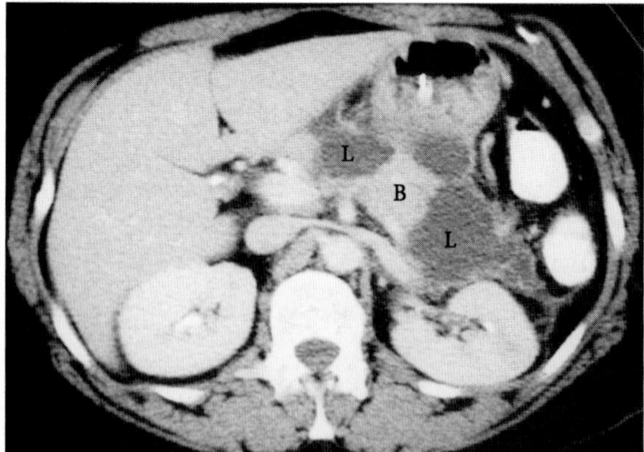

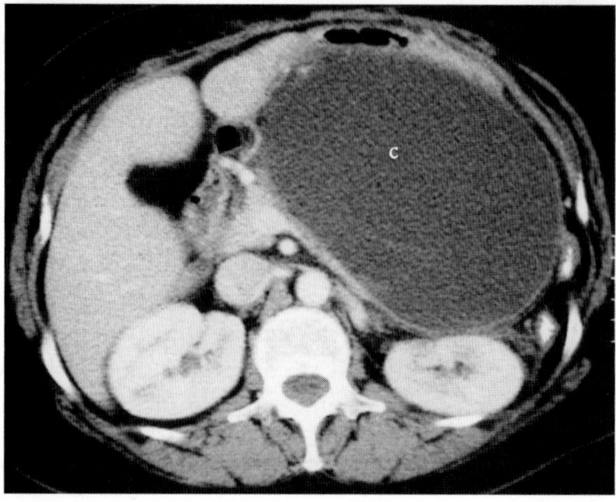

Fig. 4.11a,b. Gallstone pancreatitis in 49-year-old woman. **a** Necrosis with liquefaction (*L*) affects the tail and part of the body (*B*) of the pancreas. Patient was discharged after clinical symptoms subsided. **b** Follow-up CT examination 3 months later reveals the development of a large fully encapsulated pseudocyst (*C*).

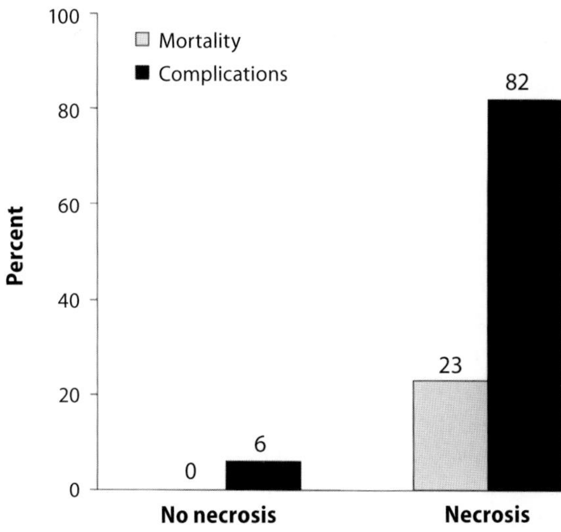

Fig. 4.12. Necrosis vs morbidity and mortality

There is general agreement that the development of pancreatic necrosis and its CT detection, should be considered the most relevant imaging feature that correlates with outcome and with severity of acute pancreatitis. It must be stressed however that while the risk of death occurs mostly in patients with pancreatic necrosis, a significant incidence of complications – 22% in our experience (BALTHAZAR et al. 1985, 1990) – should be anticipated in patients with peripancreatic fluid collections and normally enhancing pancreatic glands (Fig. 4.4). Accordingly, we have combined the heretofore described CT risk factors, into a single CT grading system which we called the CT severity index (BALTHAZAR et al. 1990).

4.8.1 CT Severity Index

CT severity index is a simple, easy to calculate, scoring system which combines the original grading system (BALTHAZAR et al. 1985) with the presence and extent of pancreatic necrosis (BALTHAZAR et al. 1990). Patients with grades A through E are assigned 0 to 4 points, to which 2 points for 30%, 4 points for up to 50% and 6 points for > 50% necrosis are added (Table 4.6). The calculated CT severity index score, divided into three broad categories (0–3, 4–6, and 7–10), better reflects the early prognostic value of CT imaging. As illustrated in Figure 4.13,

Table 4.6. Acute pancreatis CT staging CT Severity Index (CTSI)

CT grade	Points	Necrosis	Points	CTSI score
A	0	None	0	0
B	1	None	0	1
C	2	< 30%	2	4
D	3	30%–50%	4	7
E	4	> 50%	6	10

CT severity index (CTSI): CT grade + necrosis (0–10)

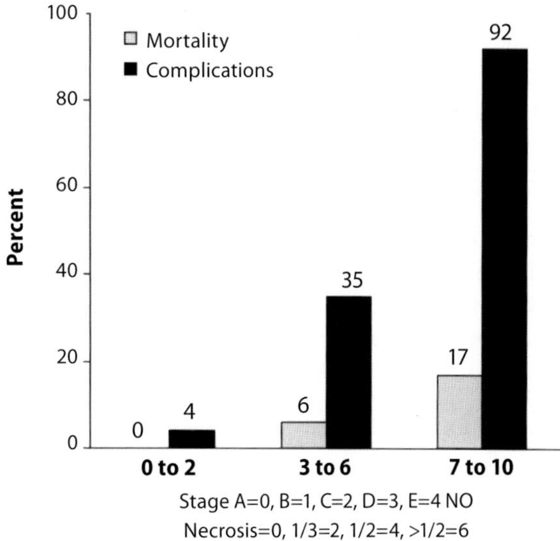

Fig. 4.13. CT severity index vs morbidity and mortality

there is a statistically relevant and steady increase in the incidence of complications and lethal attacks in these individuals. Patients with a severity index of 0 or 1 have no mortality or morbidity, whereas patients with a severity index of 2 had only a 4% morbidity. Conversely, a severity index score of 7–10 yields a 17% mortality and 92% complications rate (BALTHAZAR et al. 1990).

4.8.2 Limitations and Pitfalls of CT Staging

Several limitations and pitfalls of CT staging in acute pancreatitis have to be pointed out. First, technically inadequate examinations and particularly lack of intravenous bolus contrast administration drastically reduces the CT accuracy in staging pancreatitis. When clinically indicated, these patients will benefit by magnetic resonance (MR) imaging, using rapid gradient-echo-breath-hold techniques and fat suppression sequences. MR is an excellent alternative noninvasive modality to evaluate patients with acute pancreatitis with an accuracy generally similar to high resolution intravenous bolus CT imaging (Morgan et al. 1997; Fucher and Turner 1999).

Second, while ichemic changes are evident at the onset of an acute attack (zones of decreased attenuation), necrotic changes and liquefaction follows subsequently and become more evident within a few days. Thus, CT imaging performed 2–3 days after the initial clinical onset, has a higher accuracy in detecting and quantifying pancreatic gland necrosis (Fig. 4.11). Initially, areas of parenchymal ischemia may not be entirely depicted, or ischemia may be transitory and reversible in nature, leading to zones of liquefaction necrosis smaller or sometimes larger than expected on follow up CT examinations (Fig. 4.14). Lack of pancreatic enhancement on CT imaging is a reliable indicator of ischemia and it is usually followed by the development of necrosis, however, the extent of pancreatic necrosis is more difficult to define initially (Fig. 4.14). Patients that exhibit equivocal findings or relatively normal enhancing glands, but have large peripancreatic fluid collections or a more severe clinical course should have at least one follow up CT examination performed.

Third, the clinical implications of CT findings of necrosis depend not only on the extent of necrosis but on the location of parenchymal damage and the potential injury and disruption of the main pancreatic duct (Tann et al. 2003). Small necrotic foci located superficially or involving only the tail of the pancreas often heal spontaneously without complications (Balthazar 2002) (Fig. 4.5). They may be initially missed or misinterpreted as small intrapancreatic fluid collections. On the other hand, deep necrotic areas strategically placed in the body, neck or head of the pancreas may disrupt the integrity of the main pancreatic duct leading to large accumulations of extravasated pancreatic enzymes and the expected complications that follows (Tann et al. 2003) (Fig. 4.14). Increasing amount of fluid collections accumulating later after the onset of acute pancreatitis, should be viewed with suspicion and should be considered related most likely to focci of necrosis even when the initial CT findings are equivocal.

Fourth, the extravasation of activated pancreatic enzymes produces a severe retroperitoneal inflammatory reaction, extensive peripancreatic fat necrosis and injuries to the adjacent intestinal segments, as well as capillary network, inducing hemorrhage. This phenomena which may occur in patients without recognizable parenchymal injury, interferes with the absorption of retroperitoneal fluid and explains the development of complications in this subset of patients. CT can not accurately detect nor can it quantify the extent of retroperitoneal fat necrosis. For this reason, all residual lingering, partially encapsulated peripancreatic fluid collections, should be deemed suspicious for representing at least partially fat necrosis.

Finally, the CT features of prognostic significance – parenchymal injury and peripancreatic heterogeneous fluid collections – reflect the presence of severe pancreatitis and correlate well with the development of local complication and incidence of death in this population. The correlation with the type and extent of systemic failure and distal organ dysfunction is however, tenuous. At this time a single comprehensive scoring system combining the systemic manifestations with the local morphologic changes depicted by CT, is not available.

4.9 Complications of Acute Pancreatitis

As previously stated, most life-threatening complications of acute pancreatitis occur almost exclusively in patients with pancreatic necrosis (Steinberg and Tenner 1994; Mann et al. 1994; McKay et al. 1999; Lowham et al. 1999; Talamini et al. 1996; Mutinga et al. 2000; Balthazar 2002). Several potential lethal complications can coexist and can occur at any time during the natural history of acute pancreatitis. Some of this complications reflect systemic toxic manifestations and are associated with multiorgan failure, while others are local pathologic changes confined mainly to the pancreas and peripancreatic tissues (Balthazar 2002). Although there is some overlap in the timing of their occurrence, a clinically useful approach is to divide complications into early, intermediate and late (Table 4.7).

Early complications develop at the onset or within the first 2–3 days of an acute attack and are mostly systemic in nature. They account for the 20%–50% of the mortality rate reported in acute pancreatitis (Steinberg and Tenner 1994; Mann et al. 1994; McKay et al. 1999; Lowham et al. 1999). The pathogenesis of early complications is multifactorial and

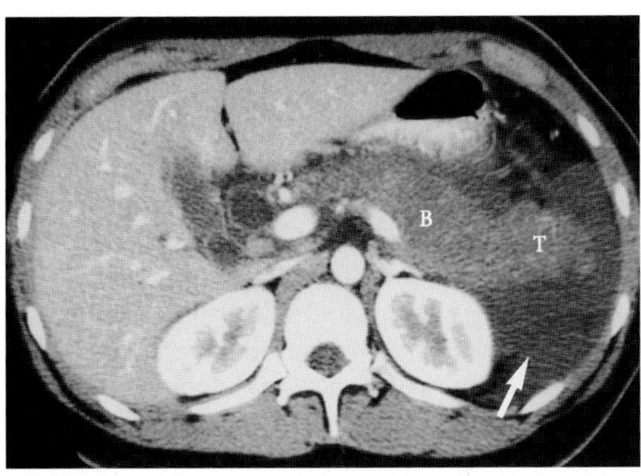

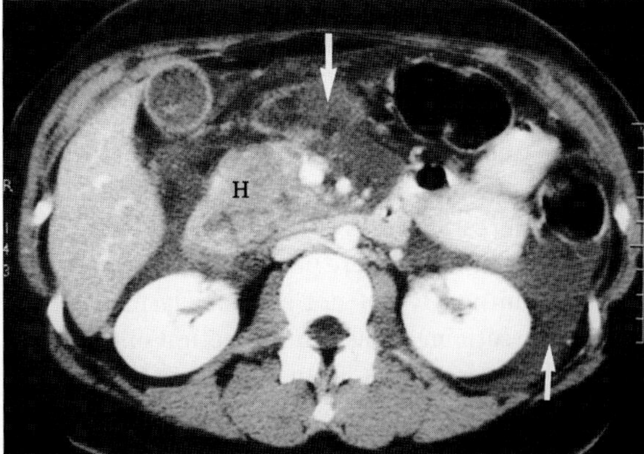

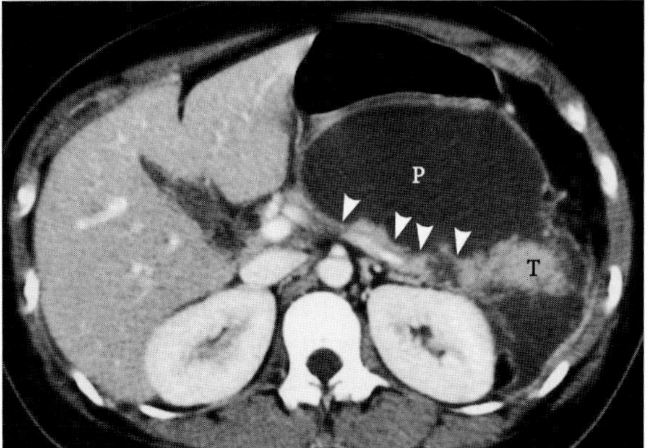

Fig. 4.14a–c. Gallstone acute pancreatitis in 18-year-old woman. **a** Pancreas is enlarged and body (*B*) and tail (*T*) of the pancreas exhibit attenuation values of 50–60 HU consistent with severe ischemia and necrosis. Large fluid collection is visualized (*arrow*). **b** Head of pancreas is enlarged (*H*) with attenuation values of 100–110 HU. Bilateral retroperitoneal fluid collections and heterogeneous collection anterior to the pancreas (*arrows*) are seen. Grade E pancreatitis, over 50% necrosis, CT severity index 10. **c** Follow-up examination reveals the development of a large pancreatic pseudocyst (*P*). Note that residual pancreatic parenchyma in the tail (*T*) and body of pancreas is still viable (*arrowheads*)

Table 4.7. Complications of acute pancreatitis

1	Early, 2–3 days: clinical manifestations of the cardiovascular, pulmonary, renal, and metabolic systems
2	Intermediate, 2–5 weeks: local retroperitoneal infections, infected necrosis, abscess, pseudocysts, gastrointestinal and biliary complications, and solid organ involvement
3	Late, months–years: vascular and hemorrhagic complications, and pancreatic ascites

Table 4.8. Systemic complications of acute pancreatitis

1	Cardiovascular: ECG: changes, cardiac, peripheral vascular failure, hypotension, and shock
2	Pulmonary: respiratory insufficiency, tachypnea, arterial hypoxemia, and adult respiratory distress syndrome
3	Renal: oliguria and anuria
4	Metabolic: coagulation factor abnormalities thrombosis or bleeding (disseminated intravascular coagulopathy), hyperglycemia, diabetic coma, and hypocalcemia

related to the presence and extent of pancreatic parenchymal injury. It has been established that the abnormal production and release in the bloodstream of various vasoactive peptides, enzymes, and inflammatory mediators are responsible for the development and the severity of cardiovascular, pulmonary, or renal functional abnormalities (Beger et al. 1997; Malfertheiner and Dominguez-Munoz 1993; Dervenis et al. 1999; Banks 1997). The clinical expression and the degree of systemic failure differ greatly from patient to patient but reflect the severity of disease in the early stages of evolution (Table 4.8). Detection of these systemic complications is made by clinical means and have lead to specific treatment options, in the attempt to decrease the early mortality in patients with acute pancreatitis.

4.9.1 Intermediate Complications

Complications that occur between the second to fifth week after an acute attack of pancreatitis are located in the abdomen and mainly in or adjacent to the pancreatic gland (Beger et al. 1985). They are associated with severe pancreatitis and they occur predominantly but not exclusively in patients with pancreatic necrosis. The detection of these local complications by CT imaging and the proper clinical management is essential, since they are responsible for >50% of the mortality reported in acute pancreatitis (Steinberg and Tenner 1994; Mann et al. 1994; McKay et al. 1999; Lowham et al. 1999).

4.9.1.1 Infected Pancreatic Necrosis

As the consequence of severe ischemic changes, devitalized pancreatic parenchyma evolves in about 20% of patients with acute pancreatitis and secondary infections develop in 5%–10% in this population (Beger et al. 1997; Malfertheiner and Dominguez-Munoz 1993). If contamination does not occur, patients remain clinically stable and the developed liquefied pancreatic collections may slowly resolve or organize into pseudocysts (Fig. 4.14). Eventually, scarring and pancreatic atrophy appears, contingent on the initial extent and severity of pancreatic injury.

Often clinically unsuspected, secondary bacterial contamination occurs in the necrotic pancreatic tissue in 40%–70% of these patients (Beger et al. 1985, 1986; Bradley and Allen 1991). It has been estimated that the incidence of secondary infections in patients with necrotizing pancreatitis is slowly increasing after an acute episode and reaches 60% after 3 weeks (Beger et al. 1985, 1986, 1997; Bradley and Allen 1991). Infected necrotic pancreatic tissue is a severe aggravating factor, increasing the mortality rate in this population (Bassi 1994). In the Beger et al. series (1997) a 67% mortality was reported with >50% infected necrosis as opposed to only 14% mortality in patients with a similar extent of sterile necrosis.

The source of contamination is probably the intestinal tract, particularly the colon. Apparently, translocation of bacteria (Escherichia coli, enterobacter, klebsiella, anaerobes, fungus) directly through the intestinal wall, via lymphatic system, hematogenous-born or due to microperforations explains this phenomenon (Bassi 1994).

Secondary infections should be suspected when sepsis (fever, chills, elevated white blood count) appears, associated with zones of nonenhancing, heterogenous partially liquefied pancreas on CT imaging (Fig. 4.15). The diagnosis can be confirmed by percutaneous needle aspirations under CT or sonography guidance and bacteriologic examination (Banks 1994, 1997; Bradley 1993; Gerzof et al. 1987). In our experience, gas bubbles depicted in the necrotic tissue, seen in about 12%–18% of cases is strongly suggestive of infected necrosis (Fig. 4.15) (Balthazar 2002). The commonly advised treatment is an aggressive surgical approach including necrosectomy, debridment, sump drainage, and lavage (Banks 1994; Beger et al. 1985). This surgical approach has been able to substantially reduce mortality rate to below 10% from previously reported 40%–80% death rate (Banks 1994; Bassi 1994).

4.9.1.2 Pancreatic Abscess

Pancreatic abscesses develop in about 3% of patients with acute pancreatitis commonly 3–4 weeks after the onset of an acute attack, in patients who had developed peripancreatic fluid collections (Banks 1997; Balthazar et al. 1994; Bittner et al. 1987; Sankaran and Walt 1975). Residual lingering fluid collections and necrotic fatty tissue undergo secondary, often polymicrobial contamination with germs of intestinal origin, forming abscesses. This complications can be defined as partially encapsulated collections of pus that appear mostly liquefied on CT (10–30 HU), located usually in proximity to, but outside of the pancreatic gland (Banks 1997; Bradley 1993) (Fig. 4.16).

The importance of differentiating infected necrosis from pancreatic abscesses has been emphasized in the literature. The mortality rate of infected necrosis is about double that of pancreatic abscesses (Bradley 1993; Bittner et al. 1987). Infected necrosis, composed of necrotic tissue and pus, has a substantially thicker content and therefore, it is more difficult to be successfully drained percutaneously. On the other hand abscesses present as mostly liquefied peripancreatic fluid collections that can be, by enlarged, effectively treated with percutaneous catheter drainage (Balthazar et al. 1994; Bittner et al. 1987; Freeny et al. 1998). An abscess appears on CT imaging, as a single or multiple poorly encapsulated

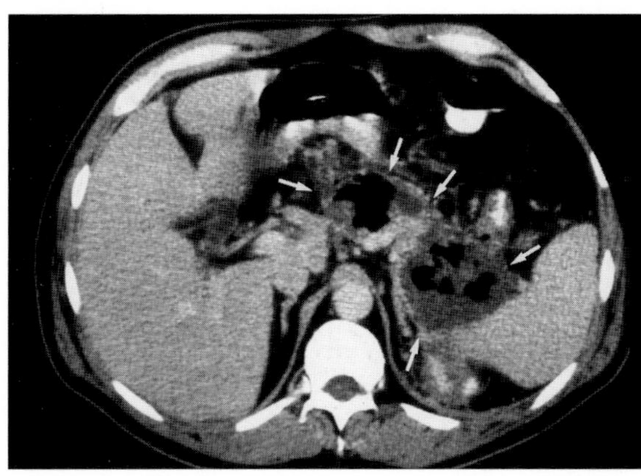

Fig. 4.15. Infected pancreatic necrosis in 65-year-old man. Entire pancreas is liquefied (*arrows*) and multiple collections of air are present in the necrotic gland

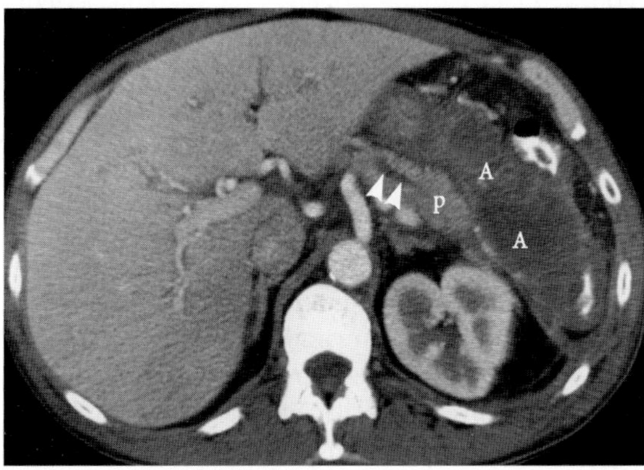

Fig. 4.16. Pancreatic abscess (*A*) in 46-year-old man that developed sepsis after repeated episodes of acute pancreatitis. Percutaneous aspiration of the poorly encapsulated fluid collection (*A*) showed E coli infected abscess. Pancreatic duct is slightly disteded (*arrowheads*). *p*: pancreas

collection of low attenuated fluid, 3–4 weeks after an acute episode of pancreatitis (Fig. 4.16). Presence of gas bubbles in these collections, although not totally specific, reinforces the clinical suspicion, in a septic patient (Balthazar et al. 1994). Confirmations of CT diagnosis requires percutaneous needle aspiration and bacteriologic examination (Gerzof et al. 1987). Small abscesses may respond to conservative broad spectrum antibiotic therapy.

4.9.1.3 Pancreatic Pseudocysts

Pancreatic pseudocysts should be separated from the ordinary fluid collections, having a dissimilar CT appearance, a different prognostic significance and requiring a different management approach. Pseudocysts are defined as completely encapsulated pancreatic fluid collections located in the pancreas or more commonly outside of the pancreatic gland, that require more than 4 weeks to evolve (Fig. 4.14) (Balthazar 2002; Sankaran and Walt 1975; Crass and Way 1981; Frey 1997). They occur in about 3%–10% of cases of acute pancreatitis (Balthazar 1989; Bradley 1979) often secondary to pancreatic necrotic foci and the development of a communicating tract with the pancreatic ductal system (Balthazar et al. 1994; Sankaran and Walt 1975; Frey 1997). In our experience most if not all pseudocysts that develop during an acute attack of pancreatitis, evolve at the site or adjacent to the site of pancreatic necrosis (Fig. 4.14). Characteristics of pseudocysts are its nonepithelialized granulation tissue wall and the very high contents of amylase in the encapsulated fluid. On CT, they appear round or oval in shape having a relative thin (1–2 mm) symmetrical capsule and a low attenuation (< 15 HU) fluid content. They can dissect fascial planes and travel away from the pancreas from the lower mediastinum to the pelvis. Pseudocysts vary greatly in size from 1 cm to 15 cm in diameter, show no septations and no intraluminal enhancement (Fig. 4.14). The developing fibrotic circumferential capsule can become slightly thicker in time and eventually it may calcify. Higher attenuation solid contents may be present in its lumen representing residual blood clots. The radiologic differential diagnosis of pseudocysts located in the pancreas, from cystic pancreatic tumors, is based on the above described morphologic features, but it can be difficult at times.

Distinguishing from chronic pseudocysts, acute pseudocysts diagnosed de novo at 4–5 weeks following an attack of pancreatitis have a totally unpredictable fate. Collected data based on sonographic examinations has shown that acute pseudocysts younger than 6 weeks had a 40% rate of resolution and a 20% incidence of complication, whereas pseudocysts older than 12 weeks tended not to resolve and had a complication rate of 67% (Bradley 1979). Similar data documenting an 18%–50% rate of serious complications has lead to an aggressive management approach of early operative drainage of most pseudocysts (Crass and Way 1981; Frey 1997; Wade 1985).

These data should be tempered however by a more recent CT investigation (Yeo et al. 1990) which suggested that the need for surgery, based on persistent abdominal pain, evidence of enlargement or complications, is more common in larger pseudocyst (>6 cm in diameter) and less common in smaller pseudocysts, 67% and 40% respectively. In the cohort of 36 symptom free patients with pseudocysts that were not drained, follow up examinations had shown complete resolution in 60%; 40% of pseudocysts remained stable or decreased in size and only one complication developed. In our institution, acute pseudocysts smaller than 5 cm in size seen in asymptomatic patients at the end of an acute episode of pancreatitis are managed nonoperatively with clinical and CT follow up examinations.

Spontaneous resolution of a pseudocyst can be explained by drainage into the pancreatic ductal system, by rupture into the peritoneal cavity and, less frequently, by spontaneous drainage into an adjacent hollow viscus such as colon or stomach (Fig. 4.17). Percutaneous drainage or surgical internal drainage is reserved for cysts larger than 5 cm in diameter and older than 6 weeks, cysts that are enlarging, symptomatic cysts (pain, outlet gastric obstruction. biliary obstruction) and infection or hemorrhage. Infection is suspected in septic patients and should be confirmed by fine-needle aspiration. The prevalence of hemorrhagic pseudocysts varies from 2% to 18% (Crass and Way 1981; Kiviluoto et al. 1989; Kelly et al. 1999) and CT findings can be helpful in detecting this complication.

Recently, the trend has been to employ a more conservative approach to the management of acute pancreatic pseudocysts. When intervention is required, percutaneus catheter drainage using sonography or CT guidance has been successful in treating over 90% of patients (VanSonnenberg et al. 1989). A retrospective study of 92 patients found similar success rates with percutaneus as compared to surgical drainage procedures of pancreatic pseudocysts (Adams et al. 1991).

4.9.2
Other Complications

Extravasation of activated pancreatic enzymes induces a chemical reaction damaging retroperitoneal vital structures adjacent to the pancreas. Segments of the upper gastrointestinal tract, colon as well as biliary ducts can be affected by variable extents and degree of injuries. Some of these abnormalities such as functional spasm, dilation, and bowel edema manifest early within the first a few days and usually resolve (Meyers and Evans 1973; Lindahl et al. 1972; Thompson et al. 1977). A more lasting, localized spasm at the splenic flexure of the colon produces a massive dilation of the proximal transverse colon, referred to as the colon cutoff sign (Price 1956). More severe and chronic inflammatory changes can manifest as stenotic intestinal or biliary lesions or can lead to the development of sinus tracts and fistulas affecting the upper gastrointestinal tract and/or colon. Inflammatory exudates can traverse fascial planes and dissect into solid organs

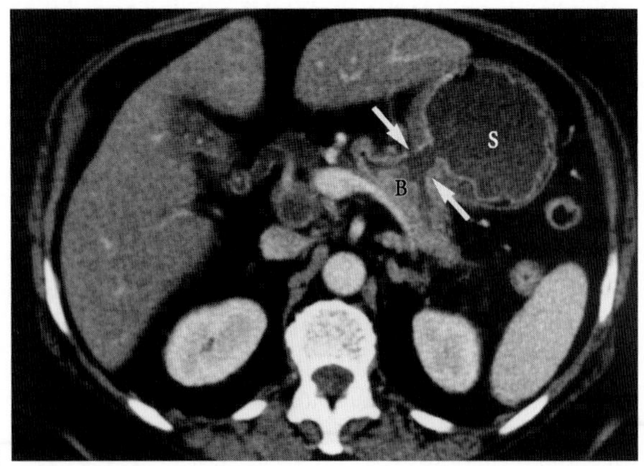

a

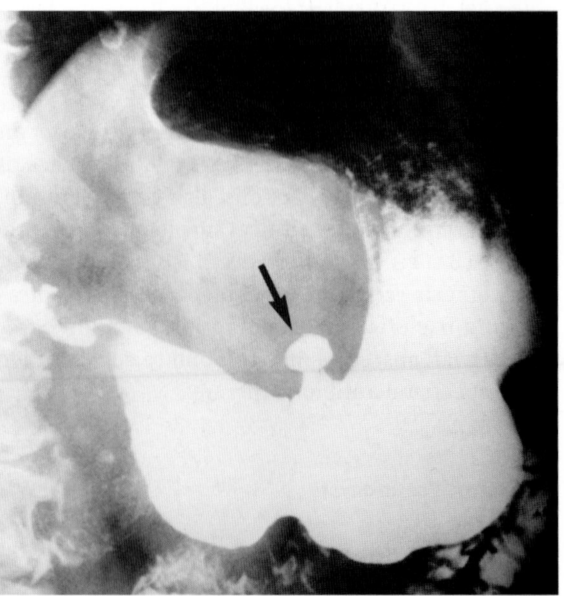
b

Fig. 4.17a,b. Spontaneous drainage of pancreatic pseudocyst into stomach in 69-year-old woman. **a** Large fistula between body of pancreas (*B*) and stomach (*S*) is clearly visualized (*arrows*). **b** Upper gastrointestinal examination shows a deep ulceration (*arrow*) at the level of the fistulous tract

such as spleen, liver or kidneys. Subcapsular or parenchymal fluid collections, intrasplenic pseudocysts, splenic infarcts and splenic hemorrhage are complications that can develop a few weeks after the onset of severe acute pancreatitis (Farman et al. 1977; Lilienfeld and Lande 1976) (Fig. 4.18).

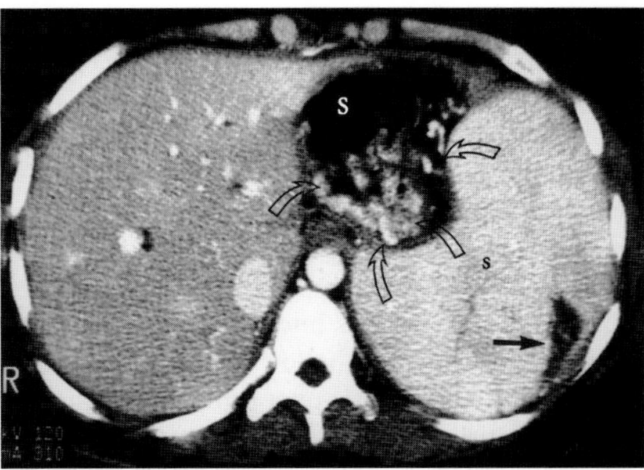

Fig. 4.18. Gastric varices in 34-year-old woman with two previous documented episodes of acute pancreatitis. Spleen (*s*) is enlarged and peripheral infarct (*black arrow*) is detected. There are many enlarged collateral veins along the posterior wall (*arrows*) of the air filled stomach (*S*)

4.10 Late Complications

4.10.1 Vascular and Hemorrhagic Complications

While some of the vascular and hemorrhagic complications may occur early, most of them are detected late within a few months to years, usually after several episodes of acute pancreatitis. These complications have an insidious clinical presentation, difficult to diagnose without a documented history of pancreatitis. CT imaging plays a predominant role in their detection and evaluation. Proteolytic enzymatic injuries produced by the autodigestive action of the extravasated fluid collections lead to the development of vascular and hemorrhagic complications affecting peripancreatic vessels (Belli et al. 1990; Cornu-Labat et al. 1997; Burke et al. 1986; Gadacz et al. 1978; Nordbach and Sisto 1989).

The most common vascular complication on the venous side is thrombosis of the splenic vein which develops in 1%–3% of patients following pancreatitis (Belli et al. 1990; Cornu-Labat et al. 1997). The thrombus may extend into the portal vein, however the rapid development of collateral circulation protects the patient until splenomegaly or gastric hemorrhage occurs. The syndrome, sometimes called isolated left-sided portal hypertension, is characterized by massive enlargement of short gastric and gastroepiploic veins with the development of gastric varices located on the posterior wall of the gastric fundus (Figs. 4.18 and 4.19) (Belli et al. 1990; Cornu-Labat et al. 1997; Madsen et al. 1986). Since the coronary vein and portal vein are patent, esophageal varices may not be seen in this condition (Madsen et al. 1986). Contrast enhanced CT imaging is an excellent noninvasive modality to diagnose this entity (Fig. 4.18).

Life – threatening abdominal hemorrhage can occur at the beginning of an acute attack of pancreatitis (Muller et al. 1999), but it is usually seen as

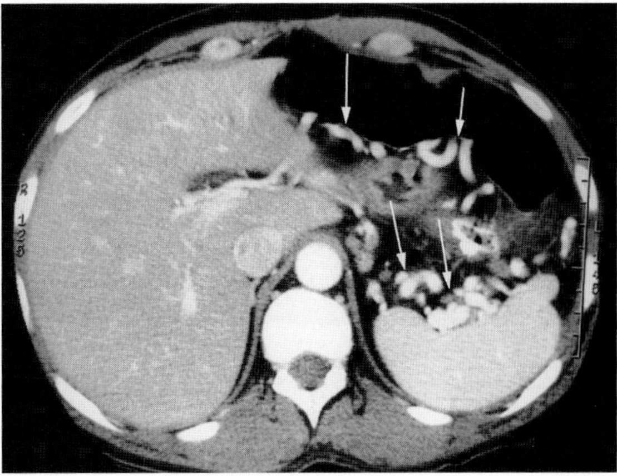

Fig. 4.19. Splenic vein thrombosis in 39-year-old man with long history of alcoholic pancreatitis. There are large collateral veins in the left upper quadrant (*arrows*) secondary to splenic vein thrombosis

a late sequela, sometimes in patients with chronic pancreatitis. It was reported to occur 1 to 9 years (median of 4 years) after the attack of pancreatitis in Bretagne et al series (Bretagne et al. 1990) and it was detected as late as 8 years, with a mean of 2–3 years after the first episode of pancreatitis in our published series (Balthazar and Fisher 2001). Most serious life threatening hemorrhagic episodes are secondary to rupture pseudoaneurysms, affecting commonly the splenic, gastroduodenal or pancreatico-duodenal arteries. Left gastric, middle colic, hepatic artery or smaller arterial branches are less commonly affected (Fig. 4.20).

The development of a pseudoaneurysm, which occurs almost exclusively on the arterial side because of higher intraluminal pressures, is apparently a relatively common complication of pancreatitis, and it is often detected in asymptomatic individuals. An incidence as high as 10% following pancreatitis was reported in an angiographic survey (White et al. 1976). Hemorrhage occurs when a slowly enlarging false aneurysm ruptures into the peritoneal cavity, erodes into an adjacent hollow viscus or communicates with the pancreatic duct producing hemosuccus pancreatitis (Balthazar and Fisher 2001).

While massive hemorrhage is mainly associated with ruptured pseudoaneurysms, bleeding pseudocysts, venous or diffuse capillary bleeding associated with pancreatic necrosis may occur (Figs. 4.21 and 4.22) (Muller et al. 1999) An incidence of 3.2% bleeding pseudoaneurysms and pseudocysts was reported in a series of 250 patients with chronic pancreatitis (Bretagne et al. 1990). In our series (Balthazar and Fisher 2001), 60% of bleeding complications were secondary to pseudoaneurysms (Fig. 4.20), 20% to hemorrhagic pseudocysts without false aneurysms (Fig. 4.21), and 20% had massive capillary bleeding related to extensive pancreatic necrosis (Fig. 4.22).

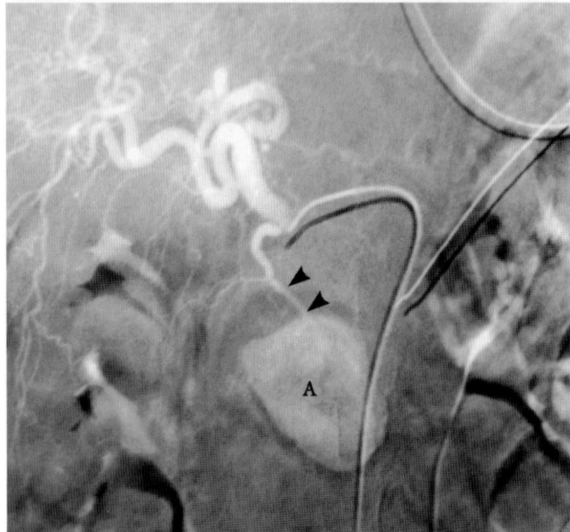

Fig. 4.20a,b. Pseudoaneurysm of the pancreatico-duodenal artery in 41-year-old man with history of pancreatitis. **a** The large oval IV contrast filled false aneurysm (*A*) is located in a fluid filled pseudocyst (*arrows*). **b** Selective angiogram shows aneurysm (*A*) arising from the superior pancreatico-duodenal artery (*arrowheads*). The aneurysm was successfully embolized

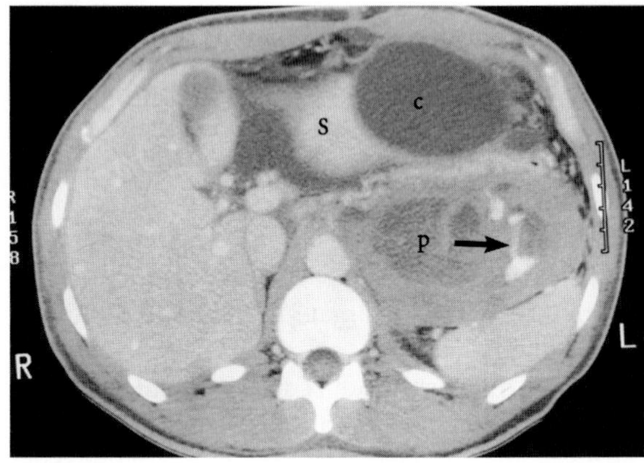

Fig. 4.21. Bleeding pseudocyst in 35-year-old with history of alcoholic pancreatis. Extravasation of IV contrast material (*arrow*) is detected within a large thick wall pseudocyst (*p*). A second thin wall uncomplicated pseudocyst is present anteriorly (*c*). S: stomach

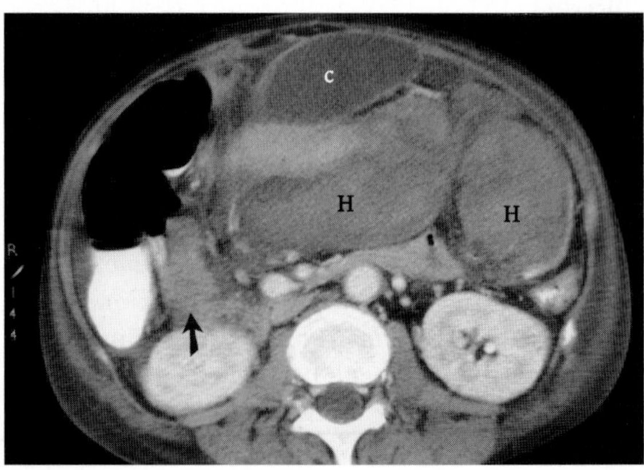

Fig. 4.22. Necrotizing pancreatitis associated with massive bleeding in 37-year- old alcoholic. Partially loculated collections of high attenuated fluid consistent with fresh hemorrhage (*H*) are depicted. Free blood is present in the right flank (*arrow*). Uncomplicated fluid filled pseudocyst (*C*) is seen arteriorly

Early detection of these potentially lethal complications by means of intravenous bolus CT imaging, followed by angiographic evaluation with embolization, and when required, an aggressive surgical approached has reduced previously recorded mortality rates from 25%–60% (Bretagne et al. 1990; Stabile et al. 1983; Vujic 1989) to about 11% (Balthazar and Fisher 2001; Stabile et al. 1983). CT imaging can identify pseudoaneurysms as sharply defined intravenous contrast filled, round or oval lesion located along or adjacent to a peripancreatic artery (Fig. 4.20). Free spill of intravenous contrast material or adjacent hemorrhage implies rupture and it is easily detected as high attenuated (40–50 HU) heterogeneous fluid collections (Figs. 4.21 and 4.22). The sensitivity of CT imaging to detect pseudoaneurysm will depend on the size of the lesion, quality of examination, and the skill of the radiologic interpretation. Small, nonbleeding false aneurysm incidentally present in asymptomatic individuals, can be easily overlooked.

4.10.2 Pancreatic Ascites

Pancreatic ascites should be defined as a syndrome, characterized by the massive, chronic accumulation of intraperintoneal pancreatic fluid associated to a permanent disruption of the main pancreatic duct and establishment of a communication between the pancreas and the peritoneal cavity (Kravetz et al. 1988; Johst et al. 1997; Weaver et al. 1982; Fernandez-Cruz et al. 1993; Fielding et al. 1989; Cameron et al. 1976; Donovitz et al. 1974). This is a rare and late development seen mainly in patients with stigmata of chronic pancreatitis, when strictures obstruct the distal pancreatic duct maintaining the pancreatic-abdominal fistula open (Fig. 4.23). It should not be confused with transitory small-volume ascites seen in patients with acute pancreatitis which occurs in about 7%–12% of cases (Balthazar et al. 1985; Johst et al. 1997).

Patients with documented long histories of pancreatitis, develop increasing abdominal girth and complain of abdominal pain and occasionally nausea and vomiting (Weaver et al. 1982). CT examination reveals massive ascites and often stigmata of chronic pancreatitis such as pancreatic atrophy, dilated pancreatic duct and ductal calcifications. Since the normal pancreas produces in excess of 1 L of exocrine secretion per day (Kravetz et al. 1988), the ascites tends to be massive. The suspected CT and clinical diagnosis can be confirmed by percutaneus needle aspiration when the protein contents in the ascitic fluid is greater than 3 g/dL and the amylase level is elevated above 1000 units (Kravetz et al. 1988).

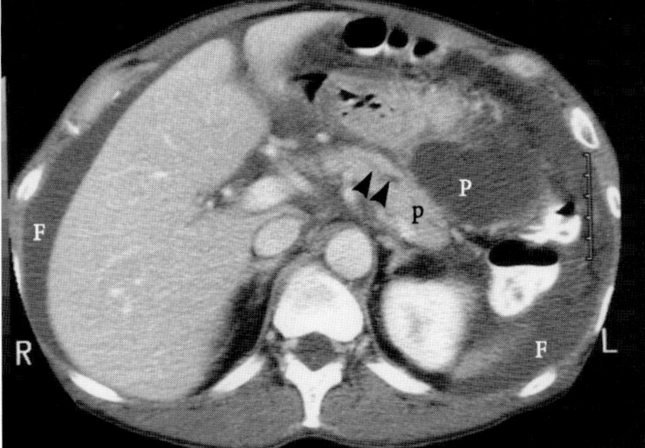

a

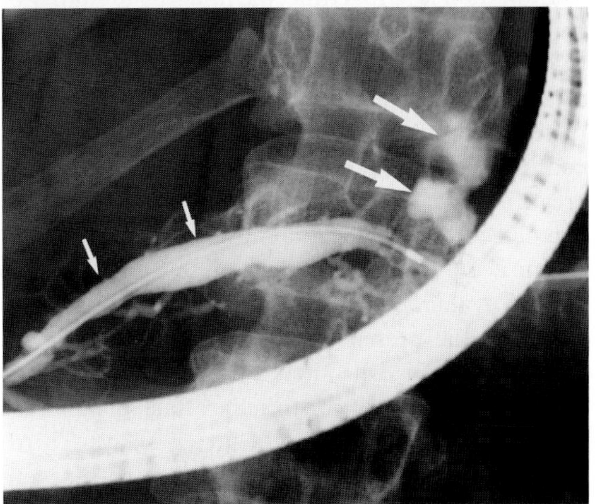
b

Fig. 4.23a,b. Pancreatic ascites in a 38-year-old man with long history of pancreatitis. **a** Pancreas (*P*) shows a dilated pancreatic duct (*arrowheads*) and free fluid is present in the peritoneal cavity (*F*). A partially loculated collection anterior to the tail of pancreas (*P*) is consistent with a ruptured pseudocyst. **b** ERCP demonstrates dilated pancreatic duct (*small arrows*), filling of secondary ductules and extravasation of contrast material from the tail of pancreas (*large arrows*)

When the initial conservative management fails, endoscopic retrograde pancreatography followed by endoscopic dilatation of strictures or stent placement is attempted (Weaver et al. 1982; Fernandez-Cruz et al. 1993; Fielding et al. 1989). Surgical segmental pancreatectomy with pancreatico-jejunostomy can be performed if endoscopic therapy is not effective. In addition it should be stressed that chronic pancreatic ascites is a serious, debilitating complication with a reported operative mortality of about 20% and recurrence rate of 15% (Cameron et al. 1976; Donovitz et al. 1974).

4.11 Summary

Helical or multidetector intravenously enhanced CT examination is at this time, the imaging modality of choice to evaluate patients with acute pancreatitis. In individuals clinically suspected of acute pancreatitis, CT has a triple role. First, by depicting specific pancreatic and retroperitoneal abnormalities, it can confirm the clinical suspicion, it can diagnose pancreatitis in patients clinically unsuspected and it can detect other acute abdominal conditions which mimic acute pancreatitis. Second, together with the clinical evaluation (mainly numerical systems), and based on the presence of pancreatic necrosis and pancreatic fluid collections (CT severity index), it can assess the severity of an acute attack of pancreatitis, at the onset or within the first 2–3 days. Third, follow up CT examinations in patients with severe pancreatitis are essential in detecting local intermediate (infected necrosis, abscesses, pseudocysts) as well as late abdominal complications (pseudoaneurysms, hemorrhage, pancreatic ascites), thus contributing to the management of these patients. CT imaging has become an indispensable diagnostic tool in the evaluation and management of patients with acute pancreatitis.

References

Adams D, Harvey T, Anderson M (1991) Percutaneous catheter drainage of pancreatic pseudocysts. Am Surg 57:29–33

Agarwal N, Pitchumoni CS (1986) Simplified prognostic criteria in acute pancreatitis. Pancreas 1:69–73

Agarwal N, Pitchumoni CS, Sivaprasad V (1990) Evaluation tests for acute pancreatitis. Am J Gastroneterol 85:356–366

Agarwal N, Pitchumoni CS (1991) Assessment of severity in acute pancreatitis. Am J Gastroenterol 86:1385–1391

Balthazar EJ (1989) CT diagnosis and staging of acute pancreatitis. Radiol Clin N Am 27:19–37

Balthazar EJ (1994) Contrast-enhanced computed tomography in severe acute pancreatitis. In Bradley EL III (ed) Acute pancreatitis: diagnosis and therapy. Raven Press, New York, pp 57–68

Balthazar EJ (2002) Acute pancreatitis: assessment of severity with clinical and CT evaluation. Radiology 223:603–613

Balthazar EJ (2002) Complications of acute pancreatitis clinical and CT evaluation. Radiol Clin N Am 40:1211–1227

Balthazar EJ (2003) Diagnosis and imaging of gallstone pancreatitis. www.pancreasweb.com/

Balthazar E, Henderson M (1973) Prominent folds on the posterior wall and lesser curvature of the stomach. A sign of acute pancreatitis. Radiology 110:319–321

Balthazar EJ, Fisher LA (2001) Hemorrhagic complications of pancreatitis: radiologic evaluation with emphasis on CT imaging. Pancreatology 1:306–313

Balthazar EJ, Freeny PC, vanSonnenberg E (1994) Imaging and intervention in acute pancreatitis. Radiology 193:297–306

Balthazar EJ, Ranson JHC, Naidich DP et al (1985) Acute pancreatitis: prognostic value of CT. Radiology 156:767–772

Balthazar EJ, Robinson DL, Megibow AJ et al (1990) Acute pancreatitis: value of CT in establishing prognosis. Radiology 174:331–336

Bank S, Wise L, Gersten M (1983) Risk factors in acute pancreatitis. Am J Gastroenterol 78:637–640

Banks PA (1993) A new classification system for acute pancreatitis. Am J Gastroenterol 89:151–152

Banks PA (1994) Acute pancreatitis: medical and surgical management. Am J Gastroenterol 89:S78–85

Banks PA (1997) Practice guidelines in acute pancreatitis. Am J Gastroenterol 92:377–386

Bassi C (1994) Infected pancreatic necrosis. Int J Pancreatol 16:1–10

Becker V, Mischke U (1991) Groove pancreatitis. Int J Pancreatol 10:173–182

Beger HG, Krautzberger W, Bittner R et al (1985) Results of surgical treatment of necrotizing pancreatitis. World J Surg 9:972–979

Beger HG, Maier W, Block S et al (1986) How do imaging methods influence the surgical strategy in acute pancreatitis? In: Malfertheiner P, Ditschuneit H (eds) Diagnostic procedures in pancreatic disease. Springer, Berlin Heidelberg New York, pp 54–60

Beger HG, Bittner R, Block S et al (1986) Bacterial contamination of pancreatic necrosis. Gastroenterol 49:433–438

Beger HG, Rau B, Mayer J et al (1997) Natural course of acute pancreatitis. World J Surg 21:130–135

Belli AM, Jennings CM, Nakielny RA (1990) Splenic and portal venous thrombosis: a vascular complication of pancreatic disease demonstrated on computed tomography. Clin Radiol 41:13–16

Berenson JE, Spitz HB, Felson B (1971) The abdominal fat necrosis sign. Radiology 100:567–571

Berk JE (1995) The management of acute pancreatitis: a critical assessment as Dr. Bockus would have wished. Am J Gastroenterol 90:696–703

Bird NC, Goodman AJ, Johnson AG (1989) Serum phospholipase A2 activity in acute pancreatitis: an early guide to severity. Br J Surg 76:731–732

Bittner R, Block S, Buchler M et al (1987) Pancreatic abscess and infected pancreatic necrosis: different local septic complications in acute pancreatitis. Dic Dis Sci 32:1082–1087

Blamey SL, Imrie CW, O'Neil J et al (1984) Prognostic factors in acute pancreatitis. Gut 25:1340–1346

Bradley EL III (1993) A clinically based classification system for acute pancreatitis. Arch Surg 128:586–590

Bradley EL III, Allen K (1991) A prospective longitudinal study of observation versus surgical intervention in the management of necrotizing pancreatitis. Am J Surg 161:1924

Bradley E III, Clements J Jr, Gonzalez A (1979) The natural history of pancreatic pseudocysts: a unified concept of management. Am J Surg 137:137–141

Bretagne JF, Heresbach D, Darnault P et al (1990) Pseudoaneurysms and bleeding pseudocysts in chronic pancreatitis; radiological findings and contribution todiagnosis in 8 cases. Gastrointest Radiol 15:9–16

Buchler M, Malfertheiner P, Schadlich H et al (1989) Role of phospholipase A2 in human acute pancreatitis. Gastroenterology 97:1521–1526

Burke JW, Erickson SJ, Kellum CD et al (1986) Pseudoaneurysms complicating pancreatitis: detection by CT. Radiology 161:447–450

Cameron JL, Kieffer RS, Anderson WJ et al (1976) Internal pancreatic fistulas: pancreatic ascites and pleural effusions. Ann Surg 183:687–693

Cappell MS, Hassan T (1993) Pancreatic diseases in AIDs – a review. J Clin Gastroenterol 17:254–263

Clavien PA, Hauser H, Meyer P et al (1988) Value of contrast-enhanced computerized tomography in the early diagnosis of acute pancreatitis. A prospective study of 202 patients. Am J Surg 155:457–466

Clavien PA, Robert J, Meyer P et al (1989) Acute pancreatitis and normoamylasemia: not an uncommon combination. Ann Surg 210:614–620

Cohen SA, Siegel JH, Kasmin FE (1996) Complications of diagnostic and therapeutic ERCP. Abdom Imaging 21:385–394

Corfield AP, Cooper MJ, Williamson RCN et al (1985) Prediction of severity in acute pancreatitis: prospective comparison of three prognostic indices. Lancet 2:403–407

Cornu-Labat G, Kasirajan K, Simon R et al (1997) Acute mesenteric vein thrombosis and pancreatitis. Int J Pancreatol 21:249–251

Cotton PB (1977) Progress report: ERCP. Gut 18:316–341

Crass RA, Way LW (1981) Acute and chronic pancreatic pseudocysts are different. Am J Surg 142:660–663

Davis S, Parbhoo SP, Gibson MJ (1980) The plain abdominal radiograph in acute pacreatitis. Clin Radiol 31:87–93

de Beaux AC, Goldie AS, Ross JA et al (1996) Serum concentration of inflammatory mediators related to organ failure with acute pancreatitis. Br J Surg 83:349–353

Denham W, Norman J (1999) The potential role of therapeutic cytokine manipulation in acute pancreatitis. Surg Clin North Am 79:767–781

Dervenis C, Johnson CD, Bassi C et al (1999) Diagnosis, objective assessment of severity, and management of acute pancreatitis. Int J Pancreatol 25:195–210

Dickson AP, Imrie CW (1984) The incidence and prognosis of body wall ecchymosis in acute pancreatitis. Sur Gynaecol Obstet 159:343–347

Dominguez-Munoz JE, Caraballo F, Garcia MJ (1991) Clinical usefulness of polymorphonuclear elastase in predicting the severity of acute pancreatitis: results of a multicentre study. Br J Surg 78:1230–1234

Donovitz M, Kerstein MD, Spiro HM (1974) Pancreatic ascites. Medicine (Baltimore) 53:183–195

Exley AR, Leese T, Holliday MP et al (1992) Endotoxaemia and serum tumor necrosis factor as prognostic markers in severe acute pancreatitis. Gut 33:1126–1128

Farman J, Dallemand S, Schneider M et al (1977) Pancreatic pseudocysts involving the spleen. Gastrointestinal Radiol 1:339–343

Feiner H (1976) Pancreatitis after cardiac surgery. Am J Surg 131:684–688

Fernandez-Cruz L, Margarona E, Llovera J et al (1993) Pancreatic ascites. Hepato-Gastroenterology 40:150–154

Fielding GA, McLatchie GR, Wilson C et al (1989) Acute pancreatitis and pancreatic fistula formation. Br J Surg 76:1126–1128

Fitz RH (1889) Acute pancreatitis: a consideration of pancreatic hemorrhage, hemorrhagic suppurative and gangrenous pancreatitis and of disseminated fat necrosis. Boston Med Surg J 120:181–187

Freeny PC (1993) Incremental dynamic bolus computed tomography of acute pancreatitis. Int J Pancreatol 13:147–158

Freeny PC, Hauptmann E, Althaus SJ et al (1998) Percutaneous CT guided catheter drainage of infected acute necrotizing pancreatitis: technique and results. AJR Am J Roentgenol 170:969–975

Frey CF (1997) Pancreatic pseudocyst operative strategy. Ann Surg 188:652–661

Fucher AS, Turner MA (1999) MR pancreatography: a useful tool for evaluating pancreatic disorders. RadioGraphics 19:5–24

Fujita N, Shirai Y, Tsukada K et al (1997) Groove pancreatis with recurrent duodenal obstruction. Int J Pancreatol 21:185–188

Gadacz TR, Trunkey D, Kieffer RF Jr (1978) Visceral vessel erosion associated with pancreatitis. Arch Surg 113:1438–1440

Gerzof SG, Banks PA, Robbins AH et al (1987) Early diagnosis of pancreatic infection by computed tomography-guided aspiration. Gastroenterol 93:1315–1320

Gross V, Leser HG, Heinisch A et al (1993) Inflammatory mediators and cytokines: new aspects of the pathophysiology and assessment of severity of acute pancreatitis. Hepatogastroenterology 40;522–531

Hill MC, Barkin J, Isikoff MB et al (1982) Acute pancreatitis: clinical vs CT findings. AJR Am J Roentgenol 139:263–269

Imre CM, Benjamin IS, McKay AJ et al (1978) A single center double blind trial of Trasyol therapy in primary acute pancreatitis. Br J Surg 65:337–341

Johst P, Tsiotos GG, Sarr MG (1997) Pancreatic ascites: a rare complications of necrotizing pancreatitis. Int J Pancreatol 22:151–154

Kelly SB, Gauhar T, Pollard R (1999) Massive intraperitoneal hemorrhage from a pancreatic pseudocysts. Am J Gastroenterol 94:3638–3641

Kemmer TP, Malfertheiner P, Buchler M et al (1991) Serum ribonuclease activity in the diagnosis of pancreatic disease. Int J Pancreatol 8:23–33

Kiviluoto T, Kivisaari L, Kivilaakso E et al (1989) Pseudocysts in chronic pancreatitis. Arch Surg 124:240–243

Kivisaari L, Somer K, Standertskjold-Nordenstam CG et al (1983) Early detection of acute fulminant pancreatitis by contrast enhanced computed tomography. Scand J Gastroenterol 18:39–41

Kloppel G (1994) Pathology of severe acute pancreatitis. In: Bradley EL III (ed) Acute pancreatitis: diagnosis and therapy. Raven, New York, NY, pp 35–46
Knaus WA, Draper EA, Wagner DP et al (1985) APACHE II: a severity of disease classification system. Crit Care Med 13:818–829
Kravetz GW, Cho KC, Baker SR (1988) Radiologic evaluation of pancreatic ascites. Radiology 13:163–166
Lankisch PG, Schirren CA, Otto J (1989) Methemalbumin in acute pancreatitis: an evaluation of its prognostic value and comparison with multiple prognostic parameters. Am J Gastroenterol 84:1391–1395
Lankisch PG, Burchard-Reckert S, Petersen M et al (1996) Etiology and age have only a limited influence on the course of acute pancreatitis. Pancreas 13:344–349
Larvin M, McMahon MJ (1989) APACHE II score for assessment and monitoring of acute pancreatitis. Lancet 2:201–204
Lee SP, Nicholls, Park HZ (1992) Biliary sludge as a cause of acute pancreatitis. N Engl J Med 326:589–593
Lilienfeld RM, Lande A (1976) A pancreatic pseudocysts presenting as thick walled renal and perinephric cysts. J Urol 115:123–125
Lindahl F, Vejlsted H, Becker OG (1972) Lesions of the colon following pancreatitis. Scand J Gastroenterol 7:375–378
London NJ, Neoptolemos JP, Lavelle J et al (1989) Contrast-enhanced abdominal computed tomography scanning and prediction of severity of acute pancreatitis: a prospective study. Br J Surg 76:268–272
Lowham A, Lavelle J, Leese T (1999) Mortality from acute pancreatitis. Int J Pancreatol 25:103–106
Madsen MS, Peterson TH, Sommer H (1986) Segmental portal hypertension. Ann Surg 204:72–77
Maier W (1987) Early objective diagnosis and staging of acute pancreatitis by contrast enhanced CT. In: Beger H, Buchler M (eds) Acute pancreatitis. Springer, Berlin hedelberg New York, pp 132–140
Malfertheiner P, Dominguez-Munoz JE (1993) Prognostic factors in acute pancreatitis. Int J Pancreatol 140:1–8
Mann DV, Hershman MJ, Hittinger R et al (1994) Multicentre audit of death from acute pancreatitis. Br J Surg 81:890–893
McKay CJ, Evans S, Sinclar M et al (1999) High early mortality rate from acute pancreatitis in Scotland, 1984–1985. Br Surg 86:1302–1306
McMahon MJ, Playforth MJ, Pickforth IR (1980) A comparative study of methods for the prediction of severity of attacks of acute pancreatitis. Br J Surg 67:22–25
Mendez G Jr, Isikoff MB, Hill MC (1980) CT of acute pancreatitis: interim assessment. AJR Am J Roentgenol 135:463–469
Meyers MA, Evans JA (1973) Effects of pancreatitis on the small bowel and colon. AJR Am J Roentgenol 119:151–165
Millward SE, Breatnach E, Simpkins KC et al (1983) Do plain films of the chest and abdomen have a role in the diagnosis of acute pancreatitis ? Clini Radiol 34:133–137
Moossa AR (1984) Diagnostic tests and procedures in acute pancreatitis. N Engl J Med 311:639–643
Morgan DE, Baron TH, Smith JK et al (1997) Pancreatic fluid collections prior to intervention: evaluation with MR imaging compared with CT and US. Radiology 203:773–778
Muller CH, Lahnert U, Schafmayer A et al (1999) Massive intraperitoneal bleeding from tryptic erosions of the splenic vein. Int J Pancreatol 26:49–52
Mutinga M, Rosenbluth A, Tenner SM et al (2000) Does mortality occur early or late in acute pancreatitis? Int J Pancreatol 28:91–95
National Center for Health Statistics (1987) Vital Statistics of the United States 1987. Vol II. Part A. Mortality. Washington, DC: Govt. Printing Office
National Hospital Discharge Survey (1989) National Hospital Discharge Survey 1987. Detailed diagnosis and procedures. Vital Health Stat [13] 100:1–304
Nevalainen TJ (1980) The role of phospholipase A in acute pancreatitis. Scand J Gastroenterol 15:641–650
Nordbach I, Sisto T (1989) Peripancreatic vascular occlusions as a complication of pancreatitis. Int Surg 74:36–39
Nordestgaard AG, Wilson SE, Williams RA (1986) Early computerized tomography as a predictor of outcome in acute pancreatitis. Am J Surg 152:127–132
Opie EL (1901) The etiology of acute hemorrhagic pancreatitis. Bull Johns Hopkins Hosp 12:182–192
Paajainen H, Laato M, Jaakkola M et al (1995) Serum tumor necrosis factor compared with C-reactive protein in assessment of severity of acute pancreatitis. Br J Surg 82:271–273
Parenti DM, Steinberg W, Kang P (1996) Infectious cases of acute pancreatitis. Pancreas 13:356–371
Pelucio MT, Rothenhaus T, Smith M et al (1995) Fatal pancreatitis as a complication of therapy for HIV infection. J Emerg Med 13:633–637
Poppel MH (1968) The roentgen manifestations of pancreatitis. Semin Roentgenol 3:227–241
Price CWR (1956) The colon cut-off sign of acute pancreatitis. Med J Aust 1:313–314
Ranson JHC (1982) Etiological and prognostic factors in human acute pancreatitis: A review. Am J Gastroenterol 77:633–638
Ranson JHC (1997) Diagnostic standards for acute pancreatitis. W J Surg 21:136–142
Ranson JHC, Rifkind KM, Roses DF et al (1974) Objective early identification of severe acute pancreatitis. Am J Gastroenterol 61:443–451
Renner IG, Savage WT, Pantoia JL et al (1985) Death due to acute pancreatitis: a retrospective analysis of 405 autopsy cases. Dig Dis Sci 30:1005–1018
Safrit HD, Rice RP (1989) Gastrointestinal complications of pancreatitis. Radiol Clin North Am 27:73–79
Saito T, Tanaka S, Yoshida H et al (2002) A case of autoimmune pancreatitis responding to steroid therapy. Pancreatol 2:550–556
Sankaran S, Walt AJ (1975) The natural and unnatural history of pancreatic pseudocysts. Br J Surg 62:37–44
Sarles H, Sarles JC, Muratore R, Guien C (1961) Chronic inflammatory sclerosis of the pancreas: an autonomous pancreatic disease? Am J Dig Dis 6:688–698
Seidlin M, Lambert JS, Dolin R et al (1992) Pancreatitis and pancreatic dysfunction in patients taking dideoxyinosine. AIDS 6:831–835
Singh SM, Simsek H (1990) Ethanol and the pancreas: current status. Gastroenterology 98:1051–1062
Spechler SJ, Dalton JW, Robbins AH et al (1983) Prevalence of normal serum amylase level in patients with acute alcoholic pancreatitis. Dig Dis Sci 28:865–869

Stabile BE, Wilson SE, Debas HT (1983) Reduced mortality from bleeding pseudocysts and pseudoaneurysms caused by pancreatitis. Arch Surg 118:45–51

Steer ML (1989) Classification and pathogenesis of pancreatitis. Surg Clin North Am 69:467–480

Stein GN, Kalser MH, Sarian NN et al (1959) An evaluation of roentgen changes in acute pancreatitis correlation with clinical findings. Gastroenterology 36:354–365

Steinberg W, Tenner S (1994) Acute pancreatitis. N Engl J Med 330:1198–1210

Stolte M, Weis M, Volkholz H, Rosch W (1982) A special form of segmental pancreatitis: „groove pancreatitis." Hepatogastroenterology 29:198–208

Talamini G, Bassi C, Falconi M et al (1996) Risk of death from acute pancreatitis. Int J Pancreatol 19:15–24

Tann M, Maglinte D, Howard TJ et al (2003) Disconnected pancreatic duct syndrome: imaging findings and therapeutic implications in 26 surgically corrected patients. J Comp Assisted Tomography 27:557–582

Tenner S, Fernandez-del Castillo C, Warshaw A et al (1997) Urinary trypsinogen activation peptide (TAP) predicts severity in patients with acute pancreatitis Int J Pancreatol 21:105–110

Thompson WM, Kelvin FM, Rice RP (1977) Inflammation and necrosis of the transverse colon secondary to pancreatitis. AJR Am J Roentgenol 128:943–948

Uhl W, Buchler M, Malfertheiner P et al (1991) Pancreatic necrosis develops within four days after the acute attack (abstr). Gastroenterology 100(5 pt 2):A302

Uhl W, Buchler M, Malfertheiner P et al (1991) PMN-elastase in comparison with CPR, antiproteases and LDH as indicators of necrosis in human acute pancreatitis. Pancreas 6:253–259

Uhl W, Isenmann R, Curti G et al (1996) Influence of etiology on the course and outcome of acute pancreatitis. Pancreas 13:335–343

VanSonnenberg E, Wittich GR, Casola G et al (1989) Percutaneous drainage of infected and noninfected pancreatic pseudocysts: experience in 101 cases. Radiology 170:757–761

Vujic I (1989) Vascular complications of pancreatitis. Radio Clin North Am 27:81–91

Wade JW (1985) Twenty-five year experience with pancreatic pseudocysts. Am J Surg 149:705–708

Warshaw AL, Lee KH (1979) Serum ribonuclease elevations and pancreatic necrosis in acute pancreatitis. Surgery 86:227–234

Weaver DW, Walt AJ, Sugawa C et al (1982) A continuing appraisal of pancreatic ascites. Surg Gyncol Obst 134:845–848

Weber CK, Adler G (2001) From acinar cell damage to systemic inflammatory response: Current concepts in pancreatitis. Pancreatology 1:356–362

White AF, Baum S, Buranasiri S (1976) Aneurysms secondary to pancreatitis. AJR Am J Roentgenol 127:393–396

WhiteT, Morgan AH, Opton D (1970) Post operative pancreatitis: a study of seventy cases. Am J Surg 120:132–137

Wilson C, Heads A, Shenkin A et al (1989) C-reactive protein, anti-proteases and complement factors as objective markers of severity in acute pancreatitis. Br J Surg 76:177–181

Wilson C, Heath DI, Imrie CW (1990) Prediction of outcome in acute pancreatitis: a comparative study of APACHE II, clinical assessment and multiple factor scoring systems. Br J Surg 77:1260–1264

Yeo CJ, Bastidas JA, Lynch-Nyhan A et al (1990) The natural history of pancreatic pseudocysts documented by computed tomography. Surg Gynecol Obstet 170:411–417

Magnetic Resonance Imaging of Acute Pancreatitis

5

Elizabeth Hecht

CONTENTS

5.1 **Introduction** *79*

5.2 **MRI Protocol** *80*
5.2.1 General Principles of MRI of the Pancreas *80*
5.2.2 Breath-hold Imaging *80*
5.2.3 Non-breath-hold Imaging *80*
5.2.4 Patient Preparation *81*
5.2.5 Protocol *81*
5.2.6 Secretin-MRCP (S-MRCP) *82*
5.2.7 Intravenous Contrast *83*

5.3 **Role of MRI of Acute Pancreatitis** *85*
5.3.1 Underlying Causes of Pancreatitis *85*

5.4 **MRI Findings in Acute Pancreatitis** *85*
5.4.1 Normal Pancreas *85*
5.4.2 Mild (Edematous) Pancreatitis *86*
5.4.3 Severe (Necrotizing) Pancreatitis and Complications *88*
5.4.4 Pancreatic Necrosis *89*
5.4.5 Hemorrhage *92*
5.4.6 Peripancreatic Collections *93*
5.4.7 Pseudocysts *94*
5.4.8 Vascular Complications *96*
5.4.9 Imaging Features of Autoimmune Pancreatitis *97*

5.5 **Emerging MRI Techniques** *100*
5.5.1 Perfusion Imaging *100*
5.5.2 MR Spectroscopy *101*
5.5.3 Diffusion-Weighted Imaging *101*
5.5.4 MR Elastography *102*

5.6 **Conclusion** *102*

References *102*

E. Hecht, MD
Department of Radiology, NYU-Langone Medical Center, 560 First Avenue, Suite HW 202, New York, NY 10016, USA

5.1 Introduction

Magnetic resonance imaging (MRI) technology and availability has rapidly improved over recent years with advances in magnet and gradient design, phased array coils and software that permit high spatial and temporal resolution imaging in a clinically practical scan time. MRI combined with MR cholangiopancreatography (MRCP) provides anatomic, physiologic and potentially biochemical information without the need for ionizing radiation or iodinated contrast agents. Compared to computed tomography (CT), MRI provides superior soft tissue contrast, direct multiplanar capability and three-dimensional (3D) data acquisition that is particularly beneficial for pancreatic imaging. Although CT has traditionally been the gold standard for imaging in acute pancreatitis, MRI is a reliable alternative for staging, assessing severity and predicting outcome in patients with acute pancreatitis (Lecesne et al. 1999; Arvanitakis et al. 2004; Arvanitakis et al. 2007; Stimac et al. 2007; Viremouneix et al. 2007). In fact, MRI is superior to CT for detection of mild acute pancreatitis, assessment of peripancreatic collections and parenchymal necrosis while secretin-MRCP (s-MRCP) provides a noninvasive method for detection of underlying anatomic and functional pancreatic duct abnormalities in the setting of acute and/or chronic pancreatitis. Finally, the addition of dynamic multiphase gadolinium chelate-enhanced MRI improves contrast resolution and provides a mechanism for assessment and quantification of parenchymal perfusion without exposure to ionizing radiation.

5.2 MRI Protocol

5.2.1 General Principles of MRI of the Pancreas

For a comprehensive assessment of the pancreas in a patient with acute pancreatitis, the MRI protocol should include (MRCP) sequences typically heavily T2-weighted, 3D volumetric or 2D thick slab projection, as well as T2-weighted fat-suppressed, T1-weighted in and opposed phase and dynamic (multiphase) gadolinium chelate contrast enhanced T1-weighted imaging in the axial and/or coronal planes. Secretin-enhanced MRCP has been advocated for assessing pancreatic function and detecting underlying anatomic abnormalities that may impair function or precipitate recurrent bouts of acute pancreatitis such as a pancreas divisum or Santorinicele. The mechanism of action of secretin, and its influence on MRI, will be discussed later in the chapter.

In general practice, all studies should be performed at 1.5 or 3.0 Tesla (T) using a phased array body coil for optimization of signal-to-noise ratio (SNR) unless the patient's body habitus is prohibitive. While 1.5 T is more widely available and more easily optimized, 3-T imaging has several advantages for pancreatic imaging including inherently higher signal-to-noise ratio that can be used to improve spatial resolution or speed up scan time and better spectral separation leading to improved fat suppression. Breath-hold imaging, fat suppression and a power contrast-agent injector are preferred for optimal dynamic contrast-enhanced imaging of the pancreas.

Phased array radiofrequency (RF) coils are composed of multiple coil elements each able to detect and route signals to separate receiver systems. Multiple coil arrays and high performance gradients are required to implement parallel imaging techniques such as SMASH (simultaneous acquisition of spatial harmonics) and SENSE (sensitivity encoding) (Sodickson and Manning 1997; Pruessmann et al. 1999). In the past, only gradients were used for spatial encoding of information but with more sophisticated RF coil technology, it is possible to under-sample phase-encoding lines in k-space and use the coil spatial information to recover the data. Parallel imaging techniques can lead to higher temporal resolution imaging without compromising spatial resolution or permit higher spatial resolution imaging without compromising temporal resolution. For example, parallel imaging is useful in MRCP imaging for high resolution 3D respiratory triggered heavily T2-weighted turbo spin echo (TSE) MRCP sequences permitting more reasonable acquisition times. Without parallel imaging such a sequence would take up to 8–12 min depending on the patient's respiratory rate but with parallel imaging, the acquisition time is decreased to 3–4 min. Parallel imaging techniques can be applied to many of the imaging sequences used in abdominal MRI for faster imaging and/or higher resolution imaging which is extremely important for pancreatic imaging as the anatomic structures are small and respiratory motion can greatly impair image quality.

5.2.2 Breath-hold Imaging

One of the keys to successful pancreatic imaging is breath-hold imaging, since it directly leads to shorter scan times, improving overall efficiency, and minimizes respiratory motion artifacts. Technicians should assess a patient's breath-holding capability when placing them in the magnet. Supplemental O_2 can be administered via a nasal cannula if needed. Acquisition time should be adjusted to an individual's breath-hold capacity to optimize image quality and compliance. End expiration has been demonstrated to be more reproducible (Holland et al. 1998). Reproducibility is critical when employing post-processing techniques such as subtraction (subtracting the unenhanced T1 data set from the contrast enhanced data set).

5.2.3 Non-breath-hold Imaging

Breath-hold sequences can be modified in several ways to reduce scan times. Spatial resolution may be modestly sacrificed by decreasing the matrix size or increasing the slice thickness. Parallel imaging techniques may also be employed. Even severely ill patients can potentially breath-hold for a short time period (5–10 s). However, if this is not possible, non-breath-hold sequences are a viable alternative. Ultra-fast sequences such as magnetization prepared T1-weighted gradient echo and half-Fourier T2-weighted single shot turbo (or fast) spin echo sequences (HASTE or SSFSE) are most useful. These sequences are obtained on a slice-by-slice basis, effectively freezing respiratory motion during acquisition. However, breathing can lead to acquisition of slices in a non-sequential manner.

There are respiratory navigated versions of the standard abdominal MRI sequences which are newly available, as well as under development. Respiratory navigator sequences track diaphragmatic motion and images are only acquired when the diaphragm is positioned at a specific elevation as chosen by the MR imager. This allows free breathing during the acquisition. The time of acquisition depends on the patient's respiratory rate and the sequence parameters defined by the technologist.

5.2.4 Patient Preparation

Patients should be fasting for at least 4 h prior to MRCP. Some authors also advocate the use of negative oral contrast (bowel "darkening") agents when evaluating biliary and pancreatic diseases. Negative oral contrast agents eliminate the high T2 signal intensity of the stomach and small bowel which can potentially obscure visualization of the biliary tree, especially on heavily T2-weighted MRCP sequences. There are a variety of commercially available negative contrast bowel agents including ferric ammonium citrate, manganese chloride, ferric particles, antacid, barium sulphate, kaolinate, pineapple juice and blueberry juice (Papanikolaou et al. 2000; Riordan et al. 2004). Some commercial products are also available such as ferumoxsil (GastroMARK, Mallinckrodt, Maryland Heights, Missouri) and diluted IV gadolinium such as gadopentetate dimeglumine (Magnevist, Berlex Laboratories, Wayne, New Jersey) (Chan et al. 2000). A combined approach using pineapple juice and a gadolinium chelate has also been proposed (Coppens et al. 2005). As a word of caution, visualization of the distal common bile duct and main pancreatic duct could be impaired in the setting of reflux of negative oral contrast material into the distal common bile duct and main pancreatic duct (Sugita and Nomiya 2002). Reflux can be seen after endoscopic sphincterotomy or surgical interventions such as a choledochoduodenostomy (Sugita and Nomiya 2002).

5.2.5 Protocol

The following protocol assumes use of a 1.5-T magnet, a dedicated phased array body coil and power injector (Table 5.1). For 3-T imaging, parameters should be slightly adjusted to compensate for expected lengthening of T1 and shortening of T2 and systemic absorption rate (SAR) limits (Lee et al. 2007). Protocol details will vary slightly depending on available technology and patient's body habitus and capabilities.

Table 5.1. Pancreas MRI/MRCP protocols with parallel imaging[a]

Sequence	TR (ms)	TE (ms)	FA (degree)	Matrix	Parallel imaging factor (R)	ST (mm)	Time (s)
Scout							
Coronal and axial SSFSE	900	90	150	320	2	4–6	20 × 2
Axial T1 GRE in/oop	180	4.8	80	256	2	8	12
Axial T2 FS TSE	3600	100	180	256	2	8	12
3D respiratory triggered T2 TSE	1300	680	180	384	3	1	120–180
2D thick slab (optional)	∞	1100	180	320		30–60	< 3
Axial 3D T1 FS GRE (VIBE) pre/post	3.2	1.3	12	256	2	2 (interpolated)	12

SSFSE, single shot fast spin echo; GRE, gradient echo; FS, fat-suppressed; TSE, turbo spin echo; VIBE, volume interpolated breath hold examination.

[a]Although the same sequences may be performed without parallel imaging, imaging times will be longer, but can still be performed in a breath-hold with the exception of the respiratory triggered sequences which depend on patient's respiratory rate (RR).

A three-plane scout should be used to ensure that the field of view is centered over the pancreas and biliary tree. A standard protocol will include Half-Fourier acquisition single shot turbo spin echo (HASTE) [or single shot fast spin echo (SSFSE)] sequences in the axial and coronal or coronal oblique plane to best visualize the biliary and pancreatic ducts. Axial dual echo T1 in- and out-of-phase images are used for detecting fat stranding, hemorrhage, fat, calcium and iron in the pancreas or in adjacent organs. Axial T2-weighted images with fat suppression, either T2-weighted fat-suppressed TSE or short tau inversion recovery (turbo STIR) are useful for detecting subtle pancreatic T2 signal abnormalities in the setting of pancreatitis.

The MRCP portion of the exam should include a thick-slab (30- to 60-mm) heavily T2-weighted sequence which can be performed in a breath-hold (single slab in < 3 s) in the coronal and at least two coronal oblique planes with approximately +/- 30 degree angulation to allow appropriate projection direction for optimal visualization of the pancreatic duct. If available, a 3D respiratory triggered, heavily T2-weighted TSE can replace the thick slab technique because of the ability to acquire a volume data set with 1-mm slice thickness which can be evaluated post hoc in 3D (Fig. 5.1).

Dynamic contrast enhanced imaging through the pancreas should be performed with a breath-hold 2D or 3D T1 fat suppressed gradient echo sequence before and following intravenous gadolinium administration. Imaging should be performed in the arterial phase, as determined by a timing run, in the venous and in delayed phases. A total of 5 s should be added to the time of peak arterial enhancement, as determined by a timing run through the aorta at the level of the pancreas, to ensure optimal pancreatic enhancement. The subsequent phases should be performed at about 60 s and 120–180 s following injection. Advantages of 3D T1-weighted imaging are thinner slice partitions, 2–3 mm, and the ability to perform arbitrary multiplanar reformations (Fig. 5.2).

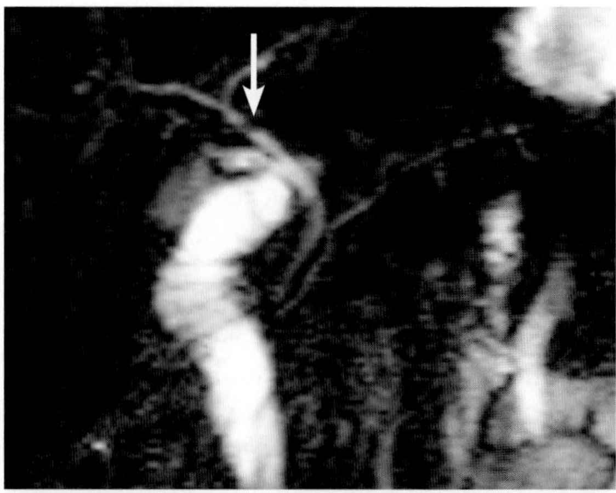
a

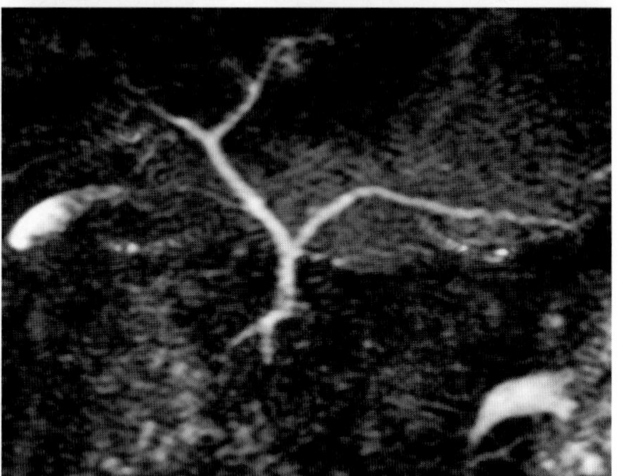
b

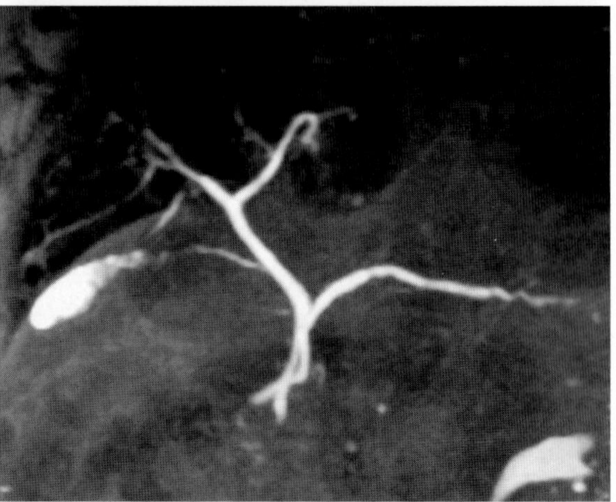
c

Fig. 5.1. **a** Coronal heavily T2W thick slab through the normal biliary tree and pancreatic duct. Note the apparent filling defect or signal loss in the common hepatic duct (*arrow*); this is a common artifact due to pulsation from the hepatic artery (not seen here). **b** Coronal heavily T2W thick slab demonstrates pancreas divisum. **c** Coronal heavily T2W 3D respiratory triggered TSE (3D-MRCP) with parallel imaging in the same patient with pancreas divisum

5.2.6 Secretin-MRCP (S-MRCP)

Secretin is a digestive enzyme that, when released in response to a meal, stimulates production of bicarbonate rich fluid by the exocrine pancreas (Cappeliez et al. 2000) and increases the tone of the sphincter of Oddi. When secretin is admin-

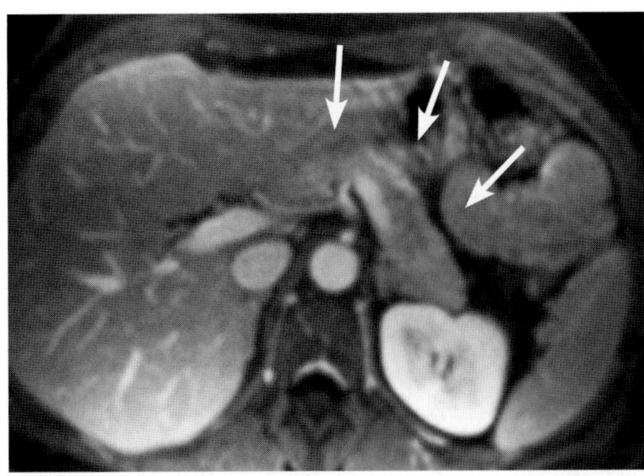

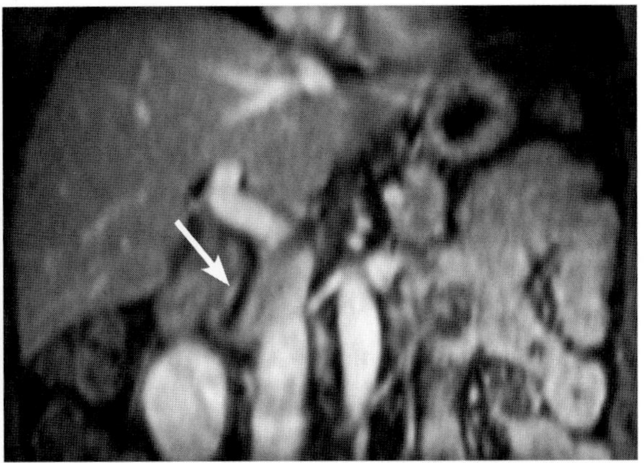

Fig. 5.2. a Axially acquired 3D T1W FS GRE (volume interpolated breath-hold examination, or VIBE) through normal body and tail of the pancreas (*arrows*). **b** Coronal reformation of the same axial images demonstrate the common bile duct (*arrow*) coursing through the pancreatic head. Note the excellent off axis resolution due to isotropic voxel size

istered intravenously, the main pancreatic duct will distend up to 3 mm from baseline and the duodenum will become progressively distended with pancreatic effluent. In healthy individuals, these effects are observed within 5 min of administration (Fig. 5.3). This physiologic response can be imaged dynamically with MR. Changes in pancreatic duct diameter may reveal underlying strictures or branch duct dilatation and quantification of pancreatic exocrine function may be assessed. In the setting of acute pancreatitis, S-MRCP may be used to identify pancreatic duct disruption and communication of the pancreatic duct with surrounding fluid collections, as well as anatomic variants such as pancreas divisum or other acquired conditions leading to sphincter of Oddi dysfunction that may be associated with recurrent bouts of acute pancreatitis (Arvanitakis et al. 2004; Manfredi et al. 2000; Delhaye et al. 2008; Matos et al. 2006).

A baseline, heavily T2-weighted thick slab MRCP in the coronal oblique plane that includes the entire main pancreatic duct, biliary tree and duodenum is required before secretin administration to determine an individual patient's response to secretin over time. It is important to eliminate any background high signal from fluid in the stomach and/or duodenum by using a negative oral contrast agent prior to administration of secretin. If high signal remains in the duodenum and stomach, it can be difficult to confidently differentiate between normal physiologic emptying of fluid from the stomach into the duodenum and pancreatic secretions into the duodenum in response to secretin infusion.

Signs of impaired response to secretin include: visualization of pancreatic side branches, delayed time to peak dilation of the pancreatic duct or delayed recovery of baseline diameter including dilation of the pancreatic duct > 3 mm at 10 min and reduced filling of the duodenum, implying impairment of functional reserve (Cappeliez et al. 2000). Progressive enhancement of pancreatic parenchyma or "acinar filling" has been observed in patients with recurrent attacks of pancreatitis likely reflecting tissue hypertension or loss of parenchymal compliance, suggestive of early chronic pancreatitis (Matos et al. 1998; Manfredi et al. 2002).

In patients with impaired pancreatic function, reduced duodenal filling alone was specific (87%) but less sensitive 72% for detection of impaired exocrine function (Cappeliez et al. 2000). S-MRCP may be of particular use in patients in whom chronic pancreatitis is suspected but no morphologic changes are evident on CT, US, MRI and even ERCP. These patients may have detectable and quantifiable functional impairment before presenting with distinct morphologic changes.

5.2.7 Intravenous Contrast

Intravenous gadolinium chelate administration is useful for assessment of pancreatic perfusion and viability as well as the vascular complications of pancreatitis such as venous thrombosis or pseudoaneurysm.

Dynamic contrast enhanced imaging through the pancreas should be performed with a breath-hold

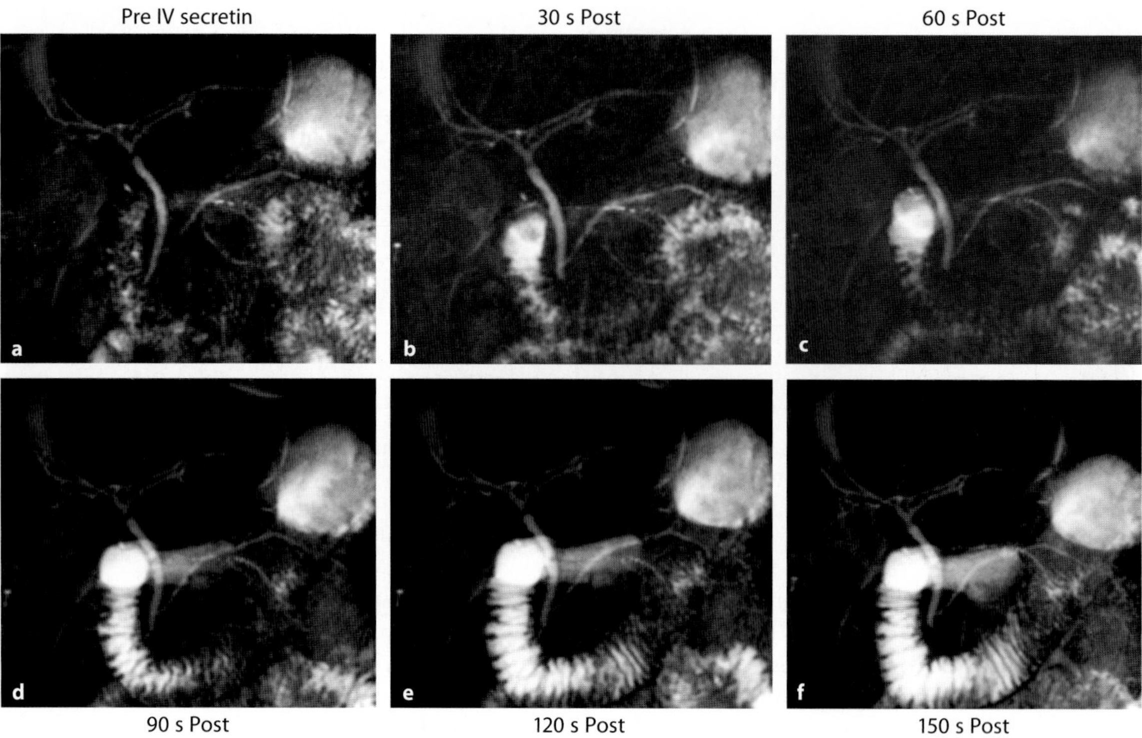

Fig. 5.3a–f. Normal response to IV administration of secretin is demonstrated on this series of 2D thick slab MRCP images before and after secretin administration with appropriate mild dilatation of the pancreatic duct demonstrating normal distensibility and prompt excretion of the pancreatic juices into the duodenum

2D or preferably 3D T1 fat suppressed gradient echo sequence before and following intravenous gadolinium administration using weight base dosing of 0.1 mmol/kg for gadolinium DTPA, although lower doses may be used if gadolinium chelate agents with higher T1 relaxivity are administered.

MRI has been advocated as an alternative to CT for imaging of patients with pancreatitis because it does not require ionizing radiation and utilizes gadolinium chelate contrast agents which are less likely to cause allergic reactions and renal toxicity and considered relatively safe in patients with renal insufficiency. However, in 2006, gadolinium chelate agents were shown to be associated with a rare debilitating and potentially fatal entity called nephrogenic systemic fibrosis (NSF), a systemic disorder with its most prominent and visible effects in the skin (Grobner and Prischl 2007). NSF almost exclusively affects patients on dialysis (peritoneal or hemodialysis) but also has been reported in patients with acute renal failure. While the exact role of gadolinium chelate agents in the development of this disease is unclear, they should be used with caution in patients with severely impaired renal function.

Gadolinium chelate agents should be avoided in patients on dialysis. In patients with eGFR < 30 mL/min/1.73m^2, gadolinium chelates should also be avoided unless the benefits of the examination outweigh the risks as determined by the clinical team.

Exogenous contrast, although helpful for assessment of pancreatic necrosis, pancreatic masses and metastases, is in fact not essential. Indeed, several studies have compared unenhanced MRI to contrast enhanced CT for staging severity and prognosis and found that both approaches are comparable (Arvanitakis et al. 2004; Arvanitakis et al. 2007; Stimac et al. 2007; Viremouneix et al. 2007; Lecesne et al. 1999). In addition, MRI has some distinct advantages over CT because of the excellent tissue contrast which will be discussed below.

5.3 Role of MRI of Acute Pancreatitis

5.3.1 Underlying Causes of Pancreatitis

There are various causes of pancreatitis with the most common being alcohol and choledocholithiasis. Other causes include abdominal trauma, infection, metabolic disorders, anatomic variants, mechanical obstruction of the pancreatic duct, vasculitis, genetic predisposition, cystic fibrosis, idiopathic, medications, ERCP and autoimmune disease. MRI can be useful for determining the underlying cause of pancreatitis particularly in the setting of a mechanical obstruction. Other causes require clinical and laboratory data for definitive diagnosis. In the acute setting, the morphologic features of pancreatitis often look similar despite the underlying causes.

As discussed above, MRI is considered comparable to multidetector CT (MDCT) in diagnosing acute pancreatitis and its complications. MRI may be superior to contrast enhanced CT for determining the composition of peripancreatic fluid collections, differentiating between pancreatic necrosis and peripancreatic fluid collections, detecting underlying duct pathology and assessing vessel patency (Ward et al. 1997; Morgan and Baron 1998; Lecesne et al. 1999; Robinson and Sheridan 2000; Amano et al. 2001; Hirota et al. 2002; Zhang et al. 2003; Arvanitakis et al. 2004). In the setting of mild acute pancreatitis, the sensitivity of MRI may even exceed that of CT with T2-weighted imaging being most useful for revealing subtle pancreatic signal changes and peripancreatic edema (Amano et al. 2001).

MRI including MRCP can provide additional information regarding the etiology of acute pancreatitis including choledocholithiasis, pancreas divisum or, more rarely, pancreatic neoplasm. Specifically, in terms of the biliary tree, it is generally agreed that an evaluation of the presence of biliary stone disease is necessary in every patient presenting with acute pancreatitis. Because of the low sensitivity of CT for detecting biliary calculi, these patients will require additional imaging, usually ultrasound, to exclude the presence of biliary stones. However, because the sensitivity of MRCP is high, a single imaging evaluation is possible for the patient referred for MRI. The sensitivity of stone detection is similar to ERCP for detection of common bile duct stones, but ERCP is associated with a failure rate of 3%–11% (Soto et al. 1996), morbidity rate of 7% and mortality rate of 1% (Reinhold and Bret 1996).

MRCP is noninvasive, requires no exogenous contrast agents, accurately assesses the diameter of ducts and permits visualization of the biliary tree in the setting of prior biliary enteric anastomosis. MRCP can help guide therapeutic intervention and determine whether a patient should undergo antegrade or retrograde cannulation of the ducts (Soto et al. 1996). The sensitivity and specificity of MRCP in detecting CBD stones is 81%–99% and 85%–99%, respectively, exceeding that of CT (45%–85% sensitivity) and US (20%–65% sensitivity) (Pedrosa and Rofsky 2003). MRCP has a high negative predictive value of 98% for detection of common bile duct stones in patients with acute gallstone pancreatitis selecting only those patients requiring stone extraction for ERCP (Makary et al. 2005).

5.4 MRI Findings in Acute Pancreatitis

5.4.1 Normal Pancreas

Normal pancreatic parenchyma demonstrates high signal intensity compared to liver parenchyma on unenhanced T1-weighted fat suppressed sequences (Fig. 5.4). This relative high signal on T1-weighted imaging is likely due to the presence of aqueous

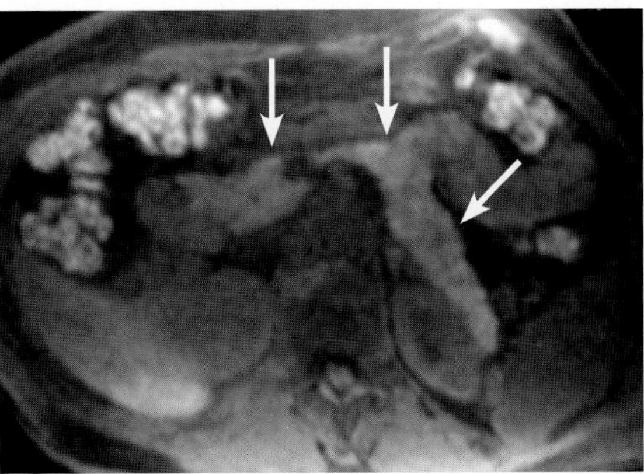

Fig. 5.4. Normal unenhanced axial T1W FS GRE image through the pancreas demonstrating the slight hyperintensity of normal pancreatic tissue (*arrows*) relative to liver and spleen

proteins in the acini of the pancreas (Semelka and Ascher 1993). Normal pancreas is isointense or slightly hypointense to normal liver on T2-weighted sequences (Fig. 5.5). Following intravenous administration of a gadolinium chelate, the normal pancreas demonstrates homogenous enhancement with maximal enhancement during the pancreatic arterial phase becoming isointense to the liver on subsequent phases of imaging (Fig. 5.6).

5.4.2 Mild (Edematous) Pancreatitis

The Balthazar CT severity index for pancreatitis can be modified and used for MRI (Table 5.2). As opposed to density measurement, changes in parenchymal T1 and T2 signal intensity may be used to provide additional information. The T1 and T2 signal intensity of the unenhanced pancreas remains normal in relation to the other abdominal viscera in mild acute pancreatitis. As the severity of the pancreatitis worsens, pancreatic parenchyma may become isointense or hypointense to hepatic parenchyma due to loss of acinar proteins. Alternatively, the pancreatic signal can become increasingly hyperintense when compared with liver parenchyma on unenhanced T1-weighted imaging due to the presence of hemorrhage (Fig. 5.7). T2 signal will increase reflecting edema. T2-weighted imaging is the most sensitive to subtle changes of edema and may reveal changes of pancreatitis in the setting of a normal CT

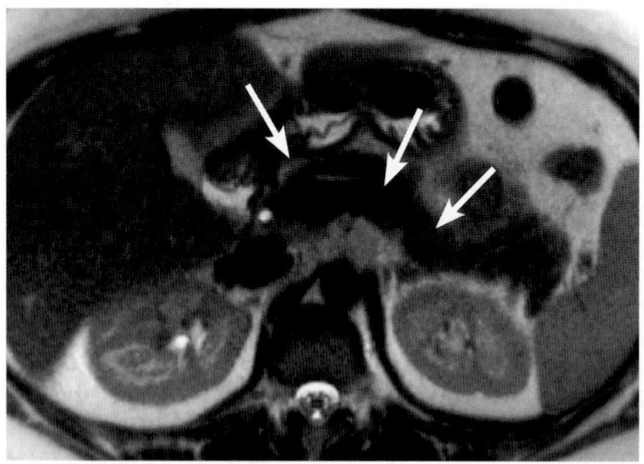

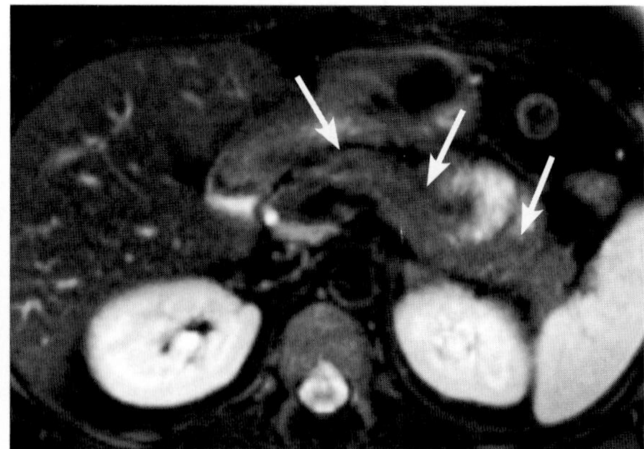

Fig. 5.5. a Axial T2W half-Fourier acquired single shot turbo spin echo (HASTE) through a normal pancreas (*arrows*). **b** Axial breath-hold T2W turbo spin echo (TSE) with parallel imaging demonstrating normal hypointensity of the pancreas (*arrows*)

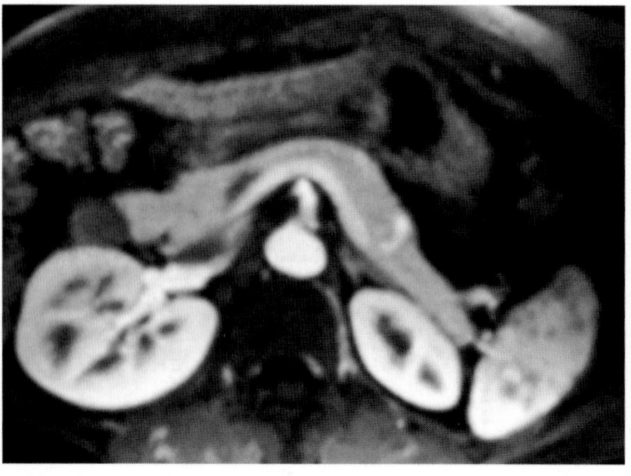

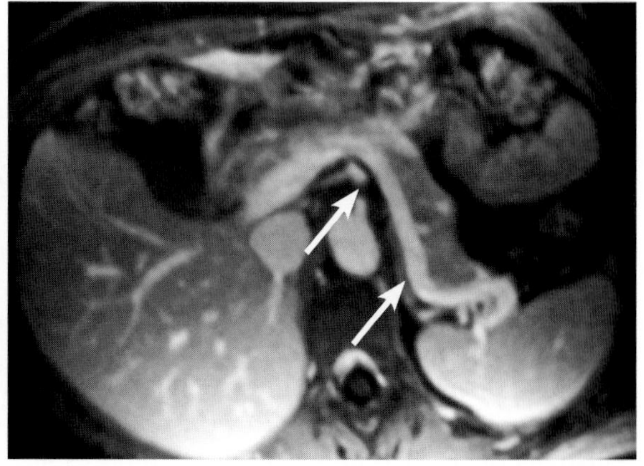

Fig. 5.6a,b. Dynamic axial T1W FS GRE image through the pancreas performed using a VIBE (volume interpolated breath-hold examination) sequence. **a** On arterial phase imaging note the maximal homogenous enhancement of the pancreas. **b** Venous phase demonstrates normal homogenous enhancement of the pancreas and a patent splenic vein (*arrows*)

Table 5.2. MRI severity index for acute pancreatitis. [Balthazar et al. (1990); Lecesne et al. (1999); Stimac et al. (2007)]

Balthazar grade	MRI findings	T1 FS	T2	Score
A	Normal pancreas	Homogenous, slightly hyperintense compared to normal liver parenchyma	Homogenous slightly hypointense to isointense to liver	0
B	Heterogeneous, and/or enlarged pancreas	Enlarged, heterogeneous, isointense to slightly hypointense compared to normal liver parenchyma	Enlarged, heterogeneous mild hyperintensity	1
C	Peripancreatic changes	As above with peripancreatic fat stranding	As above with peripancreatic hyperintensity and fat stranding	2
D	Peripancreatic collection in a single location	Homogenous or heterogeneous confluent ill-defined unencapsulated peripancreatic collection	Homogenous or heterogeneous confluent ill-defined unencapsulated peripancreatic	3
E	Two or more peripancreatic collections or retroperitoneal air	Multiple collections as above	Multiple collections as above	4
% Necrosis				
None				0
≤ 30%				2
> 30%–50%				4
> 50%				6

MRSI, MR severity index = Balthazar Score + % necrosis.

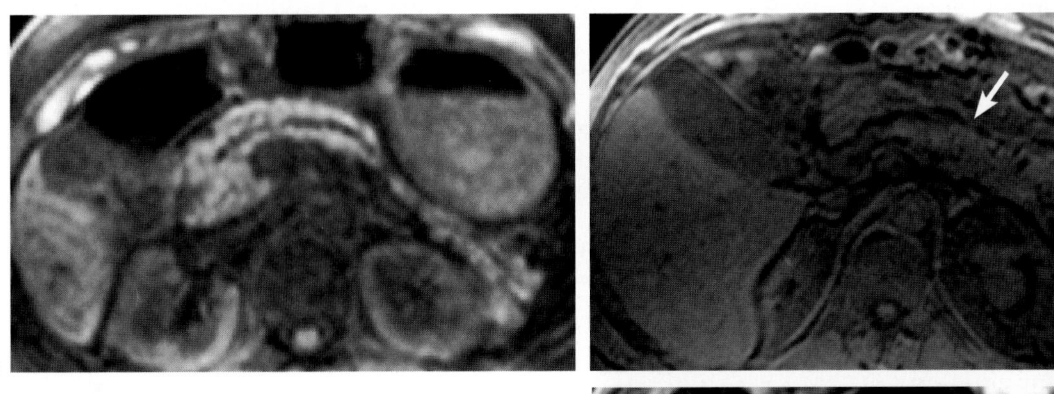

Fig. 5.7. a Axial 3D T1 GRE in a patient with mild acute pancreatitis demonstrates normal T1 hyperintensity of the pancreas. **b** Axial 3D T1 GRE image in a patient with acute on chronic pancreatitis and a pseudocyst (*P*) in the tail with loss of normal T1 hyperintensity of the pancreas (*arrow*) in the setting of acute pancreatitis. No necrosis was present. **c** In the third patient, there is patchy T1 hyperintensity in the pancreatic body and tail with severe acute pancreatitis. The areas of hyperintensity likely represent areas of hemorrhage or proteinaceous exudate and in this case correspond to regions of non-enhancement and necrosis

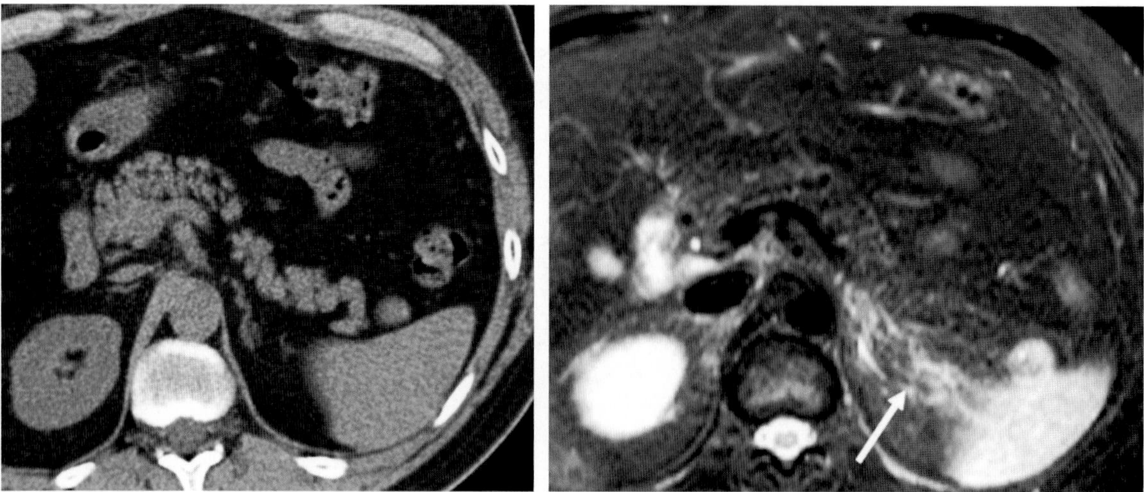

Fig. 5.8 a,b. A 40-year-old female with suspected acute pancreatitis by clinical history and laboratory data. **a** Axial image from a helical CT scan performed without IV contrast revealed no evidence of pancreatitis. **b** MRI of the pancreas performed on the same day reveals subtle T2-hyperintensity surrounding the tail of the pancreas on the axial T2W FS images compatible with peripancreatic edema (*arrow*) from acute mild pancreatitis

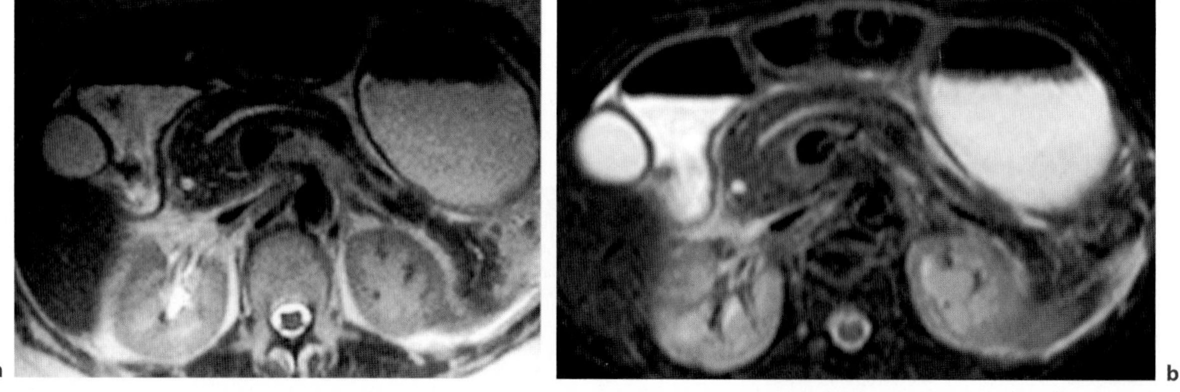

Fig. 5.9. a Axial T2W image through the pancreas demonstrates mild peripancreatic hyperintense fluid signal surrounding the pancreas which becomes more apparent on the FS T2W sequence in a patient with acute pancreatitis (**b**)

scan (Fig. 5.8). Use of fat suppression increases the conspicuity of pancreatic edema and peripancreatic fluid on T2-weighted imaging (Fig. 5.9).

With increasing disease severity, fluid accumulates in the peripancreatic space extending into the lesser sac, small bowel mesentery, anterior pararenal fascia, lateral conal fascia and track inferiorly along the retroperitoneum. Peripancreatic fat stranding likely due to inflammatory reaction can be appreciated on both T1- and T2-weighted imaging. Subtle fat stranding is often more apparent on the non-fat-suppressed T1-weighted in phase images (Fig. 5.10).

5.4.3 Severe (Necrotizing) Pancreatitis and Complications

In severe pancreatitis, more extensive peripancreatic fat necrosis and parenchymal necrosis becomes evident. In the absence of hemorrhage, T1 signal intensity becomes more heterogeneous or decreased in relation to the hepatic parenchymal signal. T2-signal intensity of the pancreatic parenchyma and peripancreatic soft tissues can increase and become closer to fluid signal intensity.

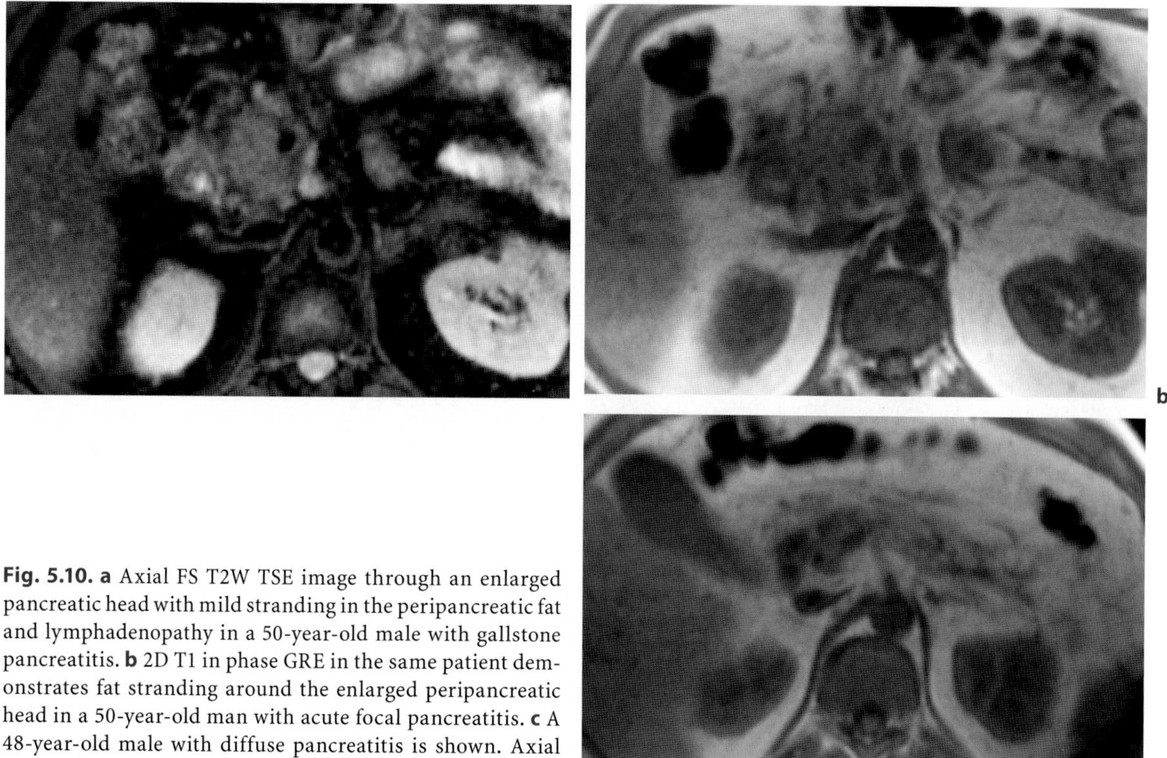

Fig. 5.10. a Axial FS T2W TSE image through an enlarged pancreatic head with mild stranding in the peripancreatic fat and lymphadenopathy in a 50-year-old male with gallstone pancreatitis. **b** 2D T1 in phase GRE in the same patient demonstrates fat stranding around the enlarged peripancreatic head in a 50-year-old man with acute focal pancreatitis. **c** A 48-year-old male with diffuse pancreatitis is shown. Axial 2D T1 in phase GRE just along the inferior margin of the pancreas demonstrates acute on chronic diffuse pancreatitis with fat stranding around the entire pancreas

5.4.4 Pancreatic Necrosis

Detection and quantification of necrosis is crucial as it is considered an important prognostic indicator in patients with acute pancreatitis (Lecesne et al. 1999; Balthazar 2002a; Balthazar 2002c). Dynamic contrast-enhanced MRI is helpful for determining the presence and extent of necrosis and for distinguishing between peripancreatic fluid collections and parenchymal necrosis. Pancreatic parenchymal enhancement may diminish or become absent in severe pancreatitis corresponding to regions of ischemia or necrosis (Fig. 5.11). However, exogenous contrast agents are not essential for detecting necrosis. In a study by Lecesne et al. (1999), areas of nonenhancing parenchyma on contrast enhanced MRI corresponded to those seen on CT. In fact, there are several studies that have compared unenhanced MRI with contrast enhanced CT for staging the severity of acute pancreatitis with both methods being equally reliable. (Lecesne et al. 1999; Viremouneix et al. 2007; Arvanitakis et al. 2007; Stimac et al. 2007). On non-contrast MRI, necrosis can be quite variable in appearance. Typically, there is focal loss of the normal acinar pattern of the pancreatic parenchyma on T1- or T2-weighted imaging with associated hyper- and/or hypointensity on T1-weighted and T2-weighted imaging (Fig. 5.12). In patients who cannot receive gadolinium contrast such as pregnant patients, non-contrast MRI offers the best alternative for detection and staging of pancreatitis.

Contrast enhanced MRI may be superior to contrast enhanced CT in differentiating necrotic foci within the pancreas from intrapancreatic fluid or hemorrhagic regions (Fig. 5.13) (Hirota et al. 2002). Small areas of necrosis can be missed on CT or misinterpreted as intraparenchymal fluid collections, particularly when imaging is performed within 12 h of onset of symptoms such that follow-up is required (Balthazar 2002c). Both MRI and CT can fail to recognize necrosis early on in the course of the disease since necrosis may not become apparent for 24–48 h after initial symptoms. However, the contrast resolution of MRI and the ability to acquire

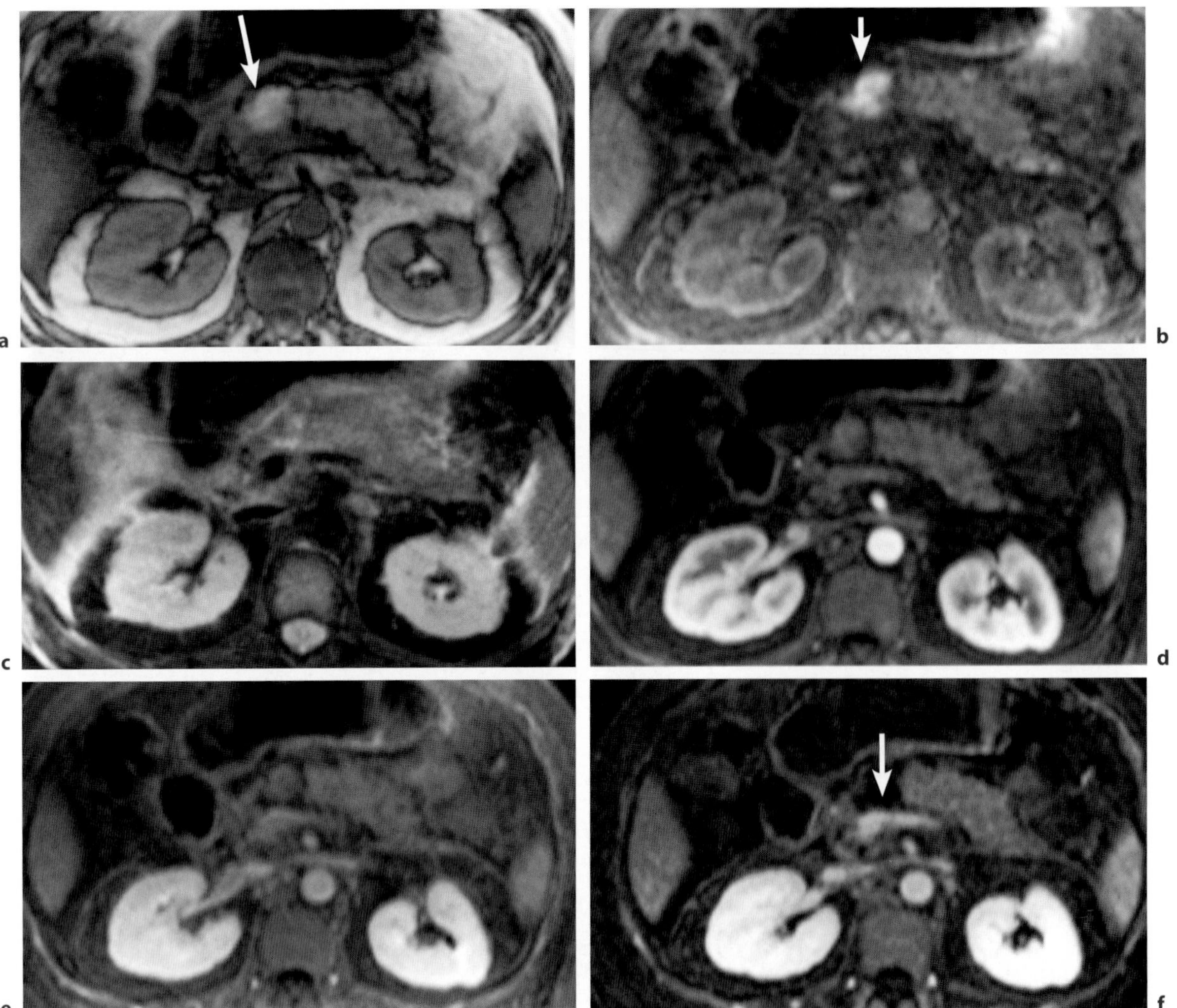

Fig. 5.11a–f. Acute pancreatitis with focal hemorrhagic necrosis in the neck of the pancreas which demonstrates T1 hyperintensity (*arrow*) on unenhanced T1W GRE images (**a**) without and (**b**) with fat suppression and (**c**) T2 hyperintensity on FS T2 FSE. There is no evidence of enhancement on the FS 3D T1W GRE (**d**) arterial and (**e**) venous phases confirmed with (**f**) subtraction (*arrow*)

Fig. 5.13a–d. 77 year old male with acute hemorrhagic necrotizing pancreatitis. **a** Contrast enhanced CT performed 10 days after the MRI shows little differentiation between necrotic pancreas and peripancreatic fluid. **b** T2W image reveals that the low density collection in the pancreatic bed represents necrotic pancreas and peripancreatic fluid with **c** T1 hyperintensity on pre contrast images and no evidence of enhancement in >90% on **d** post contrast 3D T1W FS GRE images of the pancreas confirmed with subtraction, not shown here

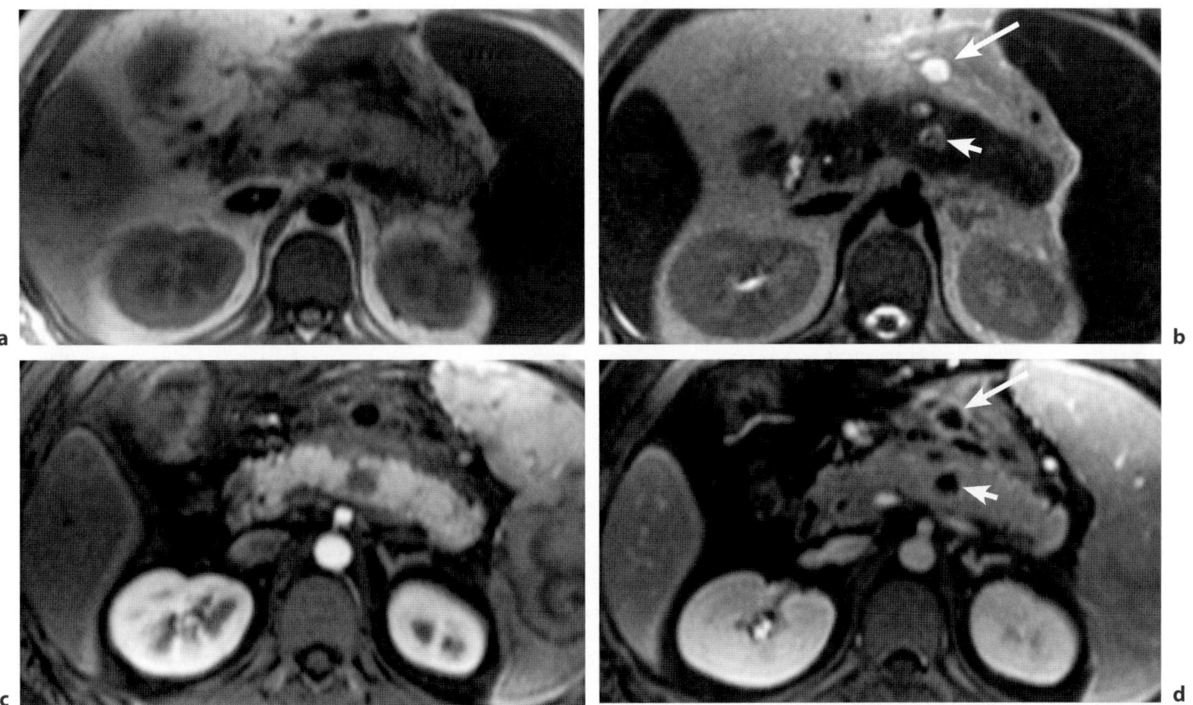

Fig. 5.12. a 2D T1W GRE images reveal extensive peripancreatic fat stranding and fluid as well has focal hypointense lesions within the pancreatic body. **b** T2W images reveal a T2 hyperintense focus in the body of the pancreas and one in the lesser sac corresponding to a focal areas of pancreatic necrosis (*short arrow*) on post contrast (**c**) arterial and (**d**) venous phase images and a small peripancreatic collection in the lesser sac (*long arrows*)

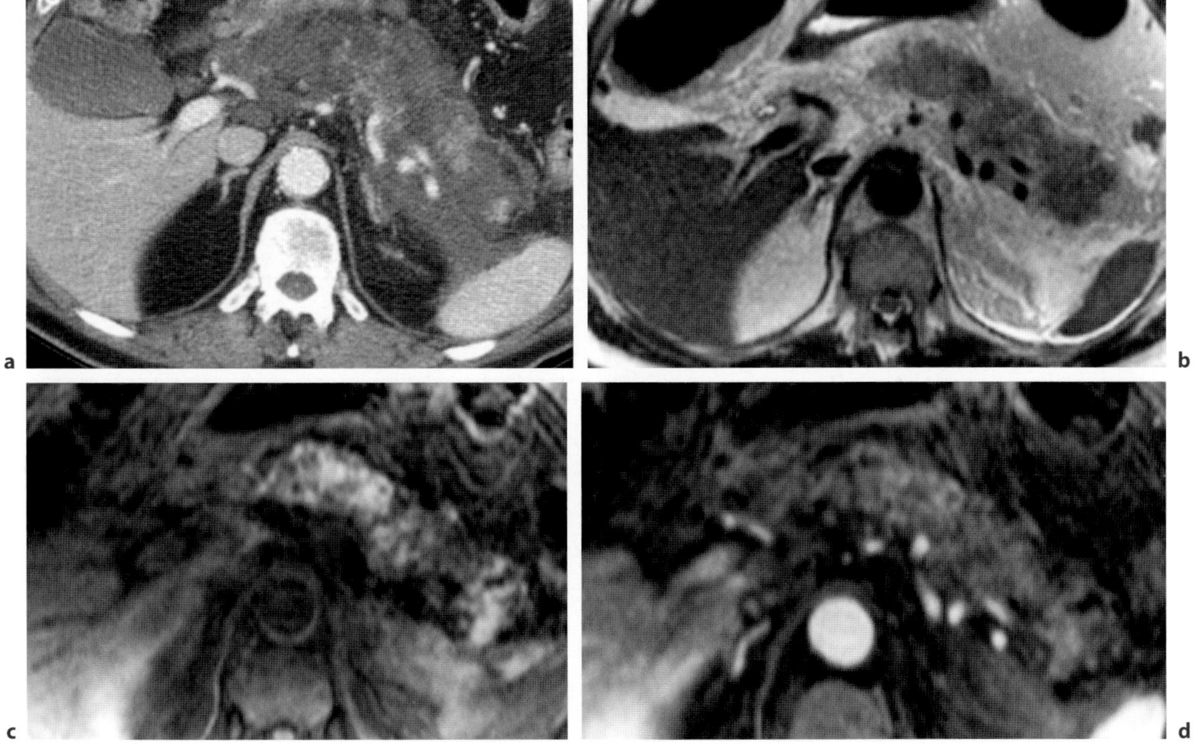

baseline and multiple post-contrast scans without increasing radiation dose allowing post-processing techniques such as subtraction make MRI superior to CT for detection of necrosis.

5.4.5 Hemorrhage

Hemorrhage and hemorrhagic fluid collections are better recognized on MR. Hemorrhage is usually hyperintense on T1-weighted imaging and should be differentiated from the normal baseline relative hyperintensity of normal pancreatic tissue. The T1 hyperintensity of hemorrhage within the pancreas decreases sensitivity for detection of enhancement and, in turn, necrosis. In cases of hemorrhagic pancreatitis, post processing with subtraction (subtracting the pre-contrast images from the post-contrast data sets) can improve sensitivity for detection of parenchymal enhancement (Fig. 5.14). On CT, it may be difficult to distinguish between peripancreatic edema and fat necrosis with hemorrhage but this is an important finding to recognize on MRI because it has been shown in a study by Martin et al. (2003) that fat necrosis with hemorrhage was associated with poor outcome (Fig. 5.15).

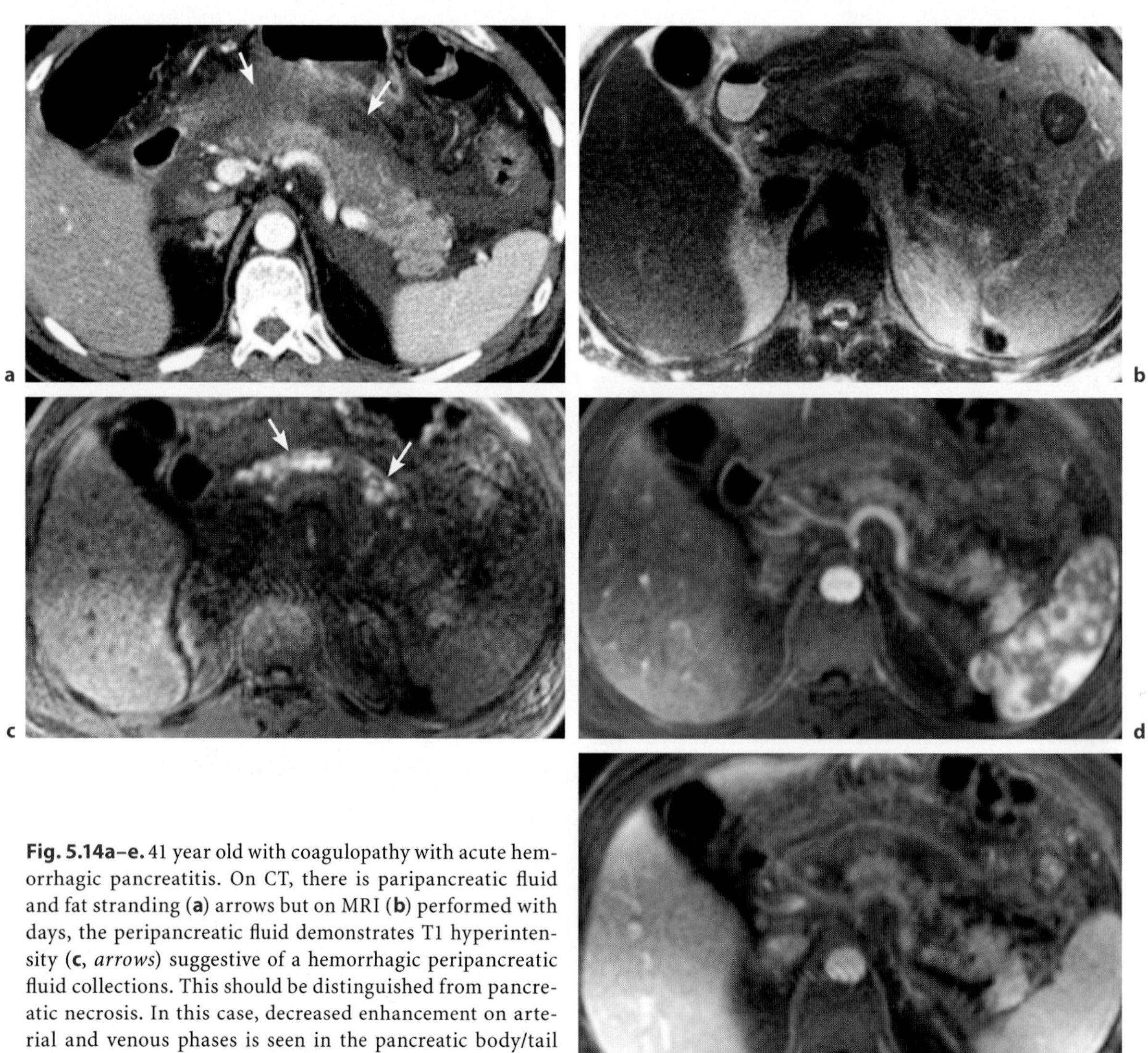

Fig. 5.14a–e. 41 year old with coagulopathy with acute hemorrhagic pancreatitis. On CT, there is paripancreatic fluid and fat stranding (**a**) arrows but on MRI (**b**) performed with days, the peripancreatic fluid demonstrates T1 hyperintensity (**c**, *arrows*) suggestive of a hemorrhagic peripancreatic fluid collections. This should be distinguished from pancreatic necrosis. In this case, decreased enhancement on arterial and venous phases is seen in the pancreatic body/tail (**d, e**) indicative of the presence of small areas of parenchymal necrosiss

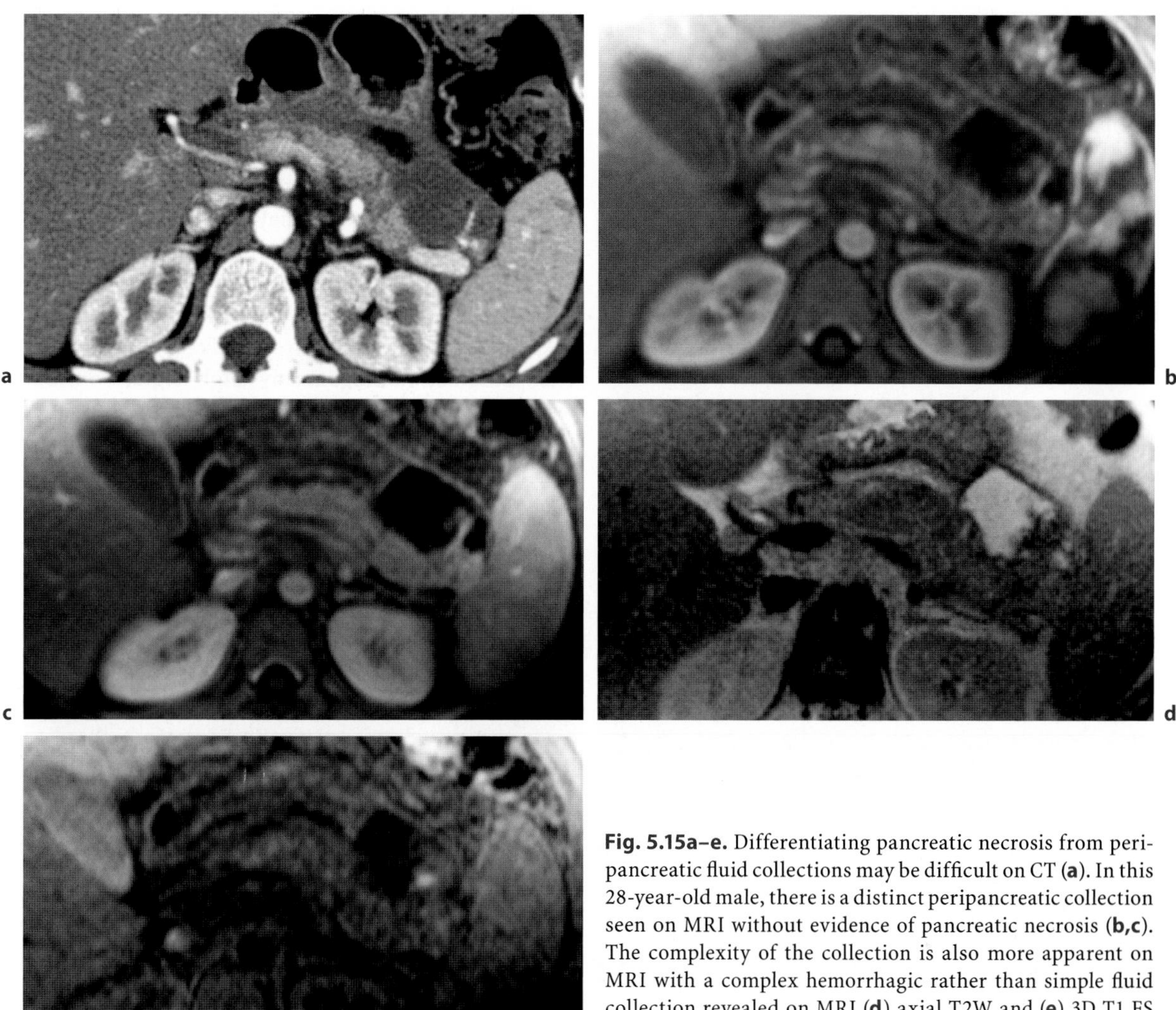

Fig. 5.15a–e. Differentiating pancreatic necrosis from peripancreatic fluid collections may be difficult on CT (**a**). In this 28-year-old male, there is a distinct peripancreatic collection seen on MRI without evidence of pancreatic necrosis (**b,c**). The complexity of the collection is also more apparent on MRI with a complex hemorrhagic rather than simple fluid collection revealed on MRI (**d**) axial T2W and (**e**) 3D T1 FS GRE image

One should recognize that correlative histopathology in acute pancreatitis is limited and, therefore, it is unclear whether the T1 hyperintensity within or surrounding the pancreas truly reflects hemorrhage since it could also reflect proteinaceous exudates. Therefore, it has been suggested to refer to these collections as "hemorrhage-like" fluid collections (Lecesne et al. 1999).

5.4.6 Peripancreatic Collections

The content of peripancreatic collections are better assessed with MRI than CT. MRI can better differentiate fluid from solid debris and thus, more accurately predict which collections would be amenable to intervention (Ward et al. 1997; Morgan and Baron 1998). T2-weighted imaging is especially useful in differentiating between the fluid and solid content of collections (Fig. 5.15). Drainage and/or aspiration of peripancreatic collections may be required, particularly when patients show signs of possible infection. Infection rate of pancreatic tissue is 7%–12 % occurring in 30%–70% of patients with necrotizing pancreatitis (Piironen 2001).

Gas, although not commonly seen in patients with infected peripancreatic collections, is a very useful sign of infection (Federle et al. 1981). Gas on MRI demonstrates a signal void on T1- and T2-weighted images with "blooming" or susceptibility effects demonstrated on long TE sequences. Gas could easily be missed on MRI or mistaken for bowel gas or calcification. In one study by Ward et al. (1997) comparing CT and MRI for pancreatitis, CT showed peripancreatic gas in 12 patients, whereas MRI prospectively detected only six patients; even after a consensus review only four of six cases with gas on CT were recognized on MRI, representing a potential limitation of MRI. Calcifications suggesting the presence of underlying chronic pancreatitis can also be missed on MRI (Fig. 5.16).

5.4.7 Pseudocysts

Pseudocysts are encapsulated collections usually located in the pancreas or adjacent to it requiring at least 4 weeks to develop after the initial episode of pancreatitis (Balthazar 2002b). If pseudocysts communicate with the main pancreatic duct, they are more likely to be detected at ERCP; however, overall, less than 50% of pseudocysts are detected at ERCP (Fayad et al. 2003). Most pseudocysts resolve spontaneously. They can vary in size and may be found in the chest, abdomen or pelvis. More often they arise at a site of necrosis or duct disruption. Location, size, complexity and number of pseudocysts should be documented.

Simple pseudocysts are typically unilocular, encapsulated, homogenously high signal on T2-weighted and low signal on T1-weighted images (Fig. 5.17). Pseudocysts can become complicated by hemorrhage, proteinaceous or necrotic debris or infection. In these cases, the cyst will appear heterogeneous on T2- and T1-weighted imaging or dem-

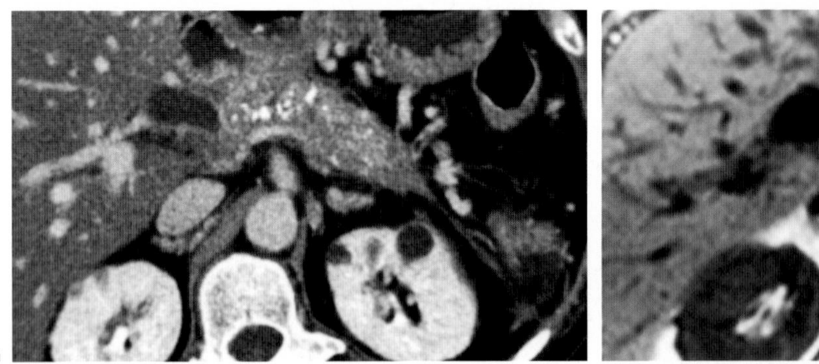

Fig. 5.16a,b. Acute on chronic pancreatitis with pancreatic calcification seen readily on (**a**) contrast enhanced CT and less well on non-enhanced T1W GRE images with relatively TE = 4.4 ms demonstrating susceptibility artifact related to calcium on the body of the pancreas

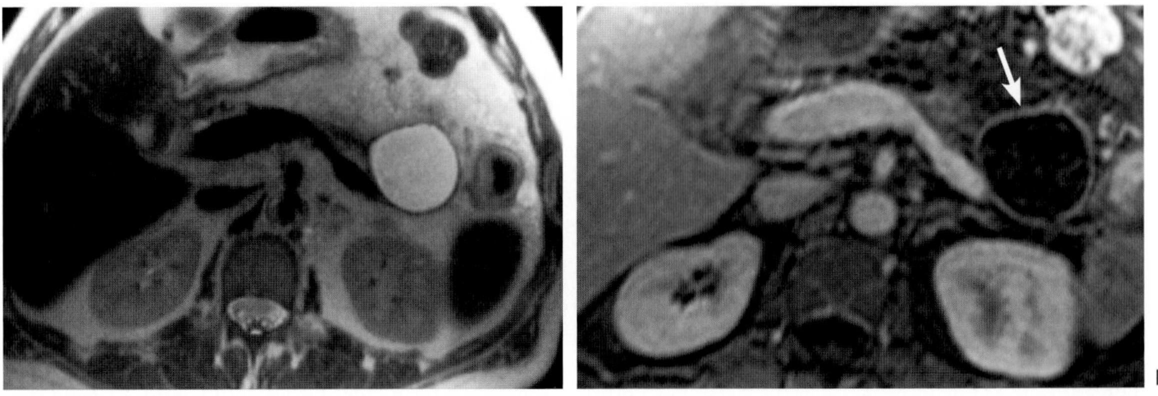

Fig. 5.17a,b. Simple pseudocyst in the tail of the pancreas with (**a**) T2 hyperintensity and (**b**) a thin smooth rim of enhancement (*arrows*) on post-contrast imaging

onstrate a hemosiderin rim on long TE sequences. Fluid levels may be present in the dependent portion of the pseudocysts. Internal debris is often irregular in shape demonstrating low signal on T2- and high signal on T1-weighted images (Fig. 5.18–5.20). Communication with main duct or side branches may be evident on heavily T2-weighted images (Fig. 5.21). A thick, irregular and/or nodular enhancing wall is not suggestive of a pseudocyst and in such cases malignancy needs to be considered. Internal enhancement would more likely favor malignancy and sampling of the mass should be performed. Contrast enhancement is usually present in the wall of the collection but internal enhancement should not be present (Fig. 5.22). Post processing with subtraction would permit optimal visualization of enhancement when evaluating a complex mass with internal T1 hyperintensity on unenhanced imaging.

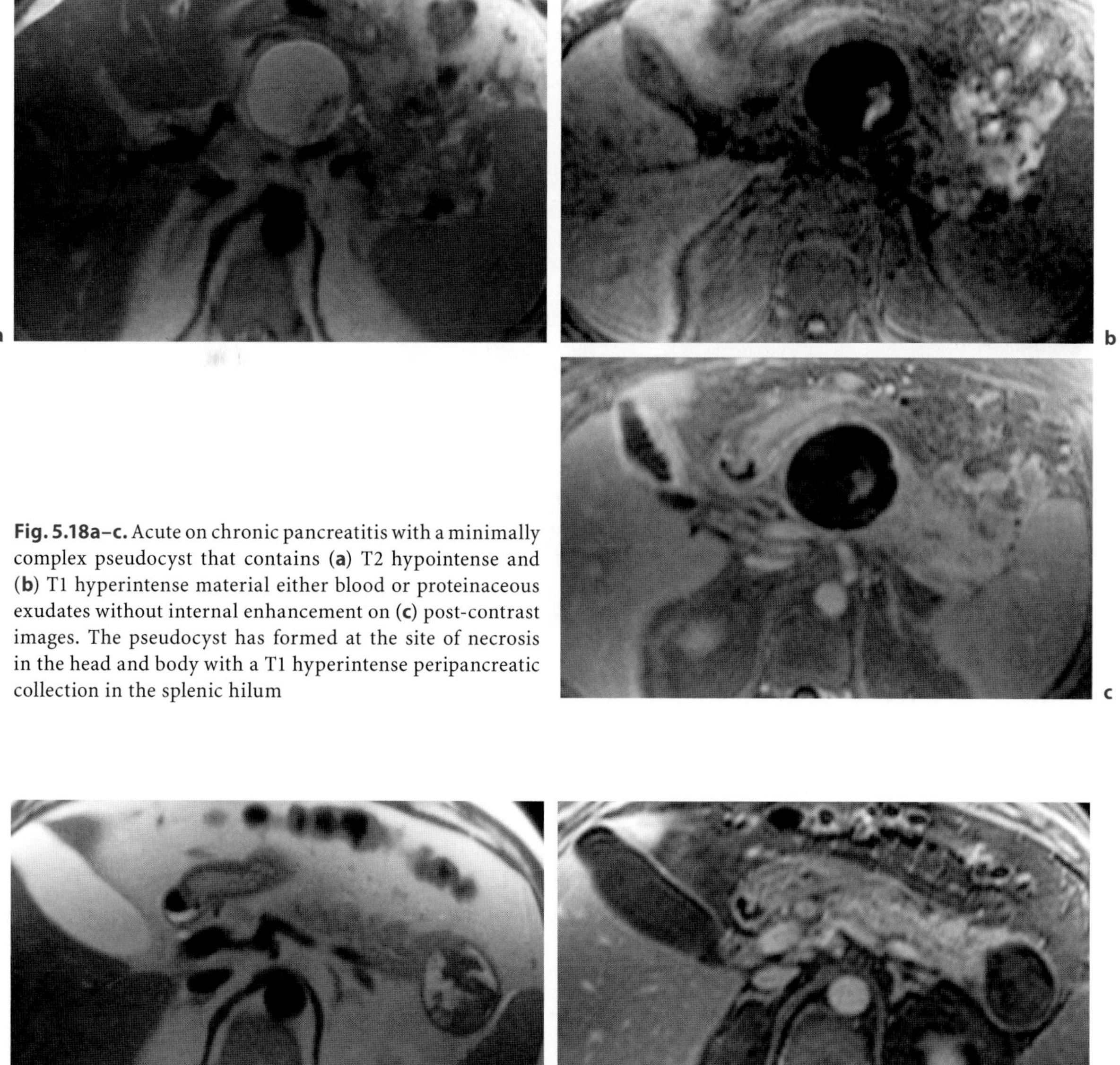

Fig. 5.18a–c. Acute on chronic pancreatitis with a minimally complex pseudocyst that contains (**a**) T2 hypointense and (**b**) T1 hyperintense material either blood or proteinaceous exudates without internal enhancement on (**c**) post-contrast images. The pseudocyst has formed at the site of necrosis in the head and body with a T1 hyperintense peripancreatic collection in the splenic hilum

Fig. 5.19a,b. Acute on chronic pancreatitis with peripancreatic fat stranding and a more complex pseudocyst with (**a**) T2 hypointense debris and (**b**) no internal enhancement on post-contrast T1W images

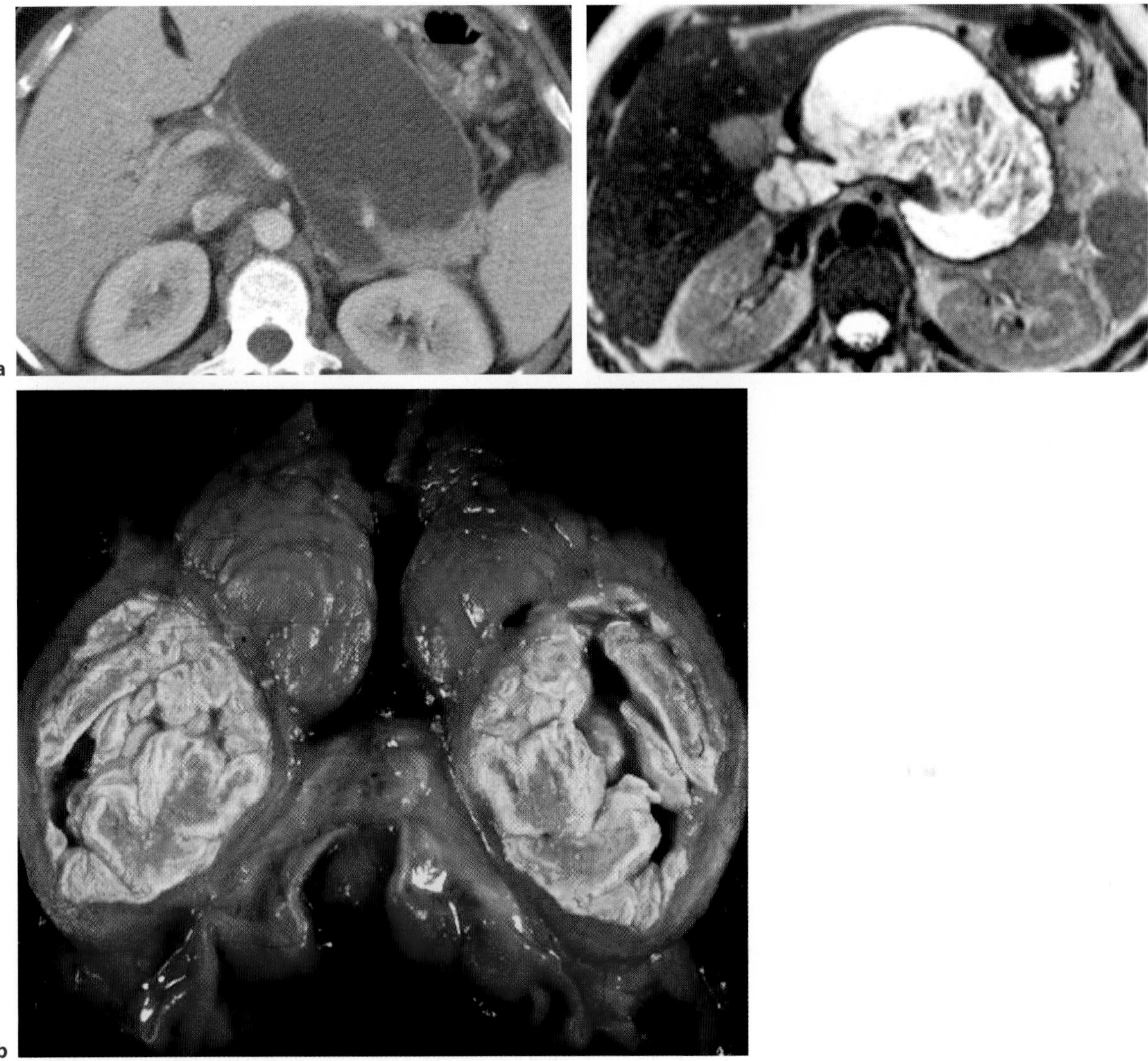

Fig. 5.20. a Contrast enhanced CT scan at the level of the pancreas shows large fluid density collection nearly replacing the entire pancreas. **b** Axial and (**c**) coronal T2W images demonstrate extensive pancreatic necrosis as seen on CT with large pseudocyst that does not represent simple fluid but rather a complex collection not amenable to percutaneous drainage. **c** Gross pathologic specimen reveals that this represents a predominately solid mass of debris

5.4.8 Vascular Complications

Vascular insults should be recognized since, although infrequent, they can result in life-threatening complications. Extravasated pancreatic enzymes can lead to loss of integrity or damage of the vessel wall resulting in inflammation and/or fibrosis with development of stricture, thrombosis, pseudoaneurysm and/or hemorrhage (Balthazar 2002b). Most commonly, splenic vein thrombosis occurs (1%–3%) (Balthazar 2002b). Thrombus can extend into the superior mesenteric vein (SMV) and portal vein. Splenic vein thrombosis leads to splenomegaly and enlargement of short gastric, left gastric veins and gastroepiploic collaterals (Fig. 5.23).

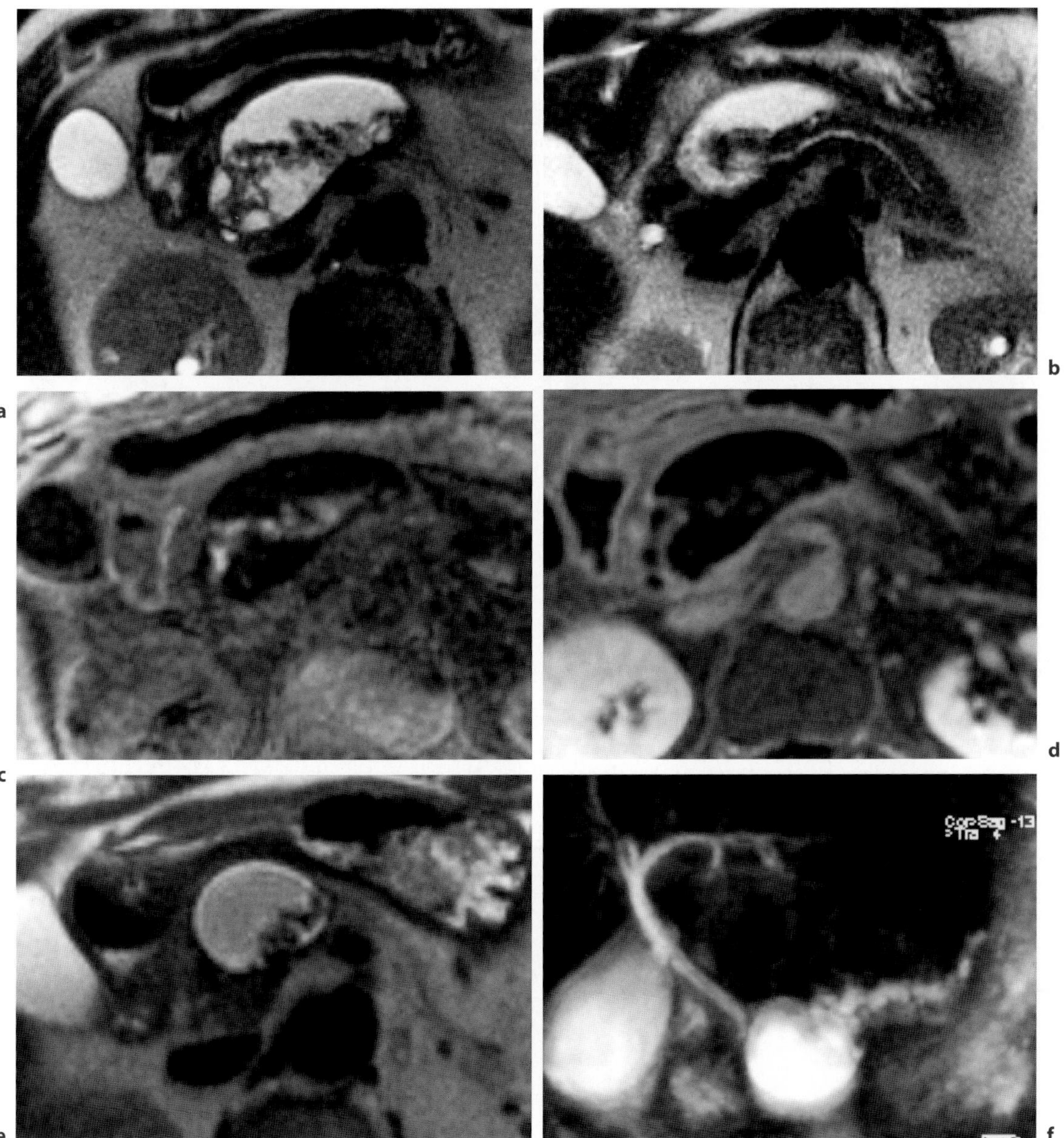

Fig. 5.21a–f. Patient with pancreas divisum and acute pancreatitis with duct disruption and large pseudocysts communicating with the main duct. **a,b** T2 HASTE images reveal a complex pseudocyst with internal debris which is (**c**) hyperintense on T1W imaging and demonstrates rim enhancement (**d**) post-contrast images. After 8 months, the pseudocyst has diminished in size as shown on the (**e**) HASTE images but disruption of the duct lead to upstream duct changes of chronic pancreatitis with main and side branch duct dilatation and irregularity seen on the (**f**) maximum intensity projection (MIP) of heavily T2W respiratory triggered 3D TSE MRCP

Pseudoaneurysms must be recognized as rupture and bleeding can develop. Most common vessels affected include splenic, gastroduodenal and pancreatico-duodenal arteries with left gastric, middle colic and hepatic artery less commonly involved (Balthazar 2002b) (Fig. 5.24).

5.4.9 Imaging Features of Autoimmune Pancreatitis

Autoimmune pancreatitis also known as primary sclerosing pancreatitis, lymphoplasmacytic sclerosing pancreatitis or nonalcoholic duct-destruc-

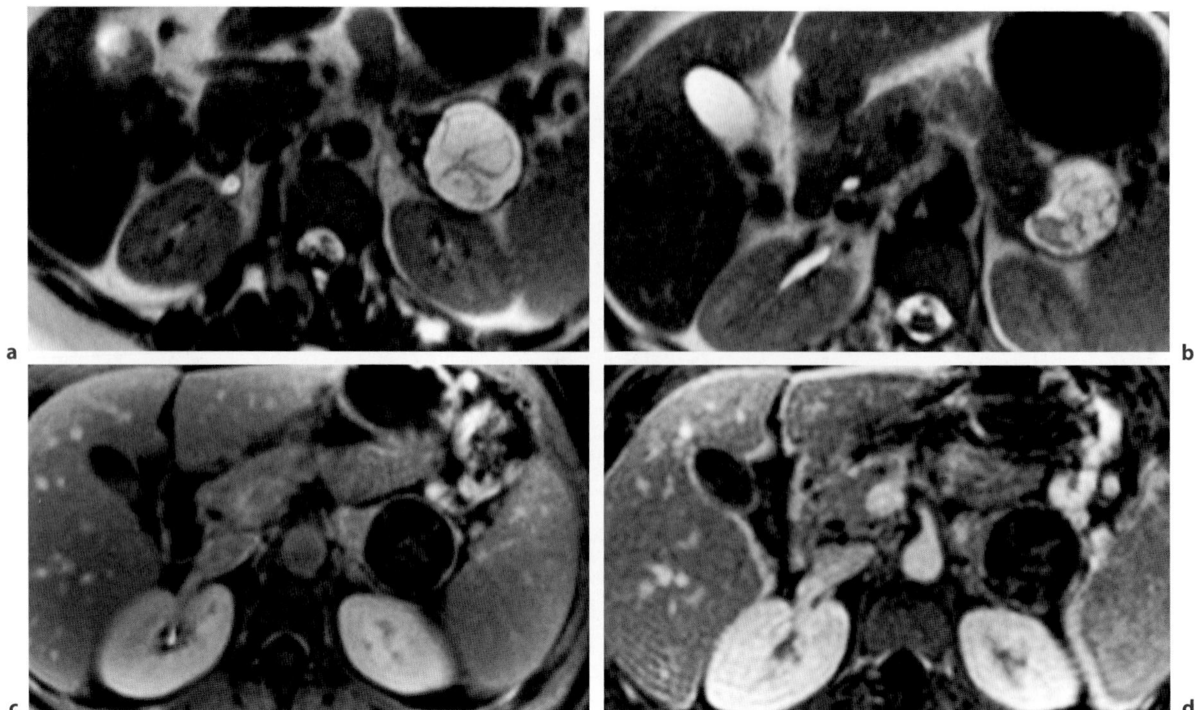

Fig. 5.22. Unilocular pancreatic tail mass predominantly (**a,b**) T2 hyperintense with linear hypointense internal architecture that (**c**) enhances on post-contrast images confirmed on (**d**) subtraction images highly suggestive of neoplasm in this patient with no history or imaging findings to suggest acute or chronic pancreatitis. This was confirmed to be a mucinous adenocarcinoma

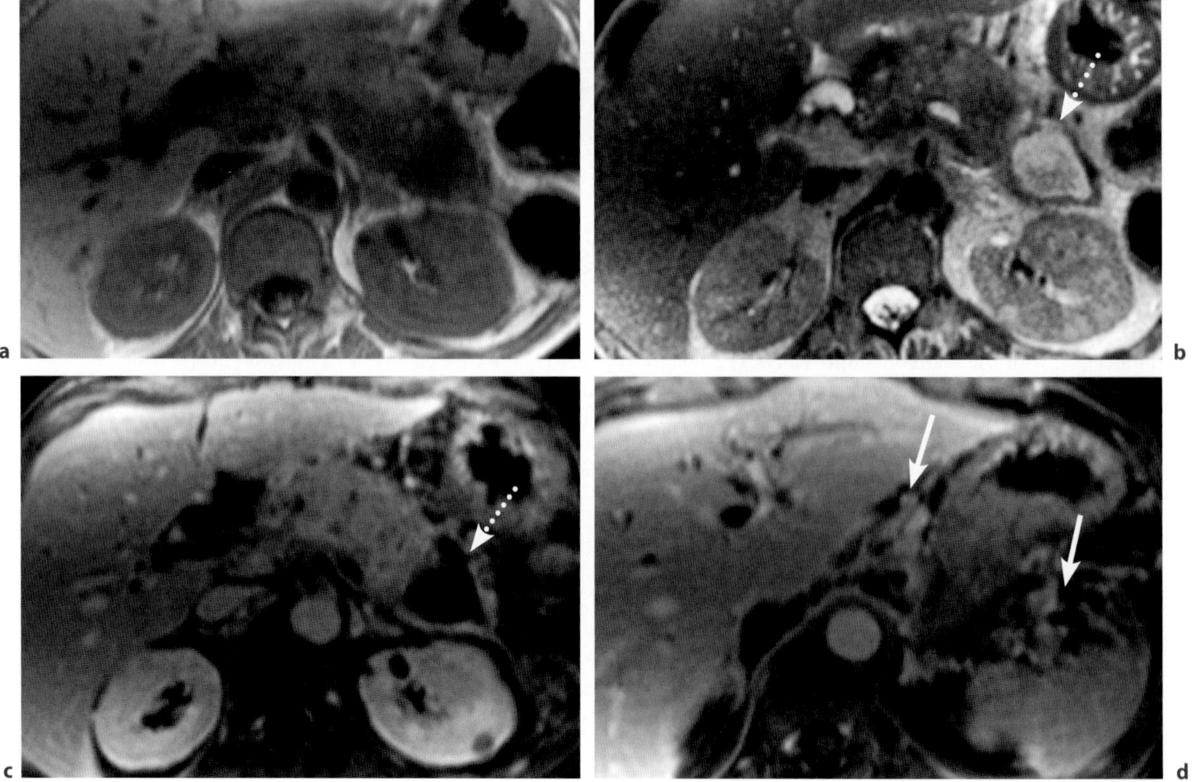

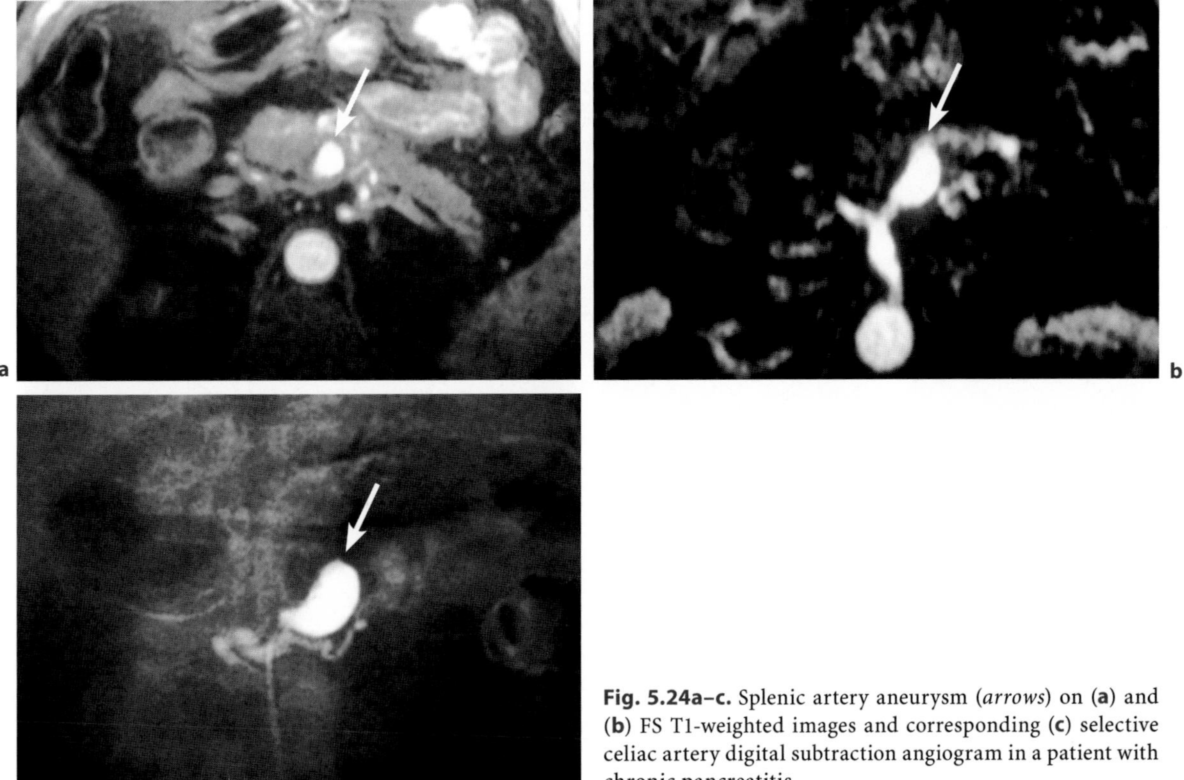

Fig. 5.24a–c. Splenic artery aneurysm (*arrows*) on (**a**) and (**b**) FS T1-weighted images and corresponding (**c**) selective celiac artery digital subtraction angiogram in a patient with chronic pancreatitis

tive chronic pancreatitis is important to recognize and to consider as a cause of pancreatitis (Sahani et al. 2004). Prognosis and management in these patients is different from other types of pancreatitis. In this subset of patients, the morphologic changes of pancreatitis are reversible and patients respond best to steroid therapy. Patients typically have no history of acute attacks of pancreatitis and no history of alcohol abuse with histopathologic specimens showing fibrotic change and lymphocyte infiltration (Irie et al. 1998). Laboratory data may reveal increased serum IgG levels and the presence of antinuclear antibodies. This entity can occur alone or in association with autoimmune diseases such as Sjögren syndrome, primary sclerosing cholangitis, ulcerative colitis and collagen vascular diseases. Imaging features include focal or diffuse (sausage-shaped) enlargement of the pancreas, pancreatic duct irregularity, homogenous but delayed enhancement and a low attenuation rim surrounding the pancreas on contrast enhanced CT corresponding to a rim of T2 and T1 hypointensity on MRI with delayed enhancement (Fig. 5.25) (Irie et al. 1998; Sahani et al. 2004; Yang et al. 2005). Interestingly, associated extrapancreatic findings may be observed including most commonly biliary strictures, salivary and submandibular gland involvement, retroperitoneal fibrosis, lymphadenopathy and renal parenchymal lesions and perirenal involvement (Irie et al. 1998; Sahani et al. 2004; Kamisawa et al. 2005; Kamisawa et al. 2006; Takahashi et al. 2007).

Fig. 5.23a–d. 49 year old male with acute on chronic alcohol related pancreatitis with **a** enlargement and loss of T1 hyperintensity in body and tail of the pancreas, peripancreatic fat stranding and a **b** T2 hyperintense collection (*dotted arrow*) replacing the tail of the pancreatic corresponding to **c** pancreatic tail necrosis and resultant fluid collection (*dotted arrow*) with **d** occlusion of the splenic vein and enlargement of perigastric (*arrows*) and perisplenic collateralss

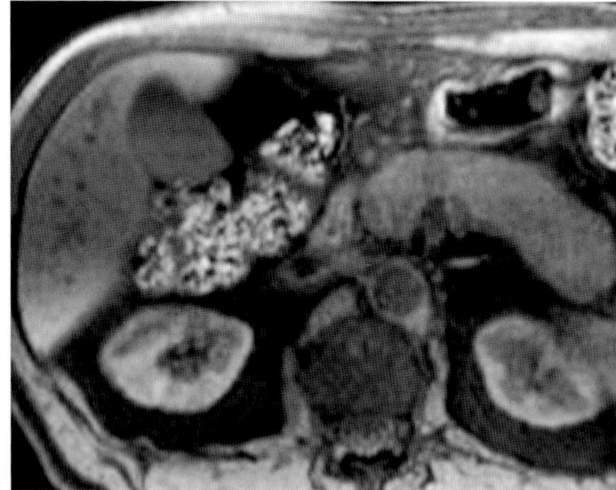
a

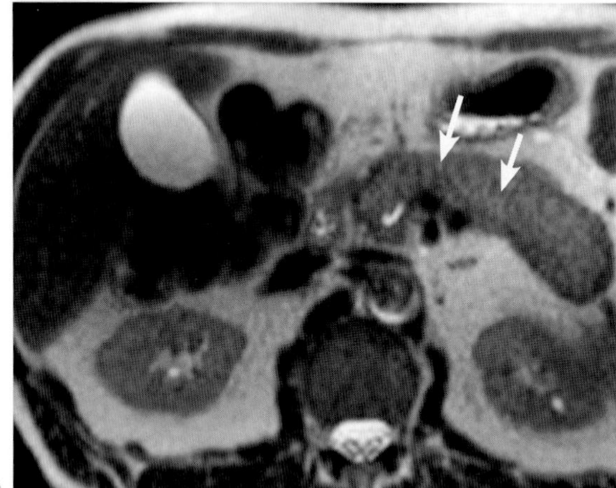
b

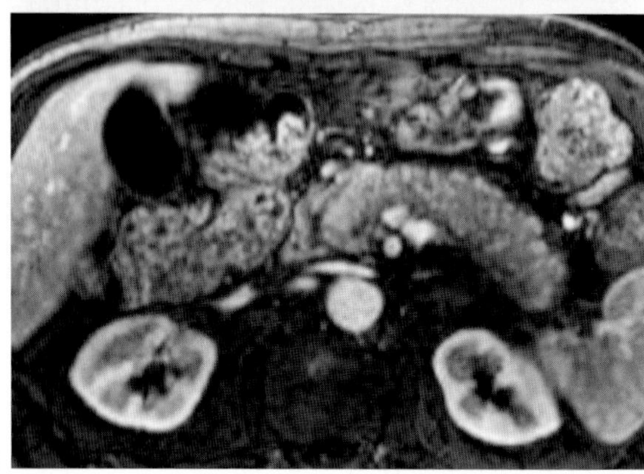
c

Fig. 5.25a–c. Autoimmune pancreatitis. **a** Axial T1 FS GRE and (**b**) axial HASTE images through the pancreas reveal diffuse enlargement of the pancreatitis with minimal peripancreatic fat stranding and (**c**) decreased enhancement of the pancreatic tail (*arrows*) in this patient with autoimmune pancreatitis

5.5 Emerging MRI Techniques

A number of MRI techniques are emerging for physiologic and tissue level characterization. These hold promise for the evaluation of both acute and chronic pancreatitis. While their implementation and future role remains speculative, the following paragraphs give a brief introduction to key promising approaches including MRI based assessment of tissue perfusion, MR spectroscopy, diffusion weighted imaging and its interpretation and MR elastography. While a complete discussion of these methods is beyond the scope of this chapter, it is hoped that a brief review will alert the interested reader to these emerging capabilities.

5.5.1 Perfusion Imaging

Perfusion describes the rate of delivery of essential nutrients (glucose and oxygen) to tissue via blood flow and thereby can serve as a marker for tissue function or viability. While adequate perfusion alone does not imply tissue viability, it can be considered a necessary but not sufficient requisite for tissue viability. In general, there are two major MRI-based approaches to assessing and measuring tissue perfusion; one uses exogenous relaxation contrast agents such as gadolinium chelates to serve as a tracer or marker for perfusion, while the other which does not use exogenous contrast agents but instead takes advantage of MRI manipulation of the intrinsic magnetic properties of blood as a mechanism of determining perfusion. Using gadolinium chelates permits the calculation of a variety of parameters related to the timing and passage of the contrast bolus. These have been variously interpreted as blood volume, blood flow, and time of arrival and transit of contrast agent, each of which may contain information indicative of hemodynamic abnormality. None of these parameters, however, is a true, quantitative measure of blood flow. Non-exogenous contrast mechanisms, such as arterial spin labeling (ASL) which magnetically tags blood water protons, can, in principle, determine blood flow quantitatively. With either approach, and indeed with quantitative or semi-quantitative methods in general, confidence in interpretation is always increased by observing predictable responsiveness in the measure upon applying a known physiological manipulation or challenge. In assessment of cardiovascular reserve, for example, hemodynamic measures are quantified pre- and post-behavioral or pharmacological stress tests.

Fortunately, for pancreatic imaging, there is a commercially available exogenous agent that can predictably alter tissue perfusion, secretin. This agent can be used to accentuate alterations in tissue perfusion from baseline in normal and abnormal pancreatic tissue.

Initially, investigators assessed pancreatic perfusion using semi-quantitative measures (Johnson and Outwater 1999; Sica et al. 2002; Zhang et al. 2003; Coenegrachts et al. 2004; Tajima et al. 2004), primarily for assessment of chronic pancreatitis. A more quantitative approach as used in liver imaging has been recently explored in normal volunteers (Bali et al. 2008). Essentially, this particular technique uses high temporal resolution dynamic contrast enhanced T1-weighted MRI sequences imaging and post processing is performed using compartmental modeling. This method may be quite sensitive for detecting, and more significantly quantifying, perfusion changes related to acute and chronic pancreatitis. More studies are needed to better understand and validate baseline pancreatic perfusion and changes that occur in response to secretin such that pathologic responses may be understood.

Recent concerns over the use of gadolinium in patients with renal dysfunction have reemphasized the need for alternative non-exogenous contrast agent enhanced imaging methods. For perfusion imaging, as an alternative to bolus tracking gadolinium chelates, arterial spin labeling (ASL) methods have been proposed and developed over the last two decades, primarily for application in the brain. They are now emerging as a potentially viable imaging technique for characterizing hemodynamics in the body. There is relatively few literature on the subject for pancreatic imaging, although a recent feasibility study is encouraging (Schrami et al. 2008).

5.5.2 MR Spectroscopy

MR spectroscopy promises regional biochemical analysis of metabolites and breakdown products. In vivo measurements are hampered by low concentrations of metabolites and respiratory, cardiac and bowel peristaltic motion. There have been some promising ex-vivo spectroscopy studies, predominantly on the bile acids and in vivo in the context of pancreatic neoplasm (Cho et al. 2005), but further investigation is warranted before clinical adoption.

5.5.3 Diffusion-Weighted Imaging

Diffusion-weighted imaging (DWI) is a unique contrast mechanism sensitive to random motion of water molecules, whether due to bulk motion or alterations in the cellular microenvironment, i.e., microscopic shifts of water protons between intra- and extracellular compartments. DWI can reflect cytotoxic edema, alterations in normal cellular density and cellular organization. While DWI has been extensively explored for neuroimaging application, only recently has DWI been feasible for body application as it is very sensitive to respiratory and bowel motion artifacts, for example. Recent advances in MRI technology permit good quality, reproducible DWI in the abdomen and pelvis. DWI has shown promise in liver imaging and is potentially useful for pancreatic imaging. DWI may be useful for assessment of pancreatic necrosis and possibly for differentiating focal pancreatitis from pancreatic carcinoma, but only preliminary data is available to date (Matsuki et al. 2007; Momtahen et al. 2008; Takeuchi et al. 2008). A recent study investigated the change in apparent diffusion coefficient (ADC) in the pancreas on DWI before and after secretin administration and found that in the pancreatic tissue of patients with risk for or known chronic pancreatitis, there was a temporal delay in the peak increase in ADC that occurs in normal control patients in response to secretin (Erturk et al. 2006). As in other abdominal organs, the apparent diffusion measured by DWI may in large part reflect intra-voxel perfusion or microscopic flow and not only true microscopic diffusion. This is of particular significance when interpreting secretin induced changes in apparent diffusion given the known perfusion effects secondary to secretin. However, the results are intriguing because DWI does not require exogenous contrast agents and may offer an alternative to contrast enhanced imaging for assessing perfusion and diffusion changes in pancreatic tissue. Generally, distinguishing between perfusion and diffusion effects is needed to better understand and measure underlying pathologic mechanisms of disease. While these two effects can be confounding they may provide complementary information relevant to studying the pathophysiology of pancreatitis.

5.5.4 MR Elastography

MR elastography is a technological approach that gives insight into tissue structure and biomechanics; it combines a mechanical vibratory stimulus (typically approximately 60 Hz) with an MRI sequence called phase contrast (PC-MRI), analogous to that used for velocity encoding in MR angiography, that is sensitive to tissue motion or vibration in at least three directions in space over time (Muthupillai et al. 1995). Complex patterns of wave propagation through a specific tissue over time can be interpreted in terms of underlying tissue properties. Alterations in the normal patterns of wave propagation may reveal underlying focal or diffuse structural or biomechanical abnormalities that may result, for example, from the presence of a benign or malignant tumor mass, tissue necrosis or fibrosis. Currently, this technique is primarily being explored for detection of liver fibrosis (Huwart et al. 2006; Rouviere et al. 2006) and in breast cancer (McKnight et al. 2002; Xydeas et al. 2005). However, preliminary work in the pancreas is ongoing with the thought that MR elastography can provide quantitative maps of shear stiffness of pancreatic tissue. Note, however, that, unlike the liver, it would appear that more complex 3D spatial modeling and temporal sampling may be warranted in the pancreas (Yin et al. 2008)

5.6 Conclusion

MRI is as effective as CT in the diagnosis and staging of acute pancreatitis and its complications. MRI offers a safe, noninvasive and reproducible method of evaluating the pancreatic parenchyma, as well as pancreatic and biliary ducts. In the setting of mild acute pancreatitis, the sensitivity of MRI exceeds that of CT (Amano et al. 2001). In severe pancreatitis, MRI is superior to contrast enhanced CT for evaluation of peripancreatic collections and degree of necrosis. Heavily T2-weighted images can provide additional information regarding the underlying cause of pancreatitis such as choledocholithiasis, pancreas divisum or, more rarely, pancreatic duct obstruction due to stricture or neoplasm.

Nonetheless, CT imaging is less expensive, faster, more readily available at any time of day, and is particularly useful in severely ill patients who are more unstable. In pediatric patients, pregnancy or patients with renal insufficiency, unenhanced MRI offers an excellent alternative.

References

Amano Y, Oish T et al. (2001) Nonenhanced magnetic resonance imaging of mild acute pancreatitis. Abdom Imaging 26:59–63

Arvanitakis M, Delhaye M et al. (2004) Computed tomography and magnetic resonance imaging in the assessment of acute pancreatitis. Gastroenterology 126:715–723

Arvanitakis M, Koustiani G et al. (2007) Staging of severity and prognosis of acute pancreatitis by computed tomography and magnetic resonance imaging – a comparative study. Dig Liver Dis 39:473–482

Bali MA, Metens T et al. (2008) Pancreatic perfusion: noninvasive quantitative assessment with dynamic contrast-enhanced MR imaging without and with secretin stimulation in healthy volunteers – initial results. Radiology 247:115–121

Balthazar EJ (2002a) Acute pancreatitis: assessment of severity with clinical and CT evaluation. Radiology 223:603–613

Balthazar EJ (2002b) Complications of acute pancreatitis: clinical and CT evaluation. Radiol Clin North Am 40:1211–1227

Balthazar EJ (2002c) Staging of acute pancreatitis. Radiol Clin North Am 40:1199–1209

Balthazar EJ, Robinson DL et al. (1990) Acute pancreatitis: value of CT in establishing prognosis. Radiology 174:331–336

Cappeliez O, Delhaye M et al. (2000) Chronic pancreatitis: evaluation of pancreatic exocrine function with MR pancreatography after secretin stimulation. Radiology 215:358–364

Chan JH, Tsui EY et al. (2000) Gadopentetate dimeglumine as an oral negative gastrointestinal contrast agent for MRCP. Abdom Imaging 25:405–408

Cho SG, Lee DH et al. (2005) Differentiation of chronic focal pancreatitis from pancreatic carcinoma by in vivo proton magnetic resonance spectroscopy. J Comput Assist Tomogr 29:163–169

Coenegrachts K, Van Steenbergen W et al. (2004) Dynamic contrast-enhanced MRI of the pancreas: initial results in healthy volunteers and patients with chronic pancreatitis. J Magn Reson Imaging 20:990–997

Coppens E, Metens T et al. (2005) Pineapple juice labeled with gadolinium: a convenient oral contrast for magnetic resonance cholangiopancreatography. Eur Radiol 15:2122–2129

Delhaye M, Matos C et al. (2008) Pancreatic ductal system obstruction and acute recurrent pancreatitis. World J Gastroenterol 14:1027–1033

Erturk SM, Ichikawa T et al. (2006) Diffusion-weighted MR imaging in the evaluation of pancreatic exocrine function before and after secretin stimulation. Am J Gastroenterol 101:133–136

Fayad LM, Kowalski T et al. (2003) MR cholangiopancreatography: evaluation of common pancreatic diseases. Radiol Clin North Am 41:97–114

Federle MP, Jeffrey RB et al. (1981) Computed tomography of pancreatic abscesses. AJR Am J Roentgenol 136:879–882

Grobner T, Prischl FC (2007) Gadolinium and nephrogenic systemic fibrosis. Kidney Int 72:260–264

Hirota M, Kimura Y et al. (2002) Visualization of the heterogeneous internal structure of so-called "pancreatic necrosis" by magnetic resonance imaging in acute necrotizing pancreatitis. Pancreas 25:63–67

Holland AE, Goldfarb JW et al. (1998) Diaphragmatic and cardiac motion during suspended breathing: preliminary experience and implications for breath-hold MR imaging. Radiology 209:483–489

Huwart L, Peeters F et al. (2006) Liver fibrosis: non-invasive assessment with MR elastography. NMR Biomed 19:173–179

Irie H, Honda H et al. (1998) Autoimmune pancreatitis: CT and MR characteristics. AJR Am J Roentgenol 170:1323–1327

Johnson PT, Outwater EK (1999) Pancreatic carcinoma versus chronic pancreatitis: dynamic MR imaging. Radiology 212:213–218

Kamisawa T, Egawa N et al. (2005) Extrapancreatic lesions in autoimmune pancreatitis. J Clin Gastroenterol 39:904–907

Kamisawa T, Tu Y et al. (2006) Involvement of pancreatic and bile ducts in autoimmune pancreatitis. World J Gastroenterol 12:612–614

Lecesne R, Taourel P et al. (1999) Acute pancreatitis: interobserver agreement and correlation of CT and MR cholangiopancreatography with outcome. Radiology 211:727–735

Lee VS, Hecht EM et al. (2007) Body and cardiovascular MR imaging at 3.0 T. Radiology 244:692–705

Makary MA, Duncan MD et al. (2005) The role of magnetic resonance cholangiography in the management of patients with gallstone pancreatitis. Ann Surg 241:119–124

Manfredi R, Costamagna G et al. (2000) Severe chronic pancreatitis versus suspected pancreatic disease: dynamic MR cholangiopancreatography after secretin stimulation. Radiology 214:849–855

Manfredi R, Costamagna G et al. (2000) Pancreas divisum and "santorinicele": diagnosis with dynamic MR cholangiopancreatography with secretin stimulation. Radiology 217:403–408

Manfredi R, Lucidi V et al. (2002) Idiopathic chronic pancreatitis in children: MR cholangiopancreatography after secretin administration. Radiology 224:675–682

Martin DR, Karabulut N et al. (2003) High signal peripancreatic fat on fat-suppressed spoiled gradient echo imaging in acute pancreatitis: preliminary evaluation of the prognostic significance. J Magn Reson Imaging 18:49–58

Matos C, Bali MA et al. (2006) Magnetic resonance imaging in the detection of pancreatitis and pancreatic neoplasms. Best Pract Res Clin Gastroenterol 20(1):157–178

Matos C, Deviere J et al. (1998) Acinar filling during secretin-stimulated MR pancreatography. AJR Am J Roentgenol 171:165–169

Matsuki M, Inada Y et al. (2007) Diffusion-weighed MR imaging of pancreatic carcinoma. Abdom Imaging 32:481–483

McKnight AL, Kugel JL et al. (2002) MR elastography of breast cancer: preliminary results. AJR Am J Roentgenol 178:1411–1417

Momtahen AJ, Balci NC et al. (2008) Focal pancreatitis mimicking pancreatic mass: magnetic resonance imaging (MRI)/magnetic resonance cholangiopancreatography (MRCP) findings including diffusion-weighted MRI. Acta Radiol 49:490–497

Morgan DE, Baron TH (1998) Practical imaging in acute pancreatitis. Semin Gastrointest Dis 9:41–50

Muthupillai R, Lomas DJ et al. (1995) Magnetic resonance elastography by direct visualization of propagating acoustic strain waves. Science 269:1854–1857

Papanikolaou N, Karantanas A et al. (2000) MR cholangiopancreatography before and after oral blueberry juice administration. J Comput Assist Tomogr 24:229–234

Pedrosa I, Rofsky NM (2003) MR imaging in abdominal emergencies. Radiol Clin North Am 41:1243–1273

Piironen A (2001) Severe acute pancreatitis: contrast-enhanced CT and MRI features. Abdom Imaging 26:225–233

Pruessmann KP, Weiger M et al. (1999) SENSE: sensitivity encoding for fast MRI. Magn Reson Med 42:952–962

Reinhold C, Bret PM (1996) MR cholangiopancreatography. Abdom Imaging 21:105–116

Riordan RD, Khonsari M et al. (2004) Pineapple juice as a negative oral contrast agent in magnetic resonance cholangiopancreatography: a preliminary evaluation. Br J Radiol 77:991–999

Robinson PJ, Sheridan MB (2000) Pancreatitis: computed tomography and magnetic resonance imaging. Eur Radiol 10:401–408

Rouviere O, Yin M et al. (2006) MR elastography of the liver: preliminary results. Radiology 240:440–448

Sahani DV, Kalva SP et al. (2004) Autoimmune pancreatitis: imaging features. Radiology 233:345–352

Schrami CMP, Schwenzer NF, Boss A, Claussen CD, Schick F (2008) Functional perfusion imaging of the pancreas using arterial spin labeling technque. Proc Intl Soc Mag Reson Med 16, Toronto, ISMRM

Semelka RC, Ascher SM (1993) MR imaging of the pancreas. Radiology 188:593–602

Sica GT, Miller FH et al. (2002) Magnetic resonance imaging in patients with pancreatitis: evaluation of signal intensity and enhancement changes. J Magn Reson Imaging 15:275–284

Sodickson DK, Manning WJ (1997) Simultaneous acquisition of spatial harmonics (SMASH): fast imaging with radiofrequency coil arrays. Magn Reson Med 38:591–603

Soto JA, Yucel EK et al. (1996) MR cholangiopancreatography after unsuccessful or incomplete ERCP. Radiology 199:91–98

Stimac D, Miletic D et al. (2007) The role of nonenhanced magnetic resonance imaging in the early assessment of acute pancreatitis. Am J Gastroenterol 102:997–1004

Sugita R, Nomiya T (2002) Disappearance of the common bile duct signal caused by oral negative contrast agent on MR cholangiopancreatography. J Comput Assist Tomogr 26:448–450

Tajima Y, Matsuzaki S et al. (2004) Use of the time-signal intensity curve from dynamic magnetic resonance imaging to evaluate remnant pancreatic fibrosis after pancreatico-jejunostomy in patients undergoing pancreatico-duodenectomy. Br J Surg 91:595–600

Takahashi N, Kawashima A et al. (2007) Renal involvement in patients with autoimmune pancreatitis: CT and MR imaging findings. Radiology 242:791–801

Takeuchi M, Matsuzaki K et al. (2008) High-b-value diffusion-weighted magnetic resonance imaging of pancreatic cancer and mass-forming chronic pancreatitis: preliminary results. Acta Radiol 49:383–386

Viremouneix L, Monneuse O et al. (2007) Prospective evaluation of nonenhanced MR imaging in acute pancreatitis. J Magn Reson Imaging 26:331–338

Ward J, Chalmers AG et al. (1997) T2-weighted and dynamic enhanced MRI in acute pancreatitis: comparison with contrast enhanced CT. Clin Radiol 52:109–114

Xydeas T, Siegmann K et al. (2005) Magnetic resonance elastography of the breast: correlation of signal intensity data with viscoelastic properties. Invest Radiol 40:412–420

Yang DH, Kim KW et al. (2005) Autoimmune pancreatitis: radiologic findings in 20 patients. Abdom Imaging 31:94–102

Yin MVS, Grimm RC, Rossman PJ, Manduca A, Ehman RL (2008) Assessment of the Pancreas with MR elastography. Proc Intl Soc Mag Reson Med 16, Toronto, ISMRM

Zhang XM, Shi H et al. (2003) Suspected early or mild chronic pancreatitis: enhancement patterns on gadolinium chelate dynamic MRI. Magnetic resonance imaging. J Magn Reson Imaging 17:86–94

Pancreatic Trauma

Pancreatic Trauma

6

ALEC J. MEGIBOW

CONTENTS

6.1 **Introduction** *107*
6.2 **Clinical Classification of Pancreatic Injury** *107*
6.3 **Imaging Diagnosis** *108*
6.3.1 Computed Tomography *108*
6.3.1.1 CT Technique *108*
6.3.1.2 CT Findings *109*
6.3.2 Magnetic Resonance Imaging *111*
6.3.3 Other Imaging Tests *113*
6.4 **Clinical Follow-Up** *113*
6.5 **Accuracy of Imaging Studies in Pancreatic Trauma** *113*
References *113*

6.1 Introduction

Traumatic injury to the pancreas occurs in approximately 5% of patients sustaining blunt abdominal trauma, 6% of patients with abdominal gunshot wounds, and 2% of patients with upper abdominal stab wounds. Pancreatic injury is associated with a 45% morbidity rate that increases to 60% if diagnosis is delayed (OLAH et al. 2003). In 70%–90 % of cases, pancreatic injuries occur in association with other injuries to surrounding vessels, organs, and viscera (BRADLEY et al. 1998; CIRILLO and KONIARIS 2002); conversely, when injuries are seen in these structures, pancreatic injury should be suspected (SUBRAMANIAN et al. 2007). Traumatic injury to the pancreas may also occur in patients who undergo endoscopic retrograde pancreatography (ERCP) (ABDEL AZIZ and LEHMAN 2007).

In a retrospective review of 16,188 trauma patients admitted to two Level I trauma hospitals over a 10-year period, 72 patients (0.4%) had pancreatic injury. Mechanism of injury was gunshot in 32 (45%), blunt in 27 (37%), and stab wound in 13 (18%). There were 18 grade I (25%), 32 grade II (45%), 16 grade III (22%), and 5 grade IV (7%) injuries. Pancreatic injury is infrequent and is most often associated with penetrating trauma (gunshot wounds and stab wounds) (AKHRASS et al. 1997).

6.2 Clinical Classification of Pancreatic Injury

The American Association for the Surgery of Trauma (AAST) proposed a five-point pancreatic organ injury scale (OIS). Severity of injury is directly related to integrity of the pancreatic duct. Hematomas and lacerations without duct injury are considered Grade I–II, whereas all lacerations associated with duct transection are graded III–V. The most severe injury is massive disruption of the pancreatic head (MOORE et al. 1990). The importance of pancreatic duct integrity has been highlighted in other large series (BRADLEY et al. 1998). Isolated pancreatic injury in the trauma patient may be difficult to detect (BUCCIMAZZA et al. 2006).

The classic clinical triad of upper abdominal pain, leukocytosis, and hyperamylasemia in the trauma patient indicative of pancreatic trauma is neither sensitive nor specific for pancreatic in-

A. J. MEGIBOW, MD, MPH, FACR
Professor, Department of Radiology, NYU-Langone Medical Center, 550 First Avenue, New York, NY 10016, USA

jury, especially immediately following the event. Serum amylase is unreliable, even reported as normal in patients with pancreatic ductal transaction (Jones 1985). Hyperamylasemia may be present when there are duodenal injuries, hepatic injuries, and in intoxicated patients (Wright and Stanski 2000).

Normal serum amylase levels may be present in 40% of cases even in the face of pancreatic duct disruption (White and Benfield 1972; Cirillo and Koniaris 2002).

ERCP-related pancreatitis is estimated to occur in 4%–8% of patients. The reported ranges from <1% to up to 40% of post-ERCP patients reflects variable diagnostic criteria for the diagnosis (Abdel Aziz and Lehman 2007). With increased awareness and more directed post-procedure monitoring, it is apparent that most cases are mild (Bhatia et al. 2006). Severe pancreatitis occurs in approximately 0.3%–0.6% of patients (Freeman and Guda 2004). Risk factors for developing post-ERCP pancreatitis include: young age, female gender, sphincter of Oddi dysfunction, and prior history of post-ERCP pancreatitis (Cheng et al. 2006). Proposed mechanisms include trauma to the papilla, hydrostatic injury, chemical or allergic injury related to the contrast material, enzymatic activation related to the introduction of a foreign substance, infection, pancreatic duct edema, and thermal injury (Freeman and Guda 2004). In terms of clinical grading, the severity of post-ERCP pancreatitis is graded by the number of days the patient requires hospitalization and on the level of intervention necessary.

6.3 Imaging Diagnosis

Most surgeons agree that imaging is crucial in the diagnosis of pancreatic injuries. Furthermore, as there is an increasing trend toward non-operative management of the trauma patient, careful imaging is required to *exclude* clinically occult pancreatic injury (Leppaniemi and Haapiainen 1999). Undiagnosed ductal disruptions produce secondary infections, fistulas, and fluid collections, requiring extended hospitalization (Subramanian et al. 2007). The imaging tests that are utilized include computed tomography (CT), ERCP and MRI, particularly with secretin stimulation (Ragozzino et al. 2003).

6.3.1 Computed Tomography

Computed tomography has an established role in the trauma patient. Almost all patients sustaining significant trauma will undergo CT scanning. Current multidetector-row CT (MDCT) technology allows almost instantaneous interrogation of the entire patient, including vessels, viscera, and musculoskeletal structures in a single acquisition (Ptak et al. 2003; Sheridan et al. 2003). Despite the excellence of current imaging technology, the signs of pancreatic injury may be subtle, missed when more dramatic findings are present, or just not visible by current techniques. A high index of suspicion and excellent CT technique are required to make the diagnosis.

6.3.1.1 CT Technique

MDCT scanners have almost totally replaced the installed base of CT in the US. These scanners have the ability to acquire thin sections composed of isotropic voxels within a short period of time. These technologic advances allow production of high resolution images that can be displayed in 3D and reduce the critical time needed to make therapeutic decisions in trauma patients (Hilbert et al. 2007).

There is no specific MDCT technique directed at evaluating pancreatic trauma; diagnoses can be made from the data sets that are generated for the overall evaluation of the patient with abdominal trauma. Oral contrast is generally not administered, particularly in cases where there is loss of consciousness. Intravenous contrast is necessary if one expects to diagnose vascular trauma and detect parenchymal laceration. As directly related to the pancreas, the increased attenuation of the pancreatic parenchyma following IV contrast facilitates visualization of the pancreatic duct. An injection rate of 3 ml/s should be considered as the absolute minimum; however, significantly improved angiographic evaluation is possible with rates at 5–6 ml/s (Miller and Shanmuganathan 2005; Venkatesh and Wan 2008). A total volume of 100–150 ml of non-ionic intravenous contrast is administered. Because of the long scan range (thorax, abdomen, and pelvis), as well as the relatively younger patient population, we choose to use a wider detector configuration (1.2–1.5 mm) that provides thin slices composed of 1.5- to 2-mm isotropic voxels.

These slices are sent to the workstation. Axial and coronal sections (4–5 mm) are automatically and simultaneously reconstructed and sent to PACS or to film. These images are combined with the 3D images created from the larger isotropic data stored on the workstation. By beginning image acquisition approximately 60–70 s following the initiation of the contrast injection, there will be high level of pancreatic parenchymal enhancement. Scanning during this phase of contrast enhancement was shown to provide maximal visualization of pancreatic duct disruption in patients with proven pancreatic injury (Wong et al. 2008)

6.3.1.2 CT Findings

The findings at MDCT parallel those outlined by in the OIS. Contusion will appear as an area of low attenuation within the affected portion of the gland. Wong and colleagues (1997) proposed the following classification of pancreatic injury: grade A, pancreatitis or superficial laceration (<50% pancreatic thickness); grade B1, deep laceration (>50% pancreatic thickness) of the pancreatic tail; grade B2, transection of the pancreatic tail; grade C1, deep laceration of the pancreatic head; grade C2, transection of the pancreatic head. It should be noted that we do not classify the injury in the formal report; rather, the above classification informs the report and helps frame appropriate management decisions.

Pancreatic laceration or fractures were the first form of pancreatic injury described in the CT literature (Jeffrey et al. 1983). Specific signs of pancreatic injury on CT include: fracture , laceration, pancreatic enlargement with edema, pancreatic hematoma, extravasation of IV contrast from peripancreatic arteries, fluid separation of the pancreas and splenic vein (Bigattini et al. 1999; Cirillo and Koniaris 2002; Gupta et al. 2004). Pancreatic fractures are most often transverse in orientation, the most common site being the body or neck of the gland (Dodds et al. 1990; Venkatesh and Wan 2008) (Fig. 6.1). High attenuation fluid representing blood may be present between the edges of the fracture. Another finding that is considered highly predictive of pancreatic injury is detection of fluid between the dorsal margin of the pancreas and the splenic vein. Although neither the precise mechanism nor the nature of fluid is known, this finding was present in 90% of patients subsequently proven to have a pancreatic injury (Lane et al. 1994).

Several authors have noted the findings that pancreatic edema and peripancreatic collections may obscure visualization of the actual pancreatic injury. Although the actual parenchymal defect in the injured pancreas may not be detected, CT findings that simulate acute pancreatitis (peripancreatic increased density, thickening of anterior renal fascia, peripancreatic fluid collections, mesocolic collections, intra- and retroperitoneal fluid) should raise the suspicion of pancreatic injury (Bigattini

a

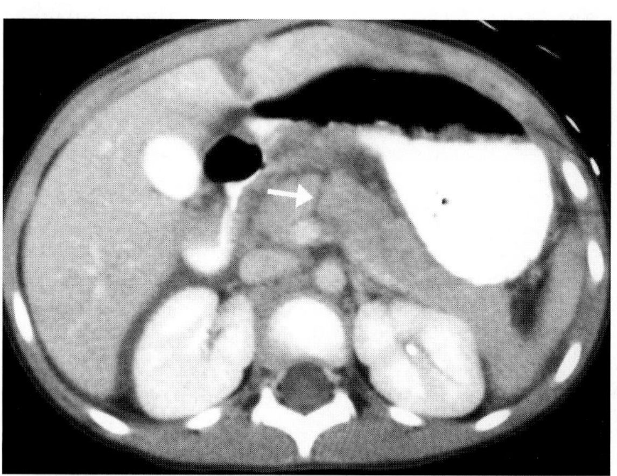

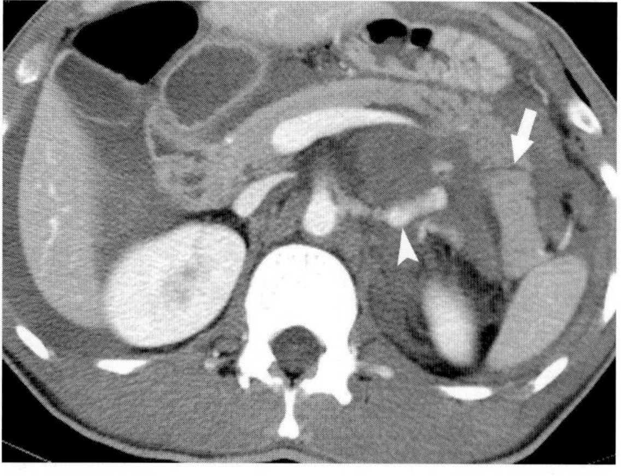

b

Fig. 6.1. a Pancreatic fracture isolated injury. The fracture line can easily be seen traversing the entire width of the gland (*arrow*). No peripancreatic abnormalities are detected. **b** Pancreatic fracture as lesser injury. MDCT image from a 33-year-old patient who sustained a stab wound to the left flank. There is extravasation of iodinated contrast from the aorta. Additionally, there is a fracture across the pancreatic body (*arrow*). The patient was taken to surgery, the aorta was repaired, and the patient survived

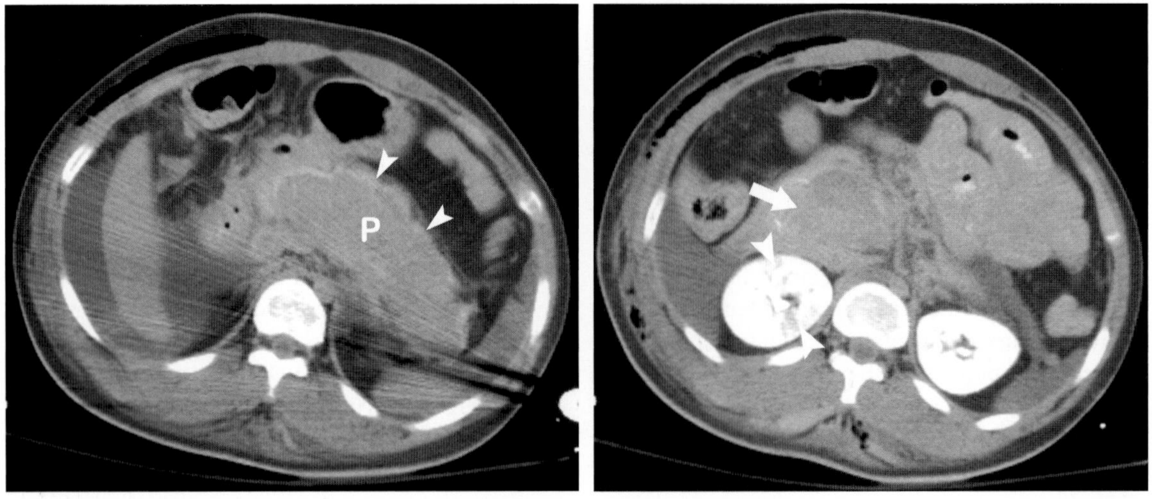

Fig. 6.2. a Diffuse pancreatic hematoma. Single image from a non-IV contrast-enhanced CT scan reveals diffuse pancreatic enlargement (*P*) in this patient who was hit by an automobile. Notice the high attenuation rim surrounding the pancreas representing blood accumulating under the capsule (*arrowheads*). **b** Diffuse pancreatic hematoma. There is a blood/fluid level in the pancreatic head (*arrow*). Peripancreatic fluid is present in the right anterior pararenal space and posterior to the pancreas on the left. Additional injuries included renal contusions (*arrowheads*) and a pelvic fracture that produced arterial injury requiring embolization

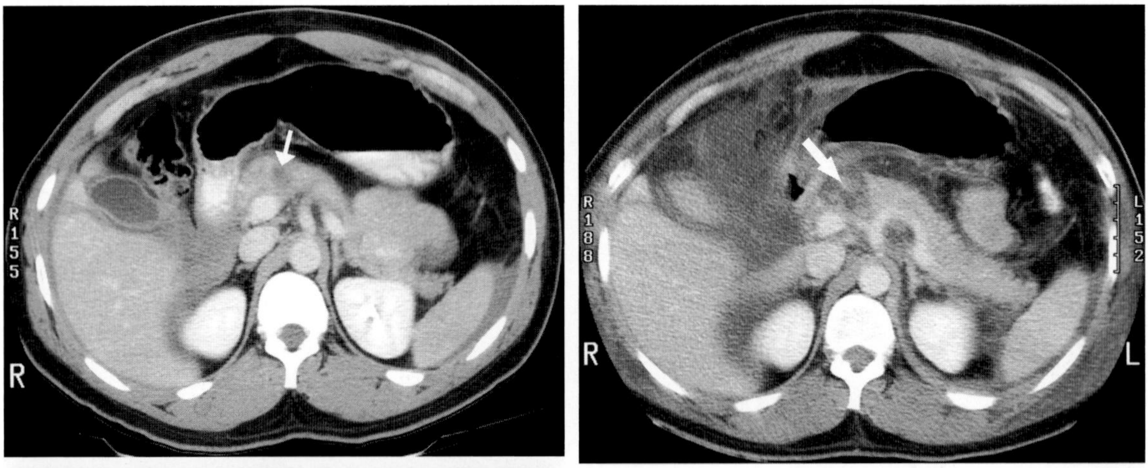

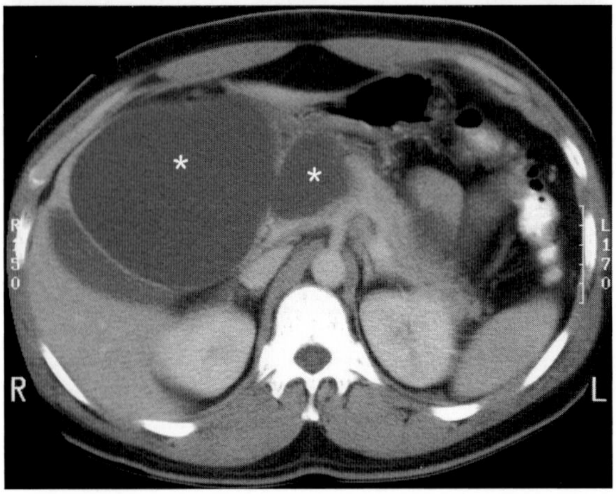

Fig. 6.3. a Evolution of pancreatic injury. CT image in 29-year-old patient who was in an automobile accident reveals a small lucency in the body of the pancreas (*arrow*). Hemoperitoneum and a liver laceration are seen. **b** Evolution of pancreatic injury. Same patient as in (**a**); CT study 3 days later. The hematoma has increased in size resulting in increasing separation of the pancreatic fragments (*arrow*). The hemoperitoneum has increased. **c** Evolution of pancreatic injury. Same patient as in (**a**) and (**b**). Study performed 2 months later. The intrapancreatic injury has increased in volume but decreased in complexity. A bilobed pseudocyst (*asterisks*) has developed. The hemoperitoneum and peripancreatic changes have resolved. The collections were percutaneously drained; the patient made an uneventful recovery

et al. 1999; Cirillo and Koniaris 2002; Gupta et al. 2004; Venkatesh and Wan 2008) (Fig. 6.2). If there is high clinical suspicion of pancreatic injury, particularly in the presence of a delayed elevation in the serum amylase, a repeated MDCT study may actually reveal the injury that was occult on the initial evaluation (Fig. 6.3) (Wright and Stanski 2000; Brestas et al. 2006).

The diagnosis of duct disruption is the single most important observation to be made in the patient sustaining a pancreatic injury (Fig. 6.4). Once duct disruption is detected, duct repair is essential; however, in patients in whom non-operative management is contemplated, it becomes important to exclude the presence of duct disruption (Cirillo and Koniaris 2002; Subramanian et al. 2007). Using current MDCT techniques, the pancreatic duct may be visualized in the majority of patients. Post-processing techniques such as minimum-intensity projection (Salles et al. 2008) and curved multi-planar reformat (Gong and Xu 2004) aid in delineation of the duct. Visualization of the duct is hampered in non-contrast scans and in patients with pancreatic edema. It is not surprising to find that the presence of duct disruption correlates with the depth of pancreatic injury (Wong et al. 1997). Currently available MDCT technology was 91% sensitive and 91% specific for identifying duct injury in 33 patients in whom operative confirmation of findings was available (Teh et al. 2007).

6.3.2 Magnetic Resonance Imaging

Most patients who have sustained upper abdominal trauma are too critically ill to undergo an MRI examination. However, MRI can be extremely useful in the detection of delayed complications related to pancreatic duct disruption (Fig. 6.5). Current MRI can produce a high quality 3D magnetic resonance cholangio-pancreatogram (MRCP). The use of secretin stimulation (S-MRCP) increases the sensitivity to detecting duct disruption (Cirillo and Koniaris 2002; Gillams et al. 2006; Hellund et al. 2007). S-MRCP has been shown to be more sensitive than ERCP for detecting duct disruption and it is non-invasive and less traumatic to fragile pancreatic tissue. Finally, S-MRCP can be safely used in the evaluation of pediatric patients (Tipnis and Werlin 2007).

The technique of S-MRCP for detection of duct disruption is no different than that used for conventional MRCP. Using parallel imaging techniques and heavily T2-weighted turbo-spin echo imaging, the entire pancreas can be evaluated in 2–4 min. The continuous acquisition will produce thin slices that can be viewed in 3D on a workstation. A 3D respiratory triggered heavily T2-weighted TSE in the coronal and coronal oblique planes with 30-degree angulation depending on the orientation of the pancreatic duct is preferred over the thick-slab technique. The coverage is between 3–6 cm and 1-mm

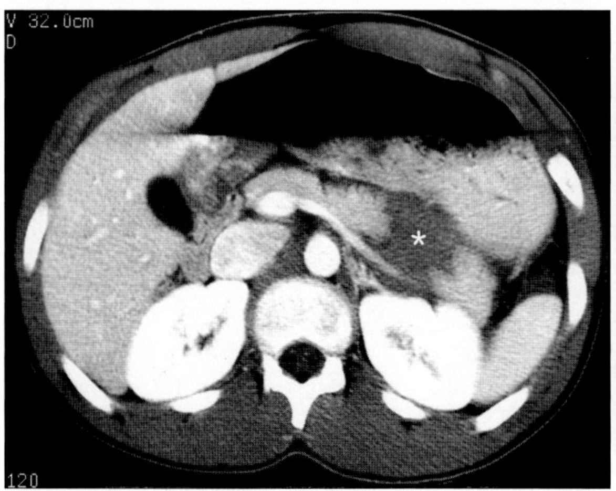

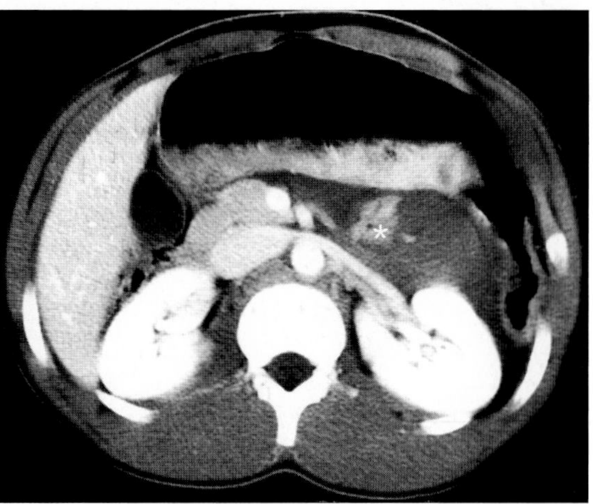

Fig. 6.4. a Intrapancreatic hematoma with pancreatic duct disruption. A high attenuation fluid collection (*asterisk*) is seen separating two fragments of enhancing pancreatic tissue in this 17-year-old male who sustained abdominal trauma. **b** Intrapancreatic hematoma with pancreatic duct disruption. Image from same study as in (**a**) reveals a portion of pancreas that is not contiguous with remainder of gland (*asterisk*). The patient developed a pseudocyst several weeks later that was percutaneously drained. Surgical resection of the pancreatic tail was required before the drainage catheters could be removed

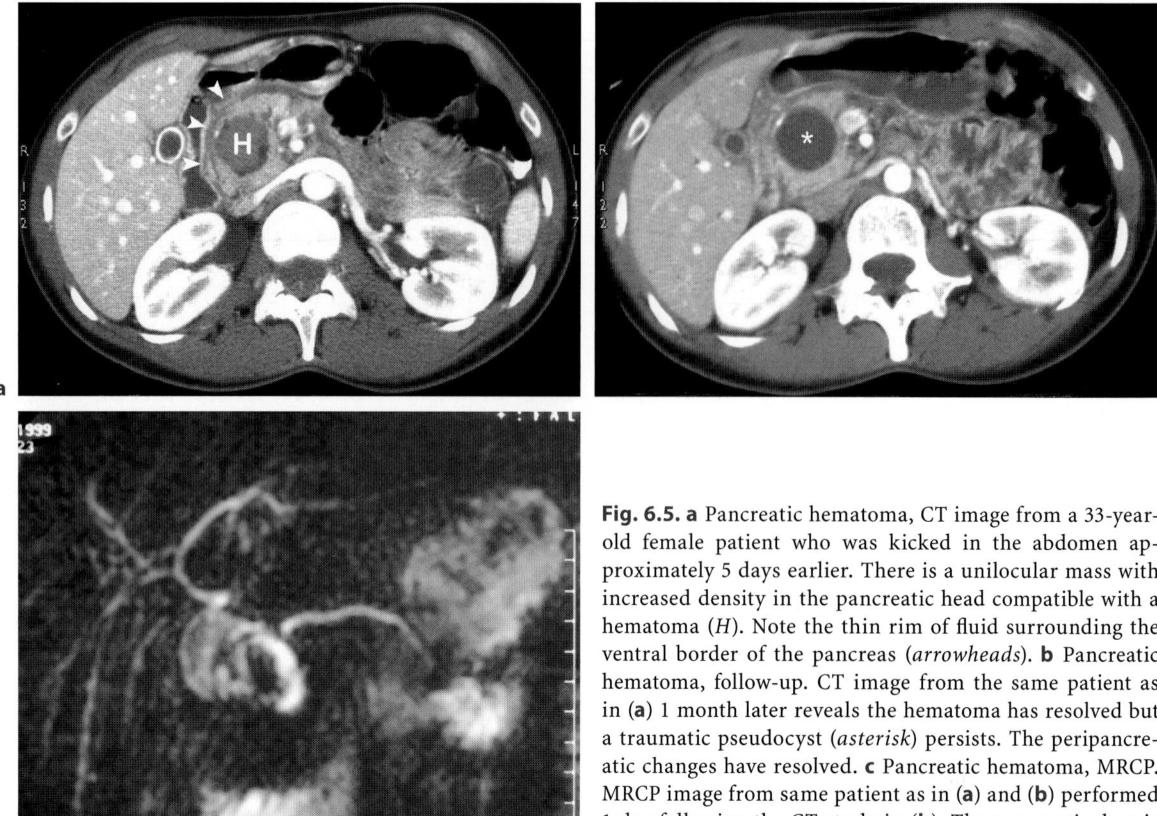

Fig. 6.5. a Pancreatic hematoma, CT image from a 33-year-old female patient who was kicked in the abdomen approximately 5 days earlier. There is a unilocular mass with increased density in the pancreatic head compatible with a hematoma (*H*). Note the thin rim of fluid surrounding the ventral border of the pancreas (*arrowheads*). **b** Pancreatic hematoma, follow-up. CT image from the same patient as in (**a**) 1 month later reveals the hematoma has resolved but a traumatic pseudocyst (*asterisk*) persists. The peripancreatic changes have resolved. **c** Pancreatic hematoma, MRCP. MRCP image from same patient as in (**a**) and (**b**) performed 1 day following the CT study in (**b**). The pancreatic duct is intact

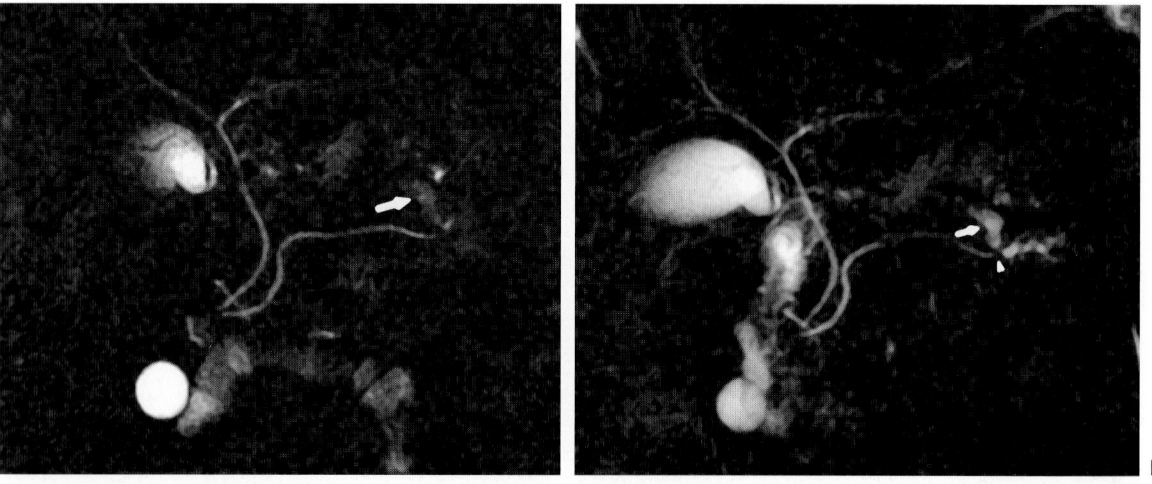

Fig. 6.6. a Peripancreatic fluid collection, value of secretin. MRCP image from patient who sustained abdominal trauma reveals a high signal focus (*arrow*) representing a fluid collection immediately superior to the tail of the pancreas. **b** Peripancreatic fluid collection, value of secretin. MRCP image in the same patient as in (**a**) reveals an increase in the size of the fluid collection (*arrow*) indicating direct communication with the main pancreatic duct. Note the upstream dilatation of the duct proximal to the disrupted and strictured main pancreatic duct (*arrowhead*). (Case courtesy of M. Fatih Akisik, MD, Indianapolis, Indiana)

slices are created. Following a slow administration of intravenous secretin at a dose of 1 ml/10-kg thick slab images are obtained at 1-min intervals over a 10-min period of observation.

S-MRCP is most useful in patients in whom there are pancreatic lacerations of >50% of the width of the gland in which duct disruption is suspected, but cannot be confirmed (Fig. 6.6).

6.3.3 Other Imaging Tests

ERCP had been used extensively in the evaluation of pancreatic duct integrity in patients having sustained blunt pancreatic trauma directly related to the fact that the major morbidity is directly associated with duct transection (Bradley et al. 1998; Phelan and Minei 2005). ERCP can show duct disruption in 75% of patients. Downstream obstruction of the pancreatic duct may prevent contrast medium from reaching the level of the disruption of the duct (Gillams et al. 2006). Most current reviews of diagnostic and management options in pancreatic trauma advocate S-MRCP, if available, to evaluate the integrity of the pancreatic duct. ERCP is reserved for patients who might benefit from pancreatic duct stenting (Wolf et al. 2005; Canlas and Branch 2007).

The focused abdominal sonogram for trauma (FAST) has gained utility among emergency physicians. While a useful technique for rapid detection of abdominal fluid collections, the FAST study is poor for localization of the source of injury (Shuster et al. 2004). In a study of 772 blunt trauma victims, 29% of abdominal injuries were missed by using FAST as the sole diagnostic technique (Chiu et al. 1997).

6.4 Clinical Follow-Up

Between 70%–85% of pancreatic injuries are OIS grade I–II and are conservatively managed; conversely, delayed treatment of severe pancreatic injury leads to a significantly increased morbidity (Cirillo and Koniaris 2002; Subramanian et al. 2007; Duchesne et al. 2008). Furthermore, it should be remembered that clinical manifestations of pancreatic injury may not appear early after the trauma, and that these findings may be difficult to detect on initial studies performed at the time of admission. Follow-up scanning several days later may finally reveal the presence of a pancreatic injury (Brestas et al. 2006).

Long-term complications of pancreatic trauma include: pancreatic fistula (23%), traumatic pancreatitis with or without abscess (6%–15%), pseudocyst formation (5%) (Figs. 6.4, 6.5), and development of duct stricture (Bradley et al. 1998). These are similar to complications seen in acute pancreatitis patients and are managed in a similar fashion.

6.5 Accuracy of Imaging Studies in Pancreatic Trauma

There has been a demonstrable improvement in the ability to detect pancreatic injury on imaging studies. The improvement is directly related to improvements in MDCT technology and in the ability to obtain rapid heavily T2-weighted MRCP images. A retrospective review of 16,188 trauma patients seen over a 10-year period and published in 1997 identified 72 patients with pancreatic injury, 17 of whom underwent initial CT. In that group, nine had a normal pancreas on the initial imaging study; all were proven to have pancreatic injuries at surgery, three of which were OIS. grade III lesions requiring distal pancreatectomy. In another patient, the CT underestimated the extent of the injury (Akhrass et al. 1996).

These results can be compared with a more recent review of 33 patients with pancreatic injuries who underwent CT scanning and subsequent laparotomy. In this group, CT was 91% specific for identification of pancreatic ductal injury (Teh et al. 2007). Finally, in a review of 35 of 120 hemodynamically stable adults who sustained low grade blunt pancreatic trauma and who underwent CT scanning, non-operative management was successful in the majority. Direct duct imaging with ERCP or MRCP was recommended to improve the analysis of the most appropriate therapeutic strategy (Duchesne et al. 2008).

References

Abdel Aziz AM, Lehman GA (2007) Pancreatitis after endoscopic retrograde cholangio-pancreatography. World J Gastroenterol 13:2655–2668

Akhrass R, Kim K et al. (1996) Computed tomography: an unreliable indicator of pancreatic trauma. Am Surg 62:647–651

Akhrass R, Yaffe MB et al. (1997) Pancreatic trauma: a ten-year multi-institutional experience. Am Surg 63:598–604

Bhatia V, Garg PK et al. (2006) Endoscopic retrograde cholangiopancreatography-induced acute pancreatitis often has a benign outcome. J Clin Gastroenterol 40:726–731

Bigattini D, Boverie J H et al. (1999) CT of blunt trauma of the pancreas in adults. Eur Radiol 9: 244–249

Bradley EL 3rd, Young PR Jr. et al. (1998) Diagnosis and initial management of blunt pancreatic trauma: guidelines from a multiinstitutional review. Ann Surg 227:861–869

Brestas PS, Karakyklas D et al. (2006) Sequential CT evaluation of isolated non-penetrating pancreatic trauma. Jop 7:51–55

Buccimazza I, Thomson SR et al. (2006) Isolated main pancreatic duct injuries spectrum and management. Am J Surg 191:448–452

Canlas KR, Branch MS (2007) Role of endoscopic retrograde cholangiopancreatography in acute pancreatitis. World J Gastroenterol 13:6314–6320

Cheng CL, Sherman S et al. (2006) Risk factors for post-ERCP pancreatitis: a prospective multicenter study. Am J Gastroenterol 101:139–147

Chiu WC, Cushing BM et al. (1997) Abdominal injuries without hemoperitoneum: a potential limitation of focused abdominal sonography for trauma (FAST). J Trauma 42:617–623; discussion 623–625

Cirillo RL Jr, Koniaris LG (2002) Detecting blunt pancreatic injuries. J Gastrointest Surg 6:587–598

Dodds WJ, Taylor AJ et al. (1990) Traumatic fracture of the pancreas: CT characteristics. J Comput Assist Tomogr 14:375–378

Duchesne JC, Schmieg R et al. (2008) Selective nonoperative management of low-grade blunt pancreatic injury: are we there yet? J Trauma 65:49–53

Freeman ML, Guda NM (2004) Prevention of post-ERCP pancreatitis: a comprehensive review. Gastrointest Endosc 59:845–864

Gillams AR, Kurzawinski T et al. (2006) Diagnosis of duct disruption and assessment of pancreatic leak with dynamic secretin-stimulated MR cholangiopancreatography. AJR Am J Roentgenol 186:499–506

Gong JS, Xu JM (2004) Role of curved planar reformations using multidetector spiral CT in diagnosis of pancreatic and peripancreatic diseases. World J Gastroenterol 10:1943–1947

Gupta A, Stuhlfaut JW et al. (2004) Blunt trauma of the pancreas and biliary tract: a multimodality imaging approach to diagnosis. Radiographics 24:1381–1395

Hellund JC, Skattum J et al. (2007) Secretin-stimulated magnetic resonance cholangiopancreatography of patients with unclear disease in the pancreatico-biliary tract. Acta Radiol 48:135–141

Hilbert P, zur Nieden K et al. (2007) New aspects in the emergency room management of critically injured patients: a multi-slice CT-oriented care algorithm. Injury 38:552–558

Jeffrey RB Jr, Federle MP et al. (1983) Computed tomography of pancreatic trauma. Radiology 147:491–494

Jones RC (1985) Management of pancreatic trauma. Am J Surg 150:698–704

Lane MJ, Mindelzun RE et al. (1994) CT diagnosis of blunt pancreatic trauma: importance of detecting fluid between the pancreas and the splenic vein. AJR Am J Roentgenol 163:833–835

Leppaniemi AK, Haapiainen RK (1999) Risk factors of delayed diagnosis of pancreatic trauma. Eur J Surg 165:1134–1137

Miller LA, Shanmuganathan K (2005) Multidetector CT evaluation of abdominal trauma. Radiol Clin North Am 43:1079–1095, viii

Moore EE, Cogbill TH et al. (1990) Organ injury scaling, II: pancreas, duodenum, small bowel, colon, and rectum. J Trauma 30:1427–1429

Olah A, Issekutz A et al. (2003) Pancreatic transection from blunt abdominal trauma: early versus delayed diagnosis and surgical management. Dig Surg 20:408–414

Phelan HA, Minei JP (2005) Pancreatic trauma: diagnostic and therapeutic strategies. Curr Treat Options Gastroenterol 8:355–363

Ptak T, Rhea JT et al. (2003) Radiation dose is reduced with a single-pass whole-body multi-detector row CT trauma protocol compared with a conventional segmented method: initial experience. Radiology 229:902–905

Ragozzino A, Manfredi R et al. (2003) The use of MRCP in the detection of pancreatic injuries after blunt trauma. Emerg Radiol 10:14–18

Salles A, Nino-Murcia M et al. (2008) CT of pancreas: minimum intensity projections. Abdom Imaging 33:207–213

Sheridan R, Peralta R et al. (2003) Reformatted visceral protocol helical computed tomographic scanning allows conventional radiographs of the thoracic and lumbar spine to be eliminated in the evaluation of blunt trauma patients. J Trauma 55:665–669

Shuster M, Abu-Laban RB et al. (2004) Focused abdominal ultrasound for blunt trauma in an emergency department without advanced imaging or on-site surgical capability. CJEM 6:408–415

Subramanian A, Dente CJ et al. (2007) The management of pancreatic trauma in the modern era. Surg Clin North Am 87:1515–1532, x

Teh SH, Sheppard BC et al. (2007) Diagnosis and management of blunt pancreatic ductal injury in the era of high-resolution computed axial tomography. Am J Surg 193:641–3; discussion 643

Tipnis NA, Werlin SL (2007) The use of magnetic resonance cholangiopancreatography in children. Curr Gastroenterol Rep 9:225–229

Venkatesh SK, Wan JM (2008) CT of blunt pancreatic trauma – a pictorial essay. Eur J Radiol 67:311–320

White PH, Benfield JR (1972) Amylase in the management of pancreatic trauma. Arch Surg 105:158–163

Wolf A, Bernhardt J et al. (2005) The value of endoscopic diagnosis and the treatment of pancreas injuries following blunt abdominal trauma. Surg Endosc 19:665–669

Wong YC, Wang LJ et al. (2008) Multidetector-row computed tomography (CT) of blunt pancreatic injuries: can contrast-enhanced multiphasic CT detect pancreatic duct injuries? J Trauma 64:666–672

Wong YC, Wang LJ et al. (1997) CT grading of blunt pancreatic injuries: prediction of ductal disruption and surgical correlation. J Comput Assist Tomogr 21:246–250

Wright MJ, Stanski C (2000) Blunt pancreatic trauma: a difficult injury. South Med J 93:383–385

Chronic Pancreatitis

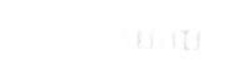

Pathophysiology of Chronic Pancreatitis

7

Giorgio Cavallini and Luca Frulloni

CONTENTS

7.1 **The Role of Alcohol in Chronic Pancreatitis: Old and New Concepts** *117*

7.2 **A Common Pathogenetic Mechanism: Ductal Obstruction** *118*

7.3 **The Causes of Ductal Obstruction: "Inflammatory Pancreatic Diseases"** *119*

7.3.1 Pancreatitis Associated with Sphincter of Oddi Dysfunctions and Biliary Lithiasis *120*

7.3.2 Pancreatitis Associated with Cystic Dystrophy of the Duodenal Wall – Groove Pancreatitis *120*

7.3.3 Autoimmune Pancreatitis *121*

7.3.4 Pancreatitis Associated with Gene Mutations *121*

7.3.5 Pancreatitis Associated with Pancreatic and Peripancreatic Anomalies *122*

7.3.6 Other Causes *123*

References *123*

Chronic pancreatitis is an inflammation of the exocrine pancreas, characterized by progressive and irreversible destruction of the whole organ, resulting in exocrine (maldigestion, steatorrhoea) and endocrine (diabetes) insufficiency.

Until a few years ago, chronic pancreatitis was considered as one individual disease; multiple hypotheses were offered as to the physiopathological mechanism without indentification of a common factor.

G. Cavallini, MD
Department of Gastroenteroloy, Internal Medicine Section C, Policlinico "GB Rossi", University of Verona, Piazzale LA Scuro 10, 37134 Verona, Italy
L. Frulloni, MD, PhD
Department of Gastroenteroloy, Policlinico "GB Rossi", Piazzale LA Scuro 10, 37134 Verona, Italy

In the 1980s and 1990s, aided by improvements in imaging techniques and genetic research, many forms of the disease have been identified that may be differentiated by their epidemiological, clinical and biochemical characteristics that therefore require different therapeutic approaches (medical, endoscopic and surgical). The unifying term "inflammatory pancreatic diseases" (Cavallini and Frulloni 2001) has been proposed for this reason.

7.1 The Role of Alcohol in Chronic Pancreatitis: Old and New Concepts

In Western industrialized countries, heavy alcohol consumption has been considered the main aetiological factor of chronic pancreatitis, on the basis of the epidemiological evidence that long-term alcohol abuse (more than 80 g of alcohol/day for more than 5 years) is reported in 70%–80% of patients (Dite et al. 2001; Dufour and Adamson 2003; Lankisch et al. 2002; Lin et al. 2001; Vaona et al. 1997).

On the basis of studies published since the beginning of the 1980s, the French school hypothesised that the underlyingpathophysiologic derangement causing CP was the precipitation of insoluble proteinic fibrillar material inside the pancreatic ducts, particularly lithostathine (LS-S) (Sarles et al. 1989a). On this proteinic matrix (protein-plug) Ca^{++} crystals were then deposited, the formation of which would be accentuated by insufficient production of LS-S. Decreased LS-S can be either genetically determined or secondary to exogenous toxic factors (alcohol, tobacco, diet, etc.). The protein (calcified) plugs would cause traumatic changes at the walls of the small ducts inducing peri-ductal inflammation and leading to stenosis of the duct and local increase in fibrosis within the adjacent pancreatic parenchyma. The upstream flow of pancreatic juice of the obstruction would be progressively impeded, with stasis of the exocrine secretion creating still further formation of the plugs and progressive secondary atrophy of the acinar structures.

In this context, alcohol accelerates LS-S degradation and decreases the solubility of Ca^{++}. This could occur through a variety of alcohol induced mechanisms, such as the increase in the concentration of proteolithic enzymes in the pancreatic juice (Sarles et al. 1971), the decrease of enzymatic inhibitors like the Pancreatic Secretory Trypsin Inhibitor (PSTI) (Rinderknecht et al. 1985) and a decrease in the pancreatic juice pH due to a decrease in the secretion of bicarbonates (Hajnal et al. 1990), or by means of direct poisoning by alcohol or its metabolites, especially acetaldehyde, of the pancreatic acinar cells with secondary reduction of lithostathine production (Pitchumoni 1988). On the basis of this hypothesis, the Marseilles-Rome 1984–1988 (Sarles et al. 1989b) classification was proposed.

There is a great deal of conflicting experimental evidence questioning the primary role of LS-S with the exception of an initial study by Sarles et al. (1971) (Pitchumoni 2001; Schneider et al. 2002; Lerch et al. 2003). For example, low levels of LS-S in patientswho abuse alcohol without CP are indistinguishable from low levels of LS-S seen in CP patients. Lastly, the levels of mRNA, the codifier of LS-S in patients with obstructive pancreatitis, were the same as those for patients with the calcified form of the disease (Cavallini et al. 1998).

The role of alcohol in chronic pancreatitis has been reconsidered from an aetiological point of view, but it still plays an important role in the pathogenesis of the disease. In cultured pancreatic rat acinar cells it has been demonstrated that ethanol metabolism follows two paths (Haber et al. 1998): (1) an oxidative path, involving alcohol dehydrogenase (ADH) type III (non saturable form of ADH) producing acetaldehyde and acetate, (2) a non oxidative path, involving fatty acid ethyl esters (FAEE) synthase and producing FAEE, in particular ethyl palmitate. FAEEs activity is 3- to 10-fold higher than in the liver.

Acetaldehyde has been shown to cause morphologic damage in the pancreas (Wilson et al. 1992; Altomare et al. 1996; Korsten et al. 1994). It has been reported to inhibit stimulated secretion from isolated pancreatic acini, probably secondary to the binding of secretagogues to their receptors or to microtubular dysfunction affecting exocytosis. During oxidation from ethanol to acetaldehyde and acetate, large quantities of hydrogen ions are released and the intracellular oxidation/reduction state is altered, leading to metabolic alteration that may contribute to acinar injury. Long-term exposure to ethanol may lead to oxidative stress in human chronic pancreatitis.

FAEE have been shown to induce pancreatic injury (Korsten et al. 1994; Haber et al. 1993, 1994). The mechanism of damage may involve the destabilization of intra-cellular membranes (in particular of lysosomal and mitochondrial), or free fatty acids released by FAEE hydrolysis, or lastly cholesteryl ester synthesis and accumulation after long-term ethanol administration.

Another potential mechanism of alcohol mediated pancreatic cellular damage could involve the activation of pancreatic stellate cells (PSC); either activated directly by ethanol (Apte and Wilson 2003; Apte et al. 2000), or indirectly by acetaldehyde/acetate (Apte et al. 2000), oxidative stress products (Gutierrez-Ruiz et al. 2002) or by pro-inflammatory cytokines released after ethanol-induced pancreatic inflammation (Haber et al. 1999; Apte et al. 1999).

Activated stellate cells produce extra-cellular matrix (ECM) and therefore contribute to progressive loss of glandular tissue and replacement with intralobular and perilobular pancreatic fibrosis.

In brief, ethanol may produce pancreatic damage by altering cellular membranes, causing metabolic alterations in acinar cells and producing oxidative stress molecules or accelerating the progression of pancreatic fibrosis by activating and stimulating PSC to directly or indirectly produce ECM.

7.2 A Common Pathogenetic Mechanism: Ductal Obstruction

Chronic pancreatitis-like lesions may be reproduced experimentally only with incomplete obstruction of the main pancreatic duct. The partial obstruction of the pancreatic duct in experimental chronic pancreatitis results in lesions of the pancreatic parenchyma that are very similar to those observed in human chronic pancreatitis (Letko et al. 1989; Tanaka et al. 1988; Pap and Boros 1989). Chronic alcoholic intake aggravates pancreatic lesions, accelerates their onset and makes them irreversible (Pap and Boros 1989).

Experimental studies have also shown that: (1) the longer the obstruction is in place, the more serious the pancreatic lesions are, (2) ductal obstruction causes the formation of pancreatic calculi in animal models (Konishi et al. 1981), (3) complete obstruction results in atrophy of pancreatic parenchyma, (4) the restoration of the pancreatic outflow prevents the formation of new calculi and slows further parenchymal damage (Runzi et al. 1993; Karanjia et al. 1994).

We may therefore assume that most aetiological factors act to produce some form of obstruction of the pancreatic duct system. The stasis of the pancreatic juice facilitates the precipitation of calcium crystals in the lumen duct, inducing calcifications that aggravate the obstruction. The acinar component undergoes severe ultra-structural changes that reduce the enzyme production and stimulate an inflammatory process and fibrosis involving all the glands above the stricture.

In the presence of lithogenetic factors, such as alcohol abuse and cigarette smoking (Sarles and Berger 1989; Cavallini et al. 1994), the process may be accelerated, with the early onset of calcifications and of exocrine and endocrine insufficiency. Regardless of the cause (aetiology) of the ductal obstruction, the consequences are always the same, i.e. inflammation, fibrosis and loss of pancreatic exocrine and endocrine tissue.

The most recent concept in the pathogenesis of chronic pancreatitis is that acute pancreatitis may recur over multiple episodes becoming chronic (Kloppel and Maillet 1992; Ammann et al. 1996). This was demonstrated in hereditary pancreatitis and in pancreatitis associated with mutations of the CFTR gene (Frullini et al. 2003) and PRSS1 gene (Whitcomb 2001), but some authors have hypothesised this as a common factor seen in all patients suffering from chronic pancreatitis (Kloppel and Maillet 1992). The main consequence of this hypothesis is not to use the terms acute recurrent and chronic pancreatitis, but to introduce the more general term "pancreatitis" for patients suffering from recurrent episodes of pancreatitis.

We can conclude that: (1) chronic pancreatitis is the advanced stage of an inflammatory process of the pancreas; (2) in an early stage of the disease we are more likely to identify the cause (aetiology) of the pancreatitis, whereas this is more difficult in a more advanced stage; (3) removing the cause of the disease in an early stage may lead to complete recovery of pancreatic function, whereas alterations are irreversible in an advanced stage.

7.3 The Causes of Ductal Obstruction: "Inflammatory Pancreatic Diseases"

There are many etiologies that lead to partial obstruction of the pancreatic ductal system with resultant episodic acute pancreatitis that, over time, progresses into CP.

The common causes of pancreatic ductal obstruction in humans are listed in Table 7.1.

Stenosis of the papilla of Vater, probably secondary to biliary lithiasis, as hypothesised at the beginning of the 20th century by Opie, is the most common cause of pancreatitis based on our experience in Verona.

Table 7.1. Causes of pancreatic ductal obstruction

Sphincter of Oddi dysfunction • Primary • Secondary to acute or chronic biliary stone disease
Cystic dystrophy of the duodenal wall (groove pancreatitis)
Autoimmune (lymphoplasmacytic) Pancreatitis
Pancreatic tumors • Adenocarcinoma • Serous cystadenoma • Intraductal papillary mucinous tumor • Neuroendocrine • Others
Pancreatic anomalies • Pancreas divisum • Annular pancreas
Genetic mutations • CFTR • SPINK1 • PRSS1 • K8 • Unknown
Necrotizing or relapsing acute pancreatitis • Pseudocysts • Parenchymal scarring • Parenchymal necrosis

Other possible causes are biliary or pancreatic tumours, pancreatic anomalies, particularly pancreas divisum, stenosis of the main pancreatic duct secondary to severe (necrotizing) or relapsing acute pancreatitis. Several genetic mutations have been described in patients suffering from chronic pancreatitis, particularly mutations of the CFTR gene (cystic fibrosis gene), as well as mutations of the gene $PRSS_1$ (cationic trypsinogen gene), the $SPINK_1$ gene (pancreatic secretory trypsin inhibitor – PSTI – gene) and the K_8 gene (keratin 8 gene).

7.3.1 Pancreatitis Associated with Sphincter of Oddi Dysfunctions and Biliary Lithiasis

The abnormalities of sphincter of Oddi contractility (sphincter of Oddi dysfunction – SOD) may be related to the biliary and/or pancreatic portions of the sphincter. Two types of pancreatic SOD have been hypothesised (Corazziari et al. 1999): (1) stenosis is a chronic inflammatory process, probably secondary to biliary lithiasis or microlithiasis, that produces fibrosis and narrows part or all of the sphincter (Corazziari et al. 1999); (2) dyskinesia is a functional alteration of the physiological motility of the sphincter that determines some delay in the passage of the pancreatic juice in duodenum (Hogan and Geenen 1988).

Preliminary data from 107 patients admitted with diagnosed recurring acute pancreatitis (defined as at least two episodes of pancreatitis before hospitalisation) and with an 8-year average follow-up, seen at our institution, shows that biliary lithiasis is the etiology in about 60% of cases. Despite therapeutic procedures (endoscopic sphincterotomy or stenting, medical therapy with bile acids), 25% of these patients developed chronic pancreatitis. The evolution toward chronic pancreatitis seems to be associated with a clinically severe pancreatitis at the first episode (pancreatic necrosis) and with the presence of genetic mutation.

From the preliminary data of the *PanCroInf-AISP* study, under the sponsorship of the Italian Association for the Study of the Pancreas (Associazione Italiana per lo Studio del Pancreas – AISP), which involves 22 Italian centres, on 500 patients suffering from chronic pancreatitis, it appears that stenosis of the sphincter of Oddi can account for approximately 40% of the causes of chronic pancreatitis.

7.3.2 Pancreatitis Associated with Cystic Dystrophy of the Duodenal Wall – Groove Pancreatitis

Cystic dystrophy of the duodenal wall (Potet and Duclert 1970; Flejou et al. 1993; Procacci et al. 1997; Rubay et al. 1999; Glaser et al. 2002), also called groove pancreatitis (Stolte et al. 1982; Becker and Mischke 1991; Fujita et al. 1997; Shudo et al. 2002; Hwang et al. 2003), is a particular kind of chronic pancreatitis that originates along the border of the entire length of the pancreas between the duodenum, the pancreas and the CBD, charaterized by the presence of inflammation or cysts.

There are two hypotheses that have been put forward to explain this unique inflammatory process. The first hypothesis (Stolte et al. 1982), supported by pathologists, maintains that the presence of ectopic pancreatic tissue inside the duodenal wall combined with the presence of an abnormal opening of the Santorini duct into the duodenum through the minor papilla alters the drainage of pancreatic secretion coming from the dorso-cranial pancreas, which would then result in a change in the direction of pancreatic flow from the minor Santorini duct towards the main duct of Wirsung. This non-physiologic flow, when associated with altered visocity of the pancreatic juice secondary to alcohol abuse, would be responsible for a functional and regional ductal obstruction producing localized CP.

The second hypothesis (Adda et al. 1984) states that the damage may be secondary to an incomplete embryologic rotation of the ventral pancreatic buds. This results in heterotopic pancreatic tissue within the duodenal wall without an efficient ductal drainage system. As the pancreatic secretion becomes altered by alcohol or other exogenous challenges, the situation of a functional obstruction to the flow of pancreatic juice results in CP. This hypothesis, would explain why, in some cases, the inflammatory/dystrophy cystic mass within the duodenal wall presents on the external face of the duodenum away from the groove.

The anatomic abnormality would initially be regional with the presence of cysts and pancreatitis only at the pancreatic head, in the groove. At a later stage, the increasing volume of inflammatory tissue and/or cysts would compress the Wirsung's duct, resulting in a stenosis and obstructive pancreatitis upstream. The process can also involve the main CBD (causing jaundice) and the duodenum (causing upper intestinal obstruction).

7.3.3 Autoimmune Pancreatitis

The possibility of an autoimmune etiology in the pathogenesis of chronic pancreatitis has been considered since the 1950s, but has never been demonstrated.

Experimentally, the instillation of tri-nitro-benzene sulfonic acid (TNBS) into the pancreatic duct of rats induced anatomic and histologic pancreatic changes similar to those observed in human chronic pancreatitis (Puig-Divi et al. 1996). TNBS acts as a hapten, alters the membranes of the epithelium and changes the antigenic profile of the pancreatic ducts. The new formatted antigen stimulates an immune T cell-mediated response, with mono- and polymorphonuclear cell infiltration in the pancreas in the first three weeks and subsequent fibrosis in more advanced stages (6 weeks) with progressive acinar atrophy. The authors used alcohol as a "barrier breaker" to facilitate the action of TNBS. Later, the same authors demonstrated that ethanol feeding aggravates the pancreatic injury in TNBS induced pancreatitis (Puig-Divi et al. 1999). The fact that the same substance can produce alterations in the biliary tree (Orth et al. 2000), the colon (Morris et al. 1989; Yamada et al. 1993) as well as the pancreas (Puig-Divi et al. 1996, 1999) may indicate a possible relationship between the immune-mediated diseases of these organs.

The biochemical finding that raises the possibility of an immune-mediated mechanism in the pathogenesis of chronic pancreatitis is the presence of antibodies against carbonic anhydrase type I and II (CA I and CA II) in patients suffering from chronic pancreatitis (Kino-Ohsaki et al. 1996; Frulloni et al. 2000). Carbonic anhydrases are a family of zinc metal enzymes that catalyze the reversible hydration of carbon dioxide to bicarbonate and hydrogen ions. The enzymes are largely distributed in the gastrointestinal tract, in particular in the salivary glands, stomach, duodenum, colon and biliary tract (Lonnerholm et al. 1985). CA II antigens are characteristically present in the pancreatic ductal epithelium (Lonnerholm et al. 1985; Parkkila et al. 1994), and therefore the presence of antibodies against this isoenzyme may provide evidence of an immune reaction to a pancreatic target antigen. Non-specific auto-antibodies, such as antinuclear antibodies, were found to be present in some patients suffering from chronic pancreatitis (Frulloni et al. 2000). Recently, serum IgG4 has been proposed as a marker of autoimmune pancreatitis. However in our experience serum IgG4 may be elevated in all pancreatic diseases.

Clinically, the association between chronic pancreatitis and assumed autoimmune diseases of the gastrointestinal tract has been widely reported in the literature (Cavallini and Frulloni 2001).

Pathological findings in patients with autoimmune pancreatitis seem to show a typical pattern (Cavallini and Frulloni 2001; Okazaki and Chiba 2002; Saito et al. 2002; Kamisawa et al. 2003; Pearson et al. 2003; Taniguchi et al. 2000). There is a rich inflammatory cellular infiltration, localised mainly around the pancreatic ducts, but also involving the other pancreatic structures (acini, vessels, nerves). Lymphocytes and granulocytes are present around the affected ducts, with rupture of the ductal basal membrane and, in some cases, complete ductal destruction (Pearson et al. 2003; Taniguchi et al. 2000; Bovo et al. 1987; Bedossa et al. 1990). Cytological material, obtained by fine needle aspiration biopsy (FNAB), may show the presence of large numbers of lymphocytes, plasma cells and granulocytes. An increased expression of the major antigen of histocompatibility type II (HLA-DR) may be observed in the epithelial cells of the pancreatic ducts that normally do not express this antigen (Bovo et al. 1987; Bedossa et al. 1990; Jalleh et al.1993).

7.3.4 Pancreatitis Associated with Gene Mutations

The discovery of a genetic mutation of cationic trypsinogen gene (PRSS1) in 1996 (Whitcomb et al. 1996) opened the chapter of "pancreatitis associated with gene mutations" and, for the first time, clinically demonstrated the relationship between acute recurrent and chronic pancreatitis. Mutations of the cystic fibrosis (CFTR) gene, the pancreatic secretory trypsin inhibitor (SPINK1) gene and the keratin 8 gene have also been described.

In the duodenum, cationic trypsin plays a central role in the digestion of dietary proteins and in activating all the others pancreatic pro-enzymes (see Chap. 1). To date, 20 genetic variants have been identified in the cationic trypsinogen gene (PRSS1) of patients with hereditary, familial, or sporadic chronic pancreatitis (Whitcomb et al. 1996; Creighton et al. 2000; Howes et al. 2001; Chen et al. 2001; Le Marechal et al. 2001; Simon et al. 2002; Pfutzer et al. 2002; Teich et al. 2004) and the assumed mechanisms involve increased activation or decreased inactivation of trypsin. Therefore, the inappropriate (intra-pancreatic) activation of trypsin, genetically determined, promotes the onset of acute recurring pancreatitis, which later develops into chronic pancreatitis.

Pancreatic Secretory Trypsin Inhibitor (PSTI) or Serine Protease Inhibitor Kazal type 1 (SPINK1), is a peptide that specifically inhibits trypsin from blocking its active site. SPINK1 is synthesized in the acinar cells and co-localized with trypsinogen into zymogen granules. It represents a defensive mechanism inside the pancreas because it prevents the premature and inappropriate activation of the trypsin in acinar cells, the interstitial space and the ductal system. Mutations of the gene coding for SPINK1 result in an intra-pancreatic activation of trypsin that, similarly to PRSS1 mutations, initially lead to acute pancreatitis and later to CP (Witt et al. 2000; Kaneko et al. 2001; Bhatia et al. 2002; Chandak et al. 2002; Drenth et al.2002; Threadgold et al. 2002; Le Marechal et al.2004).

Severe mutations in both alleles of the cystic fibrosis transmembrane conductance regulator (CFTR) gene result in the onset of clinical features of cystic fibrosis (Cavallini et al. 1994; Cohn et al. 1998; Sharer et al. 1998; Castellani et al. 1999; Arduino et al. 1999; Gomez et al. 2000; Ockenga et al. 2000; Monaghan et al. 2000; Malats et al. 2001; Bhatia et al. 2000; Castellani et al. 2001; Truninger et al. 2001; Gomez Lira et al. 2001; Kostuch et al. 2002; Gaia et al. 2002; Lee et al. 2003; Pezzilli et al. 2003; Reboul et al. 2003). The frequency of CFTR gene mutations are significantly higher in patients suffering from acute recurrent pancreatitis than in the general population. The recurrent episodes of pancreatitis lead to dilation of the main pancreatic duct and later, to the onset of pancreatic calcifications (Cavallini et al. 1994). The pathogenesis of pancreatitis in patients with cystic fibrosis may be secondary to the alteration in the composition of the pancreatic juice, with low levels of water and chloride accompanied by markedly increased water and sodium from the lumen of the pancreatic ducts. The resulting hyperconcentration of pancreatic juice faciliates the precipitation of proteins (protein plugs) causing intraductal obstruction. An alternative hypothesis involves the impairment of intraductal pH, with modifications in the transport of zymogen granules in the acinar cells and intracellular activation of proteolytic enzymes (Freedman et al. 2001).

Finally, a single mutation of the keratin 8 (K8) gene, resulting in the replacement of glycine with cysteine at amino acid position 61 (G61C), was found to be associated with chronic pancreatitis (Cavestro et al. 2003). Pancreatic epithelial cells express cytoplasmatic K8/K18 exclusively. Epithelial keratins may play a relevant role in the regulation of exocrine pancreas homeostasis and disruption of the mechanisms that normally regulate keratin expression; this may cause alteration in the processing and/or secretion of zymogen granules.

7.3.5 Pancreatitis Associated with Pancreatic and Peripancreatic Anomalies

Pancreas divisum is thought to arise from a failure of the dorsal and ventral ducts of the fetal pancreas to fuse during the second month of development. The duct of Wirsung drains the ventral pancreas and uncinate process through the major papilla, whereas the duct of Santorini drains the dorsal pancreas through the minor papilla. This leads to two separate pancreatic drainage systems.

The role of pancreas divisum as a cause of acute, recurrent pancreatitis and chronic pancreatitis is controversial (Burtin et al. 1991; Carr-Locke 1991; Cunningham 1992; Chowdhury et al. 1997; Varshney and Johnson 1999). The pathogenesis of pancreatitis associated with pancreas divisum may be secondary to functional stenosis of the dorsal duct. In pancreas divisum, most of the pancreatic secretion drains by means of the duct of Santorini through the orifice of the minor papilla that is inadequate to accommodate the volume of juice that must drain. It is unclear just how many patients with pancreas divisum eventually develop pancreatitis, because the onset of pancreatic pain is so variable, ranging anywhere from early childhood to persons in their 40s. Several investigators have reported epidemiological studies showing an increased incidence of pancreas divisum in patients undergoing investigations for unexplained pancreatitis (Cunningham 1992; Bernard et al. 1990; Dhar et al. 1996; Lu 1998).

Other anatomic anomalies such as duodenal or periampullary diverticula (Shallman and Kolts 1987; Shemesh et al. 1987; Uomo et al. 1996; Lobo et al. 1999; Naranjo-Chavez et al. 2000), santorinicele (Eisen et al. 1994; Seibert and Matulis 1995; Costamagna et al. 2000; Peterson and Slivka

2001), and choledochal cysts (SWISHER et al. 1994; RIZZO et al. 1995; SUGIYAMA et al. 1999; HIRAMATSU et al. 2001; ZHAO et al. 1999) can obstruct the pancreatic ductal orifice leading to relapsing, episodic acute pancreatitis.

Annular pancreas (PAULINO-NETTO and PAULINO 1963; AHMED et al. 1982; CHEVILLOTTE et al. 1984; GILINSKY et al. 1987; DOWSETT et al. 1989; YOGI et al. 1999) is a rare anomaly in which a band of pancreatic tissue either completely or incompletely surrounds the descending portion of the duodenum and is in continuity with the head of the pancreas. The anomaly is often discovered incidentally and/or at autopsy. Some patients with this anomaly develop duodenal stenosis, obstructive jaundice, and pancreatitis. Most individuals remain asymptomatic and the anomaly is only discovered accidentally in adulthood.

7.3.6 Other Causes

Other causes of pancreatitis secondary to obstruction of the main pancreatic duct may be the slow-growing biliary (tumour of the papilla of Vater) and pancreatic tumours (endocrine tumours, serous or mucinous cystadenoma). The pathogenic mechanism is partial obstruction of the Wirsung duct by direct compression of the tumour, causing an obstructive pancreatitis upstream of the stenosis.

We may frequently observe a sequela of acute necrotizing pancreatitis (pseudocysts, ductal stenosis, parenchymal scars). Pathogenesis may be related to direct compression of the pseudocysts on the Wirsung duct, ductal fibrosis after ductal inflammation or fibrotic retraction over the duct near the pancreatic necrotic tissue.

References

Adda G, Hannoun L, Loygue J (1984) Development of the human pancreas: variations and pathology. A tentative classification. Anat Clin 5:275–283

Ahmed A, Chan KF, Song IS (1982) Annular pancreas. J Comput Assist Tomogr 6:409–411

Altomare E, Grattagliano I, Vendemiale G, Palmieri V, Palasciano G (1996) Acute ethanol administration induces oxidative changes in rat pancreatic tissue. Gut 38:742–746

Ammann RW, Heitz PU, Kloppel G (1996) Course of alcoholic chronic pancreatitis: a prospective clinicomorphological long-term study. Gastroenterology 111:224–231

Apte MV, Wilson JS (2003) Stellate cell activation in alcoholic pancreatitis. Pancreas 27:316–320

Apte MV, Haber PS, Darby SJ, Rodgers SC, McCaughan GW, Korsten MA, Pirola RC, Wilson JS (1999) Pancreatic stellate cells are activated by proinflammatory cytokines: implications for pancreatic fibrogenesis. Gut 44:534–541

Apte MV, Phillips PA, Fahmy RG, Darby SJ, Rodgers SC, McCaughan GW, Korsten MA, Pirola RC, Naidoo D, Wilson JS (2000) Does alcohol directly stimulate pancreatic fibrogenesis? Studies with rat pancreatic stellate cells. Gastroenterology 118:780–794

Arduino C, Gallo M, Brusco A, Garnerone S, Piana MR, Di Maggio S, Gerbino Promis G, Ferrone M, Angeli A, Gaia E (1999) Polyvariant mutant CFTR genes in patients with chronic pancreatitis. Clin Genet 56:400–404

Becker V, Mischke U (1991) Groove pancreatitis. Int J Pancreatol 10:173–182

Bedossa P, Bacci J, Lemaigre G, Martin E (1990) Lymphocyte subsets and HLA-DR expression in normal pancreas and chronic pancreatitis. Pancreas 5:415–420

Bernard JP, Sahel J, Giovannini M, Sarles H (1990) Pancreas divisum is a probable cause of acute pancreatitis: a report of 137 cases. Pancreas 5:248–254

Bhatia E, Durie P, Zielenski J, Lam D, Sikora SS, Choudhuri G, Tsui LC (2000) Mutations in the cystic fibrosis transmembrane regulator gene in patients with tropical calcific pancreatitis. Am J Gastroenterol 95:3658–3659

Bhatia E, Choudhuri G, Sikora SS, Landt O, Kage A, Becker M, Witt H (2002) Tropical calcific pancreatitis: strong association with SPINK1 trypsin inhibitor mutations. Gastroenterology 123:1020–1025

Bovo P, Mirakian R, Merigo F, Angelini G, Cavallini G, Rizzini P, Bottazzo GF, Scuro LA (1987) HLA molecule expression on chronic pancreatitis specimens: is there a role for autoimmunity? A preliminary study. Pancreas 2:350–356

Burtin P, Person B, Charneau J, Boyer J (1991) Pancreas divisum and pancreatitis: a coincidental association? Endoscopy 23:55–58

Carr-Locke DL (1991) Pancreas divisum: the controversy goes on? Endoscopy 23:88–90

Castellani C, Bonizzato A, Rolfini R, Frulloni L, Cavallini GC, Mastella G (1999) Increased prevalence of mutations of the cystic fibrosis gene in idiopathic chronic and recurrent pancreatitis. Am J Gastroenterol 94:1993–1995

Castellani C, Gomez Lira M, Frulloni L, Delmarco A, Marzari M, Bonizzato A, Cavallini G, Pignatti P, Mastella G (2001) Analysis of the entire coding region of the cystic fibrosis transmembrane regulator gene in idiopathic pancreatitis. Hum Mutat 18:166

Cavallini G, Frulloni L (2001) Autoimmunity and chronic pancreatitis: a concealed relationship. JOP 2:61–68

Cavallini G, Talamini G, Vaona B, Bovo P, Filippini M, Rigo L, Angelini G, Vantini I, Riela A, Frulloni L (1994) Effect of alcohol and smoking on pancreatic lithogenesis in the course of chronic pancreatitis. Pancreas 9:42–46

Cavallini G, Bovo P, Bianchini E, Carsana A, Costanzo C, Merola M, Sgarbi D, Frulloni L, Di Francesco V, Libonati M, Palmieri M (1998) Lithostathine messenger RNA expression in different types of chronic pancreatitis. Mol Cell Biochem 185:147–152

Cavestro GM, Frulloni L, Nouvenne A, Neri TM, Calore B, Ferri B, Bovo P, Okolicsanyi L, Di Mario F, Cavallini G (2003) Association of keratin 8 gene mutation with chronic pancreatitis. Dig Liver Dis 35:416–420

Chandak GR, Idris MM, Reddy DN, Bhaskar S, Sriram PV, Singh L (2002) Mutations in the pancreatic secretory trypsin inhibitor gene (PSTI/SPINK1) rather than the cationic trypsinogen gene (PRSS1) are significantly associated with tropical calcific pancreatitis. J Med Genet 39:347–351

Chen JM, Piepoli Bis A, Le Bodic L, Ruszniewski P, Robaszkiewicz M, Deprez PH, Raguenes O, Quere I, Andriulli A, Ferec C (2001) Mutational screening of the cationic trypsinogen gene in a large cohort of subjects with idiopathic chronic pancreatitis. Clin Genet 59:189–193

Chevillotte G, Sahel J, Raillat A, Sarles H (1984) Annular pancreas. Report of one case associated with acute pancreatitis and diagnosed by endoscopic retrograde pancreatography. Dig Dis Sci 29:75–77

Chowdhury A, Chatterjee BK, Dutta P, Roy J, Chowdhury T, Das K, Goenka MK (1997) Pancreas divisum with chronic calcific pancreatitis: cause or coincidence. Trop Gastroenterol 18:172–173

Cohn JA, Friedman KJ, Noone PG, Knowles MR, Silverman LM, Jowell PS (1998) Relation between mutations of the cystic fibrosis gene and idiopathic pancreatitis. N Engl J Med 339:653–658

Corazziari E, Shaffer EA, Hogan WJ, Sherman S, Toouli J (1999) Functional disorders of the biliary tract and pancreas. Gut 45 (Suppl 2):II48–54

Costamagna G, Ingrosso M, Tringali A, Mutignani M, Manfredi R (2000) Santorinicele and recurrent acute pancreatitis in pancreas divisum: diagnosis with dynamic secretin-stimulated magnetic resonance pancreatography and endoscopic treatment. Gastrointest Endosc 52:262–267

Creighton JE, Lyall R, Wilson DI, Curtis A, Charnley RM (2000) Mutations of the cationic trypsinogen gene in patients with hereditary pancreatitis. Br J Surg 87:170–175

Cunningham JT (1992) Pancreas divisum and acute pancreatitis: romancing the stone? Am J Gastroenterol 87:802–803

Dhar A, Goenka MK, Kochhar R, Nagi B, Bhasin DK, Singh K (1996) Pancrease divisum: five years' experience in a teaching hospital. Indian J Gastroenterol 15:7–9

Dite P, Stary K, Novotny I, Precechtelova M, Dolina J, Lata J, Zboril V (2001) Incidence of chronic pancreatitis in the Czech Republic. Eur J Gastroenterol Hepatol 13:749–750

Drenth JP, Morsche R, Jansen JB (2002) Mutations in serine protease inhibitor Kazal type 1 are strongly associated with chronic pancreatitis. Gut 50:687–692

Dowsett JF, Rode J, Russell RC (1989) Annular pancreas: a clinical, endoscopic, and immunohistochemical study. Gut 30:130–135

Dufour MC, Adamson MD (2003) The epidemiology of alcohol-induced pancreatitis. Pancreas 27:286–290

Eisen G, Schutz S, Metzler D, Baillie J, Cotton PB (1994) Santorinicele: new evidence for obstruction in pancreas divisum. Gastrointest Endosc 40:73–76

Flejou JF, Potet F, Molas G, Bernades P, Amouyal P, Fekete F (1993) Cystic dystrophy of the gastric and duodenal wall developing in heterotopic pancreas: an unrecognised entity. Gut 34:343–347

Freedman SD, Kern HF, Scheele GA (2001) Pancreatic acinar cell dysfunction in CFTR (-/-) mice is associated with impairments in luminal pH and endocytosis. Gastroenterology 121:950–957

Frulloni L, Bovo P, Brunelli S, Vaona B, Di Francesco V, Nishimori I, Cavallini G (2000) Elevated serum levels of antibodies to carbonic anhydrase I and II in patients with chronic pancreatitis. Pancreas 20:382–388

Frulloni L, Castellani C, Bovo P, Vaona B, Calore B, Liani C, Mastella G, Cavallini G (2003) Natural history of pancreatitis associated with cystic fibrosis gene mutations. Dig Liver Dis 35:179–185

Fujita N, Shirai Y, Tsukada K, Kurosaki I, Iiai T, Hatakeyama K (1997) Groove pancreatitis with recurrent duodenal obstruction. Report of a case successfully treated with pylorus-preserving pancreatico-duodenectomy. Int J Pancreatol 21:185–188

Gaia E, Salacone P, Gallo M, Promis GG, Brusco A, Bancone C, Carlo A (2002) Germline mutations in CFTR and PSTI genes in chronic pancreatitis patients. Dig Dis Sci 47:2416–2421

Gilinsky NH, Lewis JW, Flueck JA, Fried AM (1987) Annular pancreas associated with diffuse chronic pancreatitis. Am J Gastroenterol 82:681–684

Glaser M, Roskar Z, Skalicky M, Krajnc I (2002) Cystic dystrophy of the duodenal wall in a heterotopic pancreas. Wien Klin Wochenschr 114:1013–1016

Gomez Lira M, Benetazzo MG, Marzari MG, Bombieri C, Belpinati F, Castellani C, Cavallini GC, Mastella G, Pignatti PF (2000) High frequency of cystic fibrosis transmembrane regulator mutation L997F in patients with recurrent idiopathic pancreatitis and in newborns with hypertrypsinemia. Am J Hum Genet 66:2013–2014

Gomez Lira M, Patuzzo C, Castellani C, Bovo P, Cavallini G, Mastella G, Pignatti PF (2001) CFTR and cationic trypsinogen mutations in idiopathic pancreatitis and neonatal hypertrypsinemia. Pancreatology 1:538–542

Gutierrez-Ruiz MC, Robles-Diaz G, Kershenobich D (2002) Emerging concepts in inflammation and fibrosis. Arch Med Res 33:595–599

Haber PS, Wilson JS, Apte MV, Pirola RC (1993) Fatty acid ethyl esters increase rat pancreatic lysosomal fragility. J Lab Clin Med 121:759–764

Haber PS, Wilson JS, Apte MV, Korsten MA, Pirola RC (1994) Chronic ethanol consumption increases the fragility of rat pancreatic zymogen granules. Gut 35:1474–1478

Haber PS, Apte MV, Applegate TL, Norton ID, Korsten MA, Pirola RC, Wilson JS (1998) Metabolism of ethanol by rat pancreatic acinar cells. J Lab Clin Med 132:294–302

Haber PS, Keogh GW, Apte MV, Moran CS, Stewart NL, Crawford DH, Pirola RC, McCaughan GW, Ramm GA, Wilson JS (1999) Activation of pancreatic stellate cells in human and experimental pancreatic fibrosis. Am J Pathol 155:1087–1095

Hajnal F, Flores MC, Radley S, Valenzuela JE (1990) Effect of alcohol and alcoholic beverages on meal-stimulated pancreatic secretion in humans. Gastroenterology 98:191–196

Hiramatsu K, Paye F, Kianmanesh AR, Sauvanet A, Terris B, Belghiti J (2001) Choledochal cyst and benign stenosis of the main pancreatic duct. J Hepatobiliary Pancreat Surg 8:92–94

Hogan WJ, Geenen JE (1988) Biliary dyskinesia. Endoscopy 20 (Suppl 1):179–183

Howes N, Greenhalf W, Rutherford S, O'Donnell M, Mountford R, Ellis I, Whitcomb D, Imrie C, Drumm B, Neoptolemos JP (2001) A new polymorphism for the RI22H mutation in hereditary pancreatitis. Gut 48:247–250

Hwang JY, Park KS, Cho KB, Hwang JS, Ahn SH, Park SK, Kwon JH (2003) Segmental groove pancreatitis: report of one case. Korean J Intern Med 18:234–237

Jalleh RP, Gilbertson JA, Williamson RC, Slater SD, Foster CS (1993) Expression of major histocompatibility antigens in human chronic pancreatitis. Gut 34:1452–1457

Kamisawa T, Funata N, Hayashi Y, Tsuruta K, Okamoto A, Amemiya K, Egawa N, Nakajima H (2003) Close relationship between autoimmune pancreatitis and multifocal fibrosclerosis. Gut 52:683–687

Kaneko K, Nagasaki Y, Furukawa T, Mizutamari H, Sato A, Masamune A, Shimosegawa T, Horii A (2001) Analysis of the human pancreatic secretory trypsin inhibitor (PSTI) gene mutations in Japanese patients with chronic pancreatitis. J Hum Genet 46:293–297

Karanjia ND, Widdison AL, Leung F, Alvarez C, Lutrin FJ, Reber HA (1994) Compartment syndrome in experimental chronic obstructive pancreatitis: effect of decompressing the main pancreatic duct. Br J Surg 81:259–264

Kino-Ohsaki J, Nishimori I, Morita M, Okazaki K, Yamamoto Y, Onishi S, Hollingsworth MA (1996) Serum antibodies to carbonic anhydrase I and II in patients with idiopathic chronic pancreatitis and Sjogren's syndrome. Gastroenterology 110:1579–1586

Kloppel G, Maillet B (1992) The morphological basis for the evolution of acute pancreatitis into chronic pancreatitis. Virchows Arch A Pathol Anat Histopathol 420:1–4

Konishi K, Izumi R, Kato O, Yamaguchi A, Miyazaki I (1981) Experimental pancreatolithiasis in the dog. Surgery 89:687–691

Korsten MA, Wilson JS, Haber PS (1994) An overview of extrapancreatic factors in the pathogenesis of alcoholic pancreatitis. Alcohol Alcohol Suppl 2:377–384

Kostuch M, Rudzki S, Semczuk A, Kulczycki L (2002) CFTR gene mutations in patients suffering from acute pancreatitis. Med Sci Monit 8:BR369–372

Lankisch PG, Assmus C, Maisonneuve P, Lowenfels AB (2002) Epidemiology of pancreatic diseases in Luneburg County. A study in a defined german population. Pancreatology 2:469–477

Le Marechal C, Bretagne JF, Raguenes O, Quere I, Chen JM, Ferec C (2001) Identification of a novel pancreatitis-associated missense mutation, R116C, in the human cationic trypsinogen gene (PRSS1). Mol Genet Metab 74:342–344

Le Marechal C, Chen JM, Le Gall C, Plessis G, Chipponi J, Chuzhanova NA, Raguenes O, Ferec C (2004) Two novel severe mutations in the pancreatic secretory trypsin inhibitor gene (SPINK1) cause familial and/or hereditary pancreatitis. Hum Mutat 23:205

Lee JH, Choi JH, Namkung W, Hanrahan JW, Chang J, Song SY, Park SW, Kim DS, Yoon JH, Suh Y, Jang IJ, Nam JH, Kim SJ, Cho MO, Lee JE, Kim KH, Lee MG (2003) A haplotype-based molecular analysis of CFTR mutations associated with respiratory and pancreatic diseases. Hum Mol Genet 12:2321–2332

Lerch MM, Albrecht E, Ruthenburger M, Mayerle J, Halangk W, Kruger B (2003) Pathophysiology of alcohol-induced pancreatitis. Pancreas 27:291–296

Letko G, Siech M, Sokolowski A, Spormann H (1989) Experimental acute pancreatitis in rats after chronic and chronic plus acute ethanol administration in combination with a pancreatic juice edema. Int Surg 74:77–80

Lin Y, Tamakoshi A, Hayakawa T, Ogawa M, Ohno Y (2001) Associations of alcohol drinking and nutrient intake with chronic pancreatitis: findings from a case-control study in Japan. Am J Gastroenterol 96:2622–2627

Lobo DN, Balfour TW, Iftikhar SY, Rowlands BJ (1999) Periampullary diverticula and pancreatico-biliary disease. Br J Surg 86:588–597

Lonnerholm G, Selking O, Wistrand PJ (1985) Amount and distribution of carbonic anhydrases CA I and CA II in the gastrointestinal tract. Gastroenterology 88:1151–1161

Lu WF (1998) ERCP and CT diagnosis of pancreas divisum and its relation to etiology of chronic pancreatitis. World J Gastroenterol 4:150–152

Malats N, Casals T, Porta M, Guarner L, Estivill X, Real FX (2001) Cystic fibrosis transmembrane regulator (CFTR) DeltaF508 mutation and 5T allele in patients with chronic pancreatitis and exocrine pancreatic cancer. PANKRAS II Study Group. Gut 48:70–74

Monaghan KG, Jackson CE, KuKuruga DL, Feldman GL (2000) Mutation analysis of the cystic fibrosis and cationic trypsinogen genes in patients with alcohol-related pancreatitis. Am J Med Genet 94:120–124

Morris GP, Beck PL, Herridge MS, Depew WT, Szewczuk MR, Wallace JL (1989) Hapten-induced model of chronic inflammation and ulceration in the rat colon. Gastroenterology 96:795–803

Naranjo-Chavez J, Schwarz M, Leder G, Beger HG (2000) Ampullary but not periampullary duodenal diverticula are an etiologic factor for chronic pancreatitis. Dig Surg 17:358–363

Ockenga J, Stuhrmann M, Ballmann M, Teich N, Keim V, Dork T, Manns MP (2000) Mutations of the cystic fibrosis gene, but not cationic trypsinogen gene, are associated with recurrent or chronic idiopathic pancreatitis. Am J Gastroenterol 95:2061–2067

Okazaki K, Chiba T (2002) Autoimmune related pancreatitis. Gut 51:1–4

Orth T, Neurath M, Schirmacher P, Galle PR, Mayet WJ (2000) A novel rat model of chronic fibrosing cholangitis induced by local administration of a hapten reagent into the dilated bile duct is associated with increased TNF-alpha production and autoantibodies. J Hepatol 33:862–872

Pap A, Boros L (1989) Alcohol-induced chronic pancreatitis in rats after temporary occlusion of biliopancreatic ducts with Ethibloc. Pancreas 4:249–255

Parkkila S, Parkkila AK, Juvonen T, Rajaniemi H (1994) Distribution of the carbonic anhydrase isoenzymes I, II, and VI in the human alimentary tract. Gut 35:646–650

Paulino-Netto A, Paulino F (1963) Annular pancreas: report of a case. Am J Dig Dis 8:448–453

Pearson RK, Longnecker DS, Chari ST, Smyrk TC, Okazaki K, Frulloni L, Cavallini G (2003) Controversies in clinical pancreatology: autoimmune pancreatitis: does it exist? Pancreas 27:1–13

Peterson MS, Slivka A (2001) Santorinicele in pancreas divisum: diagnosis with secretin-stimulated magnetic resonance pancreatography. Abdom Imaging 26:260–263

Pezzilli R, Morselli-Labate AM, Mantovani V, Romboli E, Selva P, Migliori M, Corinaldesi R, Gullo L (2003) Mutations of the CFTR gene in pancreatic disease. Pancreas 27:332–336

Pfutzer R, Myers E, Applebaum-Shapiro S, Finch R, Ellis I, Neoptolemos J, Kant JA, Whitcomb DC (2002) Novel cationic trypsinogen (PRSS1) N29T and R122C mutations cause autosomal dominant hereditary pancreatitis. Gut 50:271–272

Pitchumoni CS (2001) Pathogenesis of alcohol-induced chronic pancreatitis: facts, perceptions, and misperceptions. Surg Clin North Am 81:379–390

Pitchumoni CS, Jain NK, Lowenfels AB, DiMagno EP (1988) Chronic cyanide poisoning: unifying concept for alcoholic and tropical pancreatitis. Pancreas 3:220–322

Potet F, Duclert N (1970) Cystic dystrophy on aberrant pancreas of the duodenal wall. Arch Fr Mal App Dig 59:223–238

Procacci C, Graziani R, Zamboni G, Cavallini G, Pederzoli P, Guarise A, Bogina G, Biasiutti C, Carbognin G, Bergamo-Andreis IA, Pistolesi GF (1997) Cystic dystrophy of the duodenal wall: radiologic findings. Radiology 205:741–747

Puig-Divi V, Molero X, Salas A, Guarner F, Guarner L, Malagelada JR (1996) Induction of chronic pancreatic disease by trinitrobenzene sulfonic acid infusion into rat pancreatic ducts. Pancreas 13:417–424

Puig-Divi V, Molero X, Vaquero E, Salas A, Guarner F, Malagelada J (1999) Ethanol feeding aggravates morphological and biochemical parameters in experimental chronic pancreatitis. Digestion 60:166–174

Reboul MP, Laharie D, Amouretti M, Lacombe D, Iron A (2003) Isolated idiopathic chronic pancreatitis associated with a compound heterozygosity for two mutations of the CFTR gene. Gastroenterol Clin Biol 27:821–824

Rinderknecht H, Stace NH, Renner IG (1985) Effects of chronic alcohol abuse on exocrine pancreatic secretion in man. Dig Dis Sci 30:65–71

Rizzo RJ, Szucs RA, Turner MA (1995) Congenital abnormalities of the pancreas and biliary tree in adults. Radiographics 15:49–68; quiz 147–148

Rubay R, Bonnet D, Gohy P, Laka A, Deltour D (1999) Cystic dystrophy in heterotopic pancreas of the duodenal wall: medical and surgical treatment. Acta Chir Belg 99:87–91

Runzi M, Saluja A, Lerch MM, Dawra R, Nishino H, Steer ML (1993) Early ductal decompression prevents the progression of biliary pancreatitis: an experimental study in the opossum. Gastroenterology 105:157–164

Saito T, Tanaka S, Yoshida H, Imamura T, Ukegawa J, Seki T, Ikegami A, Yamamura F, Mikami T, Aoyagi Y, Niikawa J, Mitamura K (2002) A case of autoimmune pancreatitis responding to steroid therapy. Evidence of histologic recovery. Pancreatology 2:550–556

Sarles H (1986) Etiopathogenesis and definition of chronic pancreatitis. Dig Dis Sci 31:91S–107S

Sarles H, Berger Z (1989) Chronic calcifying pancreatitis: epidemiology and current concept of the lithogenesis. Acta Med Hung 46:225–233

Sarles H, Lebreuil G, Tasso F, Figarella C, Clemente F, Devaux MA, Fagonde B, Payan H (1971) A comparison of alcoholic pancreatitis in rat and man. Gut 12:377–388

Sarles H, Adler G, Dani R, Frey C, Gullo L, Harada H, Martin E, Norohna M, Scuro LA (1989a) Classifications of pancreatitis and definition of pancreatic diseases. Digestion 43:234–236

Sarles H, Adler G, Dani R, Frey C, Gullo L, Harada H, Martin E, Norohna M, Scuro LA (1989b) The pancreatitis classification of Marseilles-Rome 1988. Scand J Gastroenterol 24:641–642

Schneider A, Whitcomb DC, Singer MV (2002) Animal models in alcoholic pancreatitis – what can we learn? Pancreatology 2:189–203

Seibert DG, Matulis SR (1995) Santorinicele as a cause of chronic pancreatic pain. Am J Gastroenterol 90:121–123

Shallman RW, Kolts RL (1987) Duodenojejunostomy for pancreatitis secondary to periampullary duodenal diverticula. Arch Surg 122:850–851

Sharer N, Schwarz M, Malone G, Howarth A, Painter J, Super M, Braganza J (1998) Mutations of the cystic fibrosis gene in patients with chronic pancreatitis. N Engl J Med 339:645–652

Shemesh E, Friedman E, Czerniak A, Bat L (1987) The association of biliary and pancreatic anomalies with periampullary duodenal diverticula. Correlation with clinical presentations. Arch Surg 122:1055–1057

Shudo R, Yazaki Y, Sakurai S, Uenishi H, Yamada H, Sugawara K, Okamura M, Yamaguchi K, Terayama H, Yamamoto Y (2002) Groove pancreatitis: report of a case and review of the clinical and radiologic features of groove pancreatitis reported in Japan. Intern Med 41:537–542

Simon P, Weiss FU, Sahin-Toth M, Parry M, Nayler O, Lenfers B, Schnekenburger J, Mayerle J, Domschke W, Lerch MM (2002) Hereditary pancreatitis caused by a novel PRSS1 mutation (Arg-122→ Cys) that alters autoactivation and autodegradation of cationic trypsinogen. J Biol Chem 277:5404–5410

Stolte M, Weiss W, Volkholz H, Rosch W (1982) A special form of segmental pancreatitis: "groove pancreatitis". Hepatogastroenterology 29:198–208

Sugiyama M, Atomi Y, Kuroda A (1999) Pancreatic disorders associated with anomalous pancreatico-biliary junction. Surgery;126:492–497

Swisher SG, Cates JA, Hunt KK, Robert ME, Bennion RS, Thompson JE, Roslyn JJ, Reber HA (1994) Pancreatitis associated with adult choledochal cysts. Pancreas 9:633–637

Tanaka T, Ichiba Y, Fujii Y, Itoh H, Kodama O, Dohi K (1988) New canine model of chronic pancreatitis due to chronic ischemia with incomplete pancreatic duct obstruction. Digestion 41:149–155

Taniguchi T, Seko S, Okamoto M, Hamasaki A, Ueno H, Inoue F, Nishida O, Miyake N, Mizumoto T (2000) Association of autoimmune pancreatitis and type 1 diabetes: autoimmune exocrinopathy and endocrinopathy of the pancreas. Diabetes Care 23:1592–1594

Teich N, Le Marechal C, Kukor Z, Caca K, Witzigmann H, Chen JM, Toth M, Mossner J, Keim V, Ferec C, Sahin-Toth M (2004) Interaction between trypsinogen isoforms in genetically determined pancreatitis: mutation E79K in cationic trypsin (PRSS1) causes increased transactivation of anionic trypsinogen (PRSS2). Hum Mutat 23:22–31

Threadgold J, Greenhalf W, Ellis I, Howes N, Lerch MM, Simon P, Jansen J, Charnley R, Laugier R, Frulloni L, Olah A, Delhaye M, Ihse I, Schaffalitzky de Muckadell OB, Andren-Sandberg A, Imrie CW, Martinek J, Gress TM, Mountford R, Whitcomb D, Neoptolemos JP (2002) The N34S mutation of SPINK1 (PSTI) is associated with a familial pattern of idiopathic chronic pancreatitis but does not cause the disease. Gut 50:675–681

Truninger K, Malik N, Ammann RW, Muellhaupt B, Seifert B, Muller HJ, Blum HE (2001) Mutations of the cystic fibrosis gene in patients with chronic pancreatitis. Am J Gastroenterol 96:2657–2661

Uomo G, Manes G, Ragozzino A, Cavallera A, Rabitti PG (1996) Periampullary extraluminal duodenal diverticula and acute pancreatitis: an underestimated etiological association. Am J Gastroenterol 91:1186–1188

Vaona B, Armellini F, Bovo P, Rigo L, Zamboni M, Brunori MP, Dall OE, Filippini M, Talamini G, Di Francesco V, Frulloni L, Micciolo R, Cavallini G (1997) Food intake of patients with chronic pancreatitis after onset of the disease. Am J Clin Nutr 65:851–854

Varshney S, Johnson CD (1999) Pancreas divisum. Int J Pancreatol 25:135–141

Whitcomb DC (2001) Hereditary pancreatitis: a model for understanding the genetic basis of acute and chronic pancreatitis. Pancreatology 1:565–570

Whitcomb DC, Gorry MC, Preston RA, Furey W, Sossenheimer MJ, Ulrich CD, Martin SP, Gates LK Jr, Amann ST, Toskes PP, Liddle R, McGrath K, Uomo G, Post JC, Ehrlich GD (1996) Hereditary pancreatitis is caused by a mutation in the cationic trypsinogen gene. Nat Genet 14:141–145

Wilson JS, Apte MV, Thomas MC, Haber PS, Pirola RC (1992) Effects of ethanol, acetaldehyde and cholesteryl esters on pancreatic lysosomes. Gut 33:1099–1104

Witt H, Luck W, Hennies HC, Classen M, Kage A, Lass U, Landt O, Becker M (2000) Mutations in the gene encoding the serine protease inhibitor, Kazal type 1 are associated with chronic pancreatitis. Nat Genet 25:213–216

Yamada T, Sartor RB, Marshall S, Specian RD, Grisham MB (1993) Mucosal injury and inflammation in a model of chronic granulomatous colitis in rats. Gastroenterology 104:759–771

Yogi Y, Kosai S, Higashi S, Iwamura T, Setoguchi T (1999) Annular pancreas associated with pancreatolithiasis: a case report. Hepatogastroenterology 46:527–531

Zhao L, Li Z, Ma H, Zhang X, Mou X, Zhang D, Lin W, Niu A (1999) Congenital choledochal cyst with pancreatitis. Chin Med J (Engl) 112:637–640

Clinical Aspects of Chronic Pancreatitis: Features and Prognosis

8

Luca Frulloni and Giorgio Cavallini

CONTENTS

8.1 **The Different Clinical Aspects of "Inflammatory Pancreatic Diseases"** *129*
8.1.1 Pancreatitis Associated with Sphincter of Oddi Dysfunctions (Sod) and Biliary Lithiasis *130*
8.1.2 Pancreatitis Associated with Cystic Dystrophy of the Duodenal Wall (or Groove Pancreatitis) *131*
8.1.3 Autoimmune Pancreatitis *131*
8.1.4 Pancreatitis Associated with Slow-Growing Pancreatic and Biliary Tumours *131*
8.1.5 Pancreatitis Associated with Pancreatic Anomalies *132*
8.1.6 Pancreatitis Associated with Gene Mutation *132*
8.1.7 Pancreatitis Secondary to Sequelae of Acute Necrotizing Pancreatitis *133*

8.2 **Natural History of Chronic Pancreatitis and Prognosis** *133*

References *134*

The natural history of chronic pancreatitis (CP) is characterised by the appearance of clinical symptoms of acute pancreatitis, that recur and, later, develop towards the chronic more advanced phase, characterised by ductal dilatation, intraductal calcification, and clinical signs of exocrine and endocrine insufficiency.

L. Frulloni, MD, PhD
Department of Gastroenteroloy, Policlinico "GB Rossi", Piazzale LA Scuro 10, 37134 Verona, Italy
G. Cavallini, MD
Department of Gastroenterology, Internal Medicine Section C, Policlinico "GB Rossi", University of Verona, Piazzale LA Scuro 10, 37134 Verona, Italy

Pain is characteristically recurrent and relapsing (Ammann 2001; Ammann and Muellhaupt 1999; Cavallini et al. 1998). The interval between the clinical onset of pancreatitis (1st painful episode) and diagnosis of chronic pancreatitis is quite variable. It appears to be shorter (1–2 years) in patients who have a high alcohol consumption rate (Ammann and Muellhaupt 1999; Cavallini et al. 1998; Otsuki 2003) compared to those who do not drink. The chronic pancreatitis onset-diagnosis interval is considerably longer in the case of pancreatitis associated with genetic mutation (Frulloni et al. 2003).

In the advanced stage, generally 5 years after the diagnosis of chronic pancreatitis, specific signs of exocrine function failure (malabsorption and steathorroea) and endocrine function failure (diabetes) begin to appear (Ammann and Muellhaupt 1999; Cavallini et al. 1998; Otsuki 2003).

Other specific symptoms that can arise in CP may be: (1) nausea, vomiting and epigastric pain, secondary to duodenal obstruction by compression of the pancreatic head, (2) jaundice and cholestasis due to stenosis of the intra-pancreatic choledoch, (3) signs/symptoms secondary to portal hypertension, (4) signs/symptoms secondary to the formation of pseudocysts.

8.1 The Different Clinical Aspects of "Inflammatory Pancreatic Diseases"

Classification of chronic pancreatitis has always been a difficult problem. Many classification systems have been used, all based on the assumption of being able to trace all pancreatic pathologies back to one single pathogenetic mechanism (Steer et al. 1995). The most widely used classification was the Marseilles Classification of 1963 (Sarles 1965), which was then reviewed in 1984 (Singer and Sarles 1985) and again in 1988 (Sarles et al. 1989). The clinical course of the disease was therefore always described by considering the patient as a whole (Cavallini et al. 1998; Dite et al. 2001; Dani et al. 1990; Dufour and Adamson 2003). Currently, we recognize different forms of CP, each displaying somewhat unique clinical, radiological, biochemical and anatomo-pathological characteristics that also demand different therapeutic approaches (medical, endoscopic, surgical). One concept that deserves highlighting is that directly addressing the etiology, where possible, slows down the development of CP.

The clinical characteristics of the different pancreatic pathologies observed at our institution in Verona, Italy, are listed below (Table 8.1).

8.1.1 Pancreatitis Associated with Sphincter of Oddi Dysfunctions (Sod) and Biliary Lithiasis

Stenosis of the sphincter of Oddi (that may occur from a variety of causes) is the most common cause (40% of cases) of CP.

Stenosis of the sphincter of Oddi produces obstruction of the main pancreatic duct. The main pancreatic duct slowly dilates, generally in a uniform manner. As the disease progresses, secondary side branches become distended as well. The formation of intraductal calculi occurs in 36% of patients, although this is a lower frequency than in patients with CP from alcoholism (Cavallini et al. 1996, 1998; Talamini et al. 1996a; Cavallini et al. 1994; Lin et al. 2000; Talamini et al. 1996b; Talamini et al. 2000; Lin et al. 2001).

The clinical course of these patients is characterised by recurrent episodes of pancreatic-type abdominal pain, associated with elevated serum pancreatic enzymes (e.g. lipase and amylase). Biliary (micro) lithiasis is diagnosed in a large percentage of patients at the onset of pancreatitis, but a significant number of cases is not diagnosed until some years later. In these patients, endoscopic sphincterotomy therapy is effective as a method of improving the flow of pancreatic juice across the sphincter into the duodenal lumen (Rosch et al. 2002; Farnbacher et al. 2002; Binmoeller et al. 1995; Smits et al. 1996). The earlier this intervention can be performed, the more effective the result. Intraductal stones can also be removed endoscopically, effectively aided by preprocedural lithotripsy (Farnbacher et al. 2002; Brand et al. 2000).

Further relief from symptoms related to sphincter of Oddi stenosis may be obtained by endoscopically placed stents from the duodenal lumen into the main pancraetic duct. Appropriate patient selection is important to assure the procedure will be used on those who will benefit (Talamini et al. 2000; Lin

Table 8.1. Epidemiological and clinical characteristics in CP patients treated in Verona

Type of Pancreatitis	Estimated prevalence	Sex (M:F)	Alcohol and smoking	Age (onset)	Evolution into CP (Time)	Calcifications
SOD (stenosis)	30%–40%	1:1	Uncommon	30–40	5–10 years	Up to 40%
CDDW	20%–30%	All males	All drinkers and smokers	30–40	Few years	80%–100%
AIP	5%–10%	0.8:1	Rare	Variable	Unknown	Rare
SG-PBT	Less than 5%	1:1	Uncommon	Old	Depend on entity of stricture	Rare
Pancreas divisum	5–10%	0,7:1	Uncommon	20–40	Unknown	Variable
Gene mutations	5%–10%	1,25:1	Rare	10–20	3–5 years	80%–100%
Sequelae of necrotizing pancreatitis	Less than 5%	1:1	Uncommon	40–60	Depend on entity of stricture	30%

SOD = sphincter of Oddi dysphunction; CDDW = cystic dystrophy of the duodenal wall; AIP = autoimmune pancreatitis SG-PBT = slow-growing pancreato-biliary tumours; M = males; F = females

et al. 2001; Binmoeller et al. 1995; Ponchon et al. 1995; Cremer et al. 1991).

8.1.2 Pancreatitis Associated with Cystic Dystrophy of the Duodenal Wall (or Groove Pancreatitis)

CP associated with cystic dystrophy of the duodenal wall (Potet and Duclert 1970; Flejou et al. 1993; Procacci et al. 1997), also termed "groove pancreatitis" (Stolte et al. 1982; Balachandar et al. 1999; Mohl et al. 2001) or "inflammatory mass in the head of the pancreas" (Ozawa et al. 2000; Beger and Buchler 1990; Beger et al. 1990; Muranaka 1990; Eddes et al. 1996) is a distinct clinical entity.

Patients suffering from this particular form of PC are men, aged 30 to 50 years at presentation, heavy drinkers and heavy smokers. Clinically, symptoms of a duodenal obstruction (nausea, vomiting, epigastric pain) or pancreatitis can appear, as well as jaundice, due to compression of the inflammatory mass on the choledochus (CBD). Such symptoms, which are particularly severe in these patients, raise a differential diagnosis of focal pathologies of the head of the pancreas, especially tumours of the pancreatic head or of distal CBD and autoimmune pancreatitis.

Cystic dystrophy of the duodenal wall, especially the cystic form, may fully respond to therapy with octreotide or lanreotide (Rubay et al. 1999; De Parades et al. 1996; Basili et al. 2001); in patients with this form of pancreatitis in an early stage (without involvement of the body-tail of the pancreas) the radical surgery (duodeno-cephalo-pancreasectomy) may cure the disease definitively.

8.1.3 Autoimmune Pancreatitis

Patients suffering from autoimmune pancreatitis (AIP) display symptoms that are not dissimilar to CP from other causes. However, many of them will also having co-existing autoimmune diseases (Crohn's disease, ulcerative colitis, primary sclerosing cholangitis, primary biliary cirrhosis, Sjögren's syndrome); others will manifest systemic associated autoimmune diseases, (systemic lupus erythematosis, Reiter syndrome, retroperitoneal fibrosis), seen in about 50% of patients. These co-morbid conditions may be sub-clinical and should therefore be investigated during the work-up of AIP. In the majority of these patients there are none of the typical pancreatitis risk factors such as alcohol or tobacco abuse. As in other autoimmune diseases, there is a slight preponderance in females.

Clinically, the disease can present as an episode of acute pancreatitis or, more frequently, as a suspected pancreatic tumour (mass-forming pancreatitis). In the first case, the predominant symptom is pancreatic-type pain similar to that seen in mild-oedematous acute pancreatitis. In the second, the symptoms are non specific even presenting as sudden painless jaundice, similar to adenocarcinoma resulting in pancreatico-duodenectomy.

Steroid therapy is the treatment of choice for these patients. A short period (2 weeks) of high dosage steroid treatment, to then be slowly tapered, will bring the disease into complete clinical remission. For this reason the response to steroids is used as a diagnostic criterion for establishing the diagnosis of AIP.

8.1.4 Pancreatitis Associated with Slow-Growing Pancreatic and Biliary Tumours

Slow-growing pancreatic tumours [serous and mucinous cystoadenomas, endocrine tumours, intraductal mucin-producing tumours (IPMT)] may be produce CP.

In patients with these often clinically silent tumours, it is possible that the pancreatic duct obstruction, secondary to the presence of mucus inside the ducts or extrinsic compression, may produce of symptoms of pancreatitis. Misdiagnosing a cystic tumor for a retention cyst leads to the non-removal of the tumour and allows for potential degeneration. In particular, the differential diagnosis between CP and intraductal mucin-producing tumour should be carefully evaluated. The clinical characteristics of intraductal mucin-producing tumours and CP are quite different (Table 8.2).

Ductal adenocarcinomas are also associated with a peritumoral pancreatitis, probably secondary to obstruction of the pancreatic ductal system, but in these cases the predominant symptoms are obviously those related to tumour. Nevertheless, especially in patients who respond to chemo- and/or radiotherapy, it is possible that clinical pictures secondary to chronic pancreatitis also emerge (diabetes, steathorroea).

8.1.5 Pancreatitis Associated with Pancreatic Anomalies

Some congenital anomalies of the pancreas may be associated with pancreatitis. Pancreas divisum is characterised by anatomical alterations of the pancreatic ducts that results in the majority of pancreatic juice being forced to drain from the duct of Santorini into the duodenum through the minor papilla. Three variants have been described (Kleitsch 1955; Stern 1986): (1) type I, or classical divisum, in which there is total failure of fusion of the dorsal and ventral portions of the main pancreatic duct, (2) type II, in which dorsal drainage is dominant in the absence of the main pancreatic duct, (3) type III, or incomplete divisum, where a small communicating branch is present. Large autopsy series estimate pancreas divisum to be present in 5% of the population (Stimec et al. 1996; MacCarty et al. 1975).

Annular pancreas, another pancreatic anomaly, arises from two ventral buds that develop slightly caudal to the dorsal bud, and then the left bud later atrophies but rarely persists to become an annular pancreas.

The clinical significance of pancreatic anomalies, particularly the most common, pancreas divisum, has been the subject of debate for many years (Delhaye et al. 1985; Cunningham 1992; Burtin et al. 1991; Carr-Locke 1991) with opinions varying from that of an innocent congenital anomaly to a significant risk factor for the development of pancreatitis. Evidence to support pancreas divisum as a risk factor for the development of pancreatic disease derives from the observation that there is an increased incidence of the anomaly in subjects with idiopathic pancreatitis of 12%–26% (Dhar et al. 1996).

Compared with patients with pancreatitis and normal duct anatomy, patients with pancreas divisum tend to be younger, more often female, less likely to drink alcohol, and more often have a clinical pattern of recurrent acute attacks of pancreatitis (Bernard et al. 1990).

We most commonly observe an alteration in the drainage of the dorsal duct, but sometimes the ventral duct can be involved with the appearance of ductal dilatation and/or calcifications restricted to the Wirsung duct. Obviously, from a therapeutic point of view, it is very important to diagnose the precise portion of the pancreas involved since the endoscopic therapeutic approach (sphincterotomy or stent placement) can be aimed at the major (ventral duct) or minor (dorsal duct) papilla.

8.1.6 Pancreatitis Associated with Gene Mutation

In the last decade, more and more evidence has suggested that some genetic mutations can be associated with a higher frequency of pancreatitis. Comfort and Steimberg reported a family association of pancreatitis, suggesting that a genetic-type alteration should be sought (Comfort and Steimberg 1952).

That a single mutation of the CFTR gene could be a risk factor for chronic pancreatitis not associated with excessive alcohol consumption was reported in 1994 (Aygalenq et al. 1994). Following this, numerous studies have appeared in literature that confirm a greater frequency of single mutation of the CFTR gene in patients affected by recurrent acute pancreatitis and those with idiopathic chronic pancreatitis (Frulloni et al. 2003; Cohn et al. 1998; Sharer et al. 1998; Arduino et al. 1999; Bhatia

Table 8.2. Comparison of epidemiologic and clinical characteristics in CP vs. IPMT.

	Chronic pancreatitis	Intraductal mucin-producing tumours
Sex (% males)	80%	50%
Age at onset (years–mean)	40	65
Alcohol	Frequent	Rare
Cigarettes smoking	Frequent	Rare
Symptoms at onset	Pain	Diabetes, pain, steathorroea, asymptomatic
Calcifications	Frequent	Rare

et al. 2000; Gomez Lira et al. 2000; Ockenga et al. 2000; Castellani et al. 2001; Truninger et al. 2001; Nishimori and Onishi 2001).

The epidemiological and clinical characteristics of these patients are quite typical. Males seem to be more frequently affected than females, and the onset age is 19 years (Frulloni et al. 2003). Progression to CP takes about 7 years on average, with increasingly numerous episodes of acute pancreatitis 2–3 years after the initial clinical presentation. The presence of calcifications is quite rare (20%), as is exocrine and endocrine pancreatic insufficiency (diabetes and steathorroea) (Frulloni et al. 2003).

In 1996 Withcomb et al. (1996) demonstrated the presence of a mutation (R122H) of the gene that codes for cationic trypsinogen (PRSS1) in patients affected by hereditary pancreatitis, data that was later confirmed by many other studies (Gorry et al. 1997; Elitsur et al. 1998; Chen et al. 1999; Ferec et al. 1999; Ford and Whitcomb 1999; Nishimori et al. 1999; O'Reilly and Kingsnorth 2000; Applebaum-Shapiro et al. 2001; Howes et al. 2001; Le Marechal et al. 2001; Pfutzer et al. 2002; Teich et al. 2004). To date, about 20 new mutations have been described.

Genetically, hereditary pancreatitis is characterised by recessive-type genetic transmission with high penetration, due to the early onset between the age of 1 and 20 years and the really numerous reoccurrence of attacks and development towards chronic pancreatitis. At imaging, a progressive dilatation of the Wirsung duct can be observed with the appearance of a great number of intraductal and glandular calcifications in a very short period of time.

Further genetic mutations that produce CP by affecting trypsin-trypsinogen activation/deactivation are well known. These include mutations in the pancreatic secretory trypsinogen inhibitor gene (PSTI) (Witt et al. 2000; Kaneko et al. 2001; Bhatia et al. 2002; Chandak et al. 2002; Drenth et al. 2002; Threadgold et al. 2002; Le Marechal et al. 2004) and keratin 8 (K8) (Cavestro et al. 2003). We still know very little about the clinical picture associated with these gene mutations which, as with the hypotheses for the single mutation of the CFTR gene, are perhaps not enough on their own to induce the disease, as they may only be modifiers. In this way they may make people prone to the disease but not be the sole cause. Preliminary observations seem to confirm that the natural history of these patients is similar to those affected by pancreatitis associated to mutations of the CFTR gene.

8.1.7 Pancreatitis Secondary to Sequelae of Acute Necrotizing Pancreatitis

CP may arise, albeit infrequently, in patients recovering from severe necrotizing pancreatitis. In a study of 118 patients, we demonstrated the high frequency of ductal alterations in greater than 40% of patients recovering from necrotizing pancreatitis, compared with only 6% of patients affected by oedematous pancreatitis who showed these changes (Angelini et al. 1993). In those patients with necrotizing pancreatitis induced ductal scarring, 10% developed CP over a 10-year follow-up period (Angelini et al. 1993). In all, 30% of these patients with a final diagnosis of chronic pancreatitis developed pancreatic calcifications. ERCP findings in these 10 patients showed that chronic pancreatitis was secondary to stenosis of the Wirsung duct with upstream dilatation and calcification. More rarely ductal stenosis can also be caused by a pseudocyst.

8.2 Natural History of Chronic Pancreatitis and Prognosis

The natural history of CP is characterised by a progressive reduction in the painful symptoms and a parallel development towards functional insufficiency of the pancreatic gland (Steer et al. 1995; Cavallini et al. 1998; Lankisch 2001). The appearance of steathorroea occurs when the production of lipase by the pancreas falls below 10% (Dimagno et al. 1973) and is probably conditioned by numerous factors, among which diet, the production of co-lipase and biliary acids, duodenal pH, the production of extra-pancreatic lipase (lingual, gastric) (Layer and Keller 2003). The appearance of steathorroea is quite common in the advanced stages of the disease (Ammann 1990; Konzen et al. 1993; Nakamura et al. 1995; Steer et al. 1995; Nakamura and Takeuchi 1997; Cavallini et al. 1998; Nakamura et al. 1999), particularly in patients that have undergone surgery (White and Slavotinek 1979; Morrow et al. 1984; Nogueira and Dani 1985; Greenlee et al. 1990; Sakorafas et al. 2000; Hwang et al. 2001).

Diabetes develops in about 50% of patients 15 years after the onset of pancreatitis (Cavallini et al. 1998). The diabetes that appears in patients affected by chronic pancreatitis can be due to a deficit in insulin production as well as increased insulin resistance (Cavallini et al. 1993).

A large number of patients (70% at 15 years) (Cavallini et al. 1998) undergoes surgical intervention mainly due to painful symptoms (Cavallini et al. 1998; Lankisch 2001; Otsuki 2003). In the greater part of these cases the type of intervention is derivative, even if for some forms of pancreatitis, especially the one associated to cystic dystrophy of the duodenal wall, the most used surgical intervention is resection (duodeno-cephalo-pancreasectomy). Autoimmune pancreatitis deserves a separate mention, as steroid therapy would be the best choice (Pearson et al. 2003). Nonetheless, if there is doubt, these patients are often submitted to surgical resection. The 5-year follow-up of these patients reported the good course of the disease up to complete resolution of the symptoms and no relapse (Pearson et al. 2003)

Patients affected by pancreatitis secondary to organic SOD undergo endoscopic therapy (pancreatic sphincterotomy) with the reduction/disappearance of painful symptoms or, in any case, a slowing down of its natural evolution towards the chronic stage. In the more advanced phases too, endoscopic treatment allows for the removal of intraductal stones that form secondarily to the reflux obstruction of pancreatic secretion, with considerable improvement in the clinical, functional and instrumental picture.

From a prognostic point of view, patients affected by chronic pancreatitis have a mortality rate at 20 years equal to 25% (Cavallini et al. 1998), slightly inferior to that of the general population. The causes of death are mainly secondary to alcohol and tobacco correlated pathologies, particularly extra-pancreatic tumours (cancer of the lung, mouth, oesophagus and the stomach) and cardiovascular pathologies (Cavallini et al. 1998). In particular, the frequency of pancreatic adenocarcinoma is increased, possibly influenced by smoking habits (Lowenfels et al. 1993, 1999; Cavallini et al. 1998; Lankisch et al. 2002; Maisonneuve and Lowenfels 2002; Malka et al. 2002). This possibility should be suspected due to the reappearance of pancreatic pain in a patient with a long history of chronic pancreatitis that has been clinically silent for many years. The frequency of pancreatic adenocarcinoma is directly correlated to the duration of the disease (Lowenfels et al. 1993) and is therefore greater in the genetically correlated forms (Lowenfels et al. 1997, 2000).

The prognosis of patients affected by chronic pancreatitis therefore seems to be influenced by their alcohol and tobacco in-take, which also conditions their quality of life.

We are still not able to establish the natural history and the prognosis of the different types of chronic pancreatitis, even if it seems that some forms of the disease, especially the non-alcohol and tobacco correlated ones, have a more benign course.

References

Ammann RW (1990) Chronic pancreatitis in the elderly. Gastroenterol Clin North Am 19:905–914

Ammann RW (2001) The natural history of alcoholic chronic pancreatitis. Intern Med 40:368–375

Ammann RW, Muellhaupt B (1999) The natural history of pain in alcoholic chronic pancreatitis. Gastroenterology 116:1132–1140

Angelini G, Cavallini G, Pederzoli P, Bovo P, Bassi C, Di Francesco V, Frulloni L, Sgarbi D, Talamini G, Castagnini A (1993) Long-term outcome of acute pancreatitis: a prospective study with 118 patients. Digestion 54:143–147

Applebaum-Shapiro SE, Finch R, Pfutzer RH, Hepp LA, Gates L, Amann S, Martin S, Ulrich CD, Whitcomb DC (2001) Hereditary pancreatitis in North America: the Pittsburgh-Midwest Multi-Center Pancreatic Study Group Study. Pancreatology 1:439–443

Arduino C, Gallo M, Brusco A, Garnerone S, Piana MR, Di Maggio S, Gerbino Promis G, Ferrone M, Angeli A, Gaia E (1999) Polyvariant mutant CFTR genes in patients with chronic pancreatitis. Clin Genet 56:400–404

Aygalenq P, Eugene C, Fingerhut A (1994) Non-alcoholic chronic pancreatitis: should the mutation delta F508 of the CFTR gene be considered as a risk factor? Gastroenterol Clin Biol 18:907–908

Balachandar TG, Surendran R, Kannan D, Darwin P, Jeswanth S (1999) Groove pancreatitis. Trop Gastroenterol 20:78–79

Basili E, Allemand I, Ville E, Laugier R (2001) Lanreotide acetate may cure cystic dystrophy in heterotopic pancreas of the duodenal wall. Gastroenterol Clin Biol 25:1108–1011

Beger HG, Buchler M (1990) Duodenum-preserving resection of the head of the pancreas in chronic pancreatitis with inflammatory mass in the head. World J Surg 14:83–87

Beger HG, Buchler M, Bittner R (1990) The duodenum preserving resection of the head of the pancreas (DPRHP) in patients with chronic pancreatitis and an inflammatory mass in the head. An alternative surgical technique to the Whipple operation. Acta Chir Scand 156:309–315

Bernard JP, Sahel J, Giovannini M, Sarles H (1990) Pancreas divisum is a probable cause of acute pancreatitis: a report of 137 cases. Pancreas 5:248–254

Bhatia E, Choudhuri G, Sikora SS, Landt O, Kage A, Becker M, Witt H (2002) Tropical calcific pancreatitis: strong association with SPINK1 trypsin inhibitor mutations. Gastroenterology 123:1020–1025

Bhatia E, Durie P, Zielenski J, Lam D, Sikora SS, Choudhuri G, Tsui LC (2000) Mutations in the cystic fibrosis transmembrane regulator gene in patients with tropical calcific pancreatitis. Am J Gastroenterol 95:3658–3659

Binmoeller KF, Jue P, Seifert H, Nam WC, Izbicki J, Soehendra N (1995) Endoscopic pancreatic stent drainage in chronic pancreatitis and a dominant stricture: long-term results. Endoscopy 27:638–644

Brand B, Kahl M, Sidhu S, Nam VC, Sriram PV, Jaeckle S, Thonke F, Soehendra N (2000) Prospective evaluation of morphology, function, and quality of life after extracorporeal shockwave lithotripsy and endoscopic treatment of chronic calcific pancreatitis. Am J Gastroenterol 95:3428–3438

Burtin P, Person B, Charneau J, Boyer J (1991) Pancreas divisum and pancreatitis: a coincidental association? Endoscopy 23:55–58

Carr-Locke DL (1991) Pancreas divisum: the controversy goes on? Endoscopy 23:88–90

Castellani C, Gomez Lira M, Frulloni L, Delmarco A, Marzari M, Bonizzato A, Cavallini G, Pignatti P, Mastella G (2001) Analysis of the entire coding region of the cystic fibrosis transmembrane regulator gene in idiopathic pancreatitis. Hum Mutat 18:166

Cavallini G, Bovo P, Vaona B, DiFrancesco V, Frulloni L, Rigo L, Brunori MP, Andreaus MC, Tebaldi M, Sgarbi D, Angelini G, Talamini G, Procacci C, Pederzoli P, Filippini M (1996) Chronic obstructive pancreatitis in humans is a lithiasic disease. Pancreas 13:66–70

Cavallini G, Frulloni L (2001) Autoimmunity and chronic pancreatitis: a concealed relationship. JOP 2:61–68

Cavallini G, Frulloni L, Pederzoli P, Talamini G, Bovo P, Bassi C, Di Francesco V, Vaona B, Falconi M, Sartori N, Angelini G, Brunori MP, Filippini M (1998) Long-term follow-up of patients with chronic pancreatitis in Italy. Scand J Gastroenterol 33:880–889

Cavallini G, Talamini G, Vaona B, Bovo P, Filippini M, Rigo L, Angelini G, Vantini I, Riela A, Frulloni L (1994). Effect of alcohol and smoking on pancreatic lithogenesis in the course of chronic pancreatitis. Pancreas 9:42–46

Cavallini G, Vaona B, Bovo P, Cigolini M, Rigo L, Rossi F, Tasini E, Brunori MP, Di Francesco V, Frulloni L (1993) Diabetes in chronic alcoholic pancreatitis. Role of residual beta cell function and insulin resistance. Dig Dis Sci 38:497–501

Cavestro GM, Frulloni L, Nouvenne A, Neri TM, Calore B, Ferri B, Bovo P, Okolicsanyi L, Di Mario F, Cavallini G (2003) Association of keratin 8 gene mutation with chronic pancreatitis. Dig Liver Dis 35:416–420

Chandak GR, Idris MM, Reddy DN, Bhaskar S, Sriram PV, Singh L (2002) Mutations in the pancreatic secretory trypsin inhibitor gene (PSTI/SPINK1) rather than the cationic trypsinogen gene (PRSS1) are significantly associated with tropical calcific pancreatitis. J Med Genet 39:347–351

Chen JM, Mercier B, Ferec C (1999) Strong evidence that the N21I substitution in the cationic trypsinogen gene causes disease in hereditary pancreatitis. Gut 45:916

Cohn JA, Friedman KJ, Noone PG, Knowles MR, Silverman LM, Jowell PS (1998) Relation between mutations of the cystic fibrosis gene and idiopathic pancreatitis. N Engl J Med 339:653–658

Comfort MW, Steimberg AG (1952) Pedigree of a family with hereditary chronic relapsing pancreatitis. Gastroenterology 21:54–63

Cremer M, Deviere J, Delhaye M, Baize M, Vandermeeren A (1991) Stenting in severe chronic pancreatitis: results of medium-term follow-up in seventy-six patients. Endoscopy 23:171–176

Cunningham JT (1992) Pancreas divisum and acute pancreatitis: romancing the stone? Am J Gastroenterol 87:802–803

Dani R, Mott CB, Guarita DR, Nogueira CE (1990) Epidemiology and etiology of chronic pancreatitis in Brazil: a tale of two cities. Pancreas 5:474–478

De Parades V, Roulot D, Palazzo L, Chaussade S, Mingaud P, Rautureau J, Coste T (1996) Treatment with octreotide of stenosing cystic dystrophy on heterotopic pancreas of the duodenal wall. Gastroenterol Clin Biol 20:601–604

Delhaye M, Engelholm L, Cremer M (1985) Pancreas divisum: congenital anatomic variant or anomaly? Contribution of endoscopic retrograde dorsal pancreatography. Gastroenterology 89:951–958

Dhar A, Goenka MK, Kochhar R, Nagi B, Bhasin DK, Singh K (1996) Pancreas divisum: five years' experience in a teaching hospital. Indian J Gastroenterol 15:7–9

DiMagno EP, Go VL, Summerskill WH (1973) Relations between pancreatic enzyme ouputs and malabsorption in severe pancreatic insufficiency. N Engl J Med 288:813–815

Dite P, Stary K, Novotny I, Precechtelova M, Dolina J, Lata J, Zboril V (2001) Incidence of chronic pancreatitis in the Czech Republic. Eur J Gastroenterol Hepatol 13:749–750

Drenth JP, te Morsche R, Jansen JB (2002) Mutations in serine protease inhibitor Kazal type 1 are strongly associated with chronic pancreatitis. Gut 50:687–692

Dufour MC, Adamson MD (2003) The epidemiology of alcohol-induced pancreatitis. Pancreas 27:286–290

Eddes EH, Masclee AA, Lamers CB, Gooszen HG (1996) Duodenum preserving resection of the head of the pancreas in painful chronic pancreatitis. Eur J Surg 162:545–549

Elitsur Y, Chertow BC, Jewell RD, Finver SN, Primerano DA (1998) Identification of a hereditary pancreatitis mutation in four West Virginia families. Pediatr Res 44:927–930

Farnbacher MJ, Schoen C, Rabenstein T, Benninger J, Hahn EG, Schneider HAT (2002) Pancreatic duct stones in chronic pancreatitis: criteria for treatment intensity and success. Gastrointest Endosc 56:501–506

Ferec C, Raguenes O, Salomon R, Roche C, Bernard JP, Guillot M, Quere I, Faure C, Mercier B, Audrezet MP, Guillausseau PJ, Dupont C, Munnich A, Bignon JD, Le Bodic L (1999) Mutations in the cationic trypsinogen gene and evidence for genetic heterogeneity in hereditary pancreatitis. J Med Genet 36:228–232

Flejou JF, Potet F, Molas G, Bernades P, Amouyal P, Fekete F (1993) Cystic dystrophy of the gastric and duodenal wall developing in heterotopic pancreas: an unrecognised entity. Gut 34:343–347

Ford ME, Whitcomb DC (1999) Analysis of the hereditary pancreatitis-associated cationic trypsinogen gene mutations in exons 2 and 3 by enzymatic mutation detection from a single 2.2-kb polymerase chain reaction product. Mol Diagn 4:211–218

Frulloni L, Castellani C, Bovo P, Vaona B, Calore B, Liani C, Mastella G, Cavallini G (2003) Natural history of pancreatitis associated with cystic fibrosis gene mutations. Dig Liver Dis 35:179–185

Gomez Lira M, Benetazzo MG, Marzari MG, Bombieri C, Belpinati F, Castellani C, Cavallini GC, Mastella G, Pignatti PF (2000) High frequency of cystic fibrosis transmembrane regulator mutation L997F in patients with recurrent idiopathic pancreatitis and in newborns with hypertrypsinemia. Am J Hum Genet 66:2013–2014

Gorry MC, Gabbaizedeh D, Furey W, Gates LK Jr, Preston RA, Aston CE, Zhang Y, Ulrich C, Ehrlich GD, Whitcomb DC (1997) Mutations in the cationic trypsinogen gene are associated with recurrent acute and chronic pancreatitis. Gastroenterology 113:1063–1068

Greenlee HB, Prinz RA, Aranha GV (1990) Long-term results of side-to-side pancreatico-jejunostomy. World J Surg 14:70–76

Howes N, Greenhalf W, Rutherford S, O'Donnell M, Mountford R, Ellis I, Whitcomb D, Imrie C, Drumm B, Neoptolemos JP (2001) A new polymorphism for the RI22H mutation in hereditary pancreatitis. Gut 48:247–250

Hwang TL, Chen HM, Chen MF (2001) Surgery for chronic obstructive pancreatitis: comparison of end-to-side pancreatico-jejunostomy with pancreatico-duodenectomy. Hepatogastroenterology 48:270–272

Kaneko K, Nagasaki Y, Furukawa T, Mizutamari H, Sato A, Masamune A, Shimosegawa T, Horii A (2001) Analysis of the human pancreatic secretory trypsin inhibitor (PSTI) gene mutations in Japanese patients with chronic pancreatitis. J Hum Genet 46:293–297

Kleitsch W (1955) Anatomy of the pancreas: study with special reference to the duct system. Arch Surg 71:795–802

Konzen KM, Perrault J, Moir C, Zinsmeister AR (1993) Long-term follow-up of young patients with chronic hereditary or idiopathic pancreatitis. Mayo Clin Proc 68:449–453

Lankisch PG (2001) Natural course of chronic pancreatitis. Pancreatology 1:3–14

Lankisch PG, Assmus C, Maisonneuve P, Lowenfels AB (2002) Epidemiology of pancreatic diseases in Luneburg County. A study in a defined german population. Pancreatology 2:469–477

Layer P, Keller J (2003) Lipase supplementation therapy: standards, alternatives, and perspectives. Pancreas 26:1–7

Le Marechal C, Bretagne JF, Raguenes O, Quere I, Chen JM, Ferec C (2001) Identification of a novel pancreatitis-associated missense mutation, R116C, in the human cationic trypsinogen gene (PRSS1). Mol Genet Metab 74:342–344

Le Marechal C, Chen JM, Le Gall C, Plessis G, Chipponi J, Chuzhanova NA, Raguenes O, Ferec C (2004) Two novel severe mutations in the pancreatic secretory trypsin inhibitor gene (SPINK1) cause familial and/or hereditary pancreatitis. Hum Mutat 23:205

Lin Y, Tamakoshi A, Hayakawa T, Ogawa M, Ohno Y (2000) Cigarette smoking as a risk factor for chronic pancreatitis: a case-control study in Japan. Research Committee on Intractable Pancreatic Diseases. Pancreas 21:109–114

Lin Y, Tamakoshi A, Hayakawa T, Ogawa M, Ohno Y (2001) Associations of alcohol drinking and nutrient intake with chronic pancreatitis: findings from a case-control study in Japan. Am J Gastroenterol 96:2622–2627

Lowenfels AB, Maisonneuve P, Cavallini G, Ammann RW, Lankisch PG, Andersen JR, Dimagno EP, Andren-Sandberg A, Domellof L (1993) Pancreatitis and the risk of pancreatic cancer. International Pancreatitis Study Group. N Engl J Med 328:1433–1437

Lowenfels AB, Maisonneuve P, DiMagno EP, Elitsur Y, Gates LK Jr, Perrault J, Whitcomb DC (1997) Hereditary pancreatitis and the risk of pancreatic cancer. International Hereditary Pancreatitis Study Group. J Natl Cancer Inst 89:442–446

Lowenfels AB, Maisonneuve P, Lankisch PG (1999) Chronic pancreatitis and other risk factors for pancreatic cancer. Gastroenterol Clin North Am 28:673–685

Lowenfels AB, Maisonneuve P, Whitcomb DC (2000) Risk factors for cancer in hereditary pancreatitis. International Hereditary Pancreatitis Study Group. Med Clin North Am 84:565–573

MacCarty RL, Stephens DH, Brown AL Jr, Carlson HC (1975) Retrograde pancreatography in autopsy specimens. Am J Roentgenol Radium Ther Nucl Med 123:359–366

Maisonneuve P, Lowenfels AB (2002) Chronic pancreatitis and pancreatic cancer. Dig Dis 20:32–37

Malka D, Hammel P, Maire F, Rufat P, Madeira I, Pessione F, Levy P, Ruszniewski P (2002) Risk of pancreatic adenocarcinoma in chronic pancreatitis. Gut 51:849–852

Mohl W, Hero-Gross R, Feifel G, Kramann B, Puschel W, Menges M, Zeitz M (2001) Groove pancreatitis: an important differential diagnosis to malignant stenosis of the duodenum. Dig Dis Sci 46:1034–1038

Morrow CE, Cohen JI, Sutherland DE, Najarian JS (1984) Chronic pancreatitis: long-term surgical results of pancreatic duct drainage, pancreatic resection, and near-total pancreatectomy and islet autotransplantation. Surgery 96:608–616

Muranaka T (1990) Morphologic changes in the body of the pancreas secondary to a mass in the pancreatic head. Analysis by CT. Acta Radiol 1:483–488

Nakamura T, Takebe K, Kudoh K, Ishii M, Iamura K, Kikuchi H, Kasai F, Tandoh Y, Yamada N, Arai Y (1995) Steatorrhea in Japanese patients with chronic pancreatitis. J Gastroenterol 30:79–83

Nakamura T, Takeuchi T (1997) Pancreatic steatorrhea, malabsorption, and nutrition biochemistry: a comparison of Japanese, European, and American patients with chronic pancreatitis. Pancreas 14(4):323–333

Nakamura T, Tando Y, Yamada N, Watanabe T, Ogawa Y, Kaji A, Imamura K, Kikuchi H, Suda T (1999) Study on pancreatic insufficiency (chronic pancreatitis) and steatorrhea in Japanese patients with low fat intake. Digestion 60 Suppl 1:93–96

Nishimori I, Kamakura M, Fujikawa-Adachi K, Morita M, Onishi S, Yokoyama K, Makino I, Ishida H, Yamamoto M, Watanabe S, Ogawa M (1999) Mutations in exons 2 and 3 of the cationic trypsinogen gene in Japanese families with hereditary pancreatitis. Gut 44:259–263

Nishimori I, Onishi S (2001) Hereditary pancreatitis in Japan: a review of pancreatitis-associated gene mutations. Pancreatology 1:444–447

Nogueira CE, Dani R (1985) Evaluation of the surgical treatment of chronic calcifying pancreatitis. Surg Gynecol Obstet 161:117–128

Ockenga J, Stuhrmann M, Ballmann M, Teich N, Keim V, Dork T, Manns MP (2000) Mutations of the cystic fibrosis gene, but not cationic trypsinogen gene, are associated with recurrent or chronic idiopathic pancreatitis. Am J Gastroenterol 95:2061–2067

O'Reilly DA, Kingsnorth AN (2000) Hereditary pancreatitis and mutations of the cationic trypsinogen gene. Br J Surg 87:708–717

Otsuki M (2003) Chronic pancreatitis in Japan: epidemiology, prognosis, diagnostic criteria, and future problems. J Gastroenterol 38:315–326

Ozawa F, Friess H, Kondo Y, Shrikhande SV, Buchler MW (2000) Duodenum-preserving pancreatic head resection (DPPHR) in chronic pancreatitis: its rationale and results. J Hepatobiliary Pancreat Surg 7:456–465

Pearson RK, Longnecker DS, Chari ST, Smyrk TC, Okazaki K, Frulloni L, Cavallini G (2003) Controversies in clinical pancreatology: autoimmune pancreatitis: does it exist? Pancreas 27:1–13

Pfutzer R, Myers E, Applebaum-Shapiro S, Finch R, Ellis I, Neoptolemos J, Kant JA, Whitcomb DC (2002) Novel cationic trypsinogen (PRSS1) N29T and R122C mutations cause autosomal dominant hereditary pancreatitis. Gut 50:271–272

Ponchon T, Bory RM, Hedelius F, Roubein LD, Paliard P, Napoleon B, Chavaillon A (1995) Endoscopic stenting for pain relief in chronic pancreatitis: results of a standardized protocol. Gastrointest Endosc 42:452–456

Potet F, Duclert N (1970) Cystic dystrophy on aberrant pancreas of the duodenal wall. Arch Fr Mal App Dig 59:223–238

Procacci C, Graziani R, Zamboni G, Cavallini G, Pederzoli P, Guarise A, Bogina G, Biasiutti C, Carbognin G, Bergamo-Andreis IA, Pistolesi GF (1997) Cystic dystrophy of the duodenal wall: radiologic findings. Radiology 205:741–747

Rosch T, Daniel S, Scholz M, Huibregtse K, Smits M, Schneider T, Ell C, Haber G, Riemann JF, Jakobs R, Hintze R, Adler A, Neuhaus H, Zavoral M, Zavada F, Schusdziarra V, Soehendra N (2002) Endoscopic treatment of chronic pancreatitis: a multicenter study of 1000 patients with long-term follow-up. Endoscopy 34:765–771

Rubay R, Bonnet D, Gohy P, Laka A, Deltour D (1999) Cystic dystrophy in heterotopic pancreas of the duodenal wall: medical and surgical treatment. Acta Chir Belg 99:87–91

Sakorafas GH, Farnell MB, Nagorney DM, Sarr MG, Rowland CM (2000) Pancreatoduodenectomy for chronic pancreatitis: long-term results in 105 patients. Arch Surg 135:517–23; discussion 523–524

Sarles H (1965) Proposal adopted unanimously by the participants of the Symposium, Marseilles 1963. Bibl Gastroenterol 7:7–8

Sarles H, Adler G, Dani R, Frey C, Gullo L, Harada H, Martin E, Norohna M, Scuro LA (1989) The pancreatitis classification of Marseilles-Rome 1988. Scand J Gastroenterol 24:641–642

Sharer N, Schwarz M, Malone G, Howarth A, Painter J, Super M, Braganza J (1998) Mutations of the cystic fibrosis gene in patients with chronic pancreatitis. N Engl J Med 339:645–652

Singer MV GK, Sarles H (1985) Revised classification of pancreatitis: report of the Second International Symposium on the Classification of Pancreatitis in Marseille, France, March 28–30, 1984. Gastroenterology 89:683–685

Smits ME, Rauws EA, Tytgat GN, Huibregtse K (1996) Endoscopic treatment of pancreatic stones in patients with chronic pancreatitis. Gastrointest Endosc 43:556–560

Steer ML, Waxman I, Freedman S (1995) Chronic pancreatitis. N Engl J Med 332:1482–1490

Stern C (1986) A historical perspective on the discovery of the accessory duct of the pancreas, the ampulla "of Vater" and pancreas divisum. Gut 27:203–212

Stimec B, Bulajic M, Korneti V, Milosavljevic T, Krstic R, Ugljesic M (1996) Ductal morphometry of ventral pancreas in pancreas divisum. Comparison between clinical and anatomical results. Ital J Gastroenterol 28:76–80

Stolte M, Weiss W, Volkholz H, Rosch W (1982) A special form of segmental pancreatitis: "groove pancreatitis". Hepatogastroenterology 29:198–208

Talamini G, Bassi C, Falconi M, Frulloni L, Di Francesco V, Vaona B, Bovo P, Rigo L, Castagnini A, Angelini G, Vantini I, Pederzoli P, Cavallini G (1996a) Cigarette smoking: an independent risk factor in alcoholic pancreatitis. Pancreas 12:131–137

Talamini G, Bassi C, Falconi M, Sartori N, Salvia R, Di Francesco V, Frulloni L, Vaona B, Bovo P, Vantini I, Pederzoli P, Cavallini G (1996b) Pain relapses in the first 10 years of chronic pancreatitis. Am J Surg 171:565–569

Talamini G, Vaona B, Bassi C, Bovo P, Damoc T, Mastromauro M, Falconi M, Vantini I, Cavallini G, Pederzoli P (2000) Alcohol intake, cigarette smoking, and body mass index in patients with alcohol-associated pancreatitis. J Clin Gastroenterol 31:314–317

Teich N, Le Marechal C, Kukor Z, Caca K, Witzigmann H, Chen JM, Toth M, Mossner J, Keim V, Ferec C, Sahin-Toth M (2004) Interaction between trypsinogen isoforms in genetically determined pancreatitis: mutation E79K in cationic trypsin (PRSS1) causes increased transactivation of anionic trypsinogen (PRSS2). Hum Mutat 23:22–31

Threadgold J, Greenhalf W, Ellis I, Howes N, Lerch MM, Simon P, Jansen J, Charnley R, Laugier R, Frulloni L, Olah A, Delhaye M, Ihse I, Schaffalitzky de Muckadell OB, Andren-Sandberg A, Imrie CW, Martinek J, Gress TM, Mountford R, Whitcomb D, Neoptolemos JP (2002) The N34S mutation of SPINK1 (PSTI) is associated with a familial pattern of idiopathic chronic pancreatitis but does not cause the disease. Gut 50:675–681

Truninger K, Malik N, Ammann RW, Muellhaupt B, Seifert B, Muller HJ, Blum HE (2001) Mutations of the cystic fibrosis gene in patients with chronic pancreatitis. Am J Gastroenterol 96:2657–2961

Whitcomb DC, Gorry MC, Preston RA, Furey W, Sossenheimer MJ, Ulrich CD, Martin SP, Gates LK Jr, Amann ST, Toskes PP, Liddle R, McGrath K, Uomo G, Post JC, Ehrlich GD (1996) Hereditary pancreatitis is caused by a mutation in the cationic trypsinogen gene. Nat Genet 14:141–145

White TT, Slavotinek AH (1979) Results of surgical treatment of chronic pancreatitis. Report of 142 cases. Ann Surg 189:217–224

Witt H, Luck W, Hennies HC, Classen M, Kage A, Lass U, Landt O, Becker M (2000) Mutations in the gene encoding the serine protease inhibitor, Kazal type 1 are associated with chronic pancreatitis. Nat Genet 25:213–216

The Role of Ultrasound

9

Mirko D'Onofrio

CONTENTS

9.1 **Ultrasonographic Features** *139*
9.1.1 Pancreatic Gland Changes *139*
9.1.1.1 Size, Shape and Contour *139*
9.1.1.2 Echogenicity, Parenchymal Texture and Calcifications *141*
9.1.2 Pancreatic Duct Changes *141*
9.1.2.1 Caliber and Contour *141*
9.1.2.2 Intraductal Calculi *143*

9.2 **Ultrasonographic Diagnosis** *143*
9.2.1 Severity *144*
9.2.1.1 Early Stage *144*
9.2.1.2 Advanced Stage *144*
9.2.2 Etiology *145*
9.2.2.1 Obstructive Chronic Pancreatitis *145*
9.2.2.2 Non-obstructive Chronic Pancreatitis *145*

References *148*

M. D'Onofrio, MD
Department of Radiology, Policlinico "GB Rossi", University of Verona, Piazzale LA Scuro 10, 37134 Verona, Italy

9.1 Ultrasonographic Features

Pathological alterations of the pancreatic parenchyma secondary to chronic pancreatitis are characterized by non-uniform tissue scarring and focal, segmental or diffuse destruction of the parenchyma (Singer et al. 1985). These parenchymal alterations may be associated with variable degrees of main pancreatic duct dilation. Despite detailed knowledge of the pathologic changes within the pancreatic parenchyma, there is poor correlation between the anatomic alterations and clinical severity (Sarner and Cotton 1984a,b).

Ultrasonography (US) is a well established diagnostic modality that can identify the morphological alterations of the pancreatic gland characteristic of chronic pancreatitis. Current technological innovations provide a significant improvement in spatial resolution that, together with the use of harmonic frequencies and the development of compounding techniques, are responsible for the improvement in the diagnostic ability and reliability of this technique (Shapiro et al. 1998).

9.1.1 Pancreatic Gland Changes

The pancreatic alterations visible by US are secondary to alterations in size, morphology and texture of the gland.

9.1.1.1 Size, Shape and Contour

Alterations in the size of the pancreas may be seen in fewer than half of the patients affected by chronic pancreatitis (Alpern et al. 1985; Bolondi et al. 1987, 1989), the degree of change being proportional to the length of the disease. The differences between the various series on the presence and severity of size alterations of the pancreas are a result of the differences in the stage of the disease and lack of uniform criteria defining normal gland size (Lecesne et al. 1999). Early in the disease, the pancreas may appear minimally enlarged (Fig. 9.1) (Lecesne et al. 1999). This finding is non-specific; often the increased size of the pancreas is interpreted as acute pancreatitis. A variety of congenital anomalies may produce asymmetric gland enlargement. Finally, in lean young patients, the pancreatic body-tail may be bigger than the head region (Fig. 9.2). Conversely, the finding of a normal size pancreas does not exclude a diagnosis of chronic pancreatitis (Alpern et al. 1985; Lecesne et al. 1999).

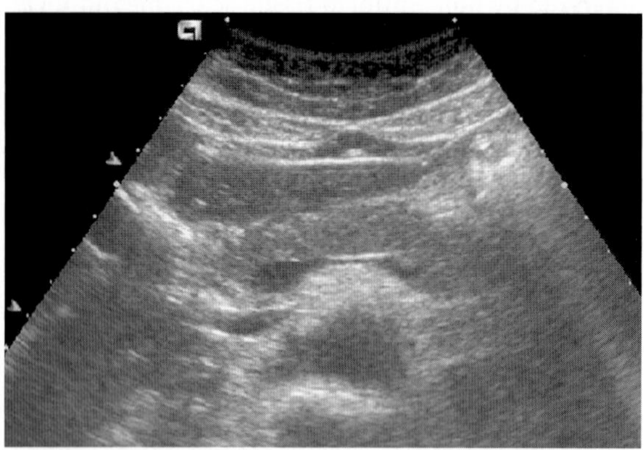

Fig. 9.1. Early stage chronic pancreatitis. US examination reveals a diffuse, slight increase in size of the pancreatic gland

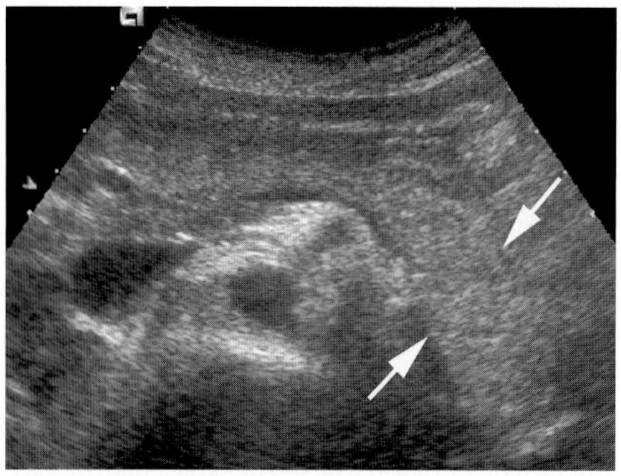

Fig. 9.2. Normal size variation in a female. At US the pancreatic body-tail (*arrows*) is bigger than the head region

Atrophy and focal alterations in size of the pancreas are more easily identified alterations (Fig. 9.3). However, these alterations of the pancreatic volume, even though easily identifiable, are expressions of advanced stages of the disease. Focal mass-like enlargement of portions of the gland in chronic pancreatitis may be difficult to differentiate from neoplasm (Fig. 9.4a). Size evaluation has therefore poor diagnostic value in the early stages of the disease and is a complementary finding in the advanced stages (Alpern et al. 1985). In the follow up of chronic pancreatitis it is critical to compare serial studies so that size changes are more readily appreciated.

In the advanced stages of the disease the glandular contours appear irregular, sharp and sometimes nodular. Because the pancreas lacks a capsule, it is difficult to appreciate these morphologic changes, particularly in obese patients even in the late stage of the disease (Lecesne et al. 1999). Careful inspection of the interface of the dorsal border of the pancreas with the splenic vein, the region of maximal sensitivity for detection of contour abnormalities resulting form chronic pancreatitis, is recommended. The poor anatomical demarcation between the pancreas and the adjacent retroperitoneal connective tissue makes the US evaluation of gross contour abnormalities extremely difficult.

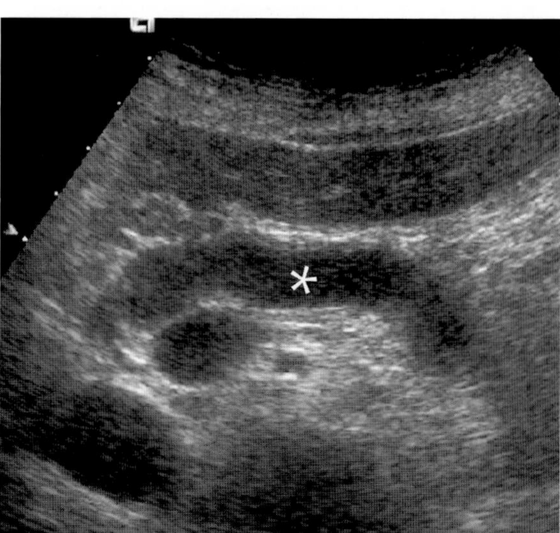

Fig. 9.3. Pancreatic atrophy in late stage chronic pancreatitis. US shows a uniform dilation of the main pancreatic duct (*asterisk*) with significant reduction of the pancreatic parenchyma

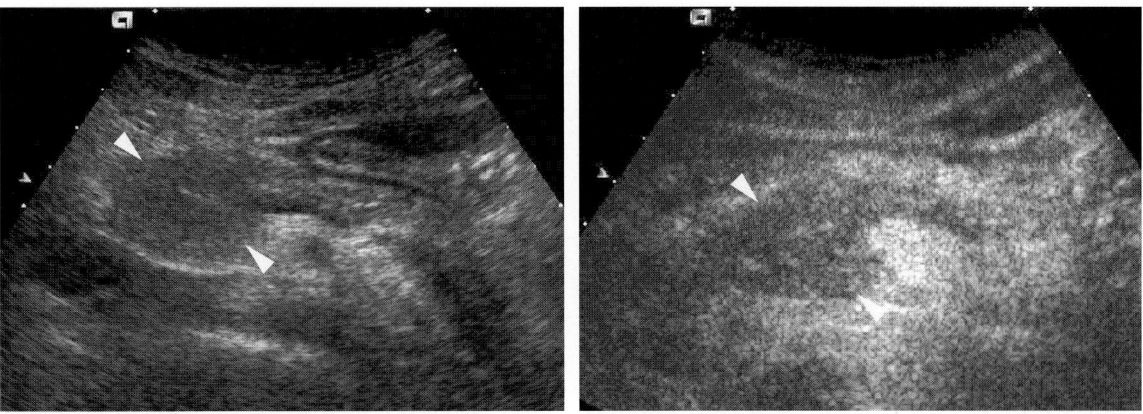

Fig. 9.4a,b. Focal enlargement of the pancreatic gland in chronic pancreatitis. **a** Baseline US demonstrates an enlarged pancreatic head (*arrowheads*) appearing slightly hypoechoic compared to the rest of parenchyma. **b** CEUS in the early phase shows enhancement (*arrowheads*) similar to that of the adjacent pancreas

9.1.1.2
Echogenicity, Parenchymal Texture and Calcifications

Echogenicity of the parenchyma is increased in chronic pancreatitis due to gland atrophy with fatty replacement infiltration (Lankisch and Banks 1998a,b) and fibrosis (Husband et al. 1977; Lecesne et al. 1999; Remer and Baker 2002). Increased echogenicity, however, is not specific; it can be found in elderly and obese patients. Alteration of glandular echotexture, on the other hand, is a more specific US finding in chronic pancreatitis. Pancreatic echotexture is inhomogeneous and coarse with coexisting hyperechoic and hypoechoic foci (Fig. 9.5) representing fibrosis and inflammation (Lecesne et al. 1999; Remer and Baker 2002). These findings are present in 50%–70% of the cases (Alpern et al. 1985; Bolondi et al. 1987). In patients with severe exocrine pancreatic insufficiency, the changes in echotexture may be seen in as many as 80% (Bolondi et al. 1989). Apparent normality of the glandular echotexture in chronic pancreatitis is reported in the Literature in up to 40% of cases, and is expected in the early stages of disease (Lees et al. 1979; Foley et al. 1980; Grant and Efrusy 1981; Alpern et al. 1985). State-of-the-art US imaging is more sensitive to the subtle alterations of the glandular texture.

The Japan Pancreas Society (Homma et al. 1997), identifies the presence of pancreatic calcifications as pathognomonic of chronic pancreatitis. Pancreatic calcifications are calcium carbonate deposits forming on a protein matrix (plugs) or on interstitial necrotic areas (Ring et al. 1973; Alpern et al. 1985; Lankisch and Banks 1998a,b). At US these appear as hyperechoic spots with a posterior shadowing. Their detection is size dependant (Fig. 9.6), due to the presence of artifact from ultrasound beam refraction. The demonstration of pancreatic calcifications may be improved by the use of harmonic imaging and high resolution US (Fig. 9.7) (Balthazar 1994). Intraductal plugs with minimal or no calcium carbonate deposits appear at US as hyperechoic spots without posterior shadowing (Fig. 9.8).

9.1.2
Pancreatic Duct Changes

Ductal alterations include dilatation, changes in contour and abnormal ductal content. US is an excellent technique to evaluate the abnormal pancreatic duct.

9.1.2.1
Caliber and Contour

Pancreatic duct dilatation is a hallmark of chronic pancreatitis. The normal duct should not be more than 2 mm in width when fasting (Lawson et al. 1982; Niederau andGrendell 1985). In the normal subject, however, main duct caliber may increase

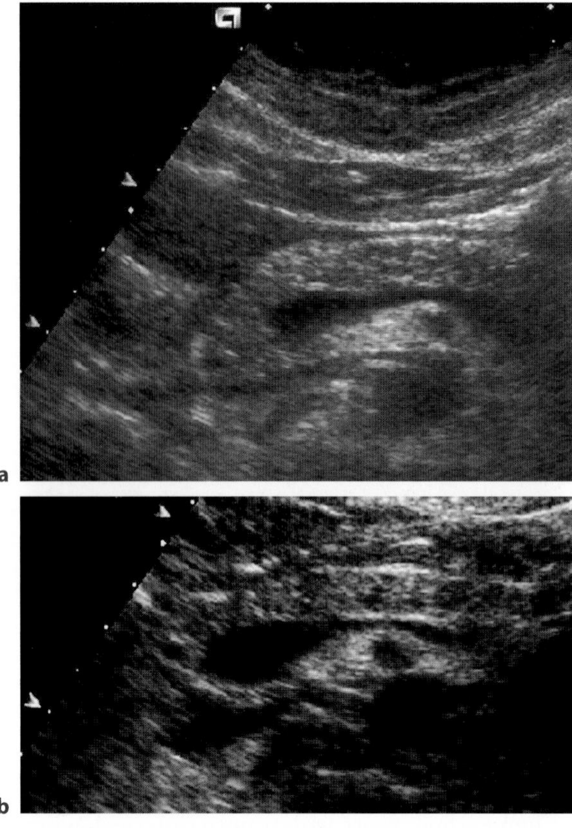

Fig. 9.5a,b. Chronic pancreatitis. **a** The US examination shows coarse echotexture of the pancreatic parenchyma produced by hyperechoic and hypoechoic foci in the parenchyma, better seen in (**b**) detailed image

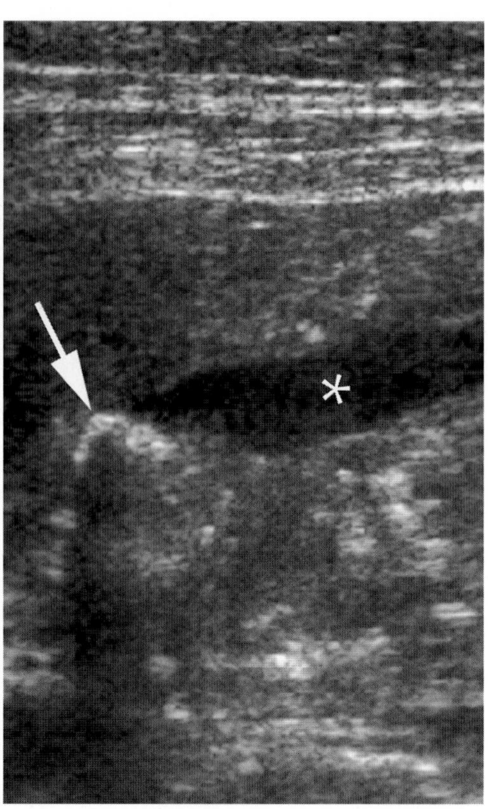

Fig. 9.7. Chronic pancreatitis. High resolution US shows a small calcification (*arrow*) with well seen posterior shadowing within the main pancreatic duct (*asterisk*)

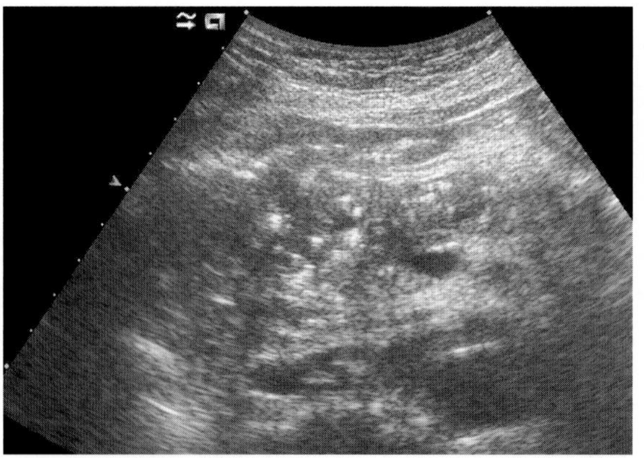

Fig. 9.6. Chronic pancreatitis. US shows increased volume of the pancreatic gland with inhomogeneous echotexture owing to the presence of variable size calcifications and ductal deposits

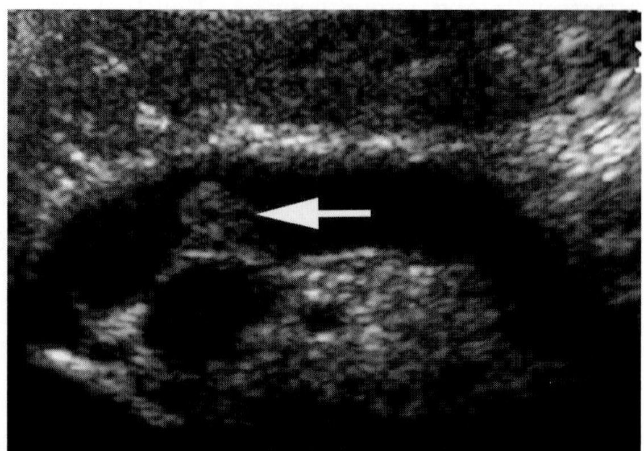

Fig. 9.8. Chronic pancreatitis. At US examination main pancreatic duct is uniformly dilated. Note the poorly shadowing endoluminal defect, presumably a protein plug or caste (*arrow*)

in physiologic conditions such as following meals (Brogna et al. 1991). The main pancreatic duct is considered as dilated when its caliber is wider than 3 mm (Remer and Baker 2002).

In chronic pancreatitis, main pancreatic duct dilation is the most easily identified US finding (Fig. 9.3). US has a sensitivity between 60%–70% (Niederau and Grendell 1985; Bolondi et al. 1987) for detecting ductal dilatation and a specificity between 80%–90% (Niederau and Grendell 1985; Hessel et al. 1982; Bolondi et al. 1987). The lower sensitivity reflects the lesser degree of duct dilation in the early stages of chronic pancreatitis, where the duct calibre may be normal (Lecesne et al. 1999). Chronic pancreatitis may also manifest with a marked narrowing of the main pancreatic duct (Fig. 9.9a), as seen in autoimmune pancreatitis (Furukawa et al. 1998). Because the inflammation may be segmental, especially in the initial stages, duct caliber alterations may be evident only in some parts of the pancreas. Duct contour alterations reflecting chronic pancreatitis are more difficult to identify (Fig. 9.10). Ductal contour irregularity, however, may also be found upstream to a complete obstruction of the main pancreatic duct by neoplasm (Fig. 9.11).

9.1.2.2 Intraductal Calculi

Intraductal calculi are protein aggregates with calcium carbonate deposits that appear at US as round echoic particles. The degree of echogenicity (and ease of identification) is proportional to the extent of the calcium deposition (Lankisch and Banks 1998a,b). When possible, harmonic assisted high resolution US aids in the demonstration of ductal filling defects (Fig. 9.7).

9.2 Ultrasonographic Diagnosis

In chronic pancreatitis, imaging is essential for establishing the diagnosis, the severity of the disease,

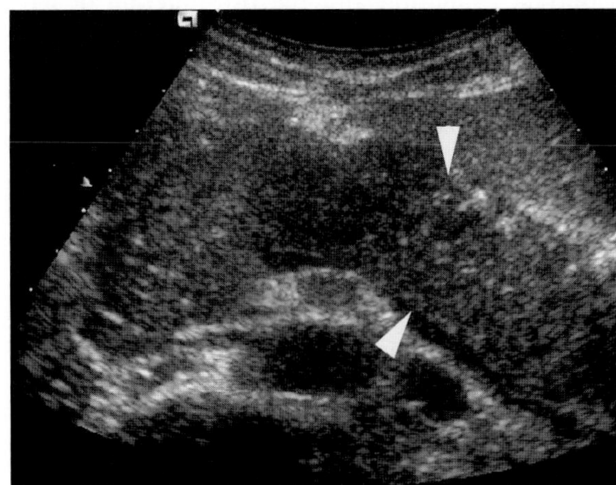

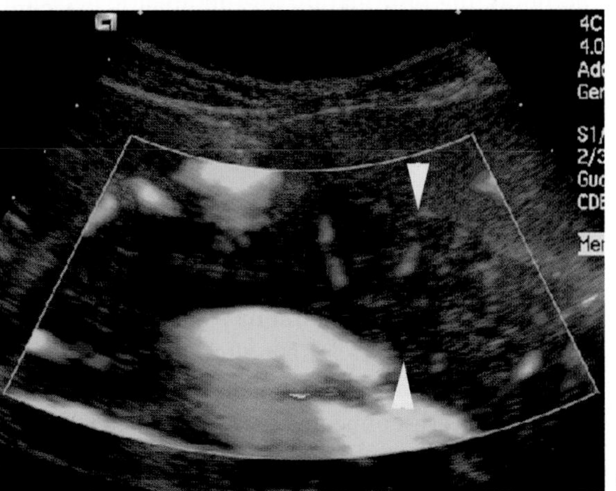

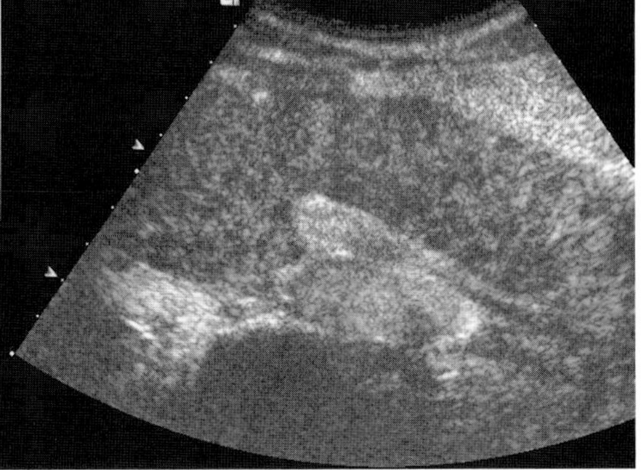

Fig. 9.9a–c. Autoimmune chronic pancreatitis. **a** At US the pancreas is diffusely hypoechoic and increased in volume (*arrowheads*) with a "sausage" appearance. The main pancreatic duct is compressed and not visible. **b** Power-Doppler US demonstrates increased vascularization of the pancreatic parenchyma (*arrowheads*). **c** CEUS better shows the intense hypervascularity of the pancreatic parenchyma (*arrowheads*)

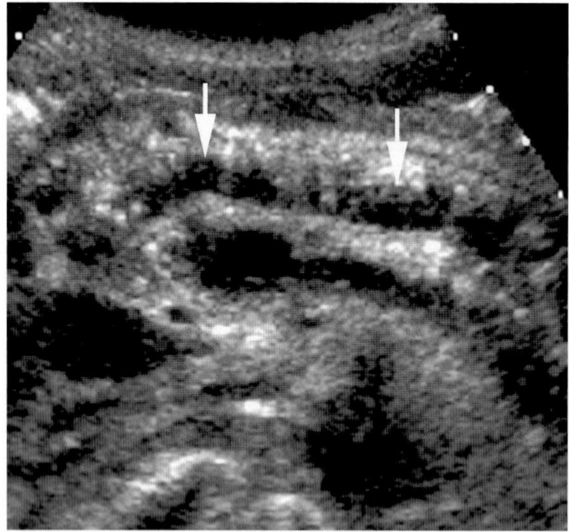

Fig. 9.10. Chronic pancreatitis. US shows inhomogeneous echotexture of the pancreatic parenchyma with microcalcifications and main pancreatic duct dilation (*arrows*) with contour irregularities

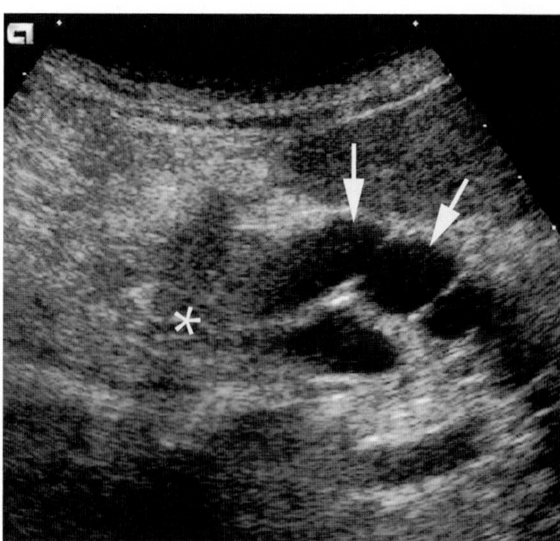

Fig. 9.11. Pancreatic ductal adenocarcinoma. At US examination a hypoechoic pancreatic head mass is visible (*asterisk*) with complete obstruction of the main pancreatic duct irregularly dilated upstream (*arrows*)

and obtaining information for therapeutic decision making. Clinical and laboratory investigation is necessary to establish the etiology in most cases.

9.2.1 Severity

Ultrasonographic diagnosis of chronic pancreatitis depends on the demonstrability of glandular parenchyma and ductal system alterations caused by chronic inflammation. Main pancreatic duct alterations are directly connected to the degree of severity of the disease. Even though there is not a direct correlation between pancreatic alterations and clinical severity of the disease, it is certainly more likely that in the advanced stages there are more prominent pancreatic alterations, improving US diagnosis. Sensitivity of 60%–70% and specificity of 80%–90% for US diagnosis of chronic pancreatitis are reported (Gowland et al. 1981; Hessel et al. 1982).

9.2.1.1 Early Stage

US ability to diagnose chronic pancreatitis in the early stages is limited, despite recent technological developments. The improvement in spatial and contrast resolution and the introduction of harmonic imaging, however, have surely improved the accuracy of US imaging in the identification of pancreatic alterations typical of the early stages of the disease (Fig. 9.5). It is possible to demonstrate the small hyperechoic (fibrosis) and hypoechoic (inflammatory) foci (Lecesne et al. 1999; Remer and Baker 2002), that are responsible for the changes in parenchymal echotexture (Fig. 9.5ab). Main pancreatic duct caliber, on the other hand, may be within a normal range in the early stages of disease (Lecesne et al. 1999). The use of secretin stimulation improves the detection of pancreatic duct alterations. Glaser et al. (1994) reported a sensitivity of 92% and a specificity of 93% for secretin enhanced US for the diagnosis of chronic pancreatitis.

9.2.1.2 Advanced Stage

In the advanced stages of chronic pancreatitis, pancreatic alterations are readily demonstrable at US (Lankisch and Banks 1998a,b). Pancreatic parenchyma is atrophic (Fig. 9.3). US shows parenchymal calcifications (Fig. 9.6) and intraductal calculi (Fig. 9.7) with a dilated main pancreatic duct (Fig. 9.10).

9.2.2 Etiology

Etiologic diagnosis is aimed at identification of the cause of the visualized pancreatic alterations, in order to define the type of chronic pancreatitis. The problem of the definition of the type of chronic pancreatitis is very important in relation to the increasing incidence of secondary forms.

9.2.2.1 Obstructive Chronic Pancreatitis

Obstructive chronic pancreatitis is characterized by a dilation of the main pancreatic duct upstream to an obstructing process, be it infiltration, invasion, compression or stenosis of the affected segment of pancreatic duct (Lankisch and Banks 1998a,b)

Neoplastic infiltration of the main duct is one of the most frequent causes of obstructive secondary chronic pancreatitis (Fig. 9.11). Obstructing neoplasms may be quite small; this possibility must be kept in mind especially when only a portion of the duct is dilated. Main pancreatic duct invasion by an intraductal papillary mucinous tumor (IPMT) causes duct dilation (Fig. 9.12a) and as a consequence secondary obstructive chronic pancreatitis (Procacci et al. 1996, 2003; Lankisch and Banks 1998a,b). At US examination, the mucin of IPMT may not be easily differentiated from the solid portions of the tumor (Fig. 9.12b). Harmonic imaging, with its better contrast resolution (Shapiro et al. 1998; Bennett and Hann 2001), may lead to the identification of the part of IPMT which is not solid (Fig. 9.12c,d). However, with US, IPMT final diagnosis by demonstrating the communication between the tumor and the pancreatic duct is difficult (Procacci et al. 2003).

Cystic dystrophy of the duodenal wall and groove pancreatitis are in a border site (groove region) between pancreas and duodenum, a site difficult to access for a correct US evaluation. However, in the presence of a unexplained main pancreatic duct dilatation at initial US (Fig. 9.13a), the groove region should be examined with high resolution US (Fig. 9.13b). The use of a high frequency probe may better evaluate the more proximal juxta-papillary portions of mainduct (Fig. 9.13b). Identification of small cystic formations in the thickened duodenal wall on the pancreatic side is a specific finding (Procacci et al. 1997) for cystic dystrophy of the duodenal wall (Fig. 9.13c).

Mass-forming focal pancreatitis has US features that may be indistinguishable from ductal adenocarcinoma (Kim et al. 2001) (Fig. 9.4a). The presence of small calcifications in the lesion (Fig. 9.14) favors chronic pancreatitis (Remer and Baker 2002). Contrast-enhanced ultrasonography (CEUS) can improve US differential diagnosis between mass forming pancreatitis and pancreatic adenocarcinoma. Specifically, ductal adenocarcinoma remains hypoechoic in all contrast-enhanced phases enhancing similar to the pancreatic parenchyma (Fig. 9.4b). Enhancement paralleling the adjacent pancreas at CEUS favors an inflammatory mass.

9.2.2.2 Non-obstructive Chronic Pancreatitis

Primary chronic pancreatitis, not caused by ductal obstruction, is the most common type of chronic pancreatitis. Alcoholism is the most common etiology (Balthazar 1994; Lankisch and Banks 1998a,b). Alcoholic chronic pancreatitis is characterized by parenchymal and ductal alterations which are readily evident on imaging studies. In the advanced phase, US can demonstrates parenchymal atrophy, main pancreatic duct dilation, pancreatic calcifications and intraductal calculi. On the basis of morphology, a US differentiation from hereditary chronic pancreatitis is difficult, even if in the latter, calcifications may be different in morphology and size from those of alcoholic chronic pancreatitis (Ring et al. 1973). Autoimmune chronic pancreatitis is a particular type of chronic pancreatitis recently recognized clinically and at histology (Furukawa et al. 1998). Autoimmune pancreatitis is characterized by periductal lymphocytic infiltration, with evolution to fibrosis (Furukawa et al. 1998). As opposed to the other forms of chronic pancreatitis, the pancreas is diffusely increased in size, with the typical "sausage" look, and main pancreatic duct is compressed or string-like (Furukawa et al. 1998). US findings are characteristic in the diffuse form when the entire gland is involved (Fig. 9.9a). Echogenicity is markedly reduced, gland volume is increased, and Wirsung duct is compressed by glandular parenchyma (Fig. 9.9a). Color- and power-Doppler may demonstrate an increase in glandular vascularization caused by inflammations (Fig. 9.9b). The peculiar vascularization of autoimmune pancreatitis is better demonstrated at CEUS (Fig. 9.9c). These findings at US may be especially useful in the study of focal forms of autoimmune chronic pancreatitis that can mimic ductal adenocarcinoma.

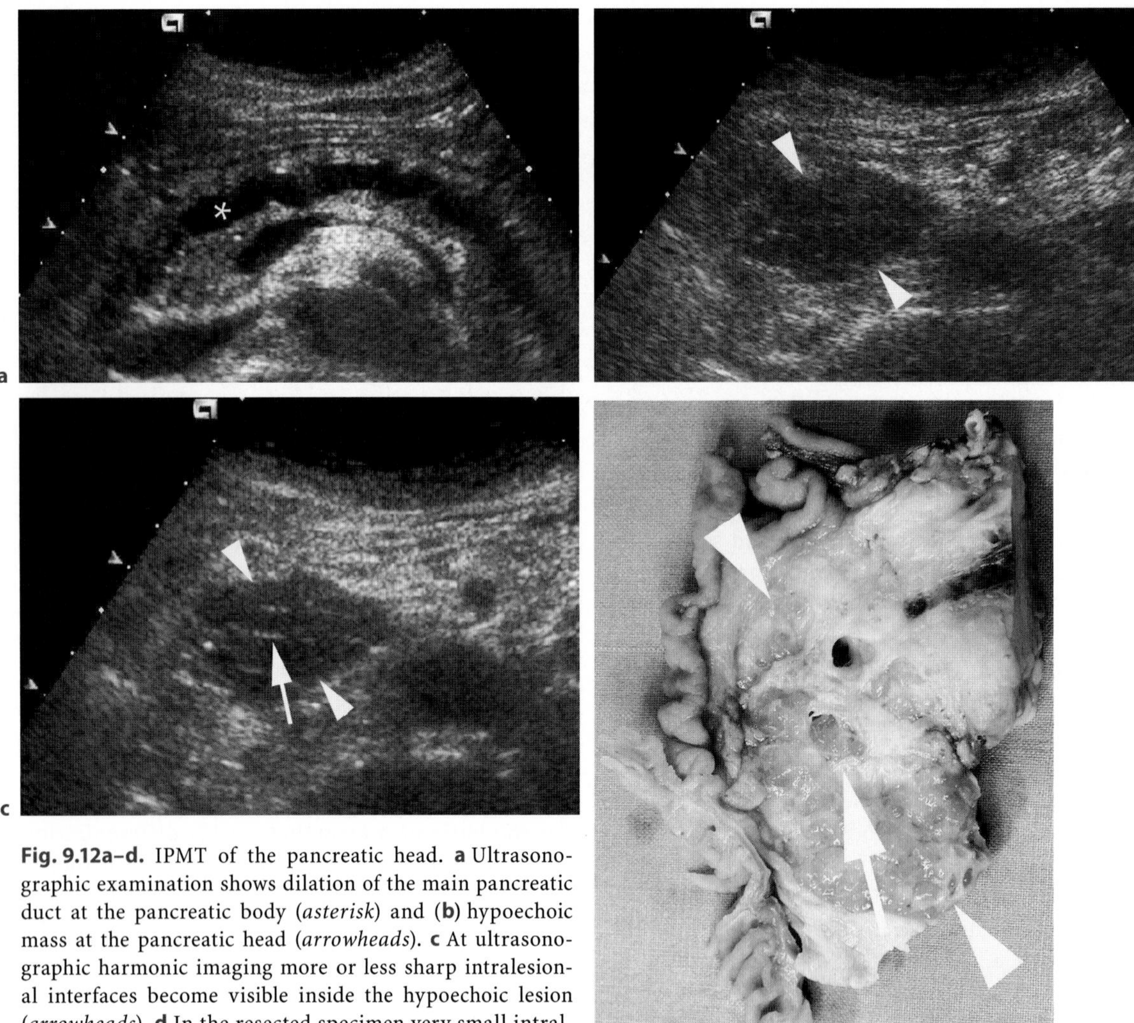

Fig. 9.12a–d. IPMT of the pancreatic head. **a** Ultrasonographic examination shows dilation of the main pancreatic duct at the pancreatic body (*asterisk*) and (**b**) hypoechoic mass at the pancreatic head (*arrowheads*). **c** At ultrasonographic harmonic imaging more or less sharp intralesional interfaces become visible inside the hypoechoic lesion (*arrowheads*). **d** In the resected specimen very small intralesional septa (*arrow*) are visible

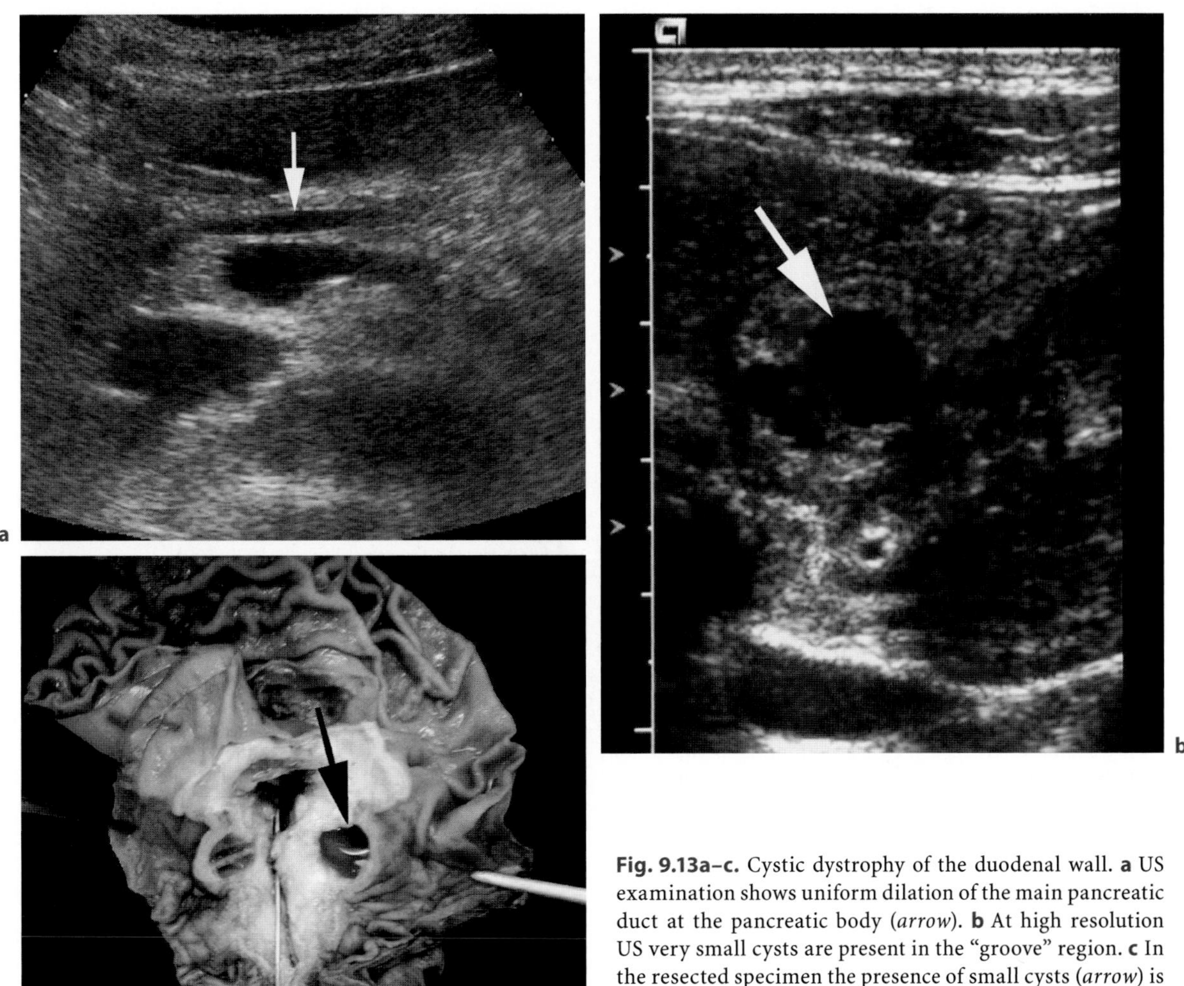

Fig. 9.13a–c. Cystic dystrophy of the duodenal wall. **a** US examination shows uniform dilation of the main pancreatic duct at the pancreatic body (*arrow*). **b** At high resolution US very small cysts are present in the "groove" region. **c** In the resected specimen the presence of small cysts (*arrow*) is diagnostic for cystic dystrophy of the duodenal wall

Fig. 9.14. Mass-forming focal chronic pancreatitis. Hypoechoic pancreatic head mass is visible at ultrasonographic examination with small calcification (*arrow*) inside the lesion. Differentiation from pancreatic neoplasm is extremely difficult prior to resection

References

Alpern MB, Sandler MA, Kellman GM, Madrazo BL (1985) Chronic pancreatitis: ultrasonic features. Radiology 155:215–219

Balthazar EJ (1994) Pancreatitis. In: Gore RM, Levine MS, Laufer I (eds) Textbook of gastrointestinal radiology. WB Saunders, pp 2132–2160

Bennett GL, Hann LE (2001) Pancreatic ultrasonography. Surg Clin North Am 81:259–281

Bolondi L, Priori P, Gullo L, Santi V, Li Bassi S, Barbara L, Labò G (1987) Relationship between morphological changes detected by ultrasonography and pancreatic esocrine function in chronic pancreatitis. Pancreas 2:222–229

Bolondi L, Li Bassi S, Gaiani S, Barbara L (1989) Sonography of chronic pancreatitis. Radiol Clin North Am 27:815

Brogna A, Bucceri AM, Catalano F, Ferrara R, Mangiameli A, Monello S, Blasi A (1991) Ultrasonographic study of the Wirsung duct caliber after meal. Ital J Gastroenterology 23:208–210

Foley WD, Stewart ET, Lawson TL, Geenan J, Loguidice J, Maher L, Unger GF (1980) Computer tomography, ultrasonography and echoscopic retrograde cholangiopancreatography in the diagnosis of pancreatic disease: a comparative study. Gastrointestinal Radiol 5:29–35

Furukawa N, Muranaka T, Yasumori K, Matsubayashi R, Hayashida K, Arita Y (1998) Autoimmune pancreatitis: radiologic findings in three histologically proven cases. J Comput Assist Tomogr 22:880–883

Glaser J, Mann O, Pausch J (1994) Diagnosis of chronic pancretitis by means of a sonographic secretin test. Int J Pancreatol 15:195–200

Gowland M, Kalantizis N, Warwick F, Braganza J (1981) Relative efficiency and predictive value of ultrasonography and endoscopic retrograde pancreatography in diagnosis of pancreatic disease. Lancet 2:190–193

Grant TH, Efrusy ME (1981) Ultrasound in the evaluation of chronic pancreatitis. JAMA 81:183–188

Hessel ST, Siegelman SS, McNeil BJ, Sanders R, Adams DF, Alderson PO, Finberg HJ, Abrams HL (1982) A prospective evaluation of computer tomography and ultrasound of the pancreas. Radiology 143:129–133

Homma T, Harada H, Koizumi M (1997) Diagnostic criteria for chronic pancreatitis by the Japan Pancreas Society. Pancreas 15:14–15

Husband JE, Meire HB, Kreel L (1977) Comparison of ultrasound and computer tomography in pancreatic diagnosis. Br J Radiol 50:855–863

Kim T, Murakami T, Takamura M, Hori M, Takahashi S, Nakamori S, Sakon M, Tanji Y, Wakasa K, Nakamura H (2001) Pancreatic mass due to chronic pancreatitis: correlation of CT and MR imaging features with pathologic findings. AJR Am J Roentgenol 177:367–371

Lankisch PG, Banks PA (1998a) Chronic pancreatitis: etiology. In: Lankisch PG, Banks PA (eds) Pancreatitis. Springer, Berlin Heidelberg New York, pp 199–208

Lankisch PG, Banks PA (1998b) Chronic pancreatitis: pathophysiology. In: Lankisch PG, Banks PA (eds) Pancreatitis. Springer, Berlin Heidelberg New York, pp 209–214

Lawson TL, Berland LL, Foley WD, Stewart ET, Geenan JE, Hogan WJ (1982) Ultrasonic visualization of the pancreatic duct. Radiology 144:865–871

Lecesne R, Laurent F, Drouillard J, Ponette E, Brys P, Van Steenbergen Van Hoe L (1999) Chronic pancreatitis. In: Baert AL, Delorme G, Van Hoe L (eds) Radiology of the pancreas, 2nd rev edn. Springer, Berlin Heidelberg New York, pp 145–180

Lees WR, Vallon AD, Denyer ME, Vahl SP, Cotton PB (1979) Prospective study of ultrasonography in chronic pancreatic disease. Br Med J 1:162–164

Niederau C, Grendell JH (1985) Diagnosis of chronic pancreatitis. Gastroenterology 88:1973–1995

Procacci C, Graziani R, Bicego E, Bergamo-Andreis IA, Mainardi P, Zamboni G, Pederzoli P, Cavallini G, Valdo M, Pistolesi GF (1996) Intraductal mucin-producing tumor of the pancreas: Imaging findings. Radiology 198:249–257

Procacci C, Graziani R, Zamboni G, Cavallini G, Pederzoli P, Guarise A, Bogina G, Biasiutti C, Carbognin G, Bergamo-Andreis IA, Pistolesi GF (1997) Cystic dystrophy of the duodenal wall: radiologic findings. Radiology 205:741–747

Procacci C, Schenal G, Della Chiara E, Fuini A, Guarise A (2003) Intraductal papillary mucinous tumors: imaging. In: Procacci C, Megibow AJ (eds) Imaging of the pancreas cystic and rare tumors. Springer, Berlin Heidelberg New York, pp 97–137

Remer EM, Baker MB (2002) Imaging of chronic pancreatitis. Radiol Clin N Am 40:1229–1242

Ring EJ, Eaton SB, Ferrucci JT, Short WF (1973) Differential diagnosis of pancreatic calcification. Am J Roentgenol Radium Ther Nucl Med 117:446–452

Sarner M, Cotton PB (1984a) Classification of pancreatitis. Gut 25:756–759

Sarner M, Cotton PB (1984b) Definitions of acute and chronic pancreatitis. Clin Gastroenterol 13:865–870

Shapiro RS, Wagreich J, Parsons RB, Stancato-Pasik A, Yeh HC, Lao R (1998) Tissue harmonic imaging sonography: evaluation of image quality compared with conventional sonography. AJR Am J Roentgenol 171:1203–1206

Singer MW, Gyr K, Sarles H (1985) Revised classification of pancretitis. Report of the Second Internetional Symposium on the Classification of Pancreatitis in Marseille, France, March 28–30, 1984. Gastroenterology 89:683–685

The Role of Computed Tomography

10

Rossella Graziani, Daniela Cenzi, Francesca Franzoso, Daniela Coser, and Marinella Neri

CONTENTS

10.1 **Relapsing Pancreatitis (RP)** *149*
10.1.1 Neoplastic Causes of RP *150*
10.1.1.1 Adenocarcinoma of the Papilla *150*
10.1.1.2 Neuroendocrine Tumors *150*
10.1.1.3 Mesenchymal Tumors *150*
10.1.2 RP Due to Congenital Malformation *150*
10.1.2.1 Pancreas Divisum *150*
10.1.2.2 Annular Pancreas *150*
10.1.2.3 Extraluminal Duodenal Diverticulum *150*
10.1.2.4 Intraluminal Duodenal Diverticulum *152*
10.1.2.5 Duodenal Duplication *152*
10.1.2.6 Choledochal Cyst-Choledochocele *152*
10.2 **Chronic Pancreatitis (CP): Early Phase** *152*
10.3 **Chronic Pancreatitis (CP): Advanced Phase** *152*
10.3.1 Obstructive Chronic Pancreatitis (OCP) *154*
10.3.1.1 CT Characterisation of OCP *154*
10.3.1.2 CT Diagnosis of Causes of OCP *156*
10.3.1.3 CT Differential Diagnosis:OCP vs Pancreatic Tumors *163*
10.3.2 Non-obstructive or Primitive Chronic Pancreatitis (PCP) *164*
10.3.2.1 CT Identification of Hereditary PCP Secondary to Genetic Mutations *164*
10.3.2.2 CT Identification of Autoimmune PCP *168*
10.3.2.3 CT Identification of PCP Associated with Toxic and Metabolic Factors *171*
10.3.2.4 CT Differential Diagnosis: PCP vs Pancreatic Tumors *176*
10.4 **Conclusions** *180*
References *180*

R. Graziani, MD; F. Franzoso, MD
D. Coser, MD; M. Neri, MD
Department of Radiology, Policlinico "GB Rossi", University of Verona, Piazzale LA Scuro 10, 37134 Verona, Italy
D. Cenzi, MD
Department of Radiology, Ospedale Borgo Trento, Piazzale Stefani 1, 37126 Verona, Italy

Continuous acquisition (either single or multidetector configuration) has a pivotal role in the evaluation of patients with chronic pancreatitis (CP) in all stages of the disease (Malfertheiner and Buchler 1989; Forsmark 2000; Brizi et al. 2001). These can be divided into an early phase of relapsing pancreatitis (RP) in which episodes of mild acute pancreatitis (MAP) or severe acute pancreatitis (SAP) repeatedly occur over a period of time, an early chronic stage, and irreversible advanced CP (Malfertheiner and Buchler 1989; Lankisch and Banks 1998).

10.1 Relapsing Pancreatitis (RP)

In patients with RP who go on to develop CP, subtle ductal abnormalities will occur that will likely not be able to be detected by current imaging. If the clinician is suspicious, altered response to secretin may be demonstrated. The morphology and dimensions of the pancreas in this phase are, in fact, normal at CT examination. Parenchymal enhancement is not affected (Figs. 10.1a and 10.2a).

The ductal structures may be normal (Figs. 10.1a and 10.2a) or dilated (Fig. 10.1f) in relation to the size of the obstruction.

The major contribution of imaging is to detect any mechanical reason that would lead to impairment of pancreatic drainage. A wide variety of etiologies may be encountered; the radiologist is advised to methodically evaluate the bile ducts for microlithiasis in the common bile duct (CBD) and/or papilla (Maione et al. 1999; Levy and Geenen 2001; Gullo et al. 2002; Levy 2002); postinflammatory papillary stenosis; a dysfunction of the sphincter of Oddi (Levy and Geenen 2001; Levy 2002); an ampullary tumor and congenital biliary anomalies (Guelrud et al. 1999; Dussaulx-Garin et al. 2000; Komuro et al. 2001); to evaluate the pancreas for congenital anomalies at the level of the pancreatic ductal system (Inamoto et al. 1983; Jadvar and Mindelzun 1999; Morgan et al. 1999; Levy and Geenen 2001; Megibow et al. 2001; Shan et al. 2002); tumors; scarring from SAP (Somogyi et al. 2001); and to evaluate the duodenum for tumors, congenital anomalies and duodenal dystrophy.

CT is excellent in elucidating neoplastic and congenital abnormalities,. Adequate treatment of such lesions can help impede any subsequent development into CP.

10.1.1
Neoplastic Causes of RP

10.1.1.1
Adenocarcinoma of the Papilla

The most common neoplastic cause of RP is adenocarcinoma of the papilla, appearing at CT as a nodular lesion with solid density located in the papilla (Pandolfo et al. 1990), slightly enhancing in the pancreatic phase of enhancement (Wise and Stanley 1984). When the duodenum is adequately distended with neutral contast, the lesion can be visualized as jutting into the lumen (Wise and Stanley 1984) (Fig. 10.1b,c). The intra- and extrahepatic biliary tracts are dilated (Fig. 10.1a), as is the main pancreatic duct (MPD) (Gmelin and Weiss 1981; Wise and Stanley 1984). This tumor is more easily recognised with MSCT (Takeshita et al. 2002) which, thanks to 3-D multiplanar capabilities (Fig. 10.1d), can localize the mass within the papilla.

10.1.1.2
Neuroendocrine Tumors

RP can be secondary to the presence of a neuroendocrine tumor, generally represented by somatostatinomas of the papilla associated with von Recklinghausen's disease (Hamissa et al. 1999), recognisable as quite small nodular lesions located in the papilla. They have a solid density and are hypervascularized in the pancreatic enhancement phase (Fig. 10.1e).

10.1.1.3
Mesenchymal Tumors

Uncommon causes of RP are ampullary mesenchymal tumors (papillary lipomas and leiomyomas, leiomyosarcoma and duodenal lymphoma) (Ferrozzi et al. 2000).

10.1.2
RP Due to Congenital Malformation

10.1.2.1
Pancreas Divisum

The most common anomaly associated with RP is pancreas divisum. The mechanism of RP is insufficient size of the minor papilla to allow drainage of pancreatic juice from the Santorini duct. Rarely, a mechanical obstruction at the minor papilla will be found (Hsu et al. 2001; Procacci et al. 2001b; Somogyi et al. 2001). The relationship of pancreas divisum and RP is controversial, as most patients with the anomaly are asymtptomatic. If, through provactive test such as assessing drainage following a secretin challenge, the causal relationship is established, then minor papilla stenting or sphincterotomy will retard progression to CP (Soulen et al. 1989; Hsu et al. 2000).

MDCT will demonstrate the normal pancratic duct in the majority of cases, especially using 3-D techniques. It is therefore possible to detect pancreas divisum on most current CT examinations (Fig. 10.1f); MRCP is reserved for doubtful cases (Megibow et al. 2001).

10.1.2.2
Annular Pancreas

A less frequent congenital cause of RP is annular pancreas. CT examination shows the presence of gastric dilatation and stenosis of the second portion of the duodenum. At the level of the narrowing, one recognizes soft tissue attenuating material that enhances identically to pancratic parenchyma. The annulus may be total or partial (Inamoto et al. 1983; England et al. 1995; Rizzo et al. 1995; Jadvar and Mindelzun 1999) (Fig. 10.2a). This obstructs the main pancreatic duct because of oedema of the duodenal wall caused by the continual traumatic difficulty of passing digested material.

10.1.2.3
Extraluminal Duodenal Diverticulum

RP associated with the presence of extraluminal duodenal diverticulum is seldom encountered. The diverticula are generally located on the mesenteric side of the second portion of the duodenum adjacent to the ampulla of Vater and at the pancreatic head, which may distend due to torsion, inflammation or obstruction by food, thus causing RP by compression of the biliary and pancreatic ducts.

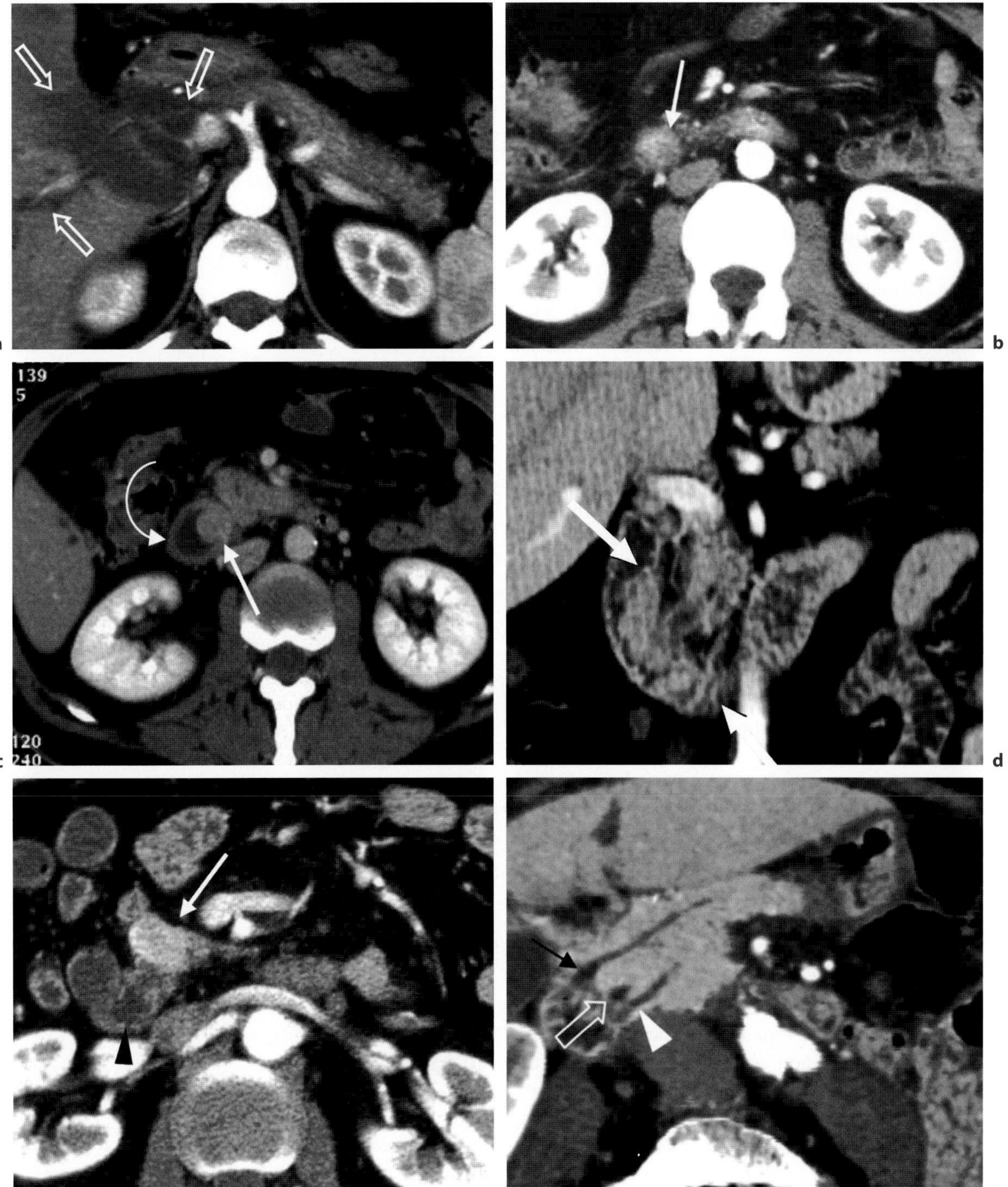

Fig. 10.1 a–f. Relapsing pancreatitis (RP): Contrast enhanced CT – axial images – (**a–c**, **e**); coronal (**d**) and curvilinear (**f**) reconstructions. **a–e** Ampullary tumors. Papillary adenocarcinoma (**a–d**). The pancreas shows normal morphology and size, preserved parenchymal enhancement, dilatation of the intrahepatic biliary tracts (**a**), gallbladder and common bile duct (*clear arrows*); there is a small mass (*arrow*) in the papillary region (**b**), jutting into the water distended duodenal lumen (**c**) (*curved arrow*). The mass has soft tissue attenuation and minimally enhances in the pancreatic phase following CM (**b**) but is hypodense in the venous phase (**c**). Solid mass (*black arrow*) in the papillary region, projecting into the duodenal lumen visualized on coronal MDCT (**d**). Neuroendocrine papillary tumor (**e**). Small mass (*arrow*) in the juxtapapillary area (*arrowhead*) with soft tissue, hypervascularized in the pancreatic phase (somatostatinoma). **f** Congenital lesions. Pancreas divisum. The outlet of the dorsal pancreatic duct (*arrow*) separate from that of the common bile duct (*empty arrow*) and the ventral pancreatic duct (*arrowhead*) in the curvilinear MDCT reconstruction.

CT examination identifies the presence of a rounded thin walled air containing mass, that may also contain oral contrast medium or debris (Fig. 10.2b,c) It is also sometimes possible to see the thin neck that connects the lesion to the medial portion of the duodenal sweep.

10.1.2.4 Intraluminal Duodenal Diverticulum

Intraluminal duodenal diverticulum, rarer still than the extraluminal forms, can increase in size as it becomes filled with food. This size increase will cause episodes of pain, vomiting (Fidler et al. 1998), jaundice and RP (Fidler et al. 1998), from by papillary compression and obstruction (Fidler et al. 1998).

If the diverticulum collapses, it appears at CT as a low density "flap" inside the duodenal lumen, which is distended by water or orally administered opaque contrast medium (Fidler et al. 1998). If the diverticulum is distended and its neck patent, the water or opaque oral CM fills the diverticular lumen. A rounded mass will then be recognisable within the lumen contrasted by water or oral CM and circumscribed by a thin, hypodense diverticular wall, which, in turn, is surrounded by a film of oral CM contained within the real duodenal lumen (Fidler et al. 1998).

10.1.2.5 Duodenal Duplication

CT examination reveals the presence of a cystic-type mass (Procacci et al. 1988), adjacent to the second and third portions of the duodenum, imbedded in the duodenal wall. The mass appears rounded or oval, is sometimes lobulated, has a thick wall and is usually not larger than 7–8 cm (Procacci et al. 1988). Its density depends on the type of duplication (Procacci et al. 1988). The non-communicating form often contains fluid and therefore has a fluid density with typical internal parallel and thin septa due to folds in the mucous covering (Procacci et al. 1988), while the communicating form, in the emptying phase, can have a solid density (Procacci et al. 1988). They can result in RP by extrinsic compression of the main pancreatic duct in the head of the gland.

10.1.2.6 Choledochal Cyst-Choledochocele

Type III choledochocyst or choledochocele is a herniation of the bileduct into the duodenal lumen. This malformation can cause repeated episodes of RP, even SAP (Fig. 10.2d) because of the intermittent obstruction of the biliary and main pancreatic ducts, although most patients with choledochocele are asymptomatic. If large enough, choledochocele appears at CT as a fluid mass located at the papilla, jutting into the duodenal lumen (Fig. 10.2e,f). The MRCP examination shows a "club-like" appearance of the intramural portion of the distal CBD jutting into the duodenal lumen (Fig. 10.2g).

10.2 Chronic Pancreatitis (CP): Early Phase

In time, repeated episodes of RP lead to the establishment of irreversible anatomic changes in the parenchyma and ductal structures. The earliest changes recognizable on a macroscopic level are cystic ectasia of the branch ducts and subtle irregularity of the contour of the main pancreatic duct. Direct visualization of the pancreatic duct with endoscopic retrograde cholangiopancreatography (ERCP), is the only method capable of detecting these changes in situ.

State-of-the-art MDCT (Kahl et al. 2002) cannot recognize these subtle ductal changes. CT imaging is employed to exclude neoplasm (Etemad and Whitcomb 2001) and anomaly in the same way as described for RP.

10.3 Chronic Pancreatitis (CP): Advanced Phase

In advanced CP, the irreversible parenchymal destruction and gross ductal abnormalities are easily recognized. CT is performed to distinguish between obstructive CP (OCP) and non-obstructive or primitive CP (PCP). In patients with OCP, MDCT can further demonstrate the etiology. MDCT also attempts to differentiate CP from a neoplastic pancreatic pathology, thus helping the clinician to make the correct therapeutic choice (Elmas 2001). This latter differentiation is a major challenge to imaging.

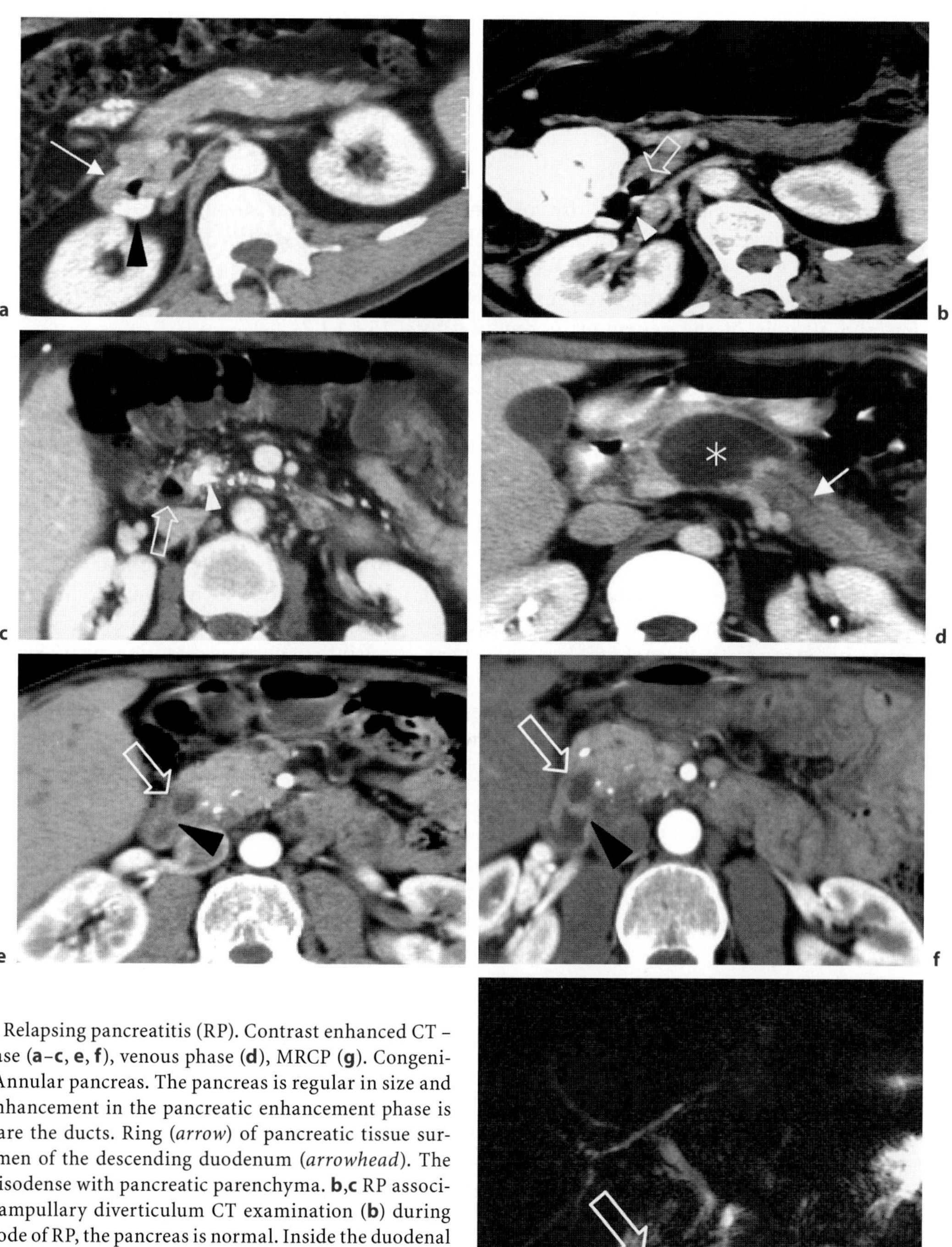

Fig. 10.2 a–g. Relapsing pancreatitis (RP). Contrast enhanced CT – pancreatic phase (**a–c**, **e**, **f**), venous phase (**d**), MRCP (**g**). Congenital lesions. **a** Annular pancreas. The pancreas is regular in size and volume; the enhancement in the pancreatic enhancement phase is preserved, as are the ducts. Ring (*arrow*) of pancreatic tissue surrounds the lumen of the descending duodenum (*arrowhead*). The attenuation is isodense with pancreatic parenchyma. **b,c** RP associated with periampullary diverticulum CT examination (**b**) during the initial episode of RP, the pancreas is normal. Inside the duodenal lumen (*arrowhead*) a small (*clear arrow*) rounded gas collection is visible (periampullary duodenal diverticulum). CT study in same patient 5 years later (**c**), after repeated episodes of RP, the small periampullary duodenal diverticulum persists (*clear arrow*). The pancreas is atrophic. A ductal stone (*arrowhead*) at the uncinate process is visible (sign of OCP). **d–g** RP associated with choledochocele. (**d**), after repeated episodes of RP there is a pseudocyst (*asterisk*) in the body of the pancreas, producing obstruction on the main pancreatic duct in the body-tail (*arrow*). The patient underwent pseudocyst-jejuno-anastomosis. At 8 years later (**e**), appearance of CP with duct stones in the pancreatic head. A small fluid density mass (*clear arrow*) can be seen near the papilla (*arrowhead*), initially interpreted as a retention cyst. At 6 months later (**f**), CT examination shows an increase in the number of tiny ductal stones in the head of the gland and the persistence of the small peri-papillary fluid formation (*clear arrow*), referable at MRCP examination (**g**) to a small choledochal cyst (*clear arrow*)

10.3.1 Obstructive Chronic Pancreatitis (OCP)

10.3.1.1 CT Characterisation of OCP

CT examination identifies OCP by recognizing characteristic alterations in both the parenchyma and the ducts. In these patients, one sees dilatation of the pancreatic ducts at the level of the obstruction and atrophy of the acinar cells, replaced by uniform and diffuse fibrosis within the pancreatic parenchyma (Elmas 2001; Etemad and Whitcomb 2001; Sakorafas et al. 2001).

10.3.1.1.1 Parenchyma

Morphology

The size of the pancreatic gland, initially normal, becomes progressively smaller (Figs. 10.3 and 10.4) due to an increasing parenchymal atrophy characterized as uniform and diffuse (Elmas 2001) (Figs. 10.3 and 10.4). In extreme cases, the parenchyma may not be visible (Procacci et al. 1998).

The unaffected pancreatic parenchyma downstream to the obstruction (Sakorafas et al. 2001) appears normal (Fig. 10.5f). This finding is unusual, however, since, in the majority of cases, the obstruction is located in the head of the pancreas and consequently involves the whole gland (Procacci et al. 1998).

Structure

On unenhanced MDCT studies the only visible pancreatic abnormality is the presence of calcifications (Figs. 10.3a and 10.4a,b), the commonest and most specific CT manifestation of chronic pancreatitis (Kim et al. 2001).

Calcifications are the consequence of calcium deposits in the form of endoductal protein plugs (Luetmer et al.1989; Procacci et al. 1998). By completely occupying the lumen of the smaller peripheral side ducts, they may appear to have an intraparenchymal location (Fig. 10.4c).

Following CM administration the parenchyma affected by CP shows reduced enhancement in the pancreatic phase (Kusano et al. 1999), thus hypodense compared to the normal parenchyma (Fig. 10.3b,e–g). This is exactly the *reverse* enhancement pattern of normal pancreatic parenchyma at this stage.

In the portal venous phase, the parenchyma becomes progressively hyperdense (Fig. 10.3c); if further delayed imaging is performed, the hyperdensity (Kusano et al. 1999) within the fibrotic areas becomes even more striking (Fig. 10.3d). This finding is more evident in the case of focal fibrosis where areas of fibrosis alternate with areas of normal tissue in the gland itself (Procacci et al. 1998).

10.3.1.1.2 Ducts

The ductal changes in OCP, present from the initial phases of the disease, are described as uniform and regular dilatation.

The branch ducts are generally undamaged (Manfredi et al. 2001). Later in the disease, the branch ducts dilate secondary to stenoses exacerbated by stone formation (Pavone et al. 1999) resulting in multi-lobulated cystic spaces (Fig. 10.4f), until they become retention cysts (Fig. 10.4g).

On dual acquisition CT studies, ductal dilatation is best evaluated in the pancreatic phase where it can reach diameters between 2–3 cm. (Fig. 10.3e,f).

In OCP, there may be stones inside the lumen of the main duct (Figs. 10.3a–f and 10.4a,b), sometimes the Santorini duct (Fig. 10.4d–e) and the minor ducts (Figs. 10.3g and 10.4c,f,g). These stones arise from calcium deposits along the intraductal protein plugs (Procacci et al. 1998; Manfredi et al. 2001). These are recognisable as small, hyperdense ductal filling defects (Fig. 10.6a,c,e,f). However, in the obstructive form, stones are less frequent compared to hereditary or primary forms of the disease (Procacci et al. 1998, 2001b).

CT examination easily recognises stones (Homma 1998; Berrocal et al. 1999), especially on unenhanced studies Care should be taken to not interpret splenic artery calcification as intraductal calculi (Luetmer et al. 1989). The stones are hyperdense, small punctate (Fig. 10.4c–d) or rounded foci (Fig. 10.3a–d). The larger ones have a "casted" or irregular morphology (Figs. 10.3f,g and 10.4a,b), are widely distributed or concentrated in groups or clusters (Fig. 10.3g).

Their number and size are variable (Procacci et al. 2001b; Cavallini and Frulloni 2002) in relation to the stage of the disease. They can remain unchanged but generally tend to increase with time (Fig. 10.4a,b).

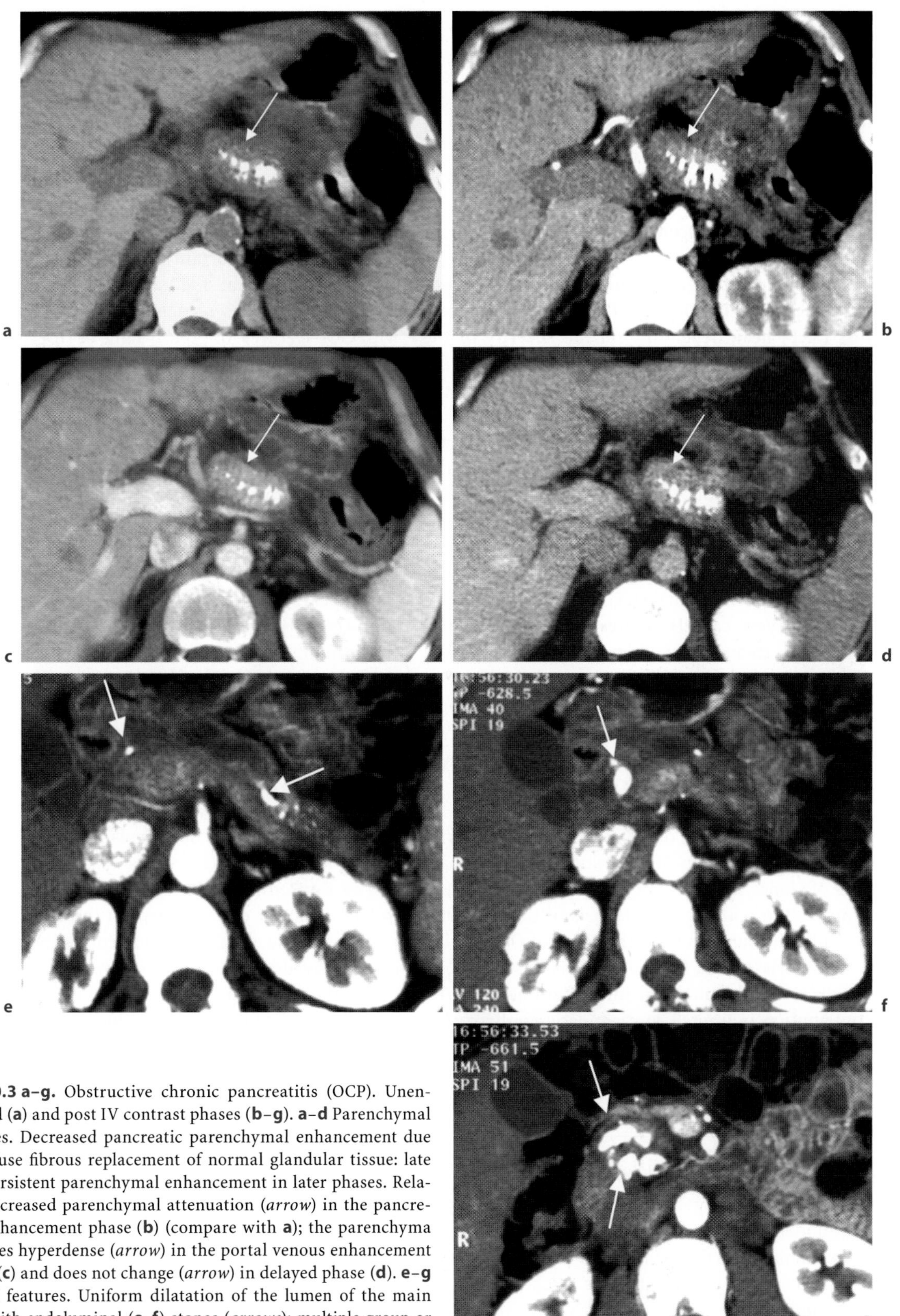

Fig. 10.3 a–g. Obstructive chronic pancreatitis (OCP). Unenhanced (**a**) and post IV contrast phases (**b–g**). **a–d** Parenchymal features. Decreased pancreatic parenchymal enhancement due to diffuse fibrous replacement of normal glandular tissue: late and persistent parenchymal enhancement in later phases. Relative decreased parenchymal attenuation (*arrow*) in the pancreatic enhancement phase (**b**) (compare with **a**); the parenchyma becomes hyperdense (*arrow*) in the portal venous enhancement phase (**c**) and does not change (*arrow*) in delayed phase (**d**). **e–g** Ductal features. Uniform dilatation of the lumen of the main duct with endoluminal (**e, f**) stones (*arrows*); multiple group or "cluster" of stones in the branch ducts of the uncinate process (**g**)

10.3.1.2
CT Diagnosis of Causes of OCP

MDCT makes a significant contribution to patient management by identifying the specific cause of OCP, leading to optimal therapy.

10.3.1.2.1
Scarring from Severe Acute Pancreatitis (SAP)

As necrotic parenchymal regions and extraglandular collections (Fig. 10.5a–c) of severe acute pancreatitis (SAP) heal, depending on the severity of the insult, variable regions of intrapancreatic scarring develop a component which can result in stenosis of the main duct. Over time, the result will be OCP.

At MDCT examination the pancreas upstream of the obstruction demonstrates uniform dilatation of the main duct, extending from the site of the duct obstruction. The branch ducts are undamaged, but there is significant parenchymal atrophy (Fig. 10.5d,e). The pancreas downstream of the obstruction appears normal (Fig. 10.5f).

Pseudocysts, can also be responsible for significant ductal stenosis that can persist at the site of the origin even after the cyst is diminished either due to spontaneous re-absorption or drainage (Fig. 10.5g).

10.3.1.2.2
Chronic Inflammatory Stenosis of the Papilla

Chronic inflammation of the papilla, in the majority of cases following repeated trauma due to the passage of stones and/or biliary microlithiasis, can, in time, lead to scarring and stenosis of the sphincter of Oddi and, subsequently, the onset of OCP.

Diagnosis of this form of OCP is based mainly on clinical and functional investigations. MDCT's contribution is limited to diagnostic confirmation of this pathology (Fig. 10.6), as it is able to exclude other causes of the ductal obstruction.

10.3.1.2.3
Duodenal Dystrophy

Duodenal dystrophy (DD) is a primary pathology of the duodenal wall, presumably originating from the ectopic pancreatic tissue (Tio et al. 1991; Vullierme et al. 2000). It appears as fibrous thickening of the duodenal wall, often associated with chronic inflammation of the intraduodenal pancreatic tissue, and with cystic lesions located at the sub-mucous or muscular layers (Tio et al. 1991; Indinnimeo et al. 2001).

The progression of ectopic pancreatic tissue inflammation, associated with the progressive increase in cyst size within it, could lead to compression of the MPD and therefore to OCP (Indinnimeo et al. 2001).

The only radical therapeutic option to stop this process is surgical resection. For this reason the correct diagnosis is important (Yamaguchi and Tanaka 1992; Procacci et al. 1997, 2001b; Indinnimeo et al. 2001). This includes recognition at MDCT together with OCP features, of typical signs of DD, in both its cystic (CDD) or solid (SDD) variants.

Cystic Variant (CDD)

This variant is easily identifiable with MDCT examination as cysts can be seen imbedded in the thickened fibrotic duodenum wall (Procacci et al. 1997).

A specific sign of duodenal wall dystrophy (Procacci et al. 1997) is fibrous parietal thickening that appears at CT (Procacci et al. 1997) as a layer of solid tissue lying between the duodenal lumen and the head of the pancreas. It is isodense compared to the parenchyma before CM administration and hypodense compared to the surrounding parenchyma in the pancreatic enhancement phase (Procacci et al. 1997) (Figs. 10.7b,e and 10.8a). This enhancement differential is more obvious when there is less injury to the adjacent pancreas (Fig. 10.7), but less evident if the parenchyma has been replaced by fibrosis as a consequence of OCP (Fig. 10.8a–c).

The thickening within the duodenal wall tends to have a slower enhancement in the venous phase (Fig. 10.7c); the enhancement becomes more apparent if delayed acquisitions are obtained (Fig. 10.7d), due to the fibrous tissue (Procacci et al. 1997; Irie et al. 1998b; Vullierme et al. 2000). Cystic formations can be seen in the space between the pancreatic head and the first, more commonly the second (Figs. 10.7b–e and 10.8b,c) or the third duodenal segments (Fig. 10.8d,e), usually on the mesenteric side and more rarely on the anti-mesenteric side (Figs. 10.7b–e and 10.8b,c). Generally, the cystic lesions are multiple (Figs. 10.7 and 10.8) from 3 to more than 10 in number, with a 3–5 mm diameter (Irie et al. 1998b). They have a fluid density and, in contrast to pseudocysts (Fig. 10.5b,g), their morphology is elongated or multilobular (Procacci et al. 1997; Ly and Miller 2002) (Fig. 10.8e) narrowing and deforming the duodenal lumen (Figs. 10.7 and

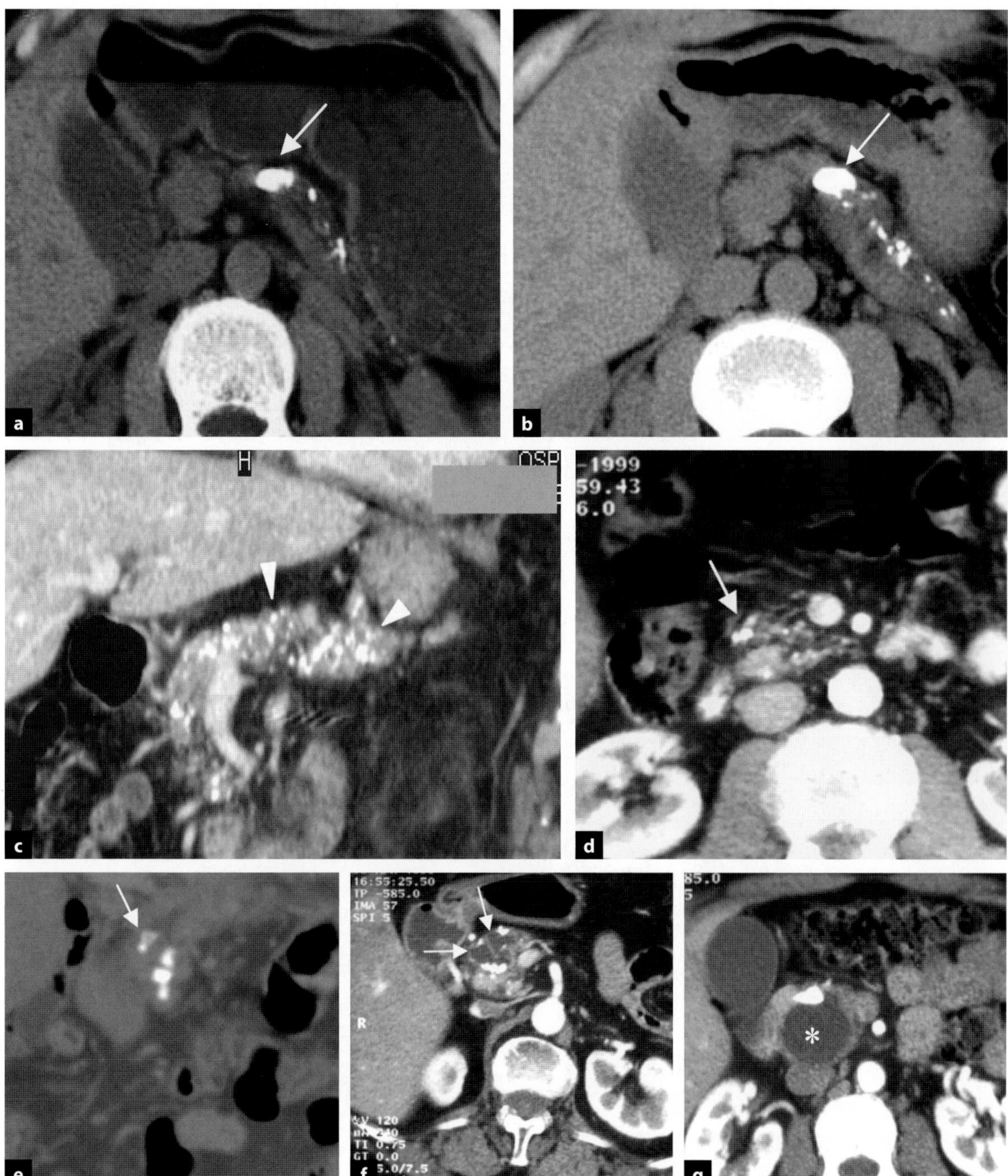

Fig. 10.4 a–g. Obstructive chronic pancreatitis (OCP). Axial CT in the pre- (**a**,**b**,**e**) and post-pancreatic enhancement phases (**d**, **f**, **g**); (**c**) coronal reconstruction. Ductal features. **a**, **b** The pancreas is atrophic, with dilatation of the main duct and intraductal calculi, varying in morphology and size (*arrow*). After 2 years (**b**), the stones in the main duct have increased in size and number. **c** Multiple small, punctate stones (*arrowhead*) in the lumen of the branch ducts of the body-tail visible with MDCT coronal reconstruction. They seem to be located within the atrophic glandular parenchyma. **d**, **e** Small rounded ductal stones in the lumen of the branch ducts of the uncinate process (**e**) and the Santorini duct (**d**, **e**: *arrow*), at the minor papilla orifice. **f**, **g** Ductal stones obstructing the lumen of several side branch ducts in the pancreatic head. These ducts are dilated and form multiple, small, cystic regions (**f**: *arrows*), or one single, large cyst (**g**: *asterisk*) with fluid density (retention cyst)

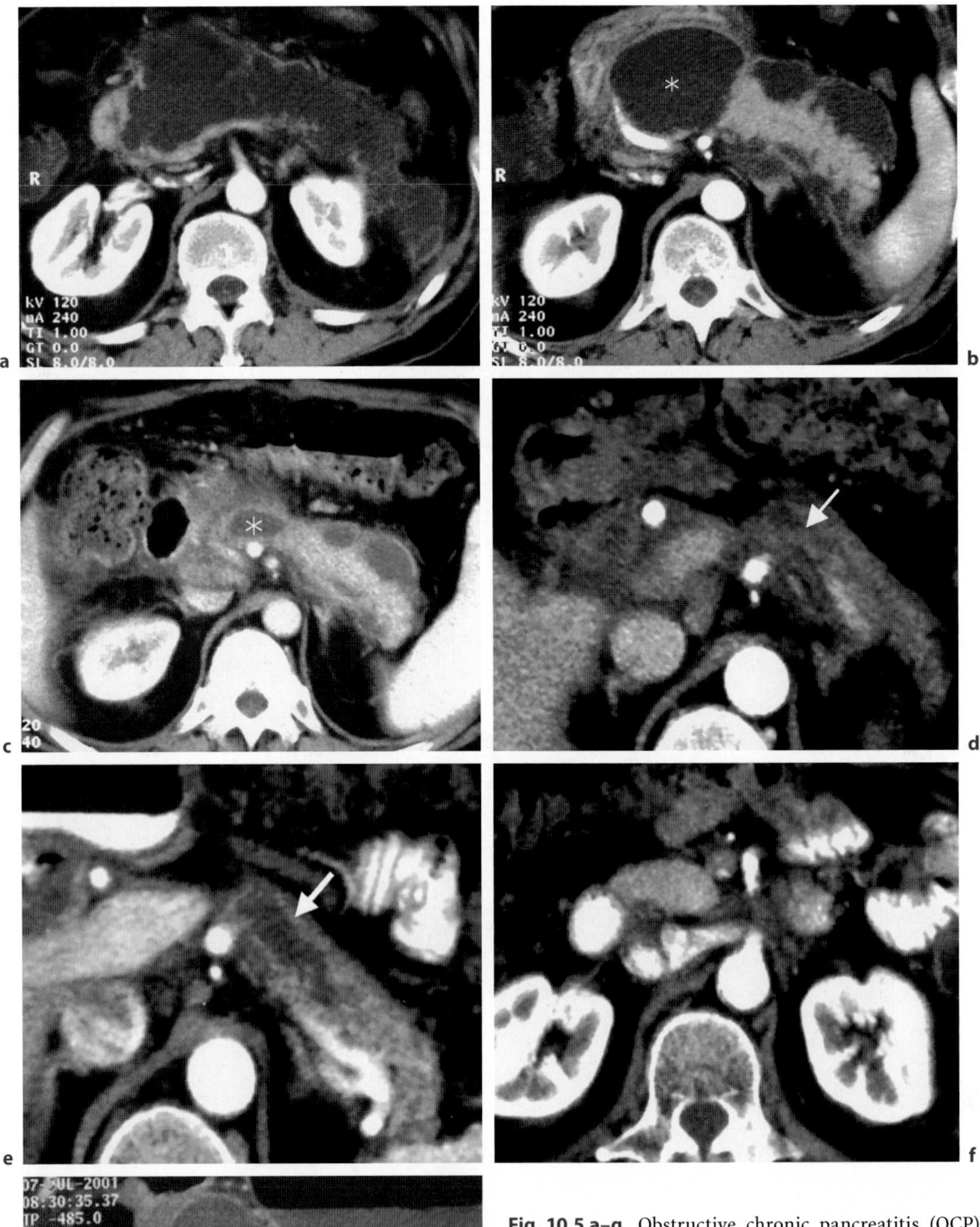

Fig. 10.5 a–g. Obstructive chronic pancreatitis (OCP) following previous SAP. CT in the pancreatic enhancement phase. Two cases (**a–f**; **g**). Widespread parenchymal necrosis with large retroperitoneal collection, following an episode of SAP (**a**); 1 month later (**b**) appearance of pseudocysts (*asterisk*) in the pancreatic isthmus becoming smaller over the next month (**c**). Same patient, 6 months later (**d**), OCP with parenchymal atrophy in the body-tail and dilatation of the MPD (*arrow*). Same patient 1 year later (**d**). The duct has increased in diameter (**e**). The head of the pancreas is normal (**f**), (post-SAP fibrotic ductal stenosis). **g** The pancreas is atrophic with uniform dilatation of the main duct at the body-tail (*arrow*), that terminates at the site of the pseudocysts (*asterisk*). Note the gastroduodenal artery which is shifted to the right (*arrowhead*)

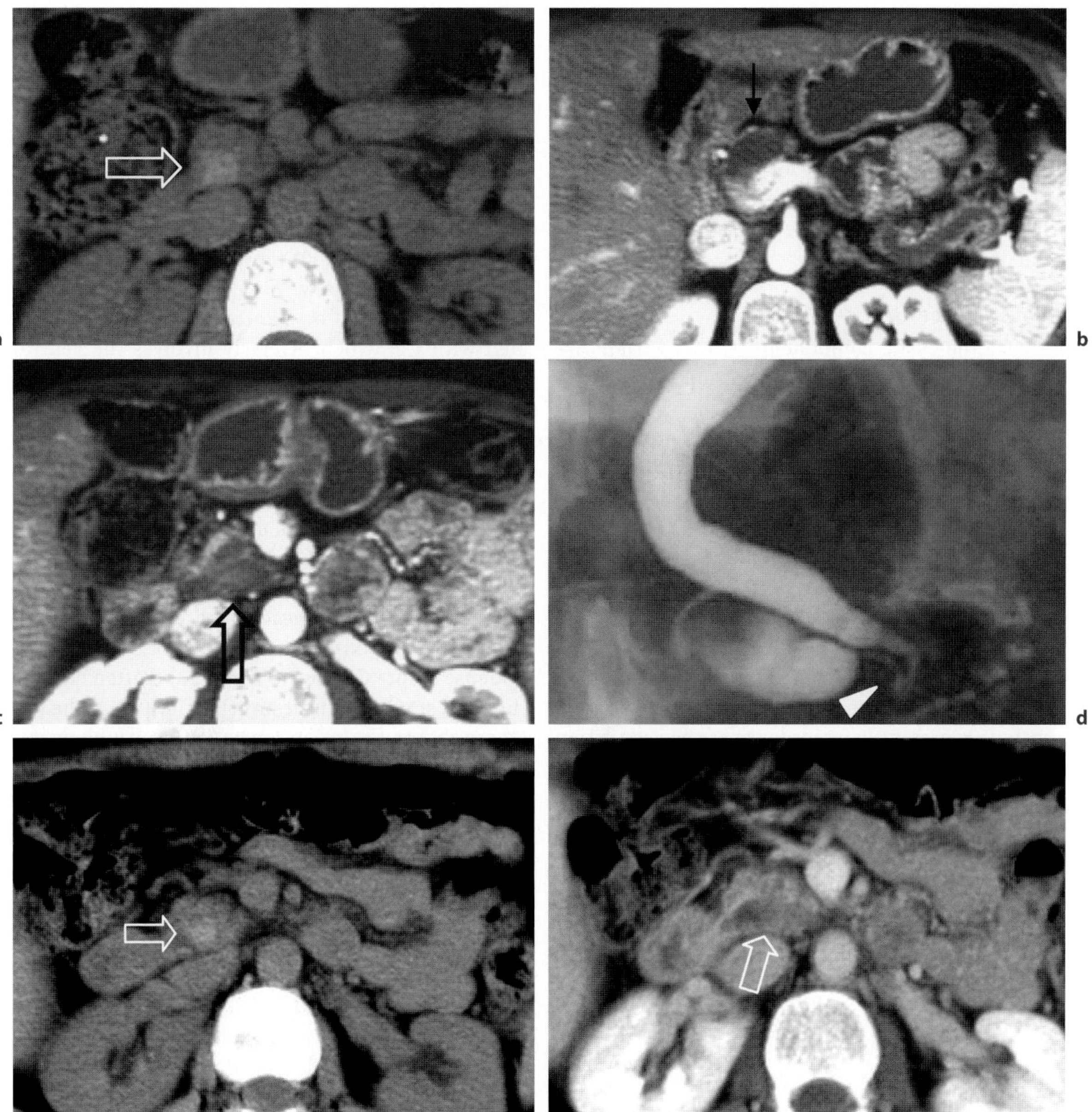

Fig. 10.6a–f. Obstructive chronic pancreatitis (OCP) due to inflammatory stenosis of the papilla. CT in the pre- (**a**,**e**) and post-intravenous contrast phases (**b**,**c**,**f**); ERCP (**d**). **a–d** At the first examination the pancreas displays total parenchymal atrophy with marked dilatation (*arrow*) of the MPD (**b**). A slightly hyperdense intraluminal filling defect (protein "plug") at the papillary region (**a**,**c**) is present. ERCP examination, 5 months later (**d**), demonstrates dilatation of the CBD, with stenosis within the intramural portion (*arrowhead*). The MPD is obstructed by stones. They were subsequently extracted endoscopically. At CT examination the following year (**e**,**f**), the protein plug has reappeared (*clear arrow*) in the distal (papillary) portion of the MPD (chronic inflammatory papillary stenosis)

10.8). There may also be gastric outlet obstruction (Itoh et al. 1994; Procacci et al. 1997; Vullierme et al. 2000; Indinnimeo et al. 2001; Procacci et al. 2001b). Lastly, since they originate in the duodenum, the cysts may displace (Procacci et al. 1997) the gastroduodenal artery forwards and to the left (Figs. 10.7a,b,e and 10.8a), precisely the opposite of what happens if the pathology originates from the head of the pancreas.

Solid Variant (SDD)

Because the cystic components of this variant are tiny and their presence "overwhelmed" by the exuberant fibrous tissue, they may be occult on imaging (Procacci et al. 1997). Therefore, this process may be easily mistaken for a solid mass (Procacci et al. 1997, 2001b).

On unenhanced MDCT, one may only observe increase in size of the pancreatic head (Fig. 10.9a). In many cases this is associated with duodenal narrowing and gastric distension. During the pancreatic phase of enhancement, the fibrous thickening of the duodenal wall is hypodense and thus distinguishable from the head of the pancreas (Fig. 10.9b), becoming progressively hyperdense as the acquisition is carried out over in portal (Fig. 10.9c) and delayed phases (Fig. 10.9d).

The cystic and solid dystrophy variants are not always separate entities but different developmental stages of one pathological process. The identification by CT examination of one or the other variant can alternate in the same patient within a short period of time (Procacci et al. 2001b) (Fig. 10.8d–f).

10.3.1.2.4 Congenital Lesions

Congenital lesions of the biliary tracts and duodenum that sustain RP, if not identified and corrected, create an increased risk for the development of OCP (Fig. 10.2b–f). Pancreas divisum is of particular importance. CT suggests the diagnosis of pancreas divisum in the rather advanced phase of OCP by recognising changes of CP affecting a single duct drainage tributary.

It is common to recognise inflammatory involvement exclusively within the dorsal pancreatic parenchyma with atrophy and dilatation of only the dorsal duct, up to its outlet into the minor papilla (Fig. 10.10a). The ventral area, corresponding to the posterior half of the head and the uncinate process, is, in contrast, perfectly normal (Procacci et al. 2001b) (Fig. 10.10b).

At the minor papilla, it is sometimes possible to observe cystic dilatation of the Santorini duct with a fluid density, jutting into the duodenal lumen (Santorinicele). According to some authors, this is the result of an obstruction associated with an acquired or congenital weakness of the distal wall of the duct (Manfredi et al. 2000) caused by functional stenosis of the minor papilla.

Less common is pancreas divisum associated with CP, which inversely involves the ventral segment while the dorsal portion is undamaged (Fig. 10.10c–e). This disease, in fact, seems to be the result of the combined effects of alcohol and biliary reflux through the ventral pancreatic duct, while the dorsal portion, which does not communicate with the biliary tree, remains uninvolved (Brinberg et al. 1998). In this case, CT examination may highlight (Soulen et al. 1989; Brinberg et al. 1998) a focal area of the pancreatic head which, in contrast to the rest of the surrounding parenchyma, remains hypodense before CM due to fibrosis and often has diffuse and small calcifications (Fig. 10.10d). If the latter are absent, the lesion can be confused with ductal adenocarcinoma (Soulen et al. 1989; Brinberg et al. 1998).

Lastly, a rare variant called inverse pancreas divisum appears on CT examination with recognisable signs of OCP involving the entire dorsal pancreas and the uncinate process except for the antero-superior portion of the head. The latter remains undamaged, and therefore demonstrates normal enhancement in the pancreatic phase, being hyperdense compared to the rest of the pancreas (Zeman et al. 1988; Silverman et al. 1989; Procacci et al. 2001b), and hypodense due to fibrosis, thus creating the image of a hypervascular pseudo-mass (Fig. 10.10f,g) in the head of the pancreas.

10.3.1.2.5 Slow-growing Tumors

Those Slow-growing pancreatic and papillary tumors which may lead to long-term obstruction of the pancreatic duct producing OCP (Maisonneuve and Lowenfels 2002) are juxtapapillary duodenal adenocarcinoma (Fig. 10.11a,b) and non-functioning pancreatic neuroendocrine tumor (Procacci et al. 1998; Levy and Ruszniewski 2002). Non-functioning neuroendocrine tumours, at CT examination, produce a large, capsulated and hypervascular mass

(Procacci et al. 1998). Sometimes there are areas of necrosis and calcifications. Because of their slow and prolonged growth, there is secondary dilatation of the MPD at the body-tail and often complete glandular atrophy (Levy and Ruszniewski 2002) (Fig. 10.11c).

The finding of OCP secondary to ductal adenocarcinoma and acinar carcinoma of the pancreas is less frequent (Yamaguchi and Tanaka 1992; Van Gulik et al. 1999; Levy and Ruszniewski 2002; Ly and Miller 2002; Schima and Fugger 2002). Downstream of the MPD dilatation and parenchymal atrophy (Procacci et al. 1998) a solid mass is visible, hypodense because of its scirrhous structure and often infiltrating the ductal structures (Procacci et al. 1998) in the ductal adenocarcinoma (Fig. 10.11d), or slightly vascularized and capsulated in the acinar carcinoma (Fig. 10.11e,f).

Other tumors responsible for OCP are cystic tumors (Levy and Ruszniewski 2002) (Fig. 10.12) of the pancreas. Among these is the serous cystoadenoma (Fig. 10.12a–d). The mucinous cystic tumor,

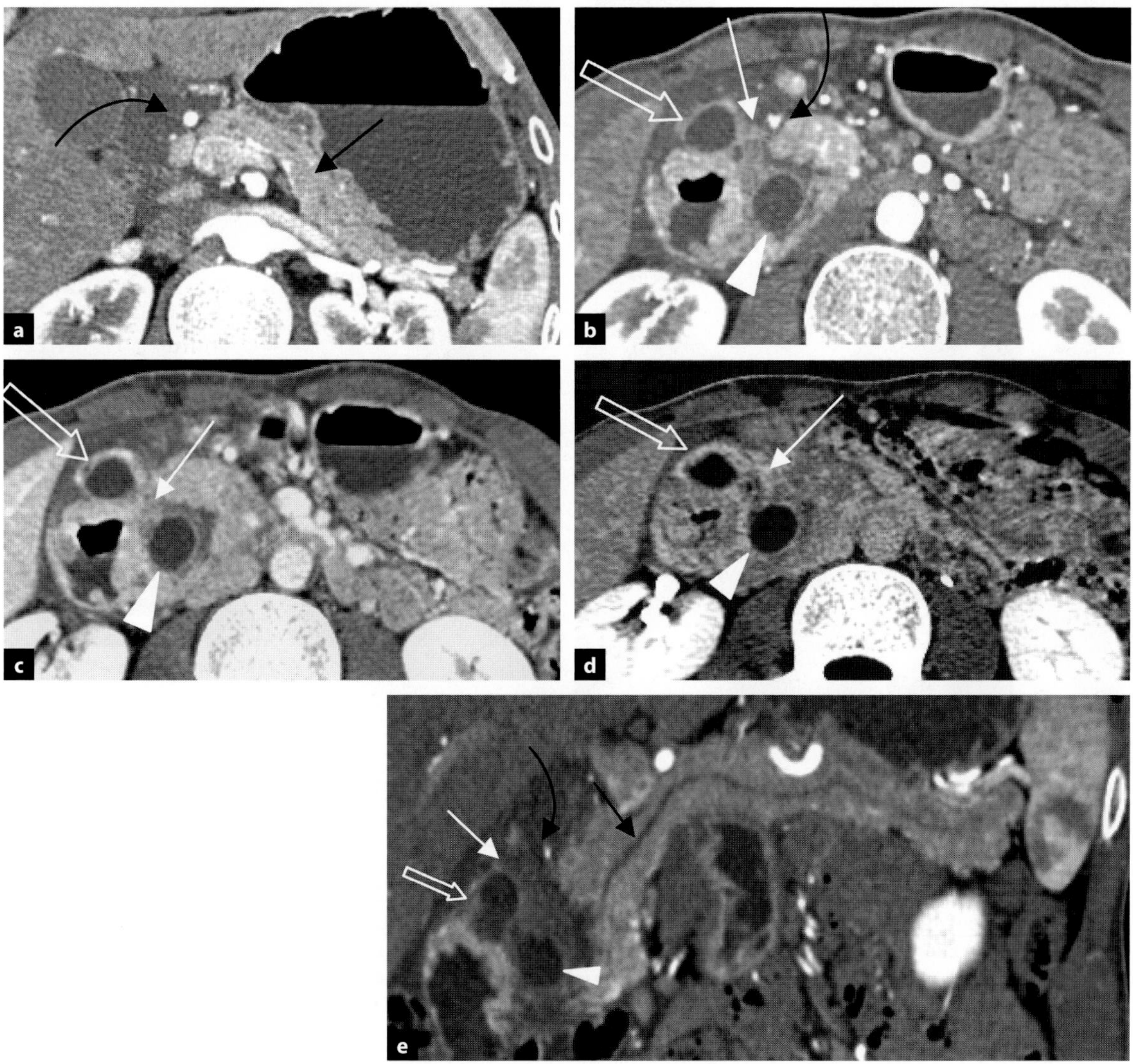

Fig. 10.7 a–e. Obstructive chronic pancreatitis (OCP) due to duodenal cystic dystrophy (CDD). MDCT: Contrast enhanced images (**a–d**), coronal curved reconstruction (**e**). Dilatation (*black arrow*) of the main duct (**a**, **e**). Thickening (*white arrow*) of the wall of the second duodenal portion, is hypodense in the pancreatic phase (**b–e**), with late and progressive enhancement in the venous (**c**) and late (**d**) phases. Within the thickened wall (**b–e**), there are two small fluid attenuation lesions. Note the anterior and left-sided displacement (**a**, **b**, **e**) of the gastro-duodenal artery (*curved arrow*)

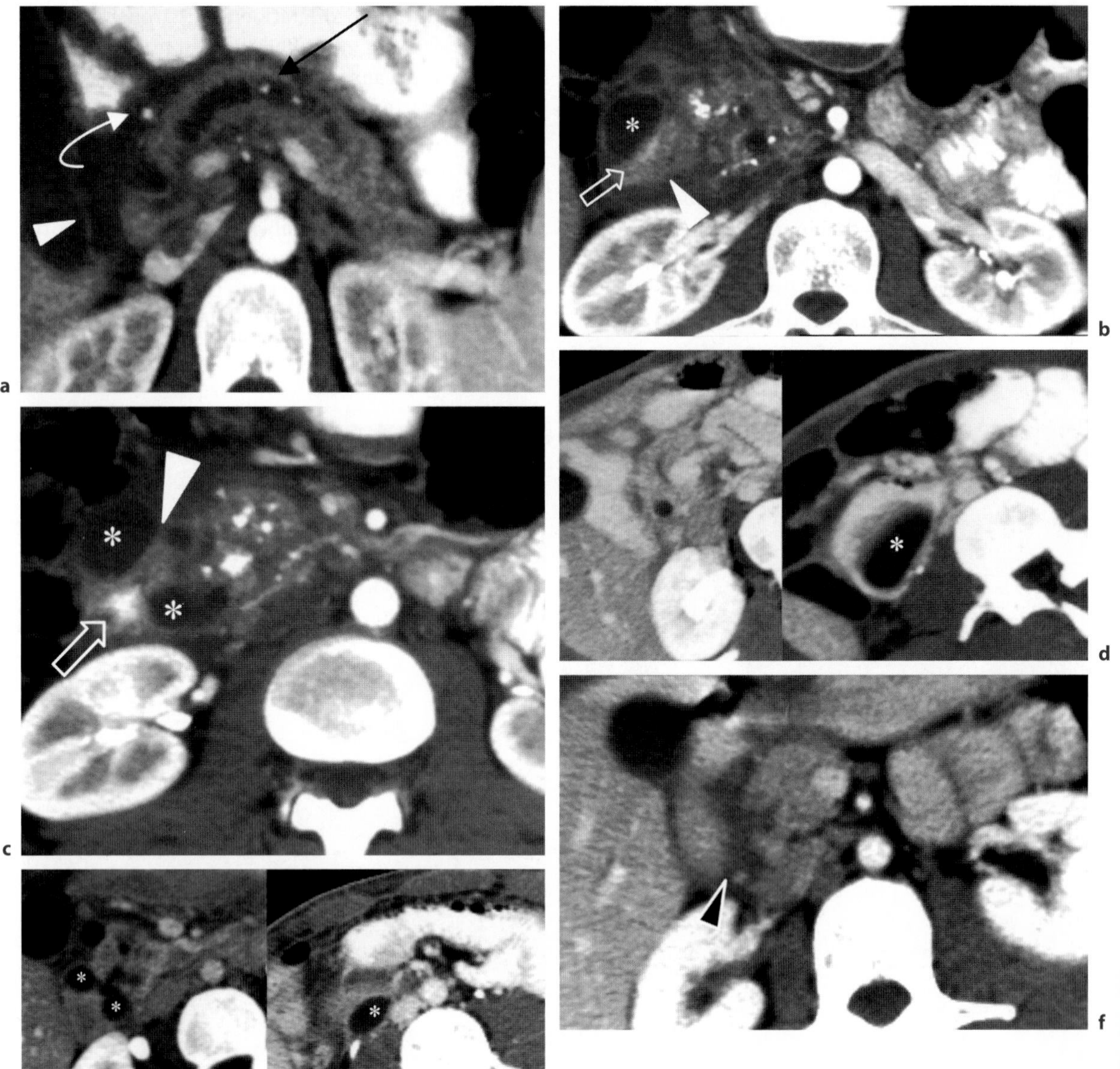

Fig. 10.8 a–f. Obstructive chronic pancreatitis (OCP) due to duodenal cystic dystrophy (CDD). Two cases of two brothers in the same family (1st case, **a–c**; 2nd case, **d–f**). CT in the pancreatic enhancement phase. **a–c** Mild atrophy of the parenchyma, uniform dilatation of the MPD (*arrow* in **a**) with multiple intraductal calculi (**a–c**). Thickening of the wall of the second portion of the duodenum (*arrowhead*), is hypodense in early contrast enhanced phases (**a–c**) with small fluid density regions inside (*asterisks*) (**b**, **c**) and narrowing (**b**, **c**) of the duodenal lumen (*clear arrow*). Note the anterior and left-sided displacement (**a**) of the gastro-duodenal artery (*curved arrow*). **d–f** Mild dilatation of the main duct and intrapancreatic portion of the CBD; fluid collection (*asterisk*) within the duodenal walls (**d**). After only 10 days (**e**), a multilocular fluid lesion has appeared in the wall of the second duodenal portion (*asterisks*), while the fluid collection in the duodenal wall has become smaller. Complete regression (**f**) of both fluid duodenal formations at the last CT examination after 30 days; thickening of the wall of the second duodenal portion still persists (*arrowhead*)

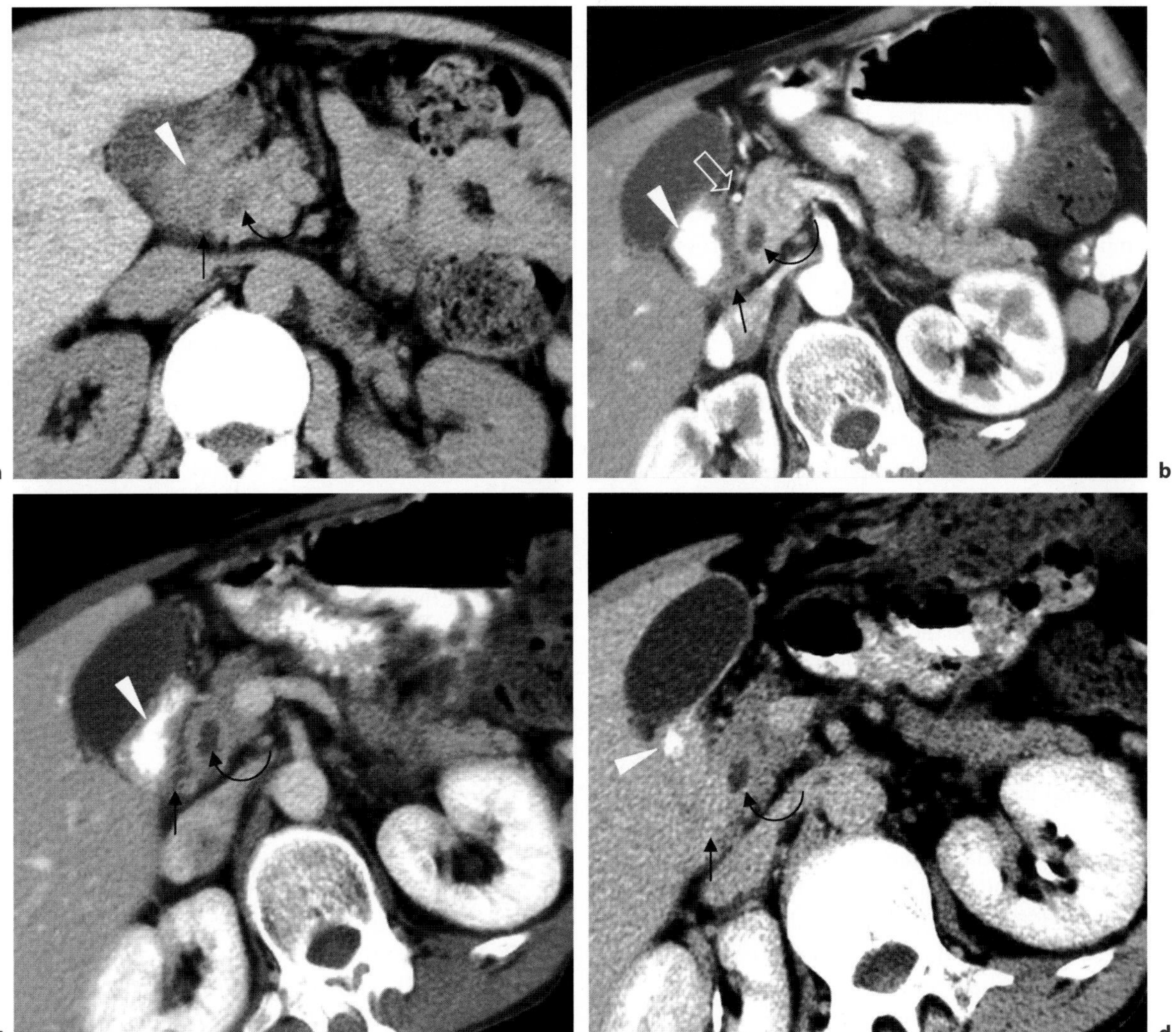

Fig. 10.9 a–d. Obstructive chronic pancreatitis (OCP) due to duodenal solid dystrophy (SDD) or grooved pancreatitis. CT in the pre- (**a**) and post-contrast enhancement phases (**b–d**). Thin sleeve of solid tissue (*arrow*), hypodense in the pre- (**a**) and post-pancreatic enhancement phases (**b**), located between the pancreatic head and the lumen (*arrowhead*) of the second duodenal portion (parietal fibrosis); note the displacement of the gastro-duodenal artery (**b**: *clear arrow*). Progressive enhancement of the peri-duodenal fibrosis, which, in the venous (**c**) and late (**d**) enhancement phases is evident. The intrapancreatic CBD is dilated (*curved arrow*)

which almost exclusively involves females and is located in the tail of the gland causes dilatation of the main duct and glandular atrophy confined to the caudal portion of the pancreas (Fig. 10.12e,f).

10.3.1.3 CT Differential Diagnosis: OCP vs Pancreatic Tumors

Once an OCP has been identified at CT examination, together with some of its potential causes, further refinements in differential diagnosis are possible (Maisonneuve and Lowenfels 2002; McNulty et al. 2001).

10.3.1.3.1 CT Differential Diagnosis: OCP vs IPMT

Intraductal papillary mucinous tumors of the pancreas (IPMT) are rare lesions (Levy and Ruszniewski 2002; Valette et al. 2001); they have a better prognosis than ductal adenocarcinoma (Ito et al. 2001;

Valette et al. 2001). Because they manifest at imaging in a very similar way to OCP (Procacci et al. 2001b; Valette et al. 2001; Irie et al. 2002; Levy and Ruszniewski 2002), it is challenging to differentiate them from OCP (Levy and Ruszniewski 2002).

Until a few years ago, the only possibility of distinguishing the two pathologies was ERCP, which could recognise the secretion of mucin from the papilla and the presence of filling defects, either mucin plugs or papillary neoplasms in the dilated ducts (Procacci et al. 2001b; Ito et al. 2001).

Current day MDCT aids in this differentiation in a larger percentage of (but not all) cases (Fig. 10.13b,c,e,f). 3-D isotropic voxels created by current MDCT technology improves the quality of multiplanar, curved-multiplanar and volume rendered images (Ito et al. 2001; McNulty et al. 2001; Nino-Murcia et al. 2001; Procacci et al. 2001b; Takeshita et al. 2002). The extent of the dilated pancreatic duct can be mapped and the adjacent atrophic pancreas assessed. Also, the presence of hyperdense ductal filling defects due to tiny papillary vegetations on the ductal wall and/or mucin filling defects inside the ductal lumen (Fig. 10.13b,e), a dilated papilla bulging into the duodenal lumen (Fig. 10.13c,f) and cystic ectasia of the branch ducts, more often in the uncinate process (Fig. 10.13f) and/or dilatation of the CBD (Procacci et al. 2001b, 2003) can be detected .

These CT signs, together with abnormal dilatation of the pancreatic duct and unexplained parenchymal atrophy that can cause an obstruction, arouse the suspicion of an intraductal tumor (Pavone et al. 1999). If IPMT cannot be distinguished from OCP, ERCP is mandatory.

10.3.1.3.2 CT Differential Diagnosis: OCP Secondary to Solid Duodenal Dystrophy (SDD) vs Ductal Adenocarcinoma of the Head of the Pancreas

Distinction between the two entities is difficult; clinically, both diseases have many common features (Procacci et al. 2001b); aspiration biopsy that fails to reveal tumor is not meaningful (Yamaguchi and Tanaka 1992; Van Gulik et al. 1999; Pugliese et al. 2001; Shams et al. 2001; Ramesh 2002). For these reasons some patients with SDD undergo surgical resection for suspected carcinoma of the head of the pancreas (Yamaguchi and Tanaka 1992; Irie et al. 1998b).

The contribution of imaging is discussed in detail in Section 10.3.1.2.3 (Fig 10.14a–g).

10.3.1.3.3 CT Differential Diagnosis: OCP Associated with Inverse Pancreas Divisum vs Neuroendocrine Tumors

As already discussed, this anomaly can be associated with phenomena of localized chronic pancreatitis within the dorsal pancreas and uncinate process, drained by the ventral duct, while the anterior and superior portion of the head of the pancreas can remain undamaged as it is drained by the dorsal duct. Because the unaffected pancreas appears hyperdense against the background of hypodense diseased gland, it is possible to mistake this condition for a neuroendocrine tumor (see Sect. 10.3.1.2.4).

10.3.2 Non-obstructive or Primitive Chronic Pancreatitis (PCP)

CT examination identifies some forms of non-obstructive, or primary, CP (PCP).

10.3.2.1 CT Identification of Hereditary PCP Secondary to Genetic Mutations

Multiple genetic mutations have been associated with the onset of CP, mostly by cystic fibrosis genes (CFTR), SPINK 1 (serine protease inhibitor Kazal type 1), α1-antitrypsin and cationic trypsinogen (Etemad and Whitcomb 2001; Bhatia et al. 2002; Mossner and Teich 2002; Teich et al. 2002; Witt and Becker 2002; Charney 2003; Frulloni et al. 2003).

CT examination is able to identify some modifications in the ductal structures and the parenchyma typical of hereditary CP.

10.3.2.1.1 Ductal Structure

In the advanced phase (Choudari et al. 2002), the main duct is dilated along its whole length (Figs. 10.15b,c and 10.16b,d), is often outlined and irregular (Hoshina et al. 1999; Procacci et al. 2001b), measures 1–2 cm diameter (Rohrmann et al. 1981). There is also associated irregular dilatation of the branch ducts (Rohrmann et al. 1981).

In the lumen of the MPD, stones can usually be recognised (Rohrmann et al. 1981; Luetmer et al. 1989; Hoshina et al. 1999), hyperdense in both pre- and post-enhancement phases (Figs. 10.15 and

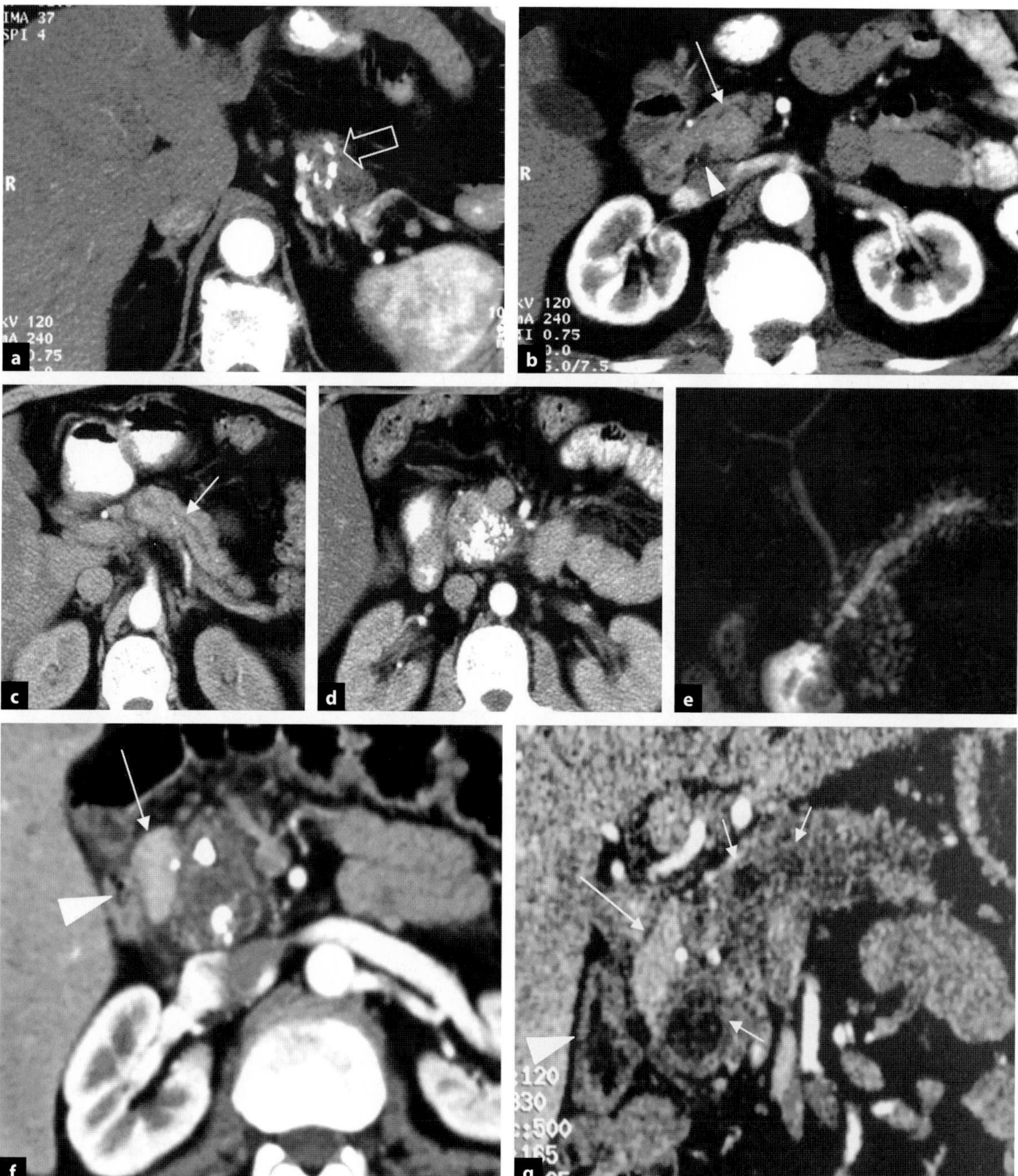

Fig. 10.10 a–g. Obstructive chronic pancreatitis (OCP) due to pancreas divisum. Axial CT in the pancreatic enhancement phase (**a–d**, **f**); coronal reconstruction (**g**); MRCP (**e**). Three cases (1st case, **a**, **b**; 2nd case, **c–e**; 3rd case, **f**,**g**). **a**, **b** Small ductal stones (*clear arrow*) in the body of the pancreas (dorsal pancreas); the dorsal pancreatic duct drains into the minor papilla (*arrow*). The posterior half of the head and the uncinate process (ventral pancreas) are normal; the CBD (**b**) is visible in the major papilla (*arrowhead*). **c–e** Mild, uniform dilatation (*arrow*) of the dorsal pancreatic duct (**c**); CP with numerous stones (**d**) in the posterior half of the head and the uncinate process (ventral pancreas); MRCP examination (**e**) demonstrates the intersection of the CBD and the dorsal pancreatic duct, confirming the presence of pancreas divisum. **f**, **g** Fibrosis of the parenchyma in the head is hypodense in the pancreatic phase, dilatation (*short arrow*) of the main duct (**g**) with stones in the pancreatic head (**f**). A solid nodule (*arrow*) between the duodenal lumen (*arrowhead*) and the pancreatic head, hyperdense in the pancreatic enhancement phase, unlike the fibrotic pancreatic parenchyma, representing an inverse pancreas divisum

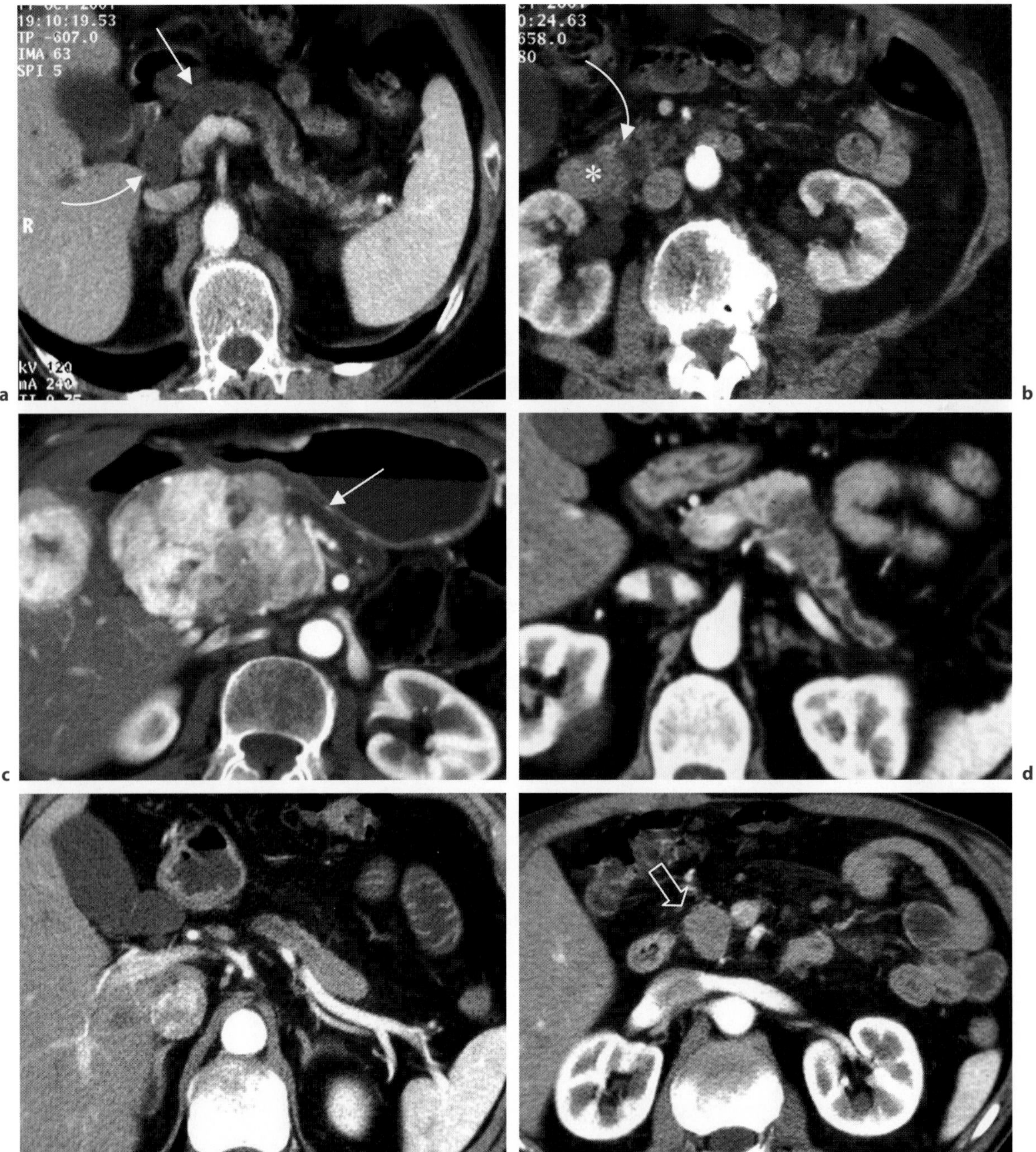

Fig. 10.11 a–f. Obstructive chronic pancreatitis (OCP) due to neoplasm. CT in the pancreatic enhancement phase. **a, b** The pancreas is atrophic, the MPD (*arrow*) is dilated due to the prolonged obstructive effect of a juxtapapillary mass. The mass has a solid, slightly vascularized (*asterisk*). Marked dilatation of the CBD (*curved arrow*) obstructed by the mass (adenocarcinoma of the papilla). **c** Total atrophy of the parenchyma, with prominent and uniform dilatation of the MPD at the body-tail (*arrow*) due to the prolonged obstructive effect of a large mass at the head of the pancreas. The mass is solid and hypervascular with necrotic central areas. Hypervascular hepatic metastases are visible (non-functioning neuroendocrine pancreatic tumor). **d** The tail of the pancreas is small and atrophic. The MPD is dilated due to the obstructive effect of a hypovascular mass (*arrow*) at the pancreatic body of the pancreas (ductal adenocarcinoma of the pancreas). **e, f** The pancreas is small and atrophic at the body-tail (**e**) while the main duct is slightly dilated due to the initial obstructive effect of a mass (**f**: *clear arrow*) with solid density (**f**), poorly vascularised and regular margins (acinar carcinoma of the pancreas)

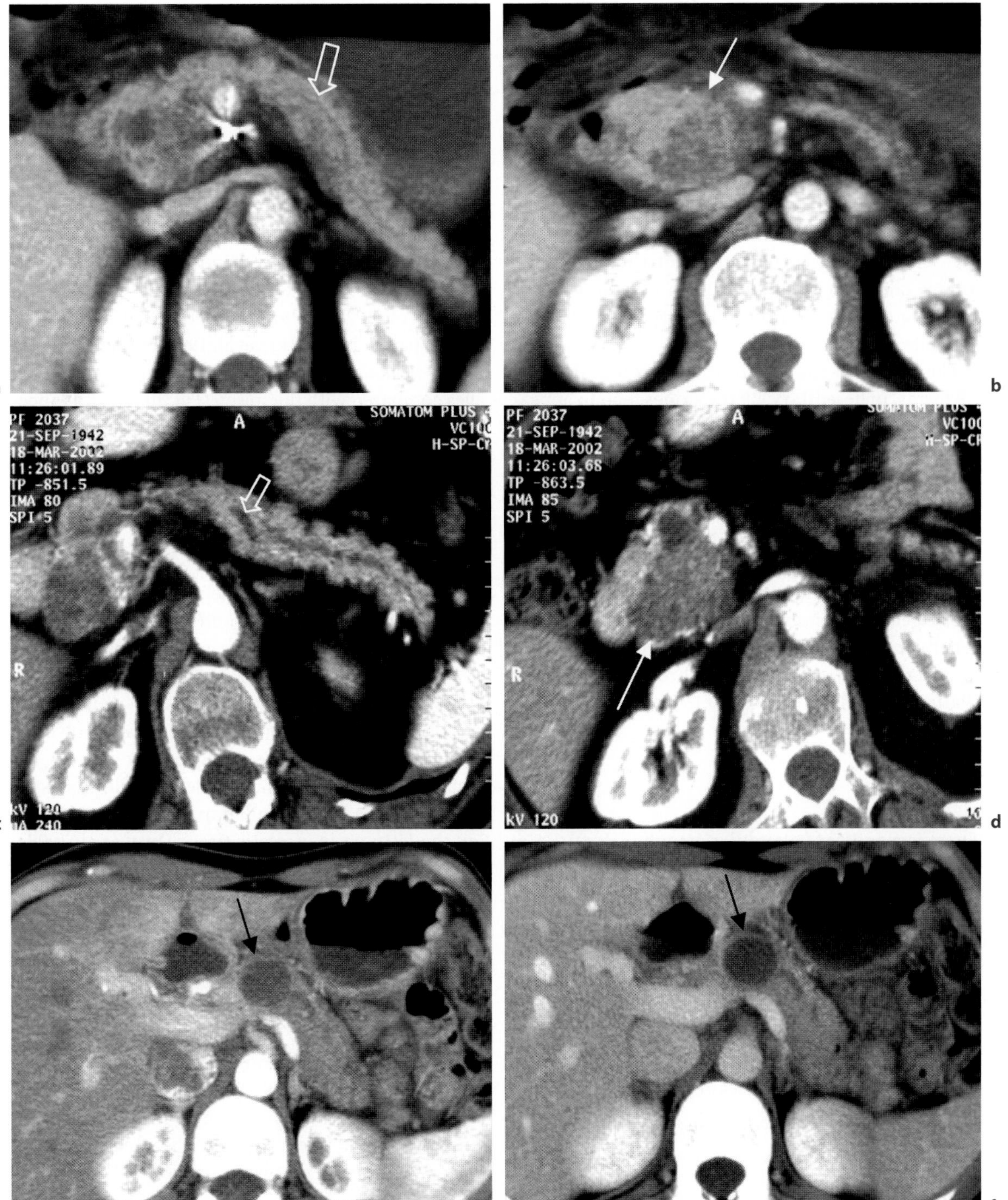

Fig. 10.12 a–f. Obstructive chronic pancreatitis (OCP) due to neoplasm. CT in the pancreatic enhancement (**a**–**e**) and venous (**f**) phases. **a**–**d** Initial parenchymal atrophy and mild dilatation of the MPD (**a**: *clear arrow*) due to the mild obstructive effect of a fluid density mass (**b**: *arrow*), with lobulated margins and multiple small cystic spaces separated by radially oriented septa. CT examination 4 years later (**c**, **d**), shows further glandular atrophy. The main duct (*clear arrow*) is progressively dilated due to the increase in the size of the lesion (*arrow*) in the head of the pancreas (serous cystoadenoma of the pancreas). **e**, **f** Slight dilatation of the MPD in the body-tail due to the initial obstructive effect of a mass in the pancreatic neck (*arrow*). The mass has a fluid density and is relatively hypodense in the pancreatic (**e**) and venous (**f**) phases (cystic papillary tumor of the pancreas).

10.16). They are fewer in the early phase, becoming more numerous later, and are widely distributed inside the dilated main duct. They are either round or oval and are often more than 2–3 cm in diameter (Figs. 10.15 and 10.16). They can have a typically hyperdense peripheral margin and a hypodense centre (Rohrmann et al. 1981; Hoshina et al. 1999) due to the lack of calcium deposits in the central core, an aspect often described by some authors as a "bull's eye" (Fig. 10.16f). Visualization of this somewhat unique characteristic of calculi in hereditary CP is accentuated by examining the images using "bone (wide level, wide width) windows".

Compared to the calcifications present in other CP forms, in hereditary CP the stones tend to appear earlier, are larger (Luetmer et al. 1989; Procacci et al. 1998) and are typically rounded, often aligned within the considerably dilated main duct (Figs. 10.15 and 10.16). Therefore, the ductal stones, numerous and large, particularly the "bull's-eye" type, are a rather characteristic finding of hereditary CP. In contrast, in hereditary CP associated with cystic fibrosis gene mutations (CFTR), the calcifications are generally smaller and tend to appear later compared to other forms of hereditary chronic pancreatitis (Frulloni et al. 2003) (Fig. 10.13d).

10.3.2.1.2 Parenchyma

There is significant glandular atrophy (Hoshina et al. 1999; Procacci et al. 2001b) and only the residual rind of tissue displays enhancement (Fig. 10.15c–f). Some parenchymal portions can be unaffected or even appear hypertrophic (Fig. 10.16e,f).

The parenchymal fibrosis often causes stenosis of the intrapancreatic portion of the CBD (Choudari et al. 2002). Moreover, in hereditary pancreatitis, the frequency of pseudocysts is higher compared to other forms of CP (Choudari et al. 2002; Charney 2003).

10.3.2.2 CT Identification of Autoimmune PCP

Identification of autoimmune PCP is important since this disease responds quickly to oral steroid therapy (Irie et al. 1998a; Pavone et al. 1999; Taniguchi et al. 2000; Etemad and Whitcomb 2001). CT examination is able to identify some unique findings that are useful for making a correct diagnosis.

Two forms of autoimmune PCP are distinguishable: diffuse and focal (Wakabayashi et al. 2002), which are probably just different stages of the same disease (Wakabayashi et al. 2002).

10.3.2.2.1 Diffuse Form

Parenchyma

The dimensions of the gland (Fig. 10.17) are increased (Horiuchi et al. 1996; Irie et al. 1998a; Eerens et al. 2001; Procacci et al. 2001a,b).

The parenchyma (Irie et al. 1998a; Procacci et al. 2001a) is isodense on non-contrast enhanced CT images compared with the spleen (Fig. 10.17c). Enhancement is late in the pancreatic phase (as opposed to the brisk enhancement seen in the normal pancreas during this phase of study), due to the presence of widespread lymphocytic infiltration. The parenchyma is hypodense compared to the spleen (Fig. 10.17d). During the subsequent venous phases it becomes less hypodense (Fig. 10.17a,b,e). In the venous phase a peripheral hyperdense band can appear known as a "capsule-like rim" (Irie et al. 1998a; Eerens et al. 2001; Procacci et al. 2001a) surrounding the gland. It has smooth and well-defined margins, probably due to inflammatory processes that involve the peripancreatic tissue. According to some authors, the "capsule-like rim" is in fact made up of fibrous tissue secondary to a chronic inflammatory process involving the fatty peripancreatic tissue (Irie et al. 1998a; Eerens et al. 2001; Etemad and Ehitcomb 2001).

In the late phase (Fig. 10.17f) the gland remains less dense compared to the spleen while the peripheral band becomes hyperdense (Irie et al. 1998a; Procacci et al. 2001a).

If no irreversible structural changes in the gland are found (Procacci et al. 2001a), regression of the inflammatory process can be expected with steroid therapy (Pavone et al. 1999). The size of the pancreas and the parenchymal enhancement return to normal and the "capsule-like rim" of peripheral enhancement disappears (Irie et al. 1998a; Eerens et al. 2001).

Ducts

The periductal inflammatory cellular infiltrate (Irie et al. 1998a) produces diffuse narrowing of the main pancreatic duct (Furukawa et al. 1998; Irie et al. 1998a; Van Hoe et al. 1998), which has irregular walls (Etemad and Whitcomb 2001). If the ductal stenosis is localized, the upstream duct is dilated (Fig. 10.17a).

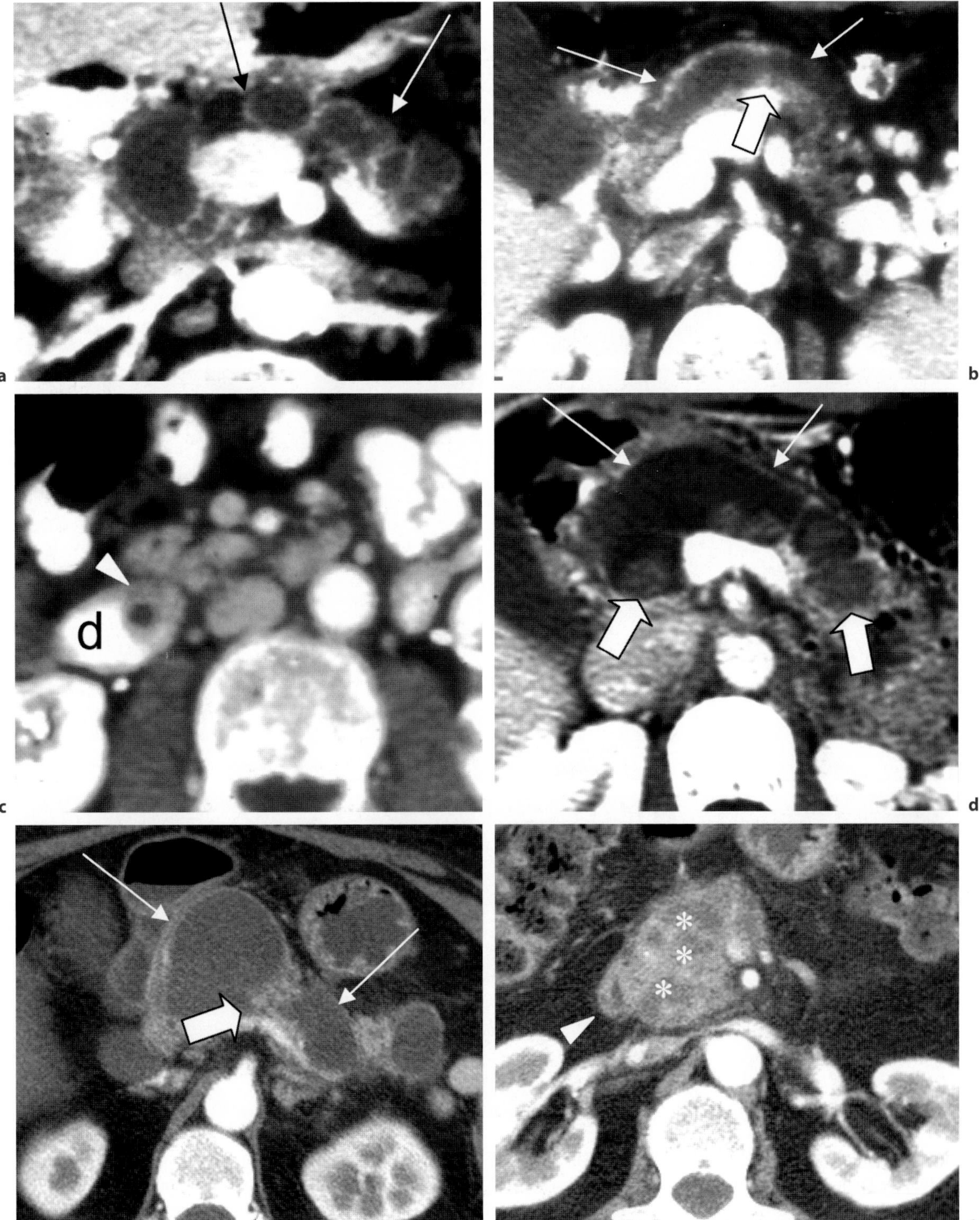

Fig. 10.13 a–f. Obstructive chronic pancreatitis (OCP) and primitive chronic pancreatitis (PCP) vs intraductal papillary mucinous tumor (IPMT). CT in the pancreatic enhancement phase. Four cases: (1st case, **a**; 2nd case, **b,c**; 3rd case, **d**; 4th case, **e,f**). Total atrophy of the parenchyma; marked and uniform dilatation (*arrows*) of the MPD (**a**, **b**, **d**, **e**). Multiple hyperdense ductal filling defects (*thick arrows*) of large size in **d** (non-calcific protein plugs), smaller in **b**, **e** (neoplastic papillary vegetations and/or mucin deposits). The side branches of the uncinate process are dilated (**f**: *asterisks*), the papilla is enlarged (*arrowhead*) and bulges into the duodenal lumen (*d* in **c**). (**a**: OCP); **d**: hereditary PCP, secondary to genetic mutation: CFTR; **b**, **c**, **e**, **f**: IPMT)

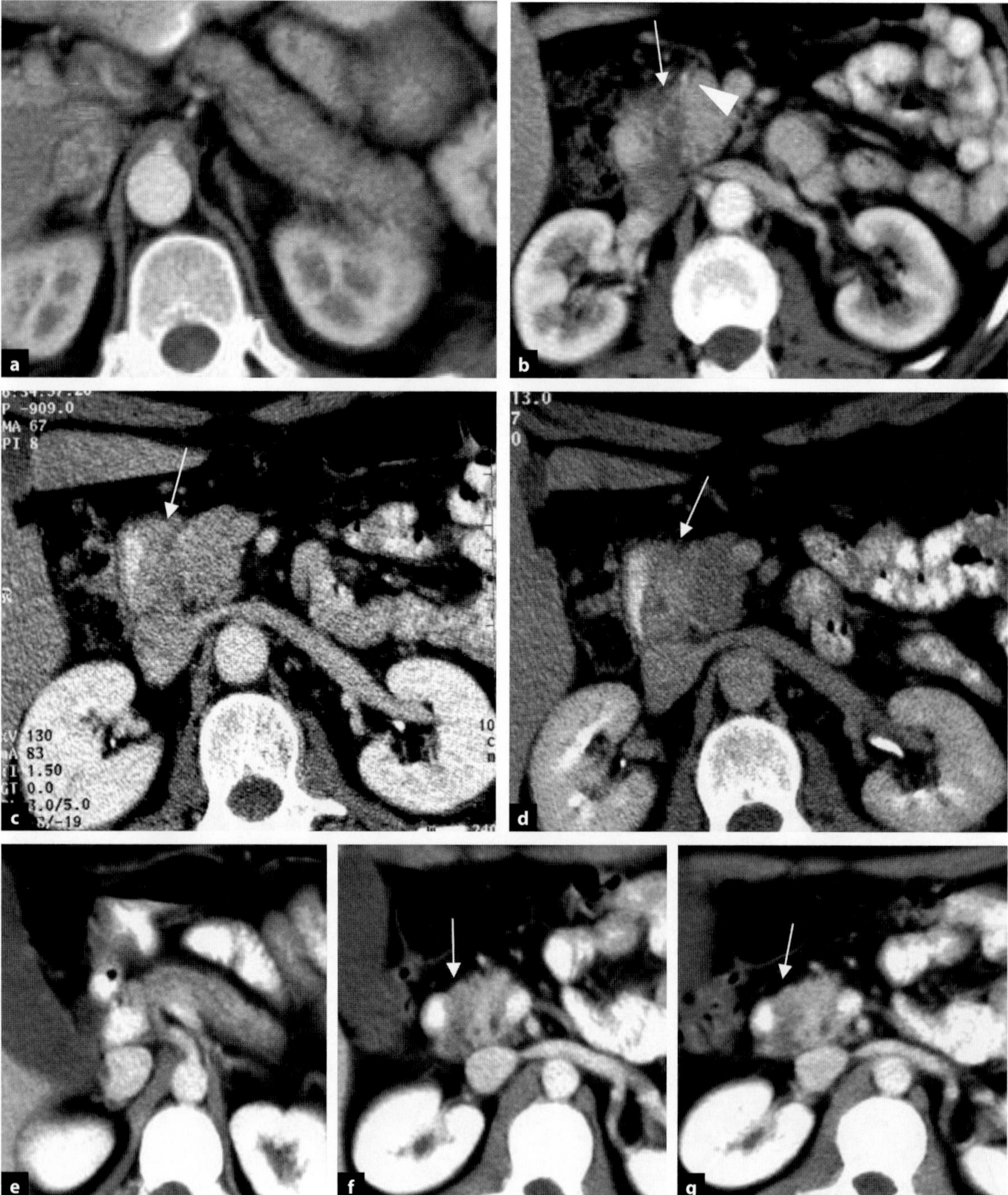

Fig. 10.14 a–g. CT differential diagnosis of obstructive chronic pancreatitis (OCP) due to solid duodenal dystrophy (SDD) vs ductal adenocarcinoma. Two cases: (1st case, **a–d** > SDD; 2nd case, **e–g** > ductal adenocarcinoma). Contrast enhanced CT. Solid tissue (*arrow*) between the pancreatic head and the lumen of the second duodenal portion; the lesion is hypodense in the pancreatic enhancement phase (**b, f**) and shows late enhancement in the venous phase (**c**), with further enhancement in the late phase (**d**), although remaining hypodense **g**. The main duct is not dilated at the body-tail in **a**, but it is dilated in **e**. The gastro-duodenal artery (*arrowhead*) is displaced anterior and to the left in **b** (**a–d**: the histological diagnosis on the resected specimen was of solid duodenal dystrophy. The patient underwent resection due to a CT misdiagnosis of pancreatic tumor; **e–g**: ductal pancreatic adenocarcinoma)

The side branch ducts show no cystic dilatation (Van Hoe et al. 1998), but, like the MPD, they are narrower or destroyed (Coyle et al. 2002). These ductal changes can also be resolved with steroid therapy (Irie et al. 1998a).

Stones are absent in most cases at presentation (Irie et al. 1998a; Van Hoe et al. 1998), but can be seen in the advanced stages of the disease where the "capsule-like rim" is not visible (Procacci et al. 2001a).

10.3.2.2.2 Focal Form

Parenchyma

There is a focal increase in the size of the pancreatic gland that may appear as a subtle localized swelling or a frank mass (Irie et al. 1998a; Eerens et al. 2001; Procacci et al. 2001a,b) (Fig. 10.18).

Before the administration of CM, the affected region is isodense to the rest of the healthy parenchyma and the spleen (Furukawa et al. 1998; Procacci et al. 2001a). There is no atrophy of the parenchyma proximal to the lesion (Van Hoe et al. 1998).

Enhancement is late in the pancreatic phase (Irie et al. 1998a) and is reduced compared to the surrounding parenchyma because of the presence of lymphocytic infiltration (Fig. 10.18a,c,e). In the venous phase (Procacci et al. 2001a) the affected parenchyma is denser than the spleen and the adjacent healthy parenchyma (that has already begun to "de-enhance") (Fig. 10.18b,f).

In the focal form the characteristic "capsule-like rim" appears in the venous phase (Irie et al. 1998a; Eerens et al. 2001; Procacci et al. 2001a) with smooth and well-defined margins (Irie et al. 1998a).

In the late phase, the affected gland remains hypodense compared to the spleen and the adjacent unaffected parenchyma while the peripheral band becomes hyperdense (Irie et al. 1998a; Procacci et al. 2001a).

If no irreversible structural changes in the gland have occurred (Procacci et al. 2001a), complete regression of the disease can be achieved with steroid therapy (Pavone et al. 1999) both clinically and at imaging (Irie et al. 1998a; Eerens et al. 2001).

Ducts

The periductal inflammatory cellular infiltrate (Irie et al. 1998a) produces a focal, irregular narrowing of the MPD (Irie et al. 1998a; Etemad and Whitcomb 2001). Depending on the various degrees of parenchymal involvement, stenosis of the MPD lumen is often found (Procacci et al. 2001a) with dilatation upstream (Fig. 10.18d). Such dilatation, when present, however, is modest, especially given the size of the inflammatory mass (Van Hoe et al. 1998). These ductal changes resolve with steroid therapy (Irie et al. 1998a).

Involvement of Adjacent Structures and Complications in Diffuse and Focal Forms

Both the focal forms, located at the head of the pancreas, and the diffuse forms, can involve the intrapancreatic portion of the CBD, causing stenosis with dilatation of the proximal biliary tracts (Furukawa et al. 1998; Irie et al. 1998a; Procacci et al. 2001a; Van Hoe et al. 1998).

The major arterial structures are not encased, nor is there venous obstruction (Irie et al. 1998a; Van Hoe et al. 1998.

10.3.2.3 CT Identification of PCP Associated with Toxic and Metabolic Factors

Hypercalcemia is a well established cause of CP although the pathogenesis is still largely unknown (Ring et al. 1973; Etemad and Whitcomb 2001). 50% of patients with hyperparathyroidism develop chronic calcific pancreatitis (Ring et al. 1973). The pancreatic stones found are non-specific in their composition and appearance.

Since CP can develop before the full clinical picture of hyperparathyroidism develops, it is important to consider the parathyroid disease every time that CT examination (Ring et al. 1973) reveals the presence of co-existent pancreatic and renal calcifications (Fig. 10.19a–c).

In patients with chronic renal failure secondary hyperparathyroidism can accelerate the development of CP and calcific CP (Etemad and Whitcomb 2001).

A relationship between alcohol and chronic pancreatitis has been proposed for more than 50 years. Alcohol is probably not a direct cause but a co-factor in the development of CP (Etemad and Whitcomb 2001). Calcific CP is present in 20%–40% of cases, usually manifesting after 5–10 years of abdominal pain attacks in patients with alcoholic chronic calcific pancreatitis.

The parenchyma, especially in the early phases of the disease, can demonstrate focal or diffuse in-

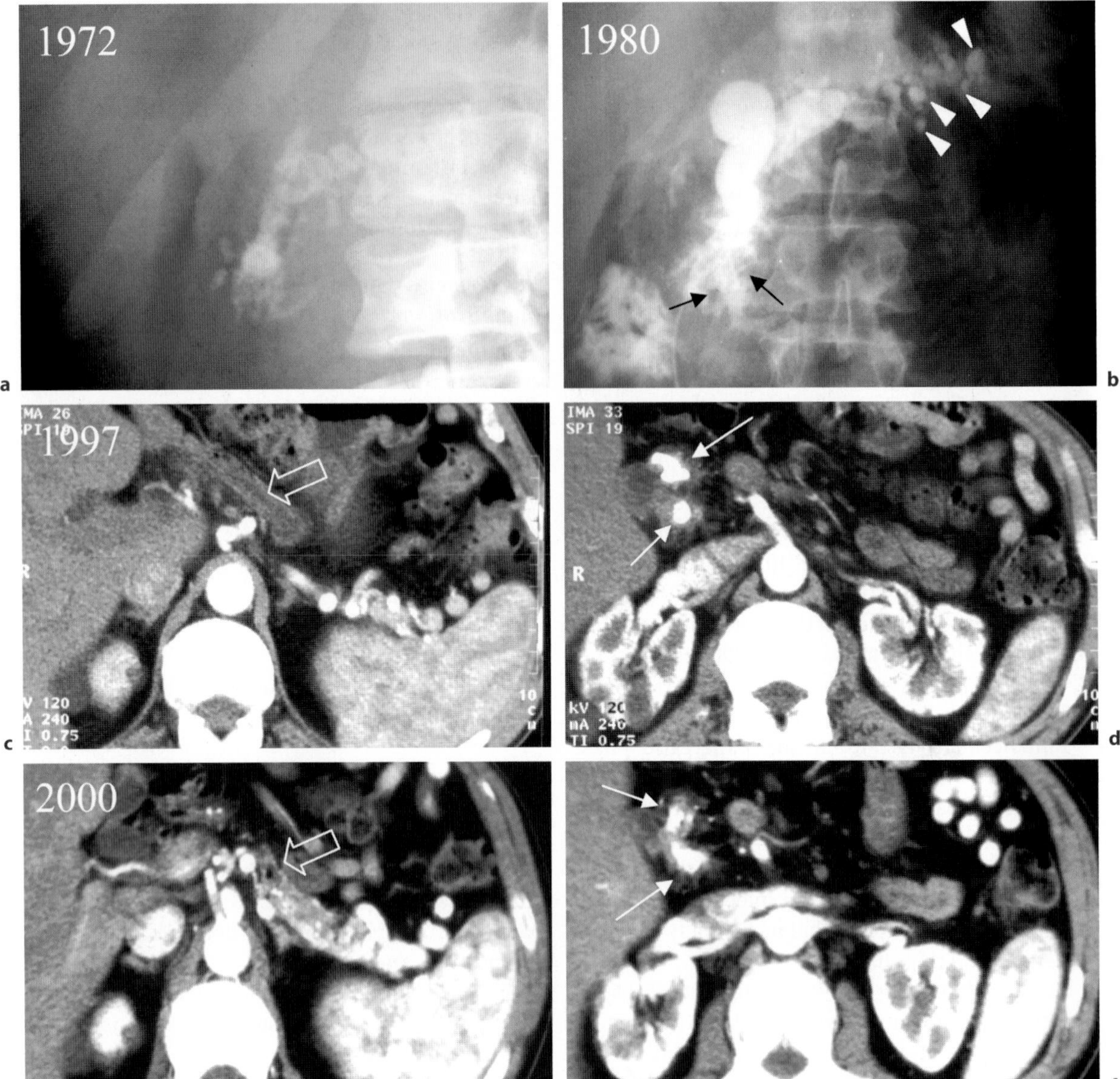

Fig. 10.15 a–f. Primary chronic pancreatitis (PCP): hereditary CP (associated genetic mutation: SPINK 1). Plain film (**a**), ERCP (**b**), CT in the enhanced phase (**c–f**). **a** CP at the onset, in early age (25 years): multiple and large calcifications in the pancreatic area at plain film. At 8 years later (**b**) the ERCP examination reported marked dilatation of the MPD with endoluminal (stones) defects (*arrows*) and dilatation of the branch ducts (*arrowheads*). At 17 years later (**c**, **d**), the pancreas is atrophic, dilatation (*clear arrow*) of the main duct (**c**) and multiple large ductal stones (*arrows* in **d**). No change is seen at CT, 3 years later (**e**, **f**)

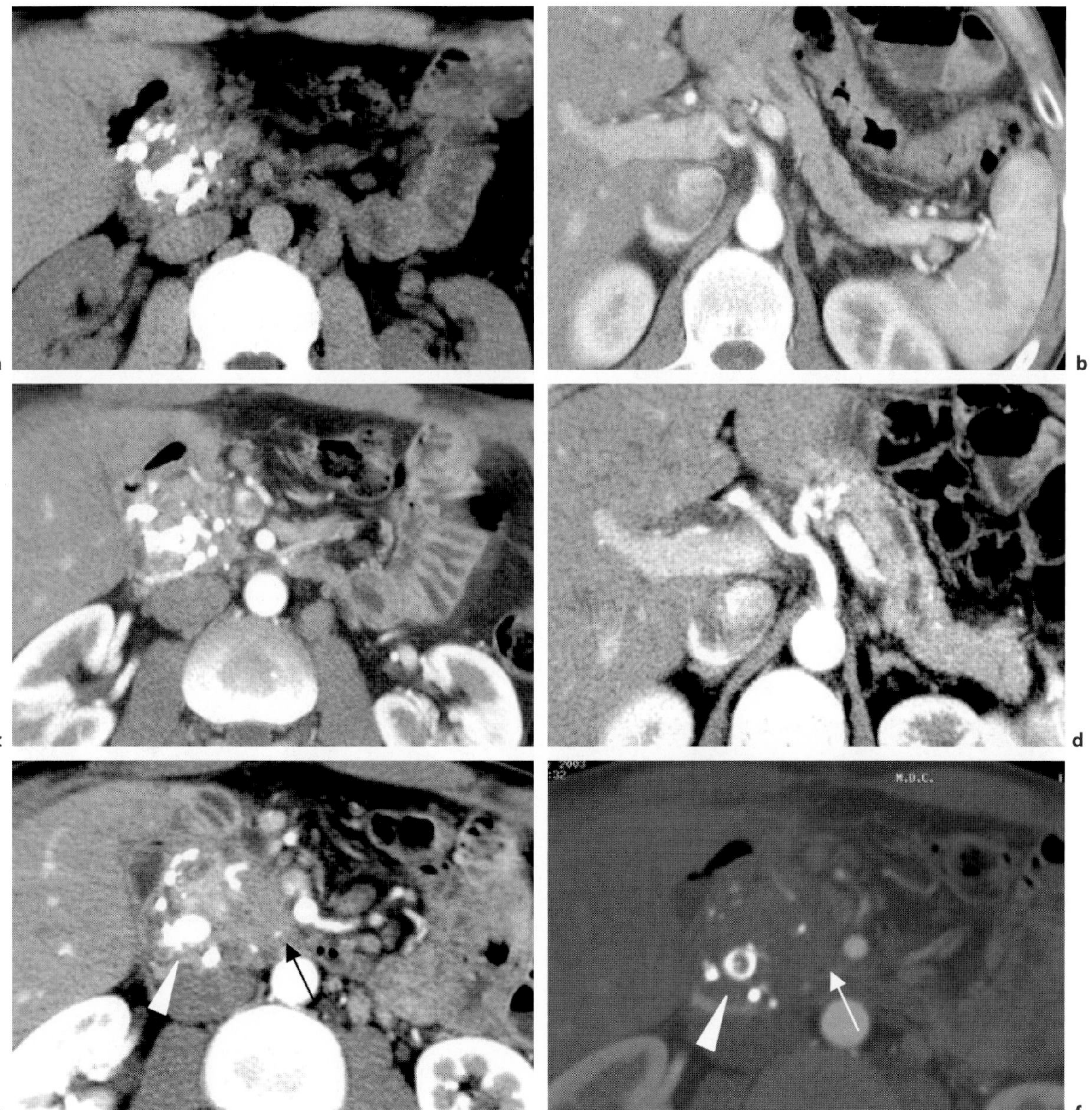

Fig. 10.16 a-f. Primary chronic pancreatitis (PCP): hereditary CP (associated genetic mutation: SPINK 1). CT pre- (**a**) and post- (**b–f**) CM administration. **a–c** CP at the onset in adult age (40 years): the pancreas is reduced in size in the body-tail, with early atrophy of the glandular parenchyma. Irregular dilatation of the MPD (**b**) and multiple and large ductal stones (**a**,**c**) in the head are seen. At 5 months later (**d–f**), dilatation of the MPD has increased (**d**); a hypodense area in the medial side of the head (**e**) has appeared (*arrow*). A ductal stone (**e**, **f**: *arrowhead*) with a central hypodense nucleus due to the lack of calcification and hyperdense peripheral rim ("bull's eye" appearance) is visible in the pancreatic head

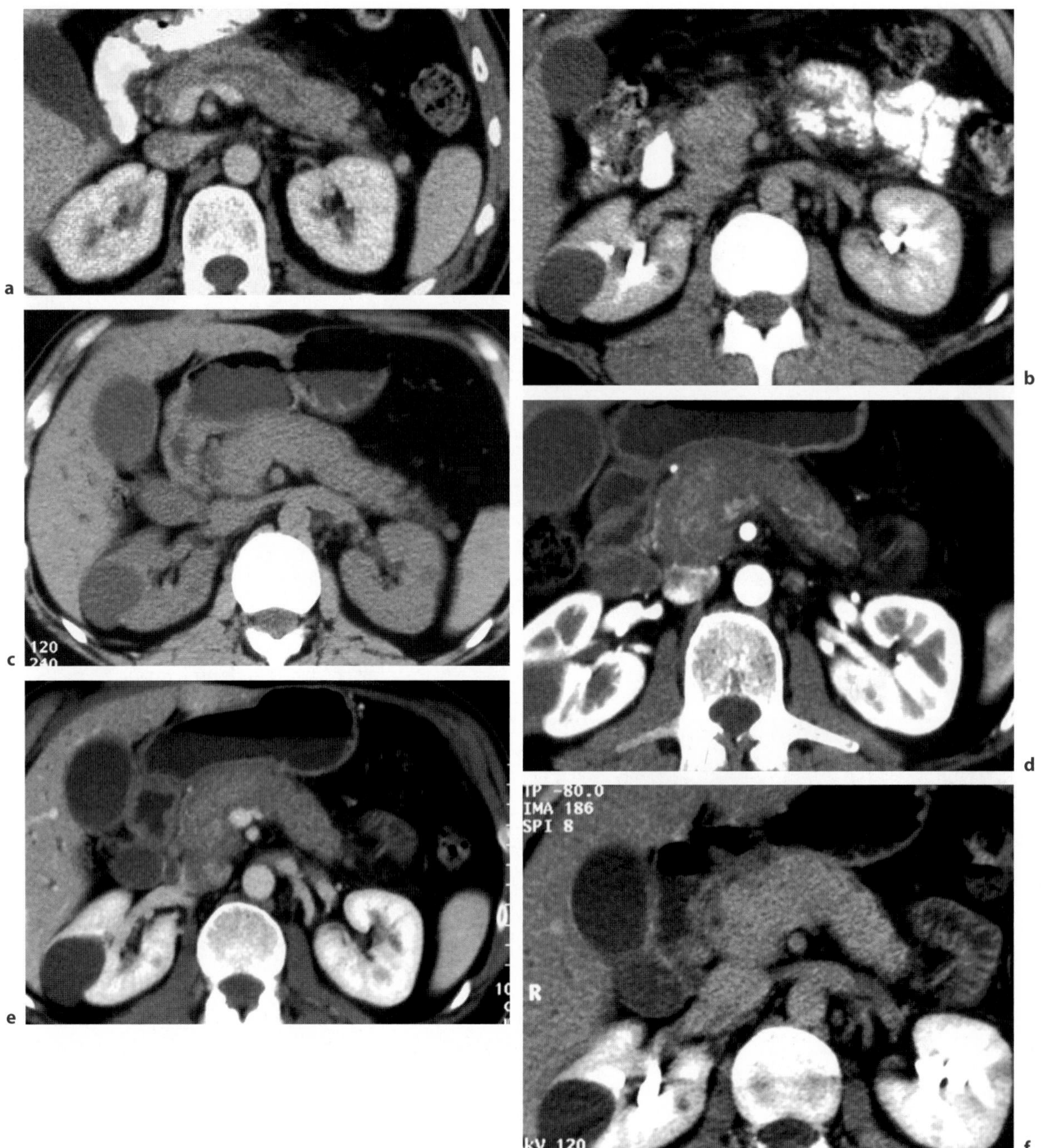

Fig. 10.17 a–f. Primary chronic pancreatitis (PCP): diffuse autoimmune CP. CT in the pre- (**c**) and post- (**a**, **b**, **d–f**) enhancement phases. **a**, **b** Mild increase in size of the pancreatic gland, with mild hyperdensity of the glandular parenchyma (venous phase), initial dilatation of the MPD (**a**) at the body-tail (autoimmune pancreatitis not recognised at the clinical onset). At 4 months later (**c–f**) there is diffuse increase in the size of the pancreas with an altered enhancement of the parenchyma, showing late and reduced enhancement of the glandular tissue, hypodense in the pancreatic enhancement phase (**d**), but progressively more hyperdense in the venous (**e**) and late (**f**) phases. The initial dilatation of the MPD (**a**) has regressed: the duct is compressed due to infiltration of inflammatory cells

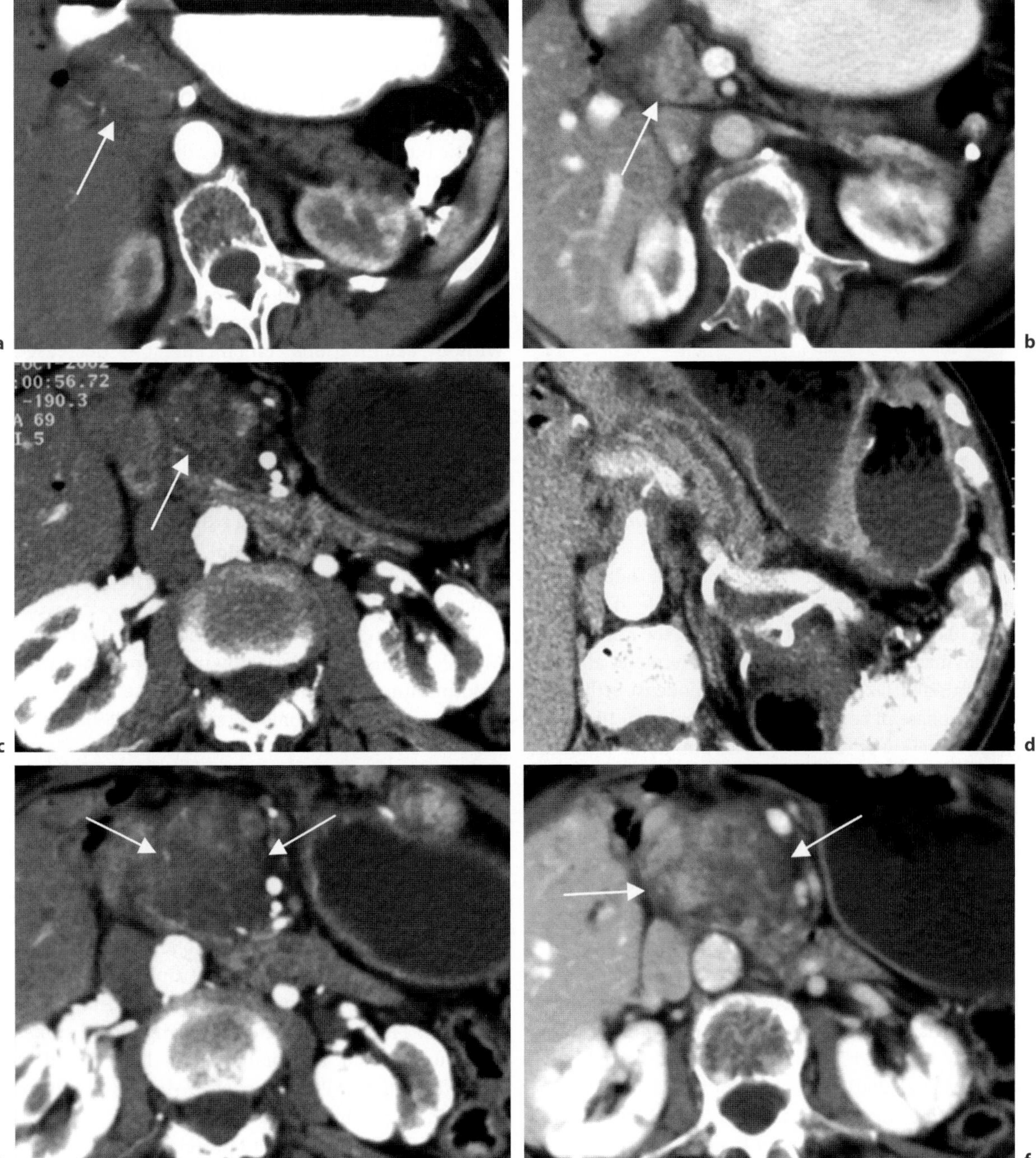

Fig. 10.18a–f. Primary chronic pancreatitis (PCP): focal autoimmune CP. Contrast enhanced CT. **a, b** At the onset, there is a mild increase in the size of the pancreatic head compared to the body and tail with altered enhancement of the parenchyma: hypodense (*arrow*) in the pancreatic enhancement phase (**a**), more hyperdense (*arrow*) in the venous phase (**b**). At 2 years later (**c**) a further increase in the size of the pancreatic head is seen. The parenchymal hypodensity has increased (*arrow*) in the contrast enhanced pancreatic phase. At the third CT examination after 6 months (**d–f**), the pancreatic head is even larger and hypodense (*arrows*) (**e**) in the pancreatic enhancement phase and clearly more hyperdense in the venous phase (**f**). The MPD has become dilated (**d**) at the body-tail. The case was diagnosed as a pancreatic tumor (intra-operative histological diagnosis of focal autoimmune CP)

crease in size and an altered enhancement after CM caused by the presence of unevenly distributed fibrotic areas within the substance of the parenchyma (Fig. 10.19d–f). In the more advanced phase, there is a fibrotic retraction of the parenchyma until atrophy occurs. The collateral ducts show ectasia that can sometimes become retention cysts. The main pancreatic duct (Ring et al. 1973) has strictures alternating with more dilated parts and the so-called "chain-of-lakes" appearance. There are multiple stones of variable size and the morphology is often irregular (Fig. 10.19d–f).

10.3.2.4 CT Differential Diagnosis: PCP vs Pancreatic Tumors

10.3.2.4.1 CT Differential Diagnosis: Autoimmune Focal PCP vs Ductal Adenocarcinoma

Focal autoimmune CP and pancreatic adenocarcinoma can be virtually indistinguishable at imaging (Fig. 10.20a–e). In each of these cases, the affected parenchyma appears hypovascular (Pavone et al. 1999; Ito et al. 2001; Ozawa et al. 2002), hypodense in the pancreatic phase of contrast enhancement (Fig. 10.20b,d), with dilatation of the MPD upstream. In autoimmune CP (Ito et al. 2001; Ozawa et al. 2002), however, the hypodensity tends to reverse in the venous phase and in the later phases (Fig. 10.20b,c) unlike adenocarcinoma (Fig. 10.20d,e). Furthermore, the margins of the autoimmune pancreatitis lesion are more sharply defined, without extrapancreatic extension (Van Hoe et al. 1998) and with preservation of major vessels.

The "capsule-like rim" sign excludes adenocarcinoma (Procacci et al. 2001a). There is no atrophy of the parenchyma as typically seen in adenocarcinoma (Yamaguchi and Tanaka 1992; Van Hoe et al. 1998; Eerens et al. 2001; Kim et al. 2001). Dilatation of the main duct is never very severe, especially in relation to the size of the lesion (Van Hoe et al. 1998).

However, CT diagnosis of autoimmune CP calls for an initial decision on the therapeutic approach and confirmation by a combination of clinical, laboratory and histologic findings.

10.3.2.4.2 CT Differential Diagnosis: Diffuse Autoimmune PCP vs Lymphoma

The CT appearance of diffuse autoimmune CP (Fig. 10.20f) can be similar (Horiuchi et al. 1996; Furukawa et al. 1998) to that of diffuse pancreatic non-Hodgkin lymphoma (NHL) (Fig. 10.20g).

30% of patients suffering from NHL show pancreatic involvement at autopsy report (Glazer et al. 1983; Webb et al. 1989), while the primary pancreatic lymphoma without other disease locations is unusual (Webb et al. 1989; Van Beers et al. 1993; Sheth and Fishman 2002).

In both pancreatic NHL and autoimmune pancreatitis (Ferrozzi et al. 2000; Remer and Baker 2002) the entire gland is increased in size. The parenchyma appears homogenous, hypodense and without calcifications. Enhancement is decreased in the pancreatic phase compared with normal patients. The pancreatic enhancement increases over time (Fig. 10.20f,g).

In contrast, the presence of lymphadenopathy located in the peripancreatic and periaortic regions (Webb et al. 1989; Horiuchi et al. 1996; Ferrozzi et al. 2000), distal to the renal veins (Sheth and Fishman 2002), is a sign of lymphoma (Fig. 10.20g).

Evaluation of the main pancreatic duct with MRCP reveals diffuse narrowing in patients with autoimmune pancreatitis, whereas the duct is of regular size in lymphoma (Webb et al. 1989).

10.3.2.4.3 CT Differential Diagnosis: Hereditary PCP from Genetic Mutations vs IPMT

Hereditary PCP associated with fibrocystic gene mutation (CFTR) in the advanced phase can appear very similar at CT examination to an IPMT. In both diseases there is parenchymal atrophy and significant dilatation of the main duct. In hereditary PCP due to CFTR mutation, late-appearing ductal stones are found which are smaller than those found in other hereditary PCPs. However, in the lumen of the MPD large, hyperdense filling defects are often present (Fig. 10.13d), due to protein aggregates that are formed because of the high level viscosity of the pancreatic juice. This is typical of cystic fibrosis (Frulloni et al. 2003; Procacci et al. 2003) appearing at CT examination like the mucin deposits and/or neoplastic papillary vegetation common to IPMTs (Fig. 10.13b,e).

For this reason, in young patients with a long history of acute pancreatitis attacks and suspected IPMT at imaging, it is advisable to carry out a study of the fibrocystic gene mutations before deciding on therapy (Frulloni et al. 2003).

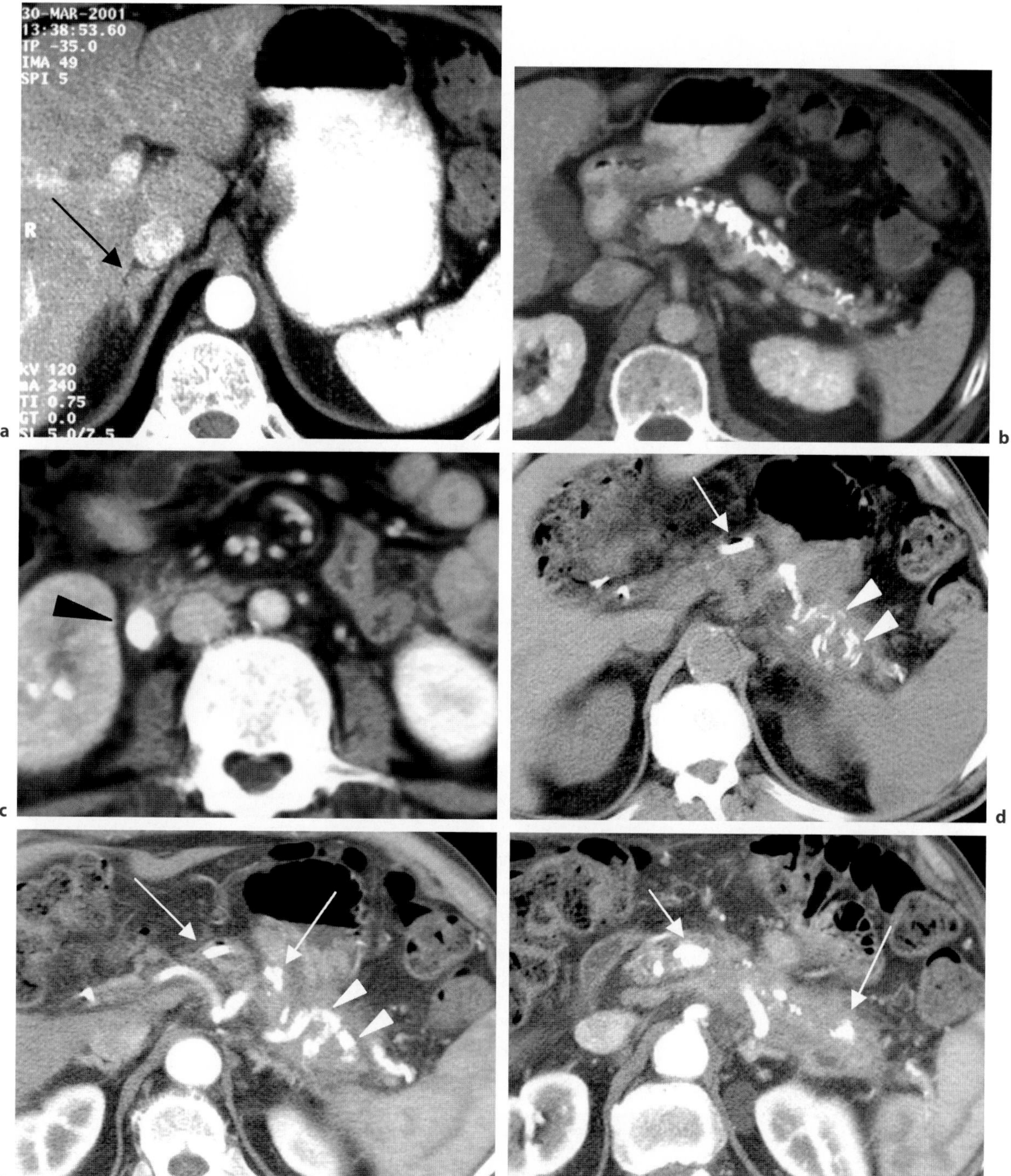

Fig. 10.19 a–f. Primary chronic pancreatitis (PCP) – metabolic causes. CT before (**d**) and after (**a–c**, **e**, **f**) CM administration. Two cases (1st case, **a–c**; 2nd case, **d–f**). **a–c** PCP associated with hypercalcemia. Total parenchymal atrophy, diffuse dilatation of the MPD, multiple and large ductal stones (**b**); small nodule (*arrow*) with solid density in the right adrenal gland (**a**: adenoma); right ureteral stones (**c**: *arrowhead*). **d–f** PCP associated with toxic causes (alcohol). Diffuse increase in the size of the pancreas, altered density with late enhancement in the pancreatic phase (**e**) due to widespread fibrosis, multiple and diffuse ductal calculi (*arrows*) with "staghorn" morphology (**e**, **f**). Lamellar calcifications of the splenic artery (**d**, **e**: *arrowheads*)

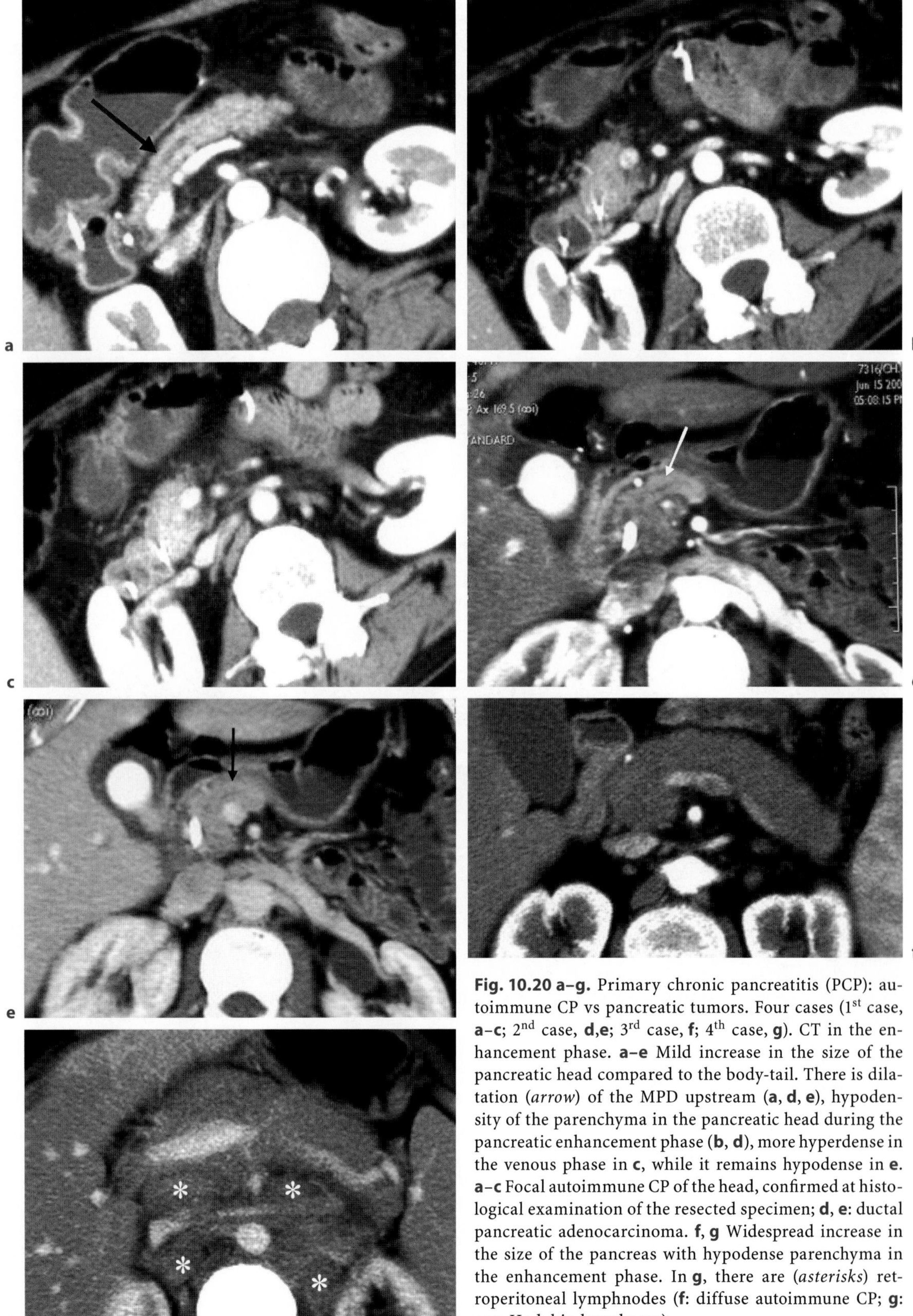

Fig. 10.20 a–g. Primary chronic pancreatitis (PCP): autoimmune CP vs pancreatic tumors. Four cases (1st case, **a–c**; 2nd case, **d,e**; 3rd case, **f**; 4th case, **g**). CT in the enhancement phase. **a–e** Mild increase in the size of the pancreatic head compared to the body-tail. There is dilatation (*arrow*) of the MPD upstream (**a**, **d**, **e**), hypodensity of the parenchyma in the pancreatic head during the pancreatic enhancement phase (**b**, **d**), more hyperdense in the venous phase in **c**, while it remains hypodense in **e**. **a–c** Focal autoimmune CP of the head, confirmed at histological examination of the resected specimen; **d**, **e**: ductal pancreatic adenocarcinoma. **f**, **g** Widespread increase in the size of the pancreas with hypodense parenchyma in the enhancement phase. In **g**, there are (*asterisks*) retroperitoneal lymphnodes (**f**: diffuse autoimmune CP; **g**: non-Hodgkin lymphoma)

10.3.2.4.4 CT Identification of Ductal Adenocarcinoma in Pre-existing CP

CP is considered as one of the risk factors for the development of pancreatic ductal adenocarcinoma (Lankisch and Banks 1998; Howes and Neoptolemos 2002; Levy and Ruszniewski 2002; Malka et al. 2002).

CT examination is limited in identifying a ductal adenocarcinoma arising in CP (Fig. 10.21) because of the decreased difference in attenuation between the cancerous lesion, which is typically hypovascularised, and the pancreatic parenchyma. Furthermore, the obstruction of the main pancreatic duct will be assumed to be secondary to CP, the offending neoplasm is not appreciated.

If the images are carefully examined, one realizes that the attenuation of the neoplasm will still be decreased compared to even the diseased parenchyma. The lesion to background difference paradoxically *increases* on delayed images as the fibrotic parenchyma retains contrast material. The onset of an adenocarcinoma in CP can sometimes be recognized by the displacement of ductal calcifications in comaprison to previous CT examinations (Elmas 2001).

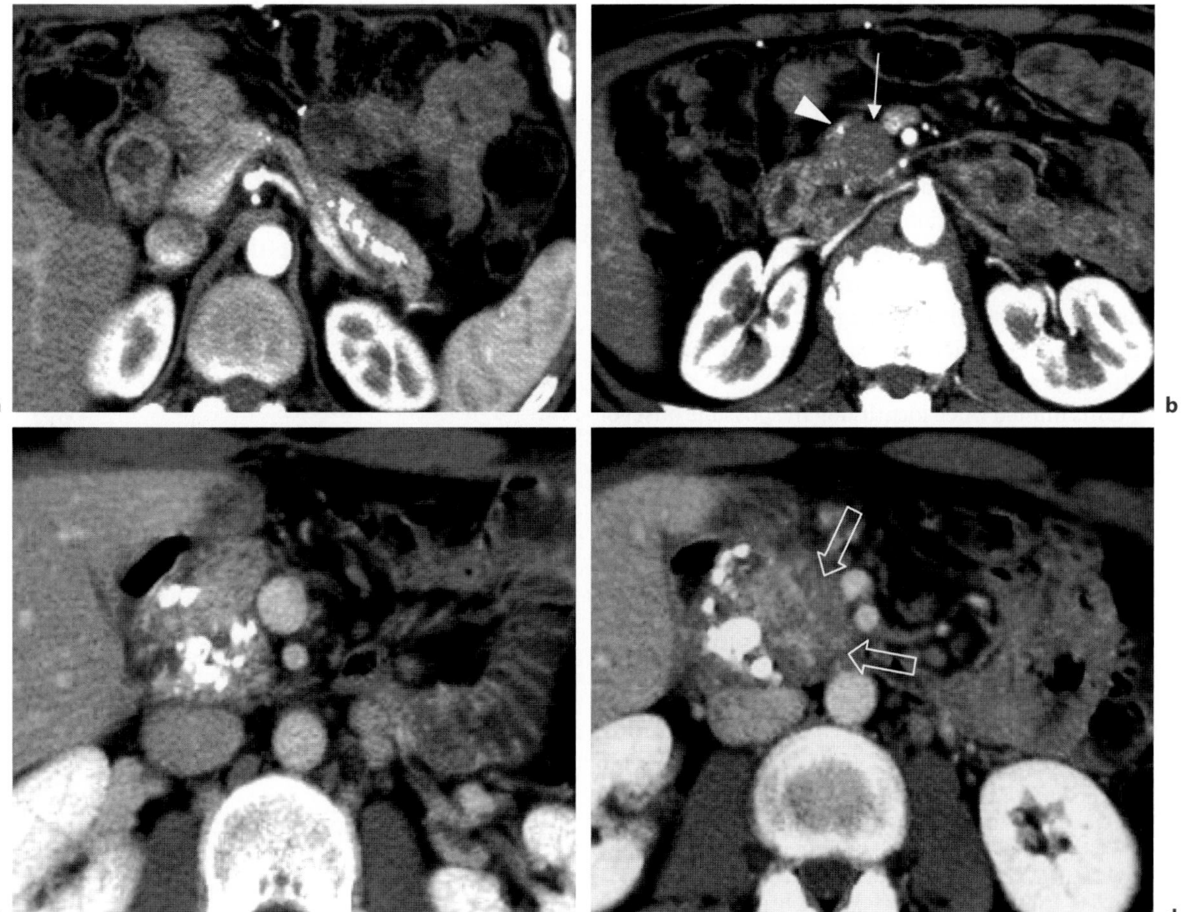

Fig. 10.21 a–d. CT differential diagnosis of CP: ductal adenocarcinoma in CP. CT in the enhancement phase. **a, b** The pancreas is small, atrophic and hypodense due to fibrosis in the pancreatic enhancement phase, with multiple ductal stones in the main duct (**a**). Small hypodense nodular area (**b**: *arrow*) of the uncinate process adherent to the superior mesenteric vein, with ventral displacement (*arrowhead*) of a small stone is seen (histological diagnosis of ductal adenocarcinoma in CP, diagnosed at intra-operative biopsy during pancreatic surgery and not recognised at CT). **c, d** Hereditary PCP (associated genetic defect SPINK 1): the pancreatic head is larger with multiple ductal stones. 5 months later (**d**), a hypodense (*clear arrows*) area appears in the pancreatic enhancement phase, responsible for displacing the stones to the right (the histological examination revealed glandular fibrosis)

10.4 Conclusions

The role of CT in diagnosing CP varies in relation to the different phases of the disease (Malfertheiner and Buchler 1989; Forsmark 2000; Brizi et al. 2001). In the early stage, CT is particularly useful for excluding other pathologies, the symptoms of which are similar to those of CP, as well as for identifying specific etiologies of obstruction which may originally cause the onset of CP. However, CT examination is not able to demonstrate the subtlest and earliest changes in the pancreatic ducts that occur in CP..

In the advanced phase, this technique is not only able to make the correct diagnosis of CP, but is also able to characterise the disease, define its aetiology and make the correct differential diagnosis between CP and tumours, as well as identify complications. In fact, CT examination easily characterises OCP where the pancreas typically appears reduced in size and there is glandular atrophy and considerable and uniform dilatation of the main duct. In many cases CT can demonstrate the cause of the obstruction (slow-growing tumours, duodenal dystrophy, pancreas divisum). CT imaging can be useful in arousing the suspicion of some unusual forms like autoimmune CP or hereditary CP.

CT is limited when identifying the possible onset of pancreatic carcinoma, of which patients with CP are more at risk than the rest of the general population.

References

Berrocal T, Torres I, Gutierrez J, Prieto C, Del Hoyo ML, Lamas M (1999) Congenital anomalies of the upper gastrointestinal tract. Radiographics 19:855–872

Bhatia E, Choudhuri G, Sikora SS, Landt O, Kage A, Becker M, Witt H (2002) Tropical calcific pancreatitis: strong association with SPINK 1 trypsin inhibitor mutations. Gastroenterology 123:1020–1025

Brinberg DE, Carr MF Jr, Premkumar A, Stein J, Green PH (1988) Isolated ventral pancreatitis in an alcoholic with pancreas divisum. Gastrointest Radiol 13:323–326

Brizi MG, Natale L, Manfredi R, Sallustio G, Vecchioli A, Marano P (2001) High resolution spiral computed tomography of the pancreas. Rays 26:111–115

Cavallini G, Frulloni L (2002) Fisiopatologia della pancreatite cronica. Argomenti di Gastroenterologia Clinica 15:203–212

Charney RM (2003) Hereditary pancreatitis. World J Gastroenterol 9:1–4

Choudari CP, Nickl NJ, Fogel E, Lehman GA, Sherman S (2002) Hereditary pancreatitis: clinical presentation, ERCP findings, and outcome of endoscopic therapy. Gastrointest Endosc 56:66–71

Coyle WJ, Pineau BC, Tarnasky PR, Knapple WL, Aabakken L, Hoffman BJ, Cunningham JT, Hawes RH, Cotton PB (2002) Evaluation of unexplained acute and acute recurrent pancreatitis using endoscopic retrograde cholangiopancreatography, sphincter of Oddi manometry and endoscopic ultrasound. Endoscopy 34:617–623

Dussaulx-Garin L, Pagenault M, Le Berre-Heresbach N, Boudjema K, Bretagne JF (2000) Obstructive pancreatitis due to mucus produced by metaplastic choledochal cyst epithelium. Gastrointest Endosc 52:787–789

Eerens I, Vanbeckevoort D, Vansteenbergen W, Van Hoe L (2001) Autoimmune pancreatitis associated with primary sclerosing cholangitis: MR imaging findings. Eur Radiol 11:1401–1404

Elmas N (2001) The role of diagnostic radiology in pancreatitis. Eur J Radiol 12:125–158

England ER, Newcomer MK, Leung JW, Cotton PB (1995) Annular pancreas divisum – a report of two cases and review of the literature. Br J Radiol 68:324–328

Etemad B, Whitcomb DC (2001) Chronic pancreatitis: diagnosis, classification, and new genetic developments. Gastroenterology 120:682–707

Ferrozzi F, Zuccoli G, Bova D, Calculli L (2000) Tumori mesenchimali del pancreas: aspetti con tomografia computerizzata. J Comput Assist Tomogr 24:622–627

Fidler JL, Saigh JA, Thompson JS, Habbe TG (1998) Demonstration of intraluminal duodenal diverticulum by computed tomography. Abdom Imaging 23:38–39

Forsmark CE (2000) The diagnosis of chronic pancreatitis. Gastrointest Endosc 52:293–298

Frulloni L, Castellani C, Bovo P, Vaona B, Calore B, Liani C, Mastella G, Cavallini G (2003) Natural history of pancreatitis associated with cystic fibrosis gene mutations. Dig Liver Dis 35:179–185

Furukawa N, Muranaka T, Yasumori K, Matsubayashi R, Hayashida K, Arita Y (1998) Autoimmune pancreatitis: radiologic findings in three histologically proven cases. J Comput Assist Tomogr 22:880–883

Glazer HS, Lee JK, Balfe DM, Mauro MA, Griffith R, Sagel SS (1983) Non-Hodgkin lymphoma: computed tomographic demonstration of unusual extranodal involvement. Radiology 149:211–217

Gmelin E, Weiss HD (1981) Tumors in the region of the papilla of Vater. Diagnosis via endoscopy, biopsy, brush cytology, ERPC and CT-scan. Eur J Radiol 1:301–306

Graf O, Boland G, Warshaw AL, Fernandez-del-Castillo C, Hahn P, Mueller P (1997) Arterial versus portal venous helical CT for revealing pancreatic adenocarcinoma: conspicuity of tumor and critical vascular anatomy. AJR Am J Roentgenol 169:119–123

Guelrud M, Morera C, Rodriguez M, Jaen D, Pierre R (1999) Sphincter of Oddi dysfunction in children with recurrent pancreatitis and anomalous pancreatico-biliary union: an etiologic concept. Gastrointest Endosc 50:194–199

Gullo L, Migliori M, Pezzilli R, Olah A, Farkas G, Levy P, Arvanitakis C, Lankisch P, Beger H (2002) An update on recurrent acute pancreatitis: data from five European countries. Am J Gastroenterol 97:1959–1962

Hamissa S, Rahmouni A, Coffin C, Wolkenstein P (1999) CT detection of an ampullary somatostatinoma in a patient with von Recklinghausen's disease. AJR Am J Roentgenol 173:503–504

Homma T (1998) Criteria for pancreatic disease diagnosis in Japan: diagnostic criteria for chronic pancreatitis. Pancreas 16:250–254

Horiuchi A, Kaneko T, Yamamura N, Nagata A, Nakamura T, Akamatsu T, Mukawa K, Kawa S, Kiyosawa K (1996) Autoimmune chronic pancreatitis simulating pancreatic lymphoma. Am J Gastroenterol 91:2607–2609

Hoshina K, Kimura W, Ishiguro T, Tominaga O, Futakawa N, Bin Z, Muto T, Makuuchi M (1999) Three generations of hereditary chronic pancreatitis. Hepatogastroenterology 46:1192–1198

Howes N, Neoptolemos JP (2002) Risk of pancreatic ductal adenocarcinoma in chronic pancreatitis. Gut 51:765–766

Hsu JT, Chen HM, Jan YY, Chen MF (2001) Chronic pancreatitis with pancreas divisum treated with pylorus-preserving pancreatoduodenectomy: a case report. Hepatogastroenterology 48:1770–1771

Inamoto K, Ishikawa Y, Itoh N (1983) CT Demonstration of annular pancreas: case report. Gastrointest Radiol 8:143–144

Indinnimeo M, Cicchini C, Stazi A, Ghini C, Laghi A, Memeo L, Iannaccone R, Teneriello FL, Mingazzini PL (2001) Duodenal pancreatic heterotopy diagnosed by magnetic resonance cholangiopancreatography: report of a case. Surg Today 31:928–931

Irie H, Honda H, Baba S, Kuroiwa T, Yoshimitsu K, Tajima T, Jimi M, Sumii T, Masuda K (1998a) Autoimmune pancreatitis: CT and MR characteristics. AJR Am J Roentgenol 170:1323–1327

Irie H, Honda H, Kuroiwa T, Hanada K, Yoshimitsu K, Tajima T, Jimi M, Yamaguchi K, Masuda K (1998b) MRI of groove pancreatitis. J Comput Assist Tomogr 22:651–655

Irie H, Honda H, Kuroiwa T, Yoshimitsu K, Aibe H, Shinozaki K, Masuda K (2002) Measurement of the apparent diffusion coefficient in intraductal mucin-producing tumor of the pancreas by diffusion-weighted echo-planar MR imaging. Abdom Imaging 27:82–87

Ito K, Koike S, Matsunaga N (2001) MR imaging of pancreatic diseases. Eur J Radiol 38:78–93

Itoh S, Yamakawa K, Shimamoto K, Endo T, Ishigaki T (1994) CT findings in groove pancreatitis: correlation with histopathological findings. J Comput Assist Tomogr 18:911–915

Jadvar H, Mindelzun RE (1999) Annular pancreas in adults: imaging features in seven patients. Abdom Imaging 24:174–177

Kahl S, Glasbrenner B, Leodolter A, Pross M, Schulz HU, Malfertheiner P (2002) EUS in the diagnosis of early chronic pancreatitis: a prospective follow-up study. Gastrointest Endosc 55:507–511

Kim T, Murakami T, Takamura M, Hori M, Takahashi S, Nakamori S, Sakon M, Tanji Y, Wakasa K, Nakamura H (2001) Pancreatic mass due to chronic pancreatitis: correlation of CT and MR imaging features with pathologic findings. AJR Am J Roentgenol 177:367–371

Komuro H, Makino SI, Yasuda Y, Ishibashi T, Tahara K, Nagai H (2001) Pancreatic complications in choledochal cyst and their surgical outcomes. World J Surg 25:1519–1523

Kusano S, Kaji T, Sugiura Y, Tamai S (1999) CT demonstration of fibrous stroma in chronic pancreatitis: pathologic correlation. J Comput Assist Tomogr 23:297–300

Lankisch PG, Banks PA (1998) Pancreatitis. Springer, Berlin Heidelberg New York, pp 199–121

Levy MJ (2002) The hunt for microlithiasis in idiopathic acute recurrent pancreatitis: should we abandon the search or intensify our efforts? Gastrointest Endosc 55:286–293

Levy MJ, Geenen JE (2001) Idiopathic acute recurrent pancreatitis. Am J Gastroenterol 96:2540–2555

Levy P, Ruszniewski P (2002) Chronic pancreatitis. Rev Prat 52:997–1000

Luetmer PH, Stephens DH, Ward EM (1989) Chronic pancreatitis: reassessment with current CT. Radiology 171:353–357

Ly JN, Miller FH (2002) MR Imaging of the pancreas. A practical approach. Radiol Clin North Am 40:1289–1306

Maione G, Guffanti E, Fontana A, Pozzi C, Baticci F, Noto S, Franzetti M (1999) Acute biliary pancreatitis. Therapeutic trends. Minerva Chir 54:843–850

Maisonneuve P, Lowenfels AB (2002) Chronic pancreatitis and pancreatic cancer. Dig Dis 20:32–37

Malfertheiner P, Buchler M (1989) Correlation of imaging and function in chronic pancreatitis. Radiol Clin North Am 27:51–64

Malka D, Hammel P, Maire F et al. (2002) Risk of pancreatic adenocarcinoma in chronic pancreatitis. Gut 51:849–852

Manfredi R, Costamagna G, Brizi MG, Spina S, Maresca G, Vecchioli A, Mutignani M, Marano P (2000) Pancreas divisum and "santorinicele": diagnosis with dynamic MR cholangiopancreatography with secretin stimulation. Radiology 217:403–408

Manfredi R, Brizi MG, Masselli G, Gui B, Vecchioli A, Marano P (2001) Imaging of chronic pancreatitis. Rays 26:143–149

McNulty NJ, Francis IR, Platt JF, Cohan RH, Korobkin M, Gebremariam A (2001) Multi-detector row helical CT of the pancreas: effect of contrast-enhanced multiphasic imaging on enhancement of the pancreas, peripancreatic vasculature, and pancreatic adenocarcinoma. Radiology 220:97–102

Megibow AJ, Lavelle MT, Rofsky NM (2001) MR imaging of the pancreas. Surg Clin North Am 81:307–320

Morgan DE, Logan K, Baron TH, Koehler RE, Smith JK (1999) Pancreas divisum: implications for diagnostic and therapeutic pancreatography. AJR Am J Roentgenol 173:193–198

Mossner J, Teich N (2002) Genetic disorders in pancreatitis: Implications in the pathogenesis of acute and chronic pancreatitis. Surgery 132:421–423

Nino-Murcia M, Jeffrey RB Jr, Beaulieu CF, Li KCP, Rubin GD (2001) Multidetector CT of the Pancreas and Bile Duct System: Value of the Curved Planar Reformations. AJR Am J Roentgenol 176:689–693

Ozawa Y, Numata K, Tanaka K, Ueno N, Kiba T, Hara K, Morimoto M, Sakaguchi T, Sekihara H, Kubota T, Shimada H, Nakatani Y (2002) Contrast-enhanced sonography of small pancreatic mass lesions. J Ultrasound Med 21:983–991

Pandolfo I, Scribano E, Blandino A, Salvi L, De Francesco F, Picciotto M, Bottari M (1990) Tumors of the ampulla diagnosed by CT hypotonic duodenography. J Comput Assist Tomogr 14:199–200

Pavone P, Panebianco V, Laghi A, Catalano C, Messina A, Lobina L, Pirillo S, Passariello R (1997) La colangiopancreatografia con risonanza magnetica nella valutazione del dotto pancreatico. Radiol Med 94:61–67

Pavone P, Laghi A, Catalano C, Panebianco V, Luccichenti G, Fraioli F, Passariello R (1999) La valutazione delle pancreatiti croniche con Risonanza Magnetica e colangiopancreatografia con RM. Radiol Med 98:373–378

Procacci C, Portuese A, Fugazzola C et al. (1988) Duodenal duplication in the adult: its relationship with pancreatitis. Gastrointest Radiol 13:315–322

Procacci C, Graziani R, Zamboni G, Cavallini G, Pederzoli P, Guarise A, Bogina G, Biasiutti C, Carbognin G, Bergamo-Andreis IA, Pistolesi GF (1997) Cystic dystrophy of the duodenal wall: radiologic findings. Radiology 205:741–747

Procacci C, Graziani R, Bicego E (1998) Trattato italiano di tomografia computerizzata. Pozzi Mucelli 845–856

Procacci C, Carbognin G, Biasiutti C, Frulloni L, Bicego E, Spoto E, el-Khaldi M, Bassi C, Pagnotta N, Talamini G, Cavallini G (2001a) Autoimmune pancreatitis: possibilities of CT characterization. Pancreatology 1:246–253

Procacci C, Graziani R, Vasori S, Venturini S (2001b) Diagnostica per immagini della pancreatite cronica. Gastroenterol Clin 5:195–205

Procacci C, Schenal G, Della Chiara E, Fuini A, Guarise A (2003) Imaging of the pancreas. Cystic Rare Tumors 97–137

Pugliese V, Pujic N, Saccomanno S, Gatteschi B, Pera C, Aste H, Ferrara GB, Nicolo G (2001) Pancreatic intraductal sampling during ERCP in patients with chronic pancreatitis and pancreatic cancer: cytologic studies and k-ras-2 codon 12 molecular analysis in 47 cases. Gastrointest Endosc 54:595–599

Ramesh H (2002) Proposal for a new grading system for chronic pancreatitis: the ABC system. J Clin Gastroenterol 35:67–70

Remer EM, Baker ME (2002) Imaging of chronic pancreatitis. Radiol Clin North Am 40:1229–1242

Ring EJ, Eaton SB Jr, Ferrucci JT Jr, Short WF (1973) Differential diagnosis of pancreatic calcification. Am J Roentgenol Radium Ther Nucl Med 117:446–452

Rizzo JR, Szucs RA, Turner MA (1995) Congenital abnormalities of the pancreas and biliary tree in adults. Radiographics 15:49–68

Rohrmann CA, Surawicz CM, Hutchinson D, Silverstein FE, White TT, Marchioro TL (1981) The diagnosis of the hereditary pancreatitis by pancreatography. Gastrointest Endosc 27:168–173

Sakorafas GH, Sarr MG, Rowland CM, Farnell MB (2001) Postobstructive chronic pancreatitis: results with distal resection. Arch Surg 136:643–648

Schima W, Függer R (2002) Evaluation of focal pancreatic masses: comparison of mangafodipir-enhanced MR imaging and contrast-enhanced helical CT. Eur Radiol 12:2998–3008

Shams J, Stein A, Cooperman AM (2001) Computed tomography for pancreatic diseases. Surg Clin North Am 81:283–306

Shan YS, Sy ED, Lin PW (2002) Annular pancreas with obstructive jaundice: beware of underlying neoplasm. Pancreas 25:314–316

Sheth S, Fishman EK (2002) Imaging of uncommon tumors of the pancreas. Radiol Clin North Am 40:1273–1287

Silverman PM, McVay L, Zeman RK, Garra BS, Grant EG, Jaffe MH (1989) Pancreatic pseudotumor in pancreas divisum: CT characteristics. J Comput Assist Tomogr 13:140–141

Somogyi L, Martin SP, Ulrich CD (2001) Recurrent acute pancreatitis. Curr Treat Options Gastroenterol 4:361–368

Soulen MC, Zerhouni EA, Fishman EK, Gayler BW, Milligan F, Siegelman SS (1989) Enlargement of the pancreatic head in patients with pancreas divisum. Clin Imaging 13:51–57

Takeshita K, Furui S, Takada K (2002) Multidetector row helical CT of the pancreas: value of three-dimensional images, two-dimensional reformations, and contrast-enhanced multiphasic imaging. J Hepatobiliary Pancreat Surg 9:576–582

Taniguchi T, Seko S, Okamoto M, Hamasaki A, Ueno H, Inoue F, Nishida O, Miyake N, Mizumoto T (2000) Association of autoimmune pancreatitis and type 1 diabetes: autoimmune exocrinopathy and endocrinopathy of the pancreas. Diabetes Care 23:1592–1594

Teich N, Bauer N, Mossner J, Keim V (2002) Mutational screening of patients with nonalcoholic chronic pancreatitis: identification of further trypsinogen variants. Am J Gastroenterol 97:341–346

Tio TL, Luiken GJ, Tytgat GN (1991) Endosonography of groove pancreatitis. Endoscopy 23:291–293

Valette O, Cuilleron M, Debelle L, Antunes L, Mosnier JF, Regent D, Veyret C (2001) Imaging of intraductal papillary mucinous tumor of the pancreas: literature review. J Radiol 82:633–645

Van Beers B, Lalonde L, Soyer P, Grandin C, Trigaux JP, De Ronde T, Dive C, Pringot J (1993) Dynamic CT in pancreatic lymphoma. J Comput Assist Tomogr 17:94–97

Van Gulik TM, Moojen TM, Van Geenen R, Rauws EA, Obertop H, Gouma DJ (1999) Differential diagnosis of focal pancreatitis and pancreatic cancer. Ann Oncol 10:85–88

Van Hoe L, Gryspeerdt S, Ectors N, Van Steenbergen W, Aerts R, Baert AL, Marchal G (1998) Nonalcoholic duct-destructive chronic pancreatitis: imaging findings. AJR Am J Roentgenol 170:643–647

Vullierme MP, Vilgrain V, Flejou JF, Zins M, O'Toole D, Ruszniewski P, Belghiti J, Menu Y (2000) Cystic dystrophy of the duodenal wall in the heterotopic pancreas: radiopathological correlations. J Comput Assist Tomogr 24:635–643

Wakabayashi T, Kawaura Y, Satomura Y, Fujii T, Motoo Y, Okai T, Sawabu N (2002) Clinical study of chronic pancreatitis with focal irregular narrowing of the main pancreatic duct and mass formation: comparison with chronic pancreatitis showing diffuse irregular narrowing of the main pancreatic duct. Pancreas 25:283–289

Webb TH, Lillemoe KD, Pitt HA, Jones RJ, Cameron JL (1989) Pancreatic lymphoma. Is surgery mandatory for diagnosis or treatment? Ann Surg 209:25–30

Wise RH Jr, Stanley RJ (1984) Carcinoma of the ampulla of vater presenting as acute pancreatitis. J Comput Assist Tomogr 8:158–161

Witt H, Becker M (2002) Genetics of chronic pancreatitis. J Pediatr Gastroenterol Nutr 34:125–136

Yamaguchi K, Tanaka M (1992) Groove pancreatitis masquerading as pancreatic carcinoma. Am J Surg 163:312–318

Zeman RK, McVay LV, Silverman PM, Cattau EL, Benjamin SB, Fleischer DF, Garra BS, Jaffe MH (1988) Pancreas divisum: thin-section CT. Radiology 169:395–398

The Role of MR Imaging in Chronic Pancreatitis

11

Lorenzo Cereser, Maria Antonietta Bali, Myriam Delhaye, and Celso Matos

CONTENTS

11.1 **Introduction** *183*

11.2 **Magnetic Resonance: Examination Technique** (See also Sect. 11.5) *184*
11.2.1 Imaging of the Pancreatic Parenchyma *184*
11.2.2 Imaging of the Ducts *186*
11.2.3 Secretin-Enhanced Magnetic Resonance Cholangiopancreatography *187*

11.3 **Magnetic Resonance: Imaging Findings** *190*
11.3.1 Diagnosis *190*
11.3.1.1 Early Chronic Pancreatitis *190*
11.3.1.2 Advanced Chronic Pancreatitis *192*
11.3.1.3 Autoimmune Pancreatitis *195*
11.3.1.4 Paraduodenal Pancreatitis *195*
11.3.2 Complication Assessment *197*
11.3.3 Differentiation Between Carcinoma and Focal Inflammatory Masses *198*
11.3.4 Road Map for Treatment Planning and Follow-Up *201*

11.4 **Work in Progress: Diffusion-Weighted Imaging** *202*
11.4.1 Differential Diagnosis Between Mass-Forming Pancreatitis and Pancreatic Carcinoma *203*
11.4.2 Exocrine Function Assessment *203*
11.4.3 Monitoring of Autoimmune Pancreatitis Treatment *203*

11.5 **Appendix** *204*

References *205*

L. Cereser, MD
M. A. Bali, MD
C. Matos, MD
Department of Radiology, MR Imaging Division, Cliniques Universitaires de Bruxelles, Hôpital Erasme, Université Libre de Bruxelles, Route de Lennik 808, 1070 Brussels, Belgium
M. Delhaye, MD, PhD
Department of Gastroenterology, Cliniques Universitaires de Bruxelles, Hôpital Erasme, Université Libre de Bruxelles, Route de Lennik 808, 1070 Brussels, Belgium

11.1 Introduction

Chronic pancreatitis is an inflammatory process leading to irreversible damage of the parenchyma and ducts, as well as to progressive exocrine and endocrine functional impairment.

Histologically, chronic pancreatitis is characterized by ductal strictures and dilatations with or without calcifications, fibrosis of the parenchyma and atrophy of acinar and islet tissue (Siddiqi and Miller 2007).

Results of recent surveys on chronic pancreatitis carried out in several countries showed that alcohol consumption is the most frequently associated risk factor (Ryu et al. 2005; Garg and Tandon 2004). Although its role in the pathogenesis of chronic pancreatitis is still unclear, alcohol seems to induce pancreatic fibrosis by stimulating pancreatic stellate cells with a subsequent activation of the downstream pathway of fibrogenesis (Talukdar et al. 2006). Other etiologies include obstruction (secondary to slow-growing tumors, severe acute pancreatitis, congenital lesions, duodenal dystrophy, chronic inflammatory stenosis of the papilla), hereditary/genetic conditions (such as cystic fibrosis) and malnutrition with a low fat and low protein diet (tropical pancreatitis). Autoimmune pancreatitis, an unusual type of chronic pancreatitis, accounts for 2%–4% of all forms of chronic pancreatitis (Pezzilli et al. 2008). According to the evidence from different surveys, between 17% and 60% of patients with chronic pancreatitis have no apparent underlying cause and are considered to have "idiopathic" chronic pancreatitis (Ryu et al. 2005; Balakrishnan et al. 2008). It is believed that many cases of idiopathic chronic pancreatitis actually have genetic bases, so this group is likely to decrease as the specific abnormalities are better understood.

There is evidence that alcoholic, paraduodenal and hereditary forms of chronic pancreatitis evolve from recurrent episodes of severe acute pancreatitis

(Klöppel and Maillet 1992; Ammann et al. 1996; Klöppel et al. 2004). This pathway has been named the "necrosis-fibrosis" sequence (Klöppel and Maillet 1993), in which the mesenchymal reaction to fat and hemorrhagic necrosis leads to fibrosis. On the other hand, obstructive and autoimmune chronic pancreatitis are not based pathogenetically on the necrosis-fibrosis sequence, and can develop without clinical pancreatitis (Klöppel 2008).

After a variable subclinical phase, chronic pancreatitis may present with chronic recurrent and intense abdominal pain. Important associated medical problems include pancreatic exocrine insufficiency, diabetes mellitus and the higher risk of pancreatic cancer.

Once pancreatic biopsies are (rarely) obtained when chronic pancreatitis is suspected, the diagnosis of chronic pancreatitis in based on clinical presentation, functional testing and cross-sectional imaging.

The main goals of imaging in the scenario of suspected chronic pancreatitis are to help the clinician in establishing the diagnosis, to assess and monitor complications, to differentiate focal inflammatory masses from pancreatic malignancy and to set up a road map for treatment planning.

From an imaging standpoint, endoscopic retrograde cholangiopancreatography (ERCP) has long been considered the diagnostic gold standard for the morphological diagnosis of chronic pancreatitis. ERCP findings of ductal abnormalities have been described in various classifications and used as criteria of severity (Cremer et al. 1976; Axon et al. 1984). Invasiveness, operator dependence and associated morbidity are the major drawbacks of this technique. Moreover, ERCP is only able to depict ductal changes.

In recent years, magnetic resonance imaging (MRI) has increasingly been utilized to diagnose pancreatic disease. Due to its capability to evaluate both duct anatomy and parenchyma of the pancreas, bile ducts and adjacent vessels, MRI allows a global assessment of morphology and function in chronic pancreatitis and can be defined as a "one-stop shop examination" (Matos et al. 2002).

11.2 Magnetic Resonance: Examination Technique

(See also Sect. 11.5)

A complete MRI examination performed in the setting of chronic pancreatitis includes:

- Imaging of the pancreatic parenchyma before and after intravenous gadolinium administration.
- Imaging of the duct system with magnetic resonance cholangiopancreatography (MRCP) without or with secretin stimulation.
- Evaluation of pancreatic exocrine function by quantifying pancreatic fluid output after secretin injection.

MRI is a sensitive means for diagnosing chronic pancreatitis even in the early phase of the disease. Due to their excellent soft-tissue contrast, cross-sectional images have high sensitivity in depicting subtle parenchymal signal intensity and enhancement abnormalities. Furthermore, secretin-enhanced MRCP can provide morphological and functional information during a single non-invasive procedure.

The major disadvantage of MRI is its lack of sensitivity in detecting calcifications, depicted as negative signal voids on both T1- and T2-weighted images and not as clearly evident as they are on computed tomography (CT). For this reason the information provided by MRI and MRCP images should be completed with a non-enhanced helical CT acquisition in the pancreatic region (Fig. 11.1a,b). Another drawback of MRI is the difficulty in detecting and determining the cause of non-calcified filling defects.

The use of MRI to investigate the pancreas has lead to significant advances in recent years, owing to the improved performance of magnets, phased array coils and gradients, as well as technical developments in terms of spatial and temporal resolution. A comprehensive MRI protocol for the pancreas combines imaging sequences of the pancreatic parenchyma and pancreatic and bile ducts along with MR angiography and secretin-enhanced MRCP.

11.2.1 Imaging of the Pancreatic Parenchyma

The protocol for imaging the pancreatic parenchyma includes a combination of turbo spin-echo (TSE) T2-weighted and gradient-echo (GRE) T1-weighted sequences.

TSE T2-weighted images are acquired during free breathing with respiratory triggering, in order to minimize the need for patient cooperation. These include the whole liver and pancreas in the axial and coronal planes. These sequences depict bile and pancreatic ducts in cross section, and may be used to guide the acquisition of MRCP scans (Fig. 11.2a–c). Fluid-filled lesions in or around the pancreas are also

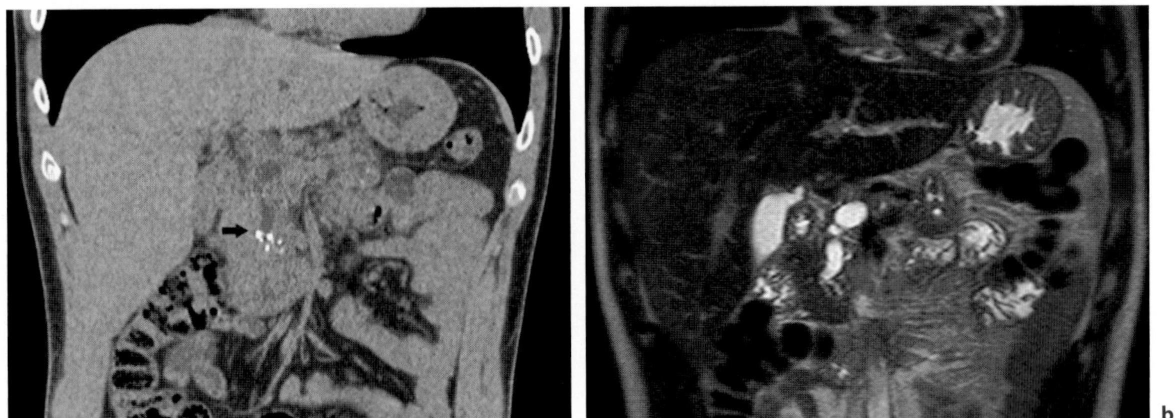

Fig. 11.1a,b. Chronic calcified pancreatitis. Coronal-reformatted non-enhanced MDCT (**a**) depicts tiny calcifications in the head of the pancreas with upstream dilation of the main pancreatic duct *(arrow)*. Comparative coronal T2-weighted TSE image of the same patient (**b**) fails to depict the intraductal calcifications and shows better the ductal dilatation

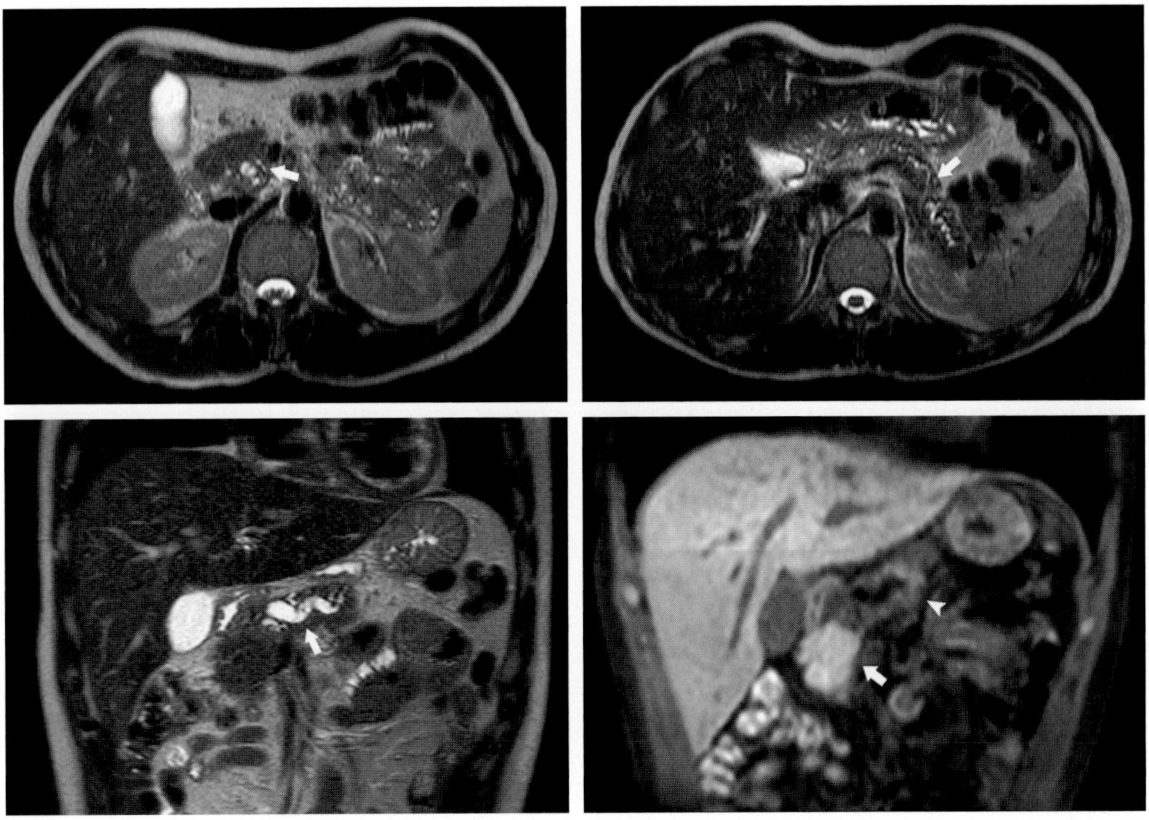

Fig. 11.2a–d. Chronic obstructive pancreatitis. Non-enhanced T2-weighted and T1-weighted sequences to evaluate the pancreatic parenchyma. Respiratory-triggered axial (**a,b**) and coronal T2-weighted TSE images (**c**) exhibit very good contrast between the abnormal ducts and the pancreas parenchyma *(arrows)*. Coronal-reformatted three-dimensional fat-sat T1-weighted GRE image (**d**) depicts normal homogeneously bright pancreas in the head *(arrow)* and reduced signal in pancreas body and tail due to the chronic inflammatory involvement *(arrowhead)*

demonstrated. When a peripancreatic exudate is suspected, a more heavily T2-weighted scan is preferred to fat suppression, the latter decreasing the conspicuity of the pancreatic contours (Matos et al. 2006).

Three-dimensional GRE fat-suppressed T1-weighted images are obtained in the axial plane during suspended respiration. Three-dimensional sequences allow improved spatial resolution and multiplanar reformatting; however, patient cooperation is required (Fig. 11.2d). Fat suppression is important in order to improve visualization of the pancreas, which appears well delineated and homogeneously bright compared with the surrounding low-intensity fat. Fat suppression is also excellent in demonstrating pancreatic masses or focal pancreatitis (less intense than normal high-intensity pancreas) and is suitable for contrast-enhanced studies (Mitchell et al. 1995). In the presence of diffuse chronic pancreatitis, the accuracy of these sequences in demonstrating focal pancreatic disease is lower, because of the homogeneous low signal intensity of the fibrotic pancreas; gadolinium-enhanced studies should therefore be performed.

After intravenous injection of gadolinium, breath-hold, three-dimensional, fat-suppressed GRE T1-weighted multiphase scans (arterial, portal venous and delayed) are acquired. The normal pancreas enhances maximally during the arterial phase and becomes isointense to the liver during the later phases (Fig. 11.3 a–d). Three-dimensional acquisition technique allows multiplanar reconstructions and multiphase angiography renderings.

11.2.2 Imaging of the Ducts

Imaging the pancreatic ducts is dependent on heavily T2-weighted MRCP images, which selectively depict static or slow-moving fluid-filled structures

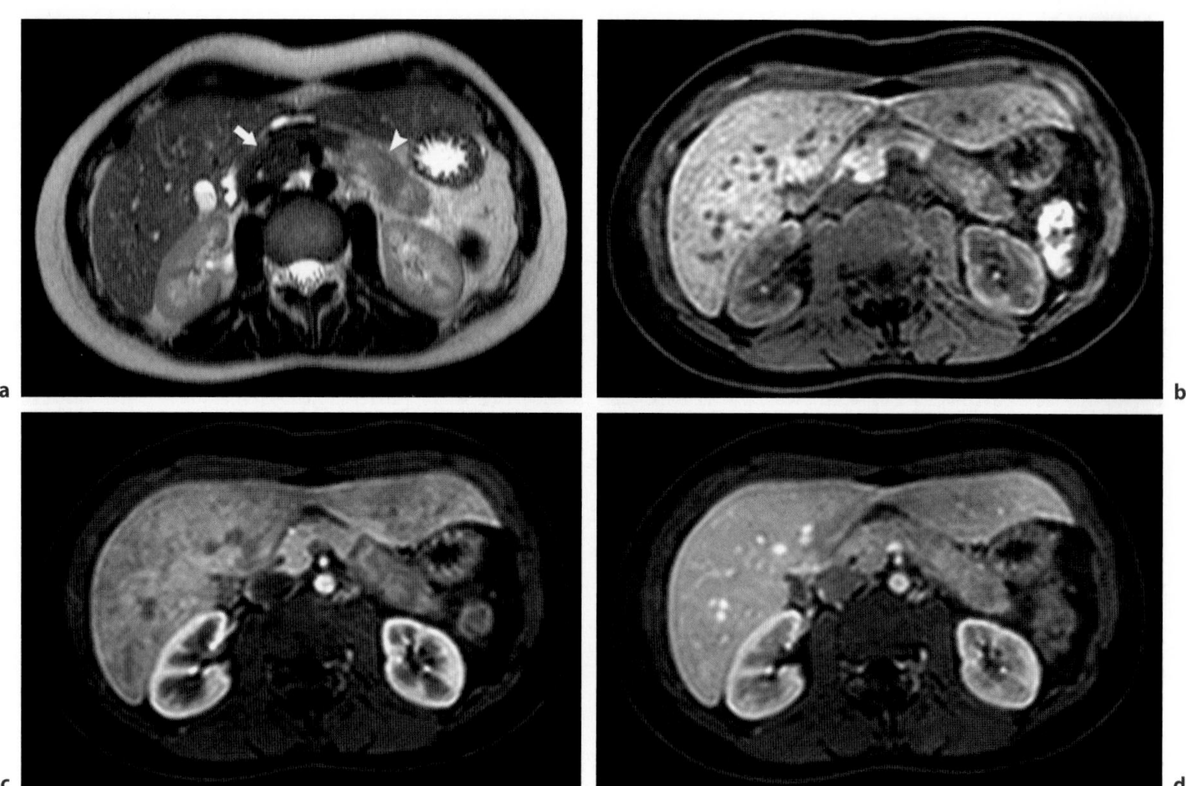

Fig. 11.3a–d. Focal chronic pancreatitis involving the body and tail. Axial T2-weighted TSE image (**a**) shows increased signal intensity involving the body and tail of the pancreas *(arrowhead)*. The head of the pancreas is of normal signal intensity *(arrow)*. Axial non-enhanced three-dimensional fat-sat T1-weighted GE image (**b**) shows decreased signal intensity involving the body and tail of the pancreas. Gadolinium-enhanced three-dimensional fat-sat T1-weighted GRE image in the arterial phase (**c**) shows reduced enhancement in the same area. Gadolinium-enhanced three-dimensional fat-sat T1-weighted GRE image in the interstitial phase (**d**) shows delayed enhancement of the affected area

(pancreatic juice, bile, residual fluid in the stomach and duodenum) with high signal intensity. Two different and complementary approaches are generally used for MRCP: the routinely adopted one consists of a thick-slab, single-shot TSE T2-weighted sequence (projective MRCP). In selected cases, a multisection thin-slab, single-shot TSE T2-weighted sequence can be added to the protocol.

Projective MRCP uses a single, 20- to 50-mm thick section that can be obtained in any desired plane with a single short breath-hold (<3 s). At least two different planes (coronal and transversal) are usually acquired, providing selective display of pancreatic and bile ducts with no respiratory artifact and a relatively good in-plane resolution (Fig. 11.4a,b). The major drawback of this technique is the possible overlap of the pancreatic ducts and other fluid-containing organs (i.e., the stomach and duodenum) (Matos et al. 2006). Adapting the section thickness, orientation and positioning of the thick slab to the anatomy of the patient can overcome these pitfalls. Moreover, patients are asked to fast at least 4 h before the examination and, if needed, a T2-negative oral contrast agent that eliminates the residual signal from overlapping fluid-containing bowel may be administrated (Hirohashi et al. 1997) (Fig. 11.5a,b).

As an alternative to the projective MRCP, three-dimensional TSE T2-weighted MRCP techniques can be applied. Thanks to recent technological refinements (i.e., parallel imaging, short interecho spacing) images with nearly isotropic voxels (≈1 mm in all three dimensions) can now be obtained in a short time (during 1.5–3 min of respiratory-triggering or in a single breath-hold) (Zhang et al. 2006). Major benefits of obtaining three-dimensional images with nearly isotropic voxels are the ability to get multiplanar and three-dimensional reconstructions (i.e., maximum intensity projection and volume rendering) and to provide better delineation of complex pancreatobiliary anatomic features and relationships. Zhang et al. (2006) compared the quality of images obtained with three-dimensional MRCP sequences and 1-mm isotropic voxels with the quality of conventional two-dimensional MRCP images. Three-dimensional images had higher relative signal intensity and contrast and delineated better the bile duct anatomy. However, no statistically significant differences between the different sequences were achieved when depiction of pancreatic ducts and confidence level in determining the presence of pancreatic ductal anomaly and pathologic changes were evaluated.

11.2.3 Secretin-Enhanced Magnetic Resonance Cholangiopancreatography

Secretin stimulation helps in filling the gap between the diagnostic capabilities of MRCP and ERCP (Hellerhoff et al. 2002). Secretin is a polypeptide hormone inducing a stimulation of the pancreatic

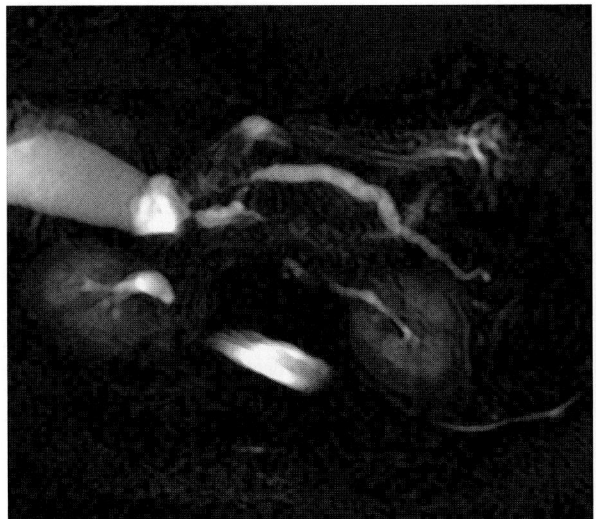

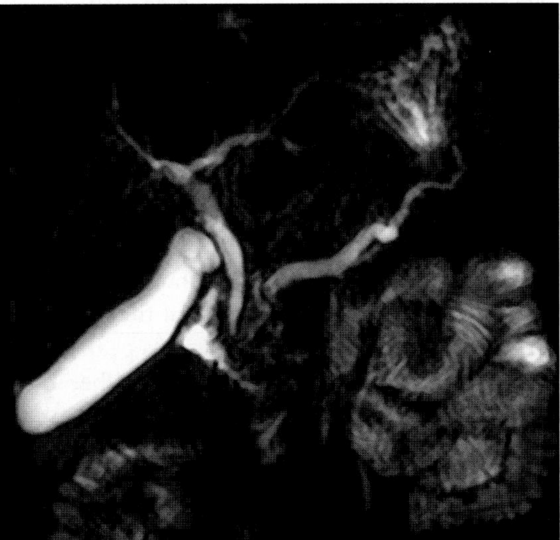

Fig. 11.4a,b. Chronic obstructive pancreatitis. Axial (**a**) and coronal (**b**) oblique thick-slab projective MRCP images show an excellent contrast between the non-flowing fluid in the ducts and bowel and the background tissues

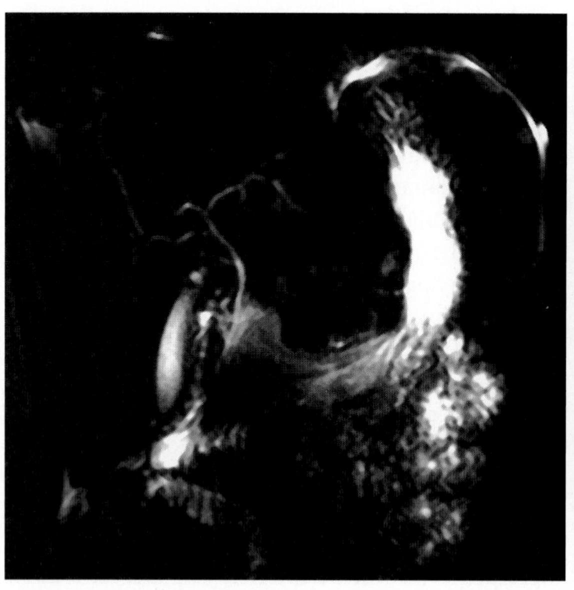
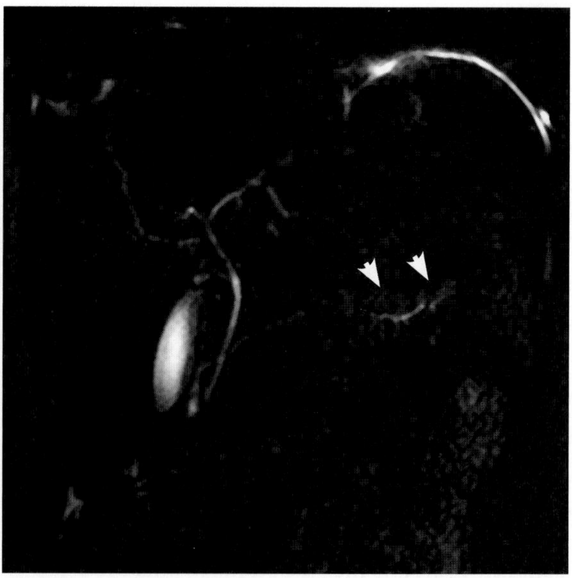

Fig. 11.5a,b. Contribution of oral negative contrast agent in a patient with focal chronic pancreatitis. After oral intake of diluted gadolinium (1 ml in 50 ml of water) complete suppression of residual fluid in the stomach and in the small bowel is achieved (**b**). This enables better depiction of the focal changes involving the pancreatic ducts in the tail of the pancreas *(arrowheads)*

secretion of bicarbonate-rich fluid and a transient increasing tone in the sphincter of Oddi. Consequently, determining an increase of the volume of fluid in the pancreatic ducts, secretin acts as a target contrast agent in MR pancreatography studies. It has been shown that its intravenous administration improves the delineation of pancreatic ducts, allows monitoring of the pancreatic duct flow dynamics and evaluation of the pancreatic exocrine function (Matos et al. 1997; Manfredi et al. 2000; Cappeliez et al. 2000; Heverhagen et al. 2001).

Once the appropriate projection MRCP image has been chosen (usually coronal oblique, displaying the full length of the MPD, the biliary tract and the duodenum), the same scan is repeated every 30 s for 10–15 min after intravenous secretin administration (0.5–1 ml/10 kg of body weight), in order to properly evaluate pancreatic flow dynamics. In normal subjects, a progressive dilatation of the MPD is observed mostly within 2–6 min, with a peak 2–3 min after secretin injection. Then the caliber of the MPD returns to the baseline value within 10 min, as pancreatic juice flows out through the papilla and progressively fills the duodenum. We consider the diameter of MPD to be abnormal when it is greater than 3 mm in the body of the gland at the end of the secretin stimulation period in patients younger than 60 years old.

Finally, secretin-enhanced MRCP (S-MRCP) can visualize the amount of pancreatic fluid excreted into the duodenum and indirectly estimate the pancreatic exocrine reserve (Matos et al. 1997) (Fig. 11.6a–c).

A semi-quantitative S-MRCP grading system for duodenal filling has been proposed:

- Grade 0: no fluid is observed.
- Grade 1: the filling remains limited to the duodenal bulb.
- Grade 2: the fluid fills the duodenal bulb and partially the duodenum up to the genu inferius.
- Grade 3: the duodenum is largely filled beyond the genu inferius.

A reduced duodenal filling volume (< grade 3) was qualitatively correlated with a reduced pancreatic exocrine reserve, calculated according to maximum bicarbonate concentration and output in a collection of pure pancreatic juice (Matos et al. 1997). This technique has been validated in a comparative study with intraductal secretin test (Cappeliez et al. 2000).

S-MRCP techniques are also feasible to obtain quantitative assessment of the pancreatic exocrine function. These techniques have been called quantitative-MRCP (Heverhagen et al. 2001; Punwani et al. 2003). It has recently been demonstrated that pancreatic fluid output measured with quantitative-

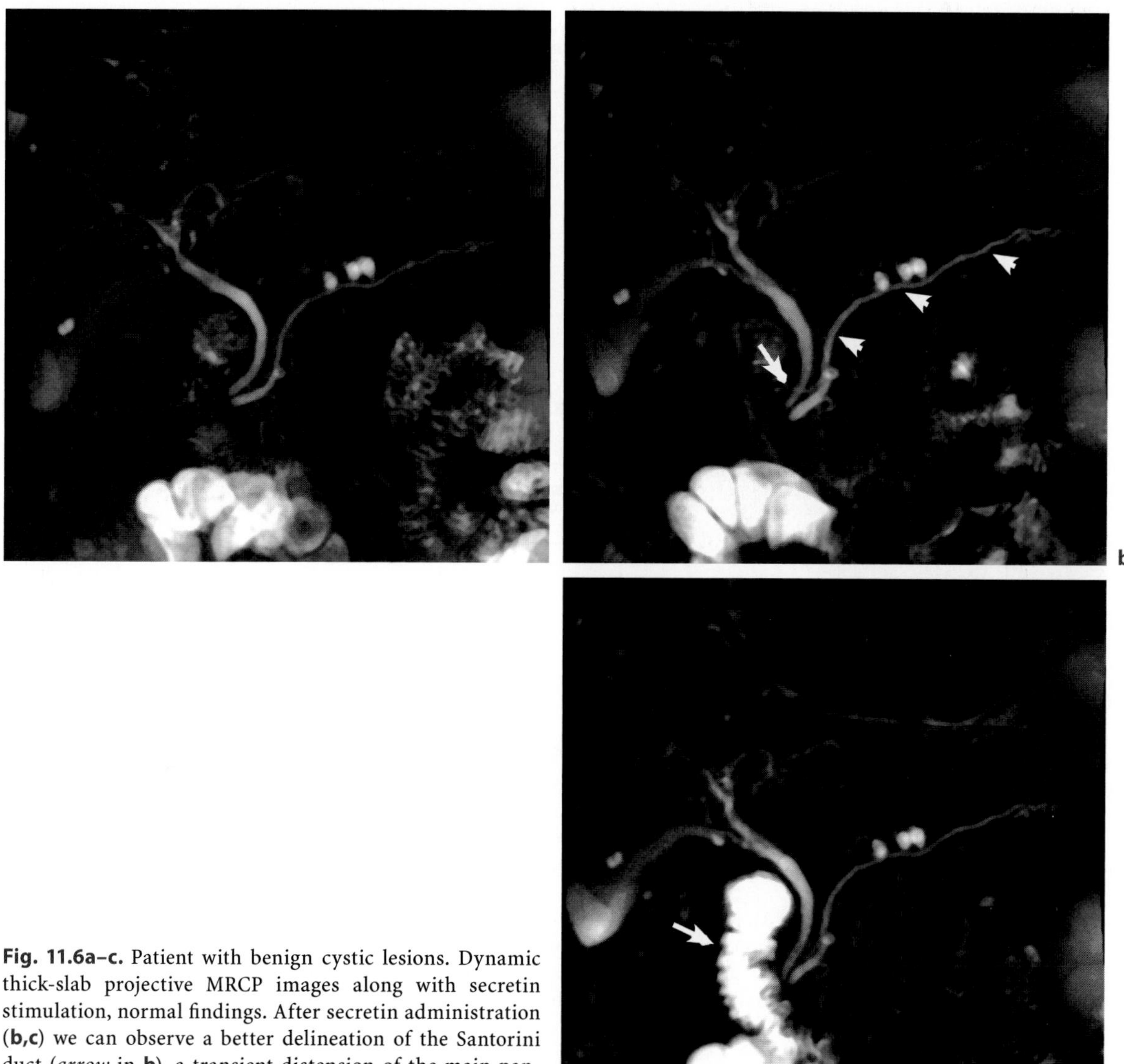

Fig. 11.6a–c. Patient with benign cystic lesions. Dynamic thick-slab projective MRCP images along with secretin stimulation, normal findings. After secretin administration (**b,c**) we can observe a better delineation of the Santorini duct (*arrow* in **b**), a transient distension of the main pancreatic duct (*arrowheads* in **b**) and a normal duodenal filling (*arrow* in **c**)

MRCP shows a good correlation with both clinical symptoms of pancreatic exocrine insufficiency (steatorrhea) and with conventional indirect function tests (urinary pancreo-lauryl and fecal elastase 1) (Gillams et al. 2008). A method to assess pancreatic function by measuring pancreatic flow output (PFO) and total excreted volume (TEV) has recently been proposed (Bali et al. 2005) (Fig. 11.7a–d). The protocol consists in a breath-hold, fat-suppressed, heavily T2-weighted coronal multislice TSE sequence (TE 850 ms; slice thickness 15–17 mm, six slices without gap) with a large field of view (350 mm). After the first dynamic acquisition, an anti-peristaltic drug and a bolus of secretin are intravenously injected. MRCP acquisitions are then repeated at intervals of 30–45 s for 15 min. By drawing an appropriate region of interest (ROI), signal intensity is then measured on each slice for all acquisitions. The ROI has to be large, covering the fluid content of stomach, duodenum, bowel and pancreas, in order to avoid any signal loss from out-flowing fluid. To calculate PFO and TEV, an individual calibration procedure is needed, based on the demonstration that there is a linear relationship between MR signal intensity and fluid volume. For this purpose, six additional acquisitions must be obtained after ingestion of 120 ml of water in six consecutive increments of 20 ml (administered at intervals of 45–60 s). The mean signal in-

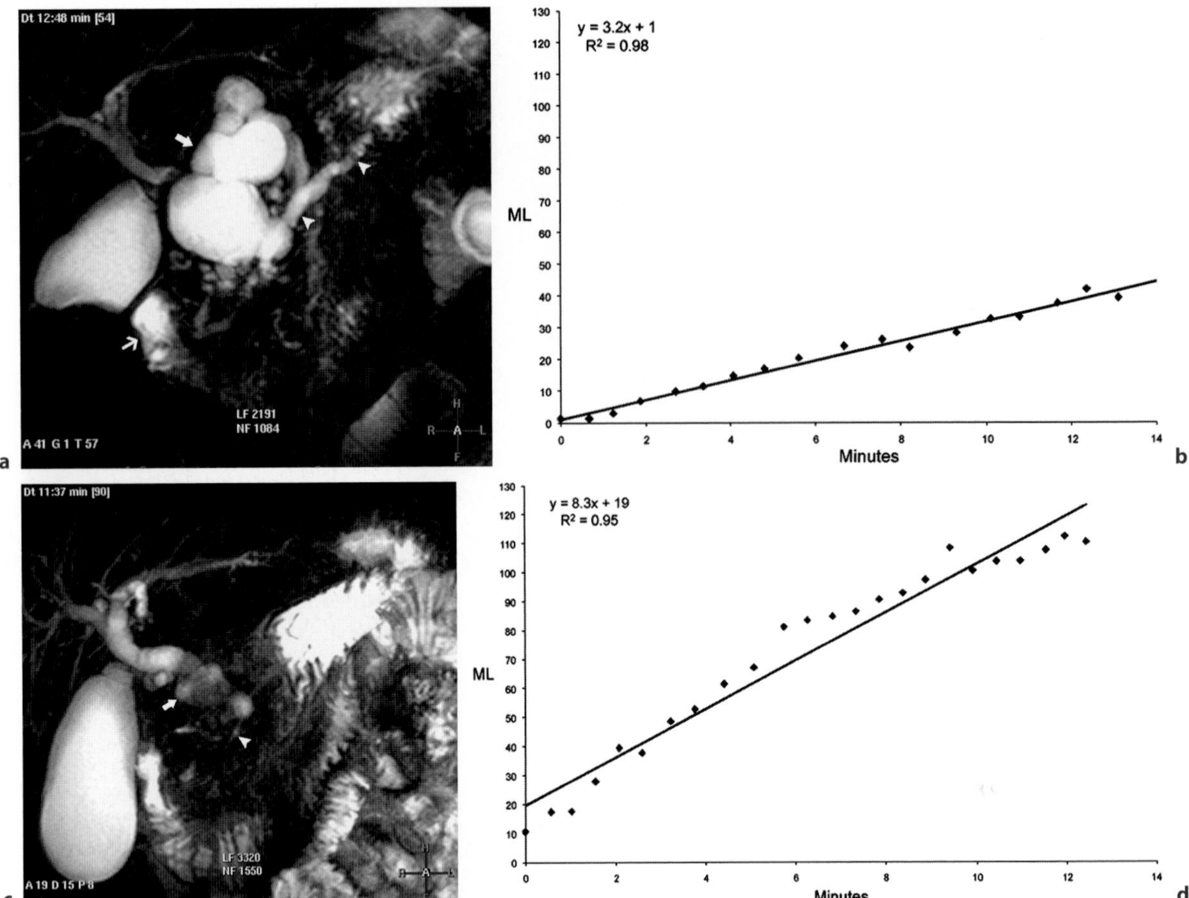

Fig. 11.7a–d. Chronic pancreatitis with pseudo cyst. Baseline examination (**a**) and quantitative secretin-enhanced MRCP (**b**) show main pancreatic duct dilatation *(arrowheads)* and multiseptated pseudo cyst *(thick arrow)*. Exocrine function is reduced *(thin arrow)* with an output of 3.2 ml/min. After endoscopic therapy (**c**,**d**) we observe a partial resolution of the pseudo cyst (*thick arrow*) and of the main pancreatic duct obstruction (*arrowhead*) along with recovery of exocrine function (output of 8.3 ml/min)

tensities measured in each of the six slices have to be plotted against the known water volume given, computing a linear regression. Combining the measurements obtained, the pancreatic exocrine volumes secreted after secretin administration are then plotted against time, defining a regression line and allowing calculating PFO (in milliliters per minute) and TEV. Gillams and Lees (2007) found that pancreatic flow rates measured at quantitative-MRCP were significantly reduced in severe chronic pancreatitis and, interestingly, also in patients with pancreatic atrophy and no other evidence for chronic pancreatitis. Quantitative-MRCP may therefore be considered as a valid technique for demonstrating chronic pancreatitis in an atrophic gland at a stage in which only impairment of excretory function is present.

11.3 Magnetic Resonance: Imaging Findings

11.3.1 Diagnosis

11.3.1.1 Early Chronic Pancreatitis

The hallmark in diagnosing chronic pancreatitis at early stage is mild beading of a few pancreatic side branches. Some authors reported that subtle mural irregularities, along with loss of the normal gentle tapering of the MPD toward the tail, may also be detected (Graziani et al. 2005; Czakó 2007).

ERCP is the most sensitive technique in depicting these subtle abnormalities of the ducts. MRCP has a lower spatial resolution and reflects the physiological condition of pancreatic ducts, thus leading to false-negative results. Therefore, when chronic pancreatitis at early stage is suspected, secretin stimulation is mandatory, since it may help in filling the gap between MRCP and ERCP.

The evaluation of MPD caliber, duodenal filling and the visualization of dilated side branches in the body and in the tail of pancreas at dynamic S-MRCP may allow a specific diagnosis of chronic pancreatitis at early stage (Fig. 11.8a–d). MANFREDI et al. (2000) performed MRCP before and after secretin administration in a group of 84 patients with clinical and/or laboratory findings suggestive of pancreatic disease and without ductal alterations detectable at ultrasonography (US) and/or CT. Secretin administration significantly improved the number of visible MPD segments (from 65% to 97%) and the visualization of side branches (from 4% to 63%), helping in the diagnosis of chronic pancreatitis at early stage and reducing the false-negative rate of MRCP. It has been recently reported that, in patients with suspected chronic pancreatitis, secretin administration not only improves the visibility of pancreatic ducts, but also the diagnostic performance of MRCP alone. Specificity of the two readers, respectively, increased from 89% to 94% and from 96% to 98%, as did positive predictive values (from 54% to 70% and from 71% to 86%, respectively) and inter-observer agreement (SCHLAUDRAFF et al. 2008). In another group of patients with suspected chronic pancreatitis (recurrent attacks of abdominal pain and increased serum levels of amylase and lipase in the absence of US or CT findings of chronic pancreatitis), SAI et al. (2008) found high specificity (92%) of S-MRCP for the diagnosis of mild chronic pancreatitis – defined according to the Cambridge classification as "more than three abnormal side branches with a normal MPD" – but lower sensitivity (56 and 63% for the two observers respectively).

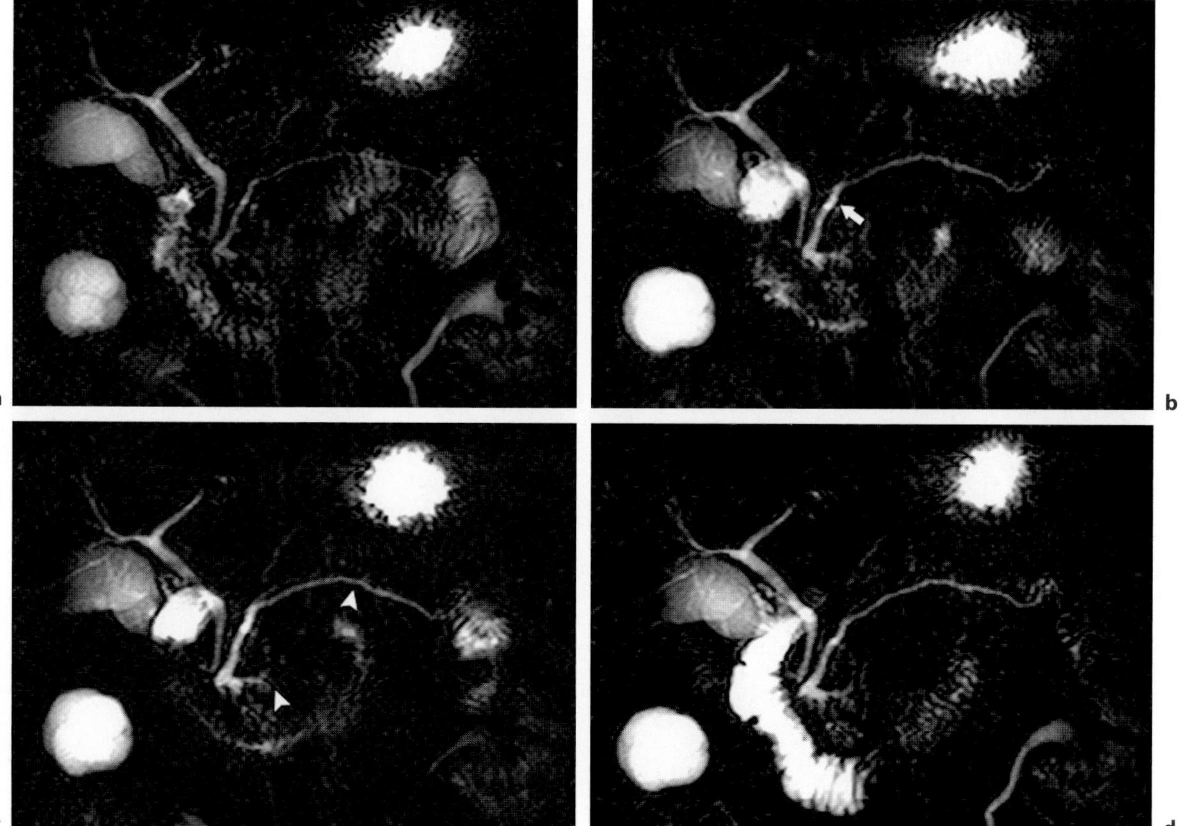

Fig. 11.8a–d. Chronic pancreatitis at early stage. Dynamic thick-slab projective MRCP images along with secretin stimulation. After secretin administration (**b,c**) better demonstration of the abnormal side branches (*arrowheads* in **c**) and main duct involvement (*arrow* in **b**) are depicted. In **d** normal duodenal filling is observed

Another probably specific although insensitive sign of chronic pancreatitis at early stage is the so-called "acinar filling" (Matos et al. 1998). It consists in a progressive hydrographic enhancement of pancreatic parenchyma in response to secretin stimulation, with morphology and distribution possibly reflecting an increased amount of free water in dilated acini (Fig. 11.9a–d). This acinar filling might be due to both outflow impairment and lack of compliance of the chronically inflamed gland, leading to ductal hypertension and subsequent fluid leakage (Laugier 1994).

No or only minor changes of the parenchyma occur in the early phase of chronic pancreatitis. In a few studies, loss of normal high signal intensity of the pancreas on T1-weighted fat-suppressed images (Kim and Pickhardt 2007) and low signal intensity ratio (signal intensity in postcontrast images divided by that in precontrast ones) in the arterial phase and/or delayed enhancement of the parenchyma (Zhang et al. 2003) have been demonstrated at this stage.

11.3.1.2 Advanced Chronic Pancreatitis

The diagnosis is easily established at MRCP by identifying structural changes involving both the MPD and the side branches, such as dilatation, narrowing or stricture formation, irregular contour and filling defects (representing deposition of calcifications, protein plugs or debris) (Fig. 11.10a,b). In alcoholic chronic pancreatitis, the severity of the duct changes depends on the extent of the surrounding

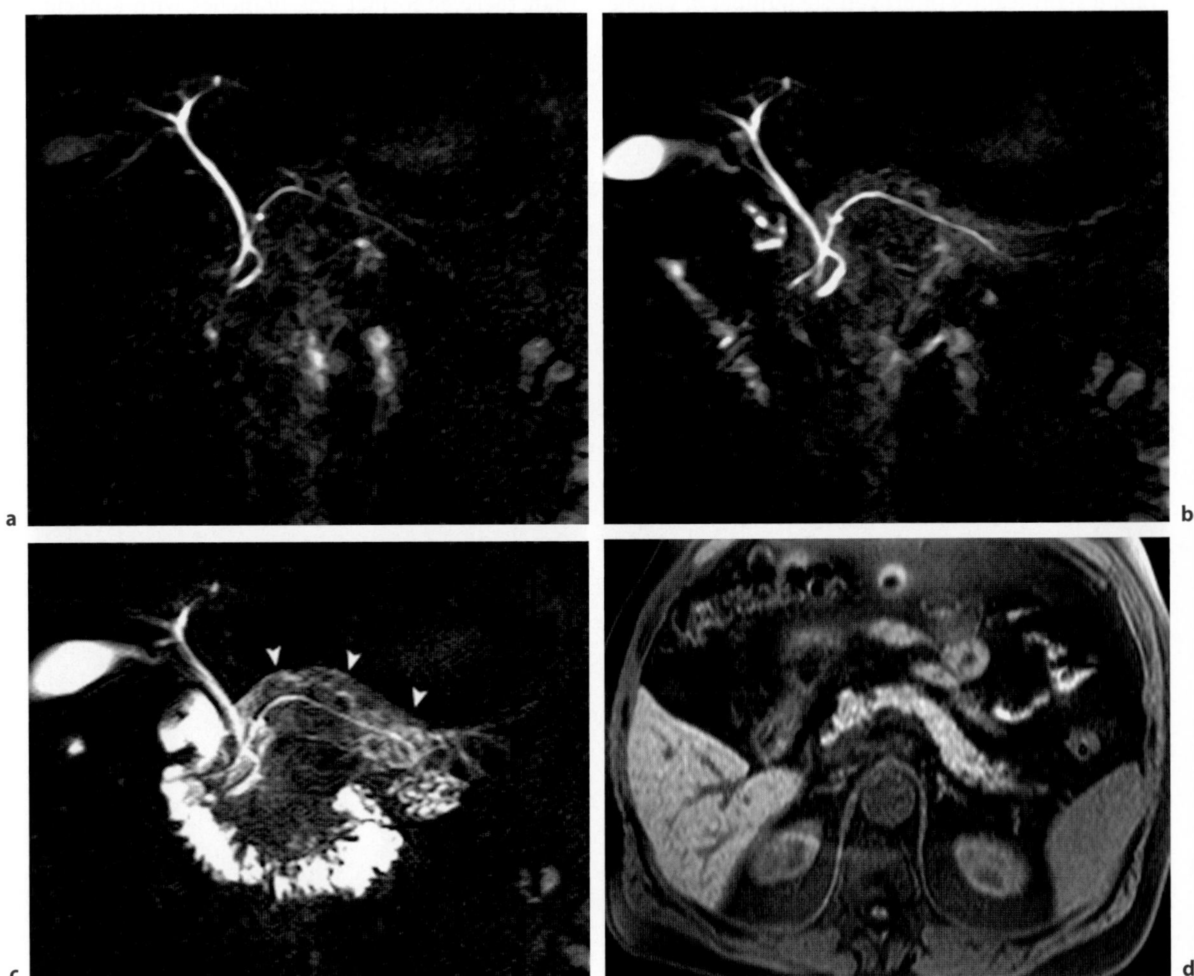

Fig. 11.9a–d. "Acinar filling" demonstration in thick-slab projective MRCP images along with secretin stimulation. Progressive enhancement of pancreatic parenchyma is observed after secretin stimulation (**b,c**) (*arrowheads* in **c**). Of interest, signal intensity of the pancreatic parenchyma is normal on fat-sat T1-weighted GRE image (**d**)

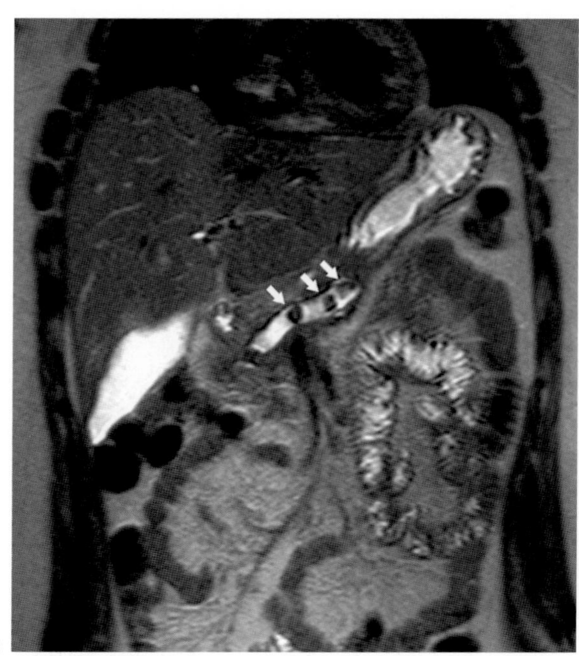

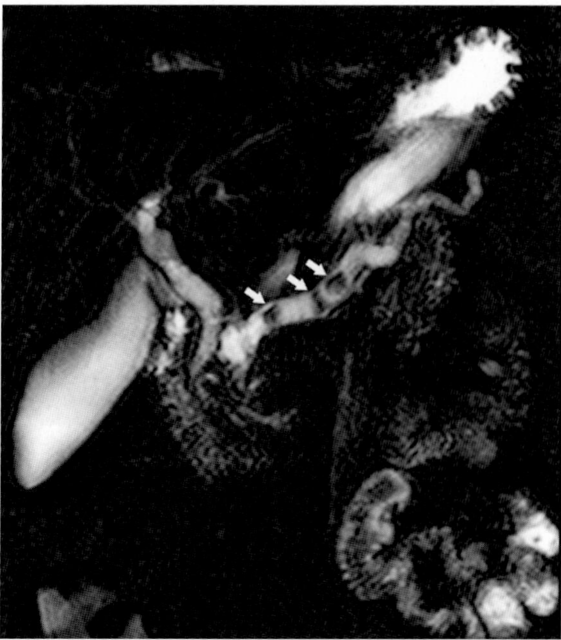

Fig. 11.10a,b. Chronic calcified pancreatitis at advanced stage. Coronal T2-weighted TSE image (**a**) and thick-slab projective MRCP (**b**) show the dilatation of the main pancreatic duct and many round hypointense filling defects corresponding to intraductal stones (*arrows*)

fibrosis. As a consequence, the MPD may be diffusely involved or only focally dilated or obstructed. Pancreatic fibrosis may also lead to a tapering stenosis of the common bile duct (CBD) (Klöppel 2008) (Fig. 11.11a,b).

Uniform dilatation of the MPD and relative sparing or only mild dilatation of branch ducts are typical features of the obstructive type of chronic pancreatitis in the advanced phase (Van Hoe et al. 2006). Later, side branches may dilate to plurilobulated cystic collections and even to true cystic formations (retention cysts) (Graziani et al. 2005) (Fig. 11.12a,b).

At this stage of chronic pancreatitis, cross-sectional MRI images depict characteristic and more prominent signal abnormalities in the parenchyma. GRE T1-weighted fat-suppressed images show a reduced signal intensity of the pancreatic parenchyma, due to decreased protein rich fluid content of the acinar cells from chronic inflammation and fibrosis (Semelka et al. 1993) (Fig. 11.2d). Complementary TSE T2-weighted images are useful to evaluate glandular atrophy and to detect calcified foci in the ducts and pseudo cysts (Fig. 11.2a–c). In obstructive chronic pancreatitis, atrophy of the parenchyma is progressive, uniform and diffuse upstream of the obstruction, most of times located at pancreatic head (Elmas 2001). An increase in glandular size and heterogeneous areas of increased signal intensity can also be detected, as a result of a superimposed focal or diffuse acute pancreatitis. On contrast-enhanced T1-weighted fat-suppressed GRE images obtained in the pancreatic phase, glandular parenchyma typically appears hypointense and heterogeneous compared to normal tissue. Then fibrotic areas tend to become more hyperintense in the venous phase and further enhanced in the late phase (Semelka et al. 1991) (Fig. 11.3b–d).

Pancreatic perfusion differences between healthy subjects and patients with moderate to severe chronic pancreatitis have been semi-quantitatively demonstrated (Coenegrachts et al. 2004). In both groups, a series of gadolinium-enhanced T1-weighted GRE sequences was acquired, and the "wash-in rate" (the maximum signal intensity slope between successive time points of the enhancement curve) and the "time-to-inflow deceleration" (duration from the onset of the signal enhancement to the point where the wash-in rate decreases to $<10\%$ of its maximal value) were calculated. In patients with chronic pancreatitis the "wash-in rate" was significantly slower compared to controls, while the "time-to-inflow deceleration" was significantly longer. It has been suggested that these perfusion differences may be re-

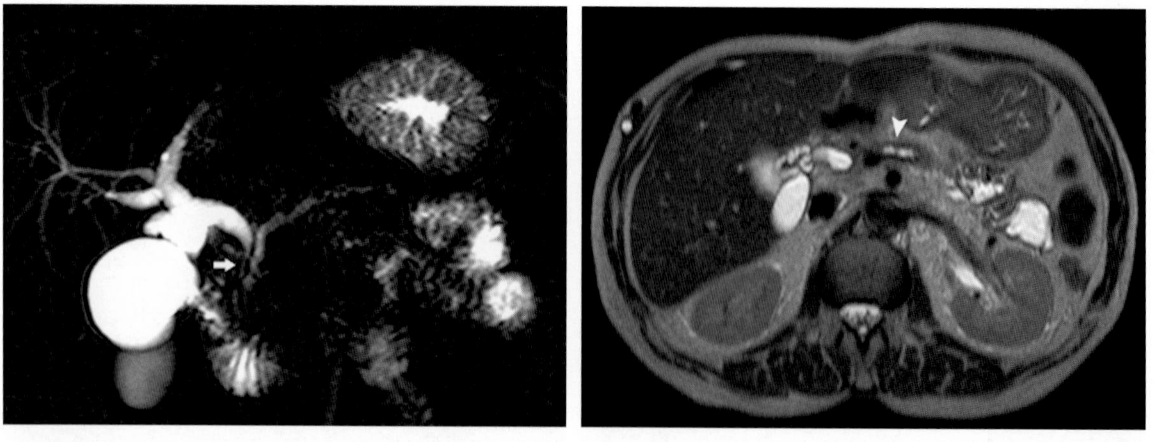

Fig. 11.11a,b. Chronic calcified pancreatitis at advanced stage with bile duct stricture. Thick-slab projective MRCP (**a**) shows moderate dilatation of the bile ducts. An incomplete stenosis of the intrapancreatic segment of the bile duct is observed (*arrow*), in addition to advanced chronic pancreatitis changes involving the main pancreatic duct. Axial T2-weighted TSE image (**b**) depicts severe atrophy of the pancreatic parenchyma (*arrowhead*)

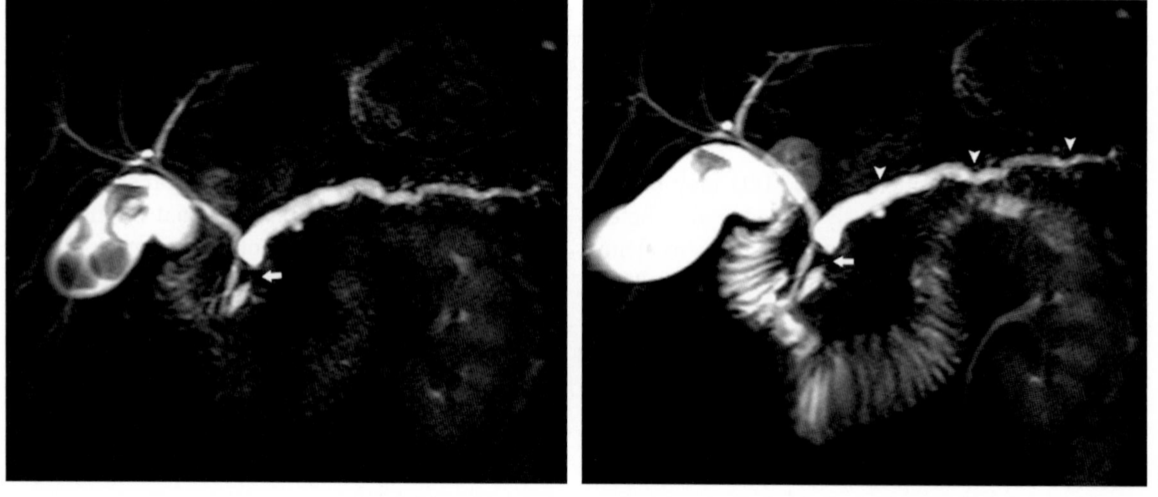

Fig. 11.12a,b. Chronic obstructive pancreatitis due to a small pancreatic carcinoma located in the head of the pancreas. Thick-slab projective MRCPs before (**a**) and after (**b**) secretin administration demonstrate a malignant stricture of the main pancreatic duct (*arrows*). Upstream dilatation of the main pancreatic duct and its side branches can also be seen (*arrowheads* in **b**). Duodenal filling is normal

lated to a combination of factors typically occurring in chronic pancreatitis, including microcirculatory disturbances and alterations in the compliance of the pancreatic parenchyma.

The evaluation of dynamic changes in MPD diameter at S-MRCP demonstrated that baseline diameter (3,6±1.7 mm vs 1.8±0.8 mm), maximum diameter (4.5±1.6 mm vs 3.0±1.7 mm) and diameter at 10 min (3.9±1.9 mm vs 1.9±0.8 mm) after secretin injection were significantly higher in patients with chronic pancreatitis than in controls with no pancreatic disease. Furthermore, in patients with chronic pancreatitis the time to reach maximum ductal diameter was longer (289±165 s vs 175±62 s), and the percentage increase in diameter was lower than in control patients (32.2±6.1% vs 66.5±47.3%, p=0.001). The significant dilatation of MPD in MRCP images before secretin administration and the poor response of MPD to secretin stimulation reflect the reduction of parenchyma's compliance in chronic pancreatitis, caused by the decrease of pancreatic juice outflow and by fibrosis (Cappeliez et al. 2000).

Several studies investigating the correlation between pancreatic function and morphological changes have led to discordant results in 12%–29% of cases (Otte 1979; Braganza et al. 1982; Malfertheiner et al. 1986; Cappeliez et al. 2000). Therefore, in chronic pancreatitis at advanced stage, this noninvasive functional test may be a valid complement to enhance characterization of the clinical stage of the disease. It has been demonstrated that grading the duodenal filling at S-MRCP can lead to a specific (87%–90%), although less sensitive (69%–72%) estimate of pancreatic exocrine function (Cappeliez et al. 2000; Schneider et al. 2006). According to these results, S-MRCP can virtually exclude a clinically relevant exocrine glandular insufficiency when dynamic filling beyond the lower duodenal flexure is seen.

Quantitative-MRCP evaluation of pancreatic exocrine function demonstrated a significantly reduced pancreatic fluid flow rate in patients with severe chronic pancreatitis (5.3±2.4 ml/min) compared to normals (7.4±2.9 ml/min). Patients with mild or moderate chronic pancreatitis showed normal flow rates, supporting the evidence that exocrine dysfunction presents late in the course of the disease (Gillams and Lees 2007).

11.3.1.3 Autoimmune Pancreatitis

Autoimmune pancreatitis is a rare form of chronic pancreatitis associated with an autoimmune inflammatory process. It is histologically characterized by a diffuse lymphoplasmacytic infiltration with acinar atrophy, marked fibrosis, obliterated phlebitis in and around the pancreas involving the portal vein and inflammatory wall thickening of bile ducts and gallbladder (Okazaki 2008).

The main age at diagnosis is over 55 years. The presenting symptoms are variable and most commonly include mild abdominal pain or discomfort, usually without acute attacks of pancreatitis. In more than half of all cases, obstructive jaundice due to intrapancreatic CBD stenosis or coexistence of sclerosing cholangitis (similar to primary sclerosing cholangitis) occurs. Other presenting symptoms can be related to other associated diseases, such as sialoadenitis, retroperitoneal fibrosis or chronic thyroiditis (Okazaki 2008).

Laboratory data showing abnormally elevated levels of serum γ-globulin, IgG/IgG4 or presence of autoantibodies support the diagnosis of autoimmune chronic pancreatitis.

According to the "Clinical Diagnostic Criteria for Autoimmune Pancreatitis" recently proposed by the Japan Pancreas Society, imaging plays a crucial role in the diagnosis of this entity (Okazaki et al. 2006).

Some typical MRI features have been described, such as focal or diffuse pancreatic enlargement with sharp borders and homogeneous though abnormal signal intensity of the parenchyma (hypointense in GRE T1-weighted and hyperintense in TSE T2-weighted images), decreased arterial enhancement and homogeneous, delayed gadolinium uptake (Sahani et al. 2004; Yang et al. 2006) (Fig. 11.13a,b). In some cases, on T2-weighted images a characteristic hypointense capsule-like smooth peripheral rim can be detected (Irie et al. 1998a). It is supposed to correspond to an inflammatory process involving peripancreatic tissues and can be associated to minimal peripancreatic stranding (Koga et al. 2002). Pancreatic calcifications are usually absent in autoimmune pancreatitis, although it has the potential to evolve to a progressive disease with pancreatic stones (Klöppel et al. 2003; Takayama et al. 2004). MRCP shows diffuse and irregular narrowing of the MPD (Fig. 11.13c), sometimes associated to narrowing of the distal CBD, the latter resembling primary sclerosis cholangitis.

Short-term follow-up MRI can be useful in assessing the response to steroid therapy. Progressive reduction in the size of the pancreatic parenchyma (both in focal and diffuse forms) and normalization of MPD abnormalities are usually demonstrated, simplifying the differential diagnosis between autoimmune pancreatitis and pancreatic adenocarcinoma.

Main differential diagnosis of diffuse autoimmune pancreatitis is pancreatic lymphoma, since both pathologies determine a diffuse enlargement of the parenchyma with similar signal intensity abnormalities. The differential diagnosis is mainly based on extra-glandular findings, such as retroperitoneal enlarged lymph nodes and/or splenic lesions (Manfredi et al. 2008).

11.3.1.4 Paraduodenal Pancreatitis

Paraduodenal pancreatitis (described under various names, such as groove pancreatitis and cystic dystrophy of heterotopic pancreas) is an uncommon type of chronic pancreatitis affecting the "groove" between the head of the pancreas, the duodenum

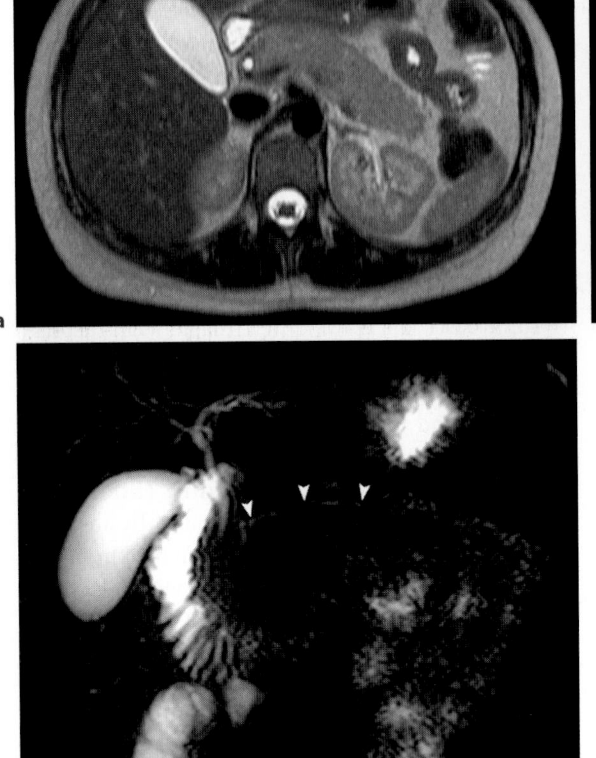

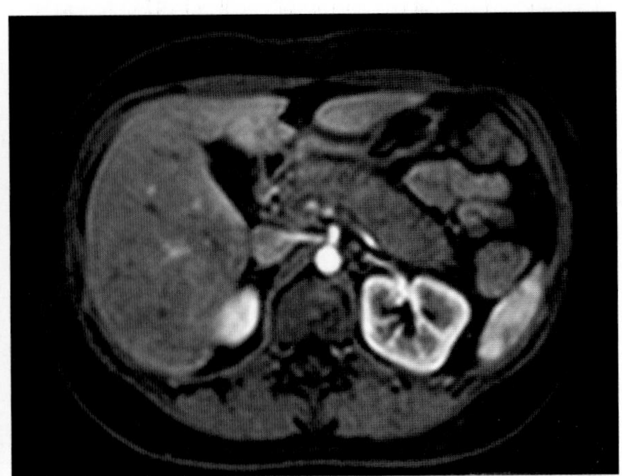

Fig. 11.13a–c. Autoimmune pancreatitis. Axial T2-weighted TSE slice (**a**) shows homogeneous hyperintense pancreas with sausage-like appearance. In the contrast-enhanced three-dimensional fat-sat T1-weighted GRE image in the arterial phase (**b**) we observe lack of enhancement of the gland. Secretin-enhanced thick-slab projective MRCP (**c**) shows a thin main pancreatic duct with strictures (*arrowheads*) due to the diffuse inflammatory process

and the common bile duct. The pancreatic parenchyma is spared (pure form), or slightly compromised (segmental form) (Stolte et al. 1982; Irie et al. 1998b). From a clinical standpoint, it is found mainly in male patients (aged 40–50 years) with a history of heavy alcohol consumption. Predominant symptoms are upper abdominal pain, weight loss and postprandial nausea and vomiting (due to stenosis of the duodenum). Paraduodenal pancreatitis is histopathologically characterized by a chronic inflammatory process with fibrosis in the pancreatico-duodenal groove, in the duodenal wall and, in the segmental form, in the superior portion of the pancreatic head, an area corresponding to the minor papilla. Cystic changes are frequently visible in the groove or in the duodenal wall and are supposed to represent cystic dystrophy of a heterotopic pancreatic tissue (Chatelain et al. 2005).

The most typical MRI finding is a sheet-like mass between the head of the pancreas and the thickened duodenal wall (Fig. 11.14a,b). This mass appears hypointense to pancreatic parenchyma on T1-weighted images and shows variable signal intensity on T2-weighted images according to the time of disease's onset, being higher in subacute phase (due to edema) and lower in chronic (due to more prominent fibrosis). After gadolinium injection a delayed contrast enhancement reflects the fibrotic content of the lesion. MRCP and cross-sectional T2-weighted images well depict the cystic changes in the groove and in the duodenal wall. Generally the cystic lesions are multiple, appear elongated or pluri-lobular rather than round (Procacci et al. 1997), and usually measure 3–5 mm in diameter (Irie et al. 1998b). Occasionally, some of the cysts may have a maximum diameter of several centimeters (Klöppel 2008), and may imprint the duodenal lumen. Shifting of the gastroduodenal artery forward and to the left is a characteristic feature that can help in differentiating pure paraduodenal pancreatitis from a pathology rising from the pancreatic head (Procacci et al. 1997). A gentle, regular tapering of the distal common bile duct with no or mild dilatation upstream may also be visible (Blasbalg et al. 2007).

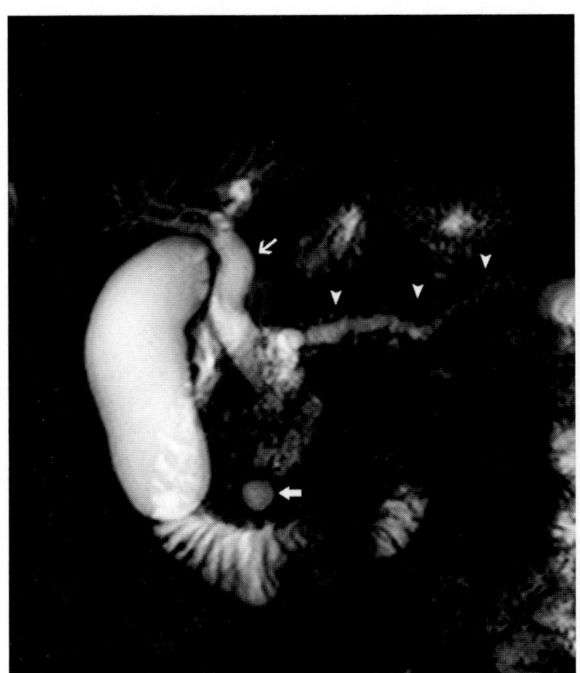

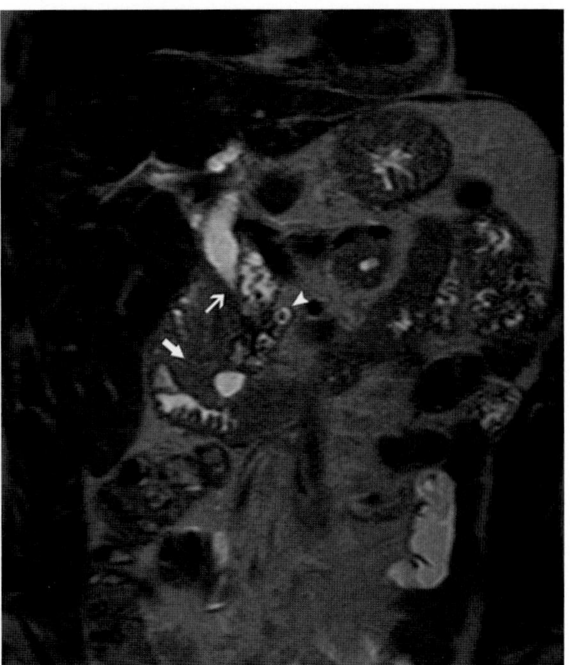

Fig. 11.14a,b. Chronic calcified pancreatitis with paraduodenal pancreatitis. Thick-slab projective MRCP (**a**) shows a widening of the pancreatico-duodenal groove between the pancreatic duct in the head and the duodenal wall, with a small cyst in the inferior part *(thick arrow)*. Associated bile duct dilatation is depicted (*thin arrow*), as well as chronic pancreatitis changes involving the main pancreatic duct and the side branches (*arrowheads*). Coronal T2-weighted TSE image (**b**) better depicts the soft tissue occupying the groove (*thick arrow*), as well as small calcifications within the side branches in the head of the pancreas (*arrowhead*) and the tapering of the distal bile duct (*thin arrow*)

11.3.2 Complication Assessment

Complications seen in chronic pancreatitis mirror the sequelae that may occur in acute pancreatitis, including pseudo cyst formation and vascular and biliary complications.

Pseudo cysts are encapsulated collections of pancreatic secretions that occur in or around the pancreas. They can be present in 30%–50% of chronic pancreatitis at early stage, commonly extrapancreatic and located in the region around the body and tail of the pancreas, and in 25%–50% of cases of chronic pancreatitis at advanced stage (Klöppel and Maillet 1991). Pseudo cysts may develop by rupture of the MPD or of a side branch, which occurs if obstruction by stones, protein plugs, or stricture is present (Fig. 11.15a–d). MRI and MRCP demonstrate their size and exact location well, particularly of non-communicating pseudo cysts that ERCP may fail to demonstrate. The MRI appearance varies according to the different components that can be found inside. Pancreatic fluid secretions typically show low signal intensity on T1-weighted images and high signal intensity on T2-weighted images. When present, pancreatic debris and sludge determine a lower signal on T2. A hemorrhagic component can be detected as hyperintense on T1-weighted images. The wall of pseudo cyst shows low signal intensity on both T1 and T2-weighted images, and may reach several millimeters thick. Due to the well-perfused granulation tissue, it may enhance after gadolinium administration (Fig. 11.16a–d). Pseudo cysts can be responsible for persistent MPD (or common bile duct) strictures due to mechanical obstruction, at the beginning, and scarring, after pseudo cyst's regression or drainage. S-MRCP may better show these strictures.

Vascular complications that may be seen on MRI include formation of arterial pseudo aneurysms, arterial bleeding and splenic or portal vein thrombosis (Miller et al. 2004). When splenic vein thrombosis occurs, the vein itself may not be visualized, and short gastric and gastro epiploic collaterals become easily detectable on gadolinium-enhanced T1-weighted images (Fig. 11.17a,b).

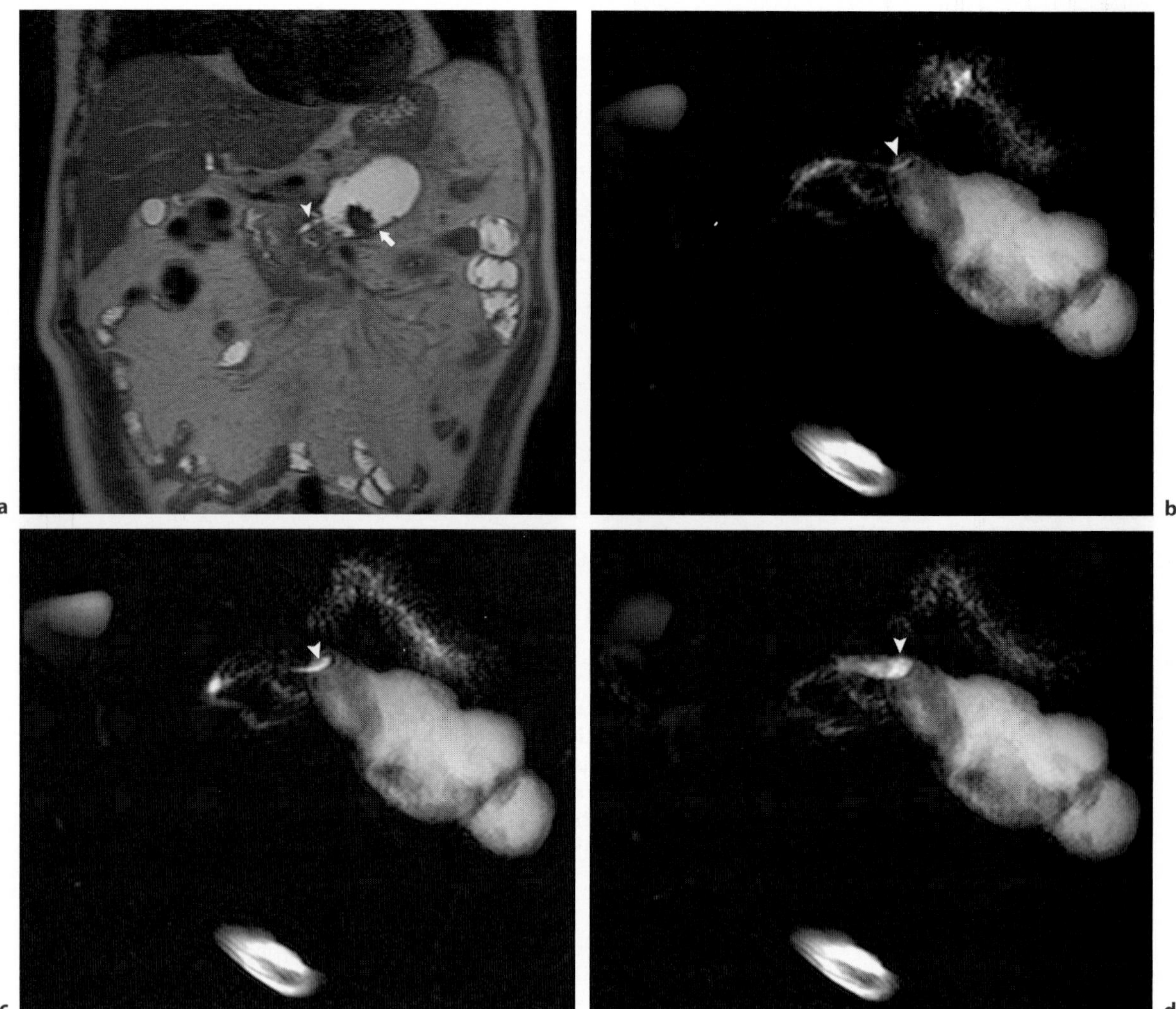

Fig. 11.15a–d. Advanced chronic pancreatitis with main pancreatic duct rupture. Coronal T2-weighted TSE image (**a**) displays a huge pseudo cyst with necrotic debris (*thick arrow*) in continuity with pancreatic duct (*arrowhead*). Axial MRCP projections along with secretin (**b–d**) demonstrate the site of the rupture as an area of progressive filling (*arrowheads*)

Choledocholithiasis, fistulas and common bile duct inflammatory strictures with upstream dilatation are the main biliary complications detectable on MRI and MRCP images (Fig. 11.17c). Gradual tapering with a funnel-like narrowed segment is the typical appearance of a common bile duct inflammatory stricture (Miller et al. 2004).

11.3.3 Differentiation Between Carcinoma and Focal Inflammatory Masses

Patients affected by chronic pancreatitis are at higher risk for the development of ductal adenocarcinoma. It has been demonstrated that the cumulative risk of pancreatic cancer in those patients in whom the duration of pancreatitis was equal or greater than 2 years was 2% at 10 years and 4% at 20 years (Lowenfels et al. 1993). In patients with hereditary pancreatitis, a chronic longstanding inflammatory process, the cumulative risk of pancreatic cancer reaches 40% by age 70 years (Lowenfels et al. 1997; Howes et al. 2004).

Clinical and imaging appearances of chronic pancreatitis in the form of a focal inflammatory mass and ductal adenocarcinoma can demonstrate significant overlap, especially at early stage, making the diagnosis difficult. Often a percutaneous CT-guided or endoscopic US-guided biopsy is needed to

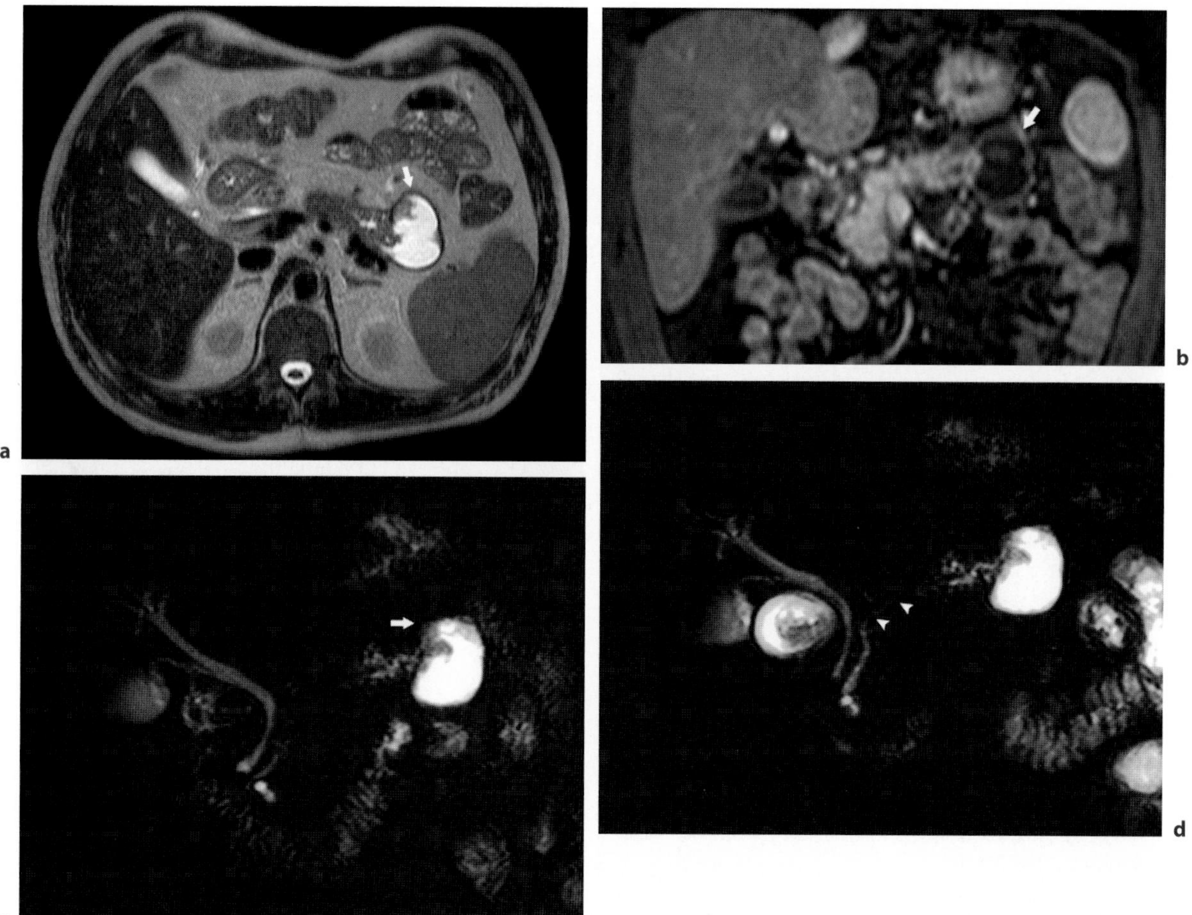

Fig. 11.16a–d. Chronic pancreatitis with pseudo cyst in the tail. Axial T2-weighted TSE image (**a**) shows a bright thin-walled collection located in the tail and containing pancreatic debris (*arrow*). Coronal-reformatted fat-sat contrast-enhanced three-dimensional T1-weighted GRE image (**b**) demonstrates the hypovascular pattern of the collection (*arrow*). Baseline (**c**) and secretin-enhanced (**d**) thick-slab projective MRCP display a benign stricture located in the main pancreatic duct in the body (*arrowheads* in **d**) with upstream chronic pancreatic changes and pseudo cyst (*arrow* in **c**)

make this differential diagnosis, but demonstration of inflammatory tissue alone cannot clarify if a malignant lesion has been missed.

From an imaging standpoint, in both conditions MRI images may depict a focal enlargement of the pancreas (often located at the head region) or a focal hypointense (due to hypovascularization and abundant fibrosis) mass with obstruction of either the pancreatic duct, the common bile duct, or both (Matos et al. 2002; Kim et al. 2002 and Pickhardt 2007). Chronic pancreatitis and pancreatic carcinoma have been considered undistinguishable on the basis of degree and time of enhancement (Johnson and Outwater 1999). Moreover, some of imaging signs that classically suggest pancreatic cancer, such as infiltration of the adjacent fat, arterial encasement and peripancreatic venous obstruction have been similarly noticed in focal inflammatory masses (Balthazar 2005; Baker 1991). It has been recently demonstrated that in patients with pancreatic mass or focal enlargement, a finding to distinguish pancreatic carcinoma from chronic pancreatitis may be the relative demarcation of the mass compared to background pancreas in the former on gadolinium-enhanced three-dimensional GRE T1-weighted sequences (Kim et al. 2007).

Pancreatic time-signal intensity curve (TIC) obtained with dynamic contrast-enhanced MRI may be another useful tool for detecting pancreatic carcinoma in patients with longstanding chronic pancreatitis. Tajima et al. (2007) demonstrated that pancreatic carcinoma tends to have a very slowly rising

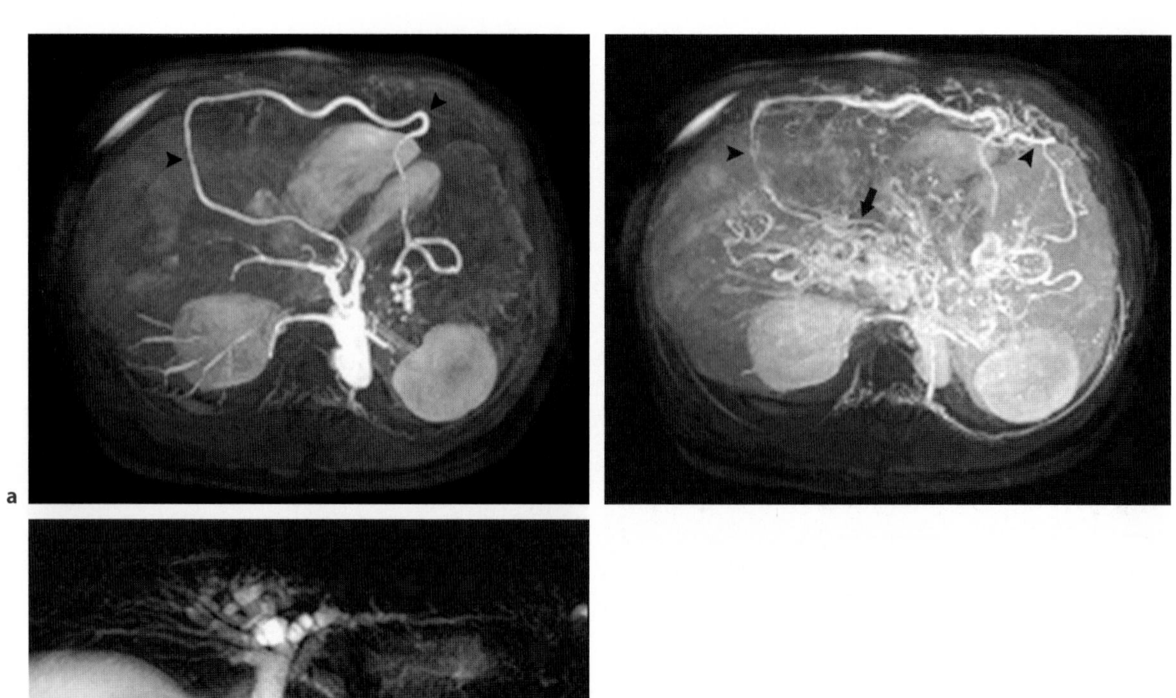

Fig. 11.17a–c. Advanced chronic pancreatitis complicated by portal and splenic vein occlusion and by bile duct stricture. Gadolinium-enhanced arterial (**a**) and venous (**b**) axial MIP images show arterial and venous gastroepiploic shunts (*arrowheads*) in association with portal venous cavernoma (*arrow*). Thick-slab projective MRCP (**c**) shows a smooth tapering of the intrapancreatic portion of the distal common bile duct (*thin arrow*) with upstream dilatation

TIC, with a peak of contrast enhancement 2–3 min after gadolinium administration, followed by a slow decline. Focal inflammatory masses tend to show less slow TIC (with peak 1 min after contrast injection), but between these two entities overlap cases exist. A differential diagnosis might be made measuring TIC in three different parts of the individual pancreas: while the TIC profile of carcinoma always shows the slowest rise to a peak among the measured TIC, the TIC profile of focal inflammatory mass is equal to at least one of the other two measured TIC (proximal or distal to the lesion) (Tajima et al. 2007).

A useful MRCP feature that suggests inflammatory pancreatic mass is the so-called "duct-penetrating sign". Defined as a normal MPD or a MPD with stenotic change and without ductal wall irregularities coursing through the mass, this sign was demonstrated in 85% of patients with inflammatory pancreatic mass and in 4% of patients with pancreatic cancer. Although a little overlap between the two entities was found, the "duct-penetrating sign" had a sensitivity of 85% and a specificity of 96% for the purpose of distinguishing focal inflammatory mass from pancreatic cancer (Ichikawa et al. 2001). In patients with chronic pancreatitis and preserved pancreatic exocrine function, S-MRCP may help demonstrate the filling dynamics of the MPD stricture and the location of the side branches at the level of the stricture (Matos et al. 2002) (Fig. 11.18a,b).

When a simultaneous dilatation of the common bile and pancreatic ducts occurs, the "double-duct sign" may be seen on MRCP (Ahualli 2007). This sign has been considered highly suggestive of but not diagnostic for pancreatic head tumor, occurring in 62%–77% of cases (Fulcher and Turner 1999). In chronic pancreatitis the narrowing of the dilated pancreatic duct or bile duct tends to be gradual in the form of a gentle tapering, while in pancreatic cancer it tends to show an abrupt interruption.

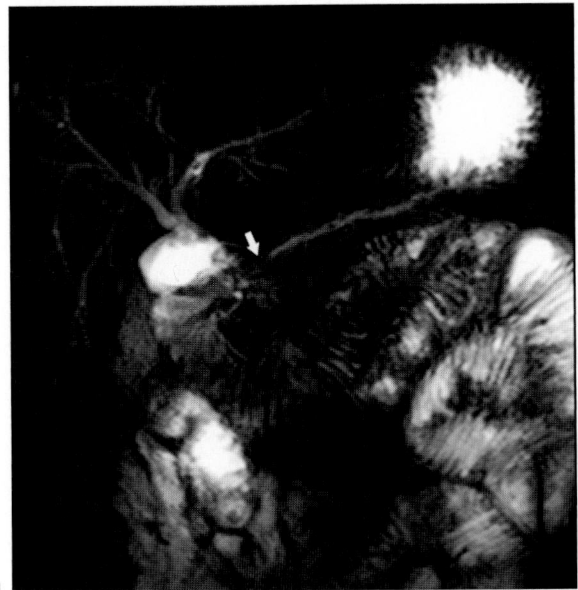

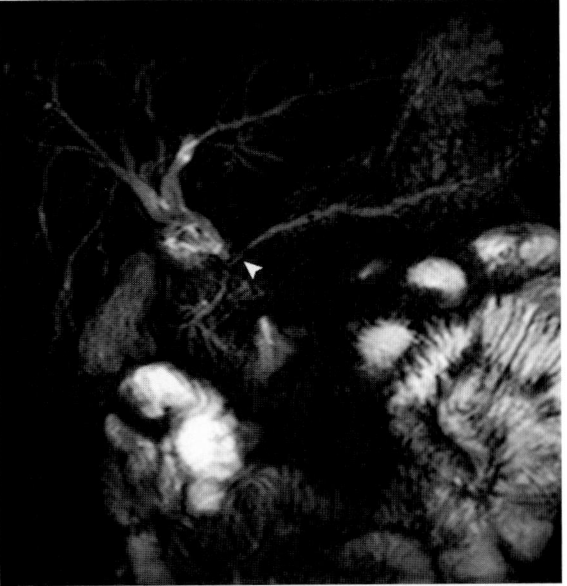

Fig. 11.18a,b. Chronic pancreatitis with a main duct stricture in the head of the pancreas. Thick-slab projective MRCP (**a**) depicts the stricture (*arrow*). Thick-slab projective MRCP along with secretin stimulation (**b**) shows filling of the stricture, compatible with an inflammatory process (*arrowhead*)

Another imaging feature that favors chronic pancreatitis is the limited parenchymal atrophy, while a neoplastic mass at the site of obstruction usually results in distal atrophy of the parenchyma.

Comparison with prior MRI or CT studies, if available, can be useful to detect follow-up changes in the appearance of the pancreas, which would raise a concern for interval development of malignancy (Kim and Pickhardt 2007).

11.3.4 Road Map for Treatment Planning and Follow-Up

In chronic pancreatitis, pain is the symptom that most often requires treatment (Steer et al. 1995). It is thought that pain may be triggered by increased pancreatic and ductal pressure secondary to an outflow obstruction, due to stones, MPD strictures or compressing pseudo cysts (Ebbehoj et al. 1990). Endoscopic treatment should therefore be applied as a first-line approach (Delhaye et al. 2003).

In addition to standard laboratory tests and plain film or CT without contrast for the detection of pancreatic calcifications, MRI is currently the noninvasive technique of choice for the selection of patients who might benefit from endotherapy (Delhaye et al. 2003).

In order to improve the access to the pancreatic duct before stone extraction or stenting, pancreatic sphincterotomy is generally performed. The preliminary execution of an MRCP (with secretin injection, if needed) can identify a dominant dorsal duct (i.e., complete or incomplete pancreas divisum), giving the clinician important anatomic information that can influence the technical approach (Matos et al. 2001) (Fig. 11.19a,b).

Endotherapy and/or extracorporeal shock-wave lithotripsy (ESWL) are the therapeutic techniques for stone extraction. MRI and S-MRCP can depict MPD strictures and assess the exocrine pancreatic function, helping the clinician in choosing the most convenient therapeutic option (Dumonceau et al. 2007). MRCP performed after stone fragmentation can also show a decrease in MPD diameter, indicating the relief of ductal obstruction.

Pancreatic stenting is indicated for dominant ductal stricture, to achieve appropriate ductal decompression (Delhaye et al. 2003). A preoperative S-MRCP can define the stricture's entity; it can also be useful during the follow-up to verify the correct positioning and the patency of the stent. It has also been shown that S-MRCP allows quantifying the secretory response before and after drainage procedures (Bali et al. 2005).

S-MRCP is suggested for the planning of pseudo cyst drainage, in order to assess the feasibility of the

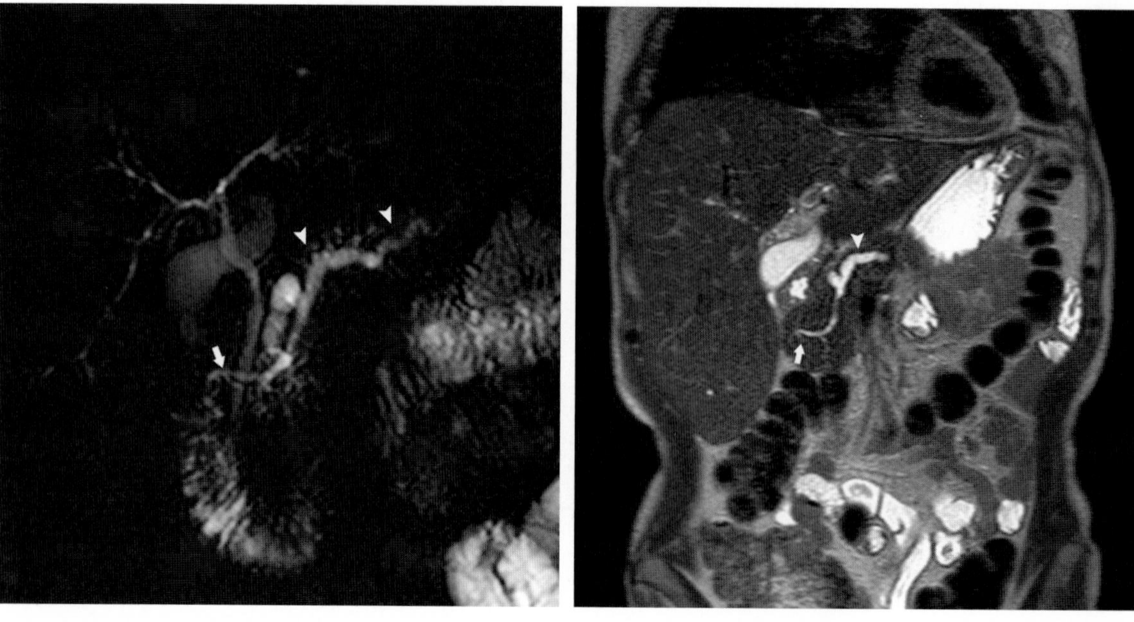

Fig. 11.19a,b. Chronic pancreatitis and dorsal dominant duct – road map before endoscopic therapy. Thick-slab projective MRCP (**a**) and coronal T2-weighted TSE image (**b**) display dorsal changes with dilatation of the main duct and side branches (*arrowheads*) and the anatomic variation (*arrows*)

procedure and to choose between the transmural and the transpapillary route. Size, number, location, proportions of fluids and necrotic debris, associated ductal lesions, connection with ductal system, associated vascular lesions (pseudo aneurysm or venous thrombosis) and compression of stomach, duodenum and CBD can be determined (Delhaye et al. 2003). Pseudo aneurysms occur in 10% of patients with pseudo cysts (Howell et al. 1998). Accurate diagnosis can be obtained with gadolinium-enhanced MRI. MRI can also be useful as follow-up imaging technique until the pseudo cysts resolves completely.

11.4 Work in Progress: Diffusion-Weighted Imaging

Diffusion-weighted imaging (DWI) explores the constant random brownian motion of water in the body (Koh and Collins 2007). DWI has recently been increasingly used to evaluate abdominal organs (Colagrande et al. 2006), although pancreatic diseases have not been widely investigated yet (Matsuki et al. 2007; Lee et al. 2008). In DWI, signal intensity reflects the water motion in the extracellular, intracellular and intravascular space (Le Bihan et al. 1988). The degree of restriction to water diffusion in tissues is correlated to their cellularity and integrity of cell membranes. In a highly cellular environment (e.g., tumor tissue), water diffusion is restricted by cell membranes, which act as barrier to water movement, and because of reduced extracellular space (Koh and Collins 2007). Water diffusion is also dependent on the amount of tissue fibrosis (Koinuma et al. 2005). From an imaging standpoint, the more water motion is restricted, the more the signal is high (compared to surrounding structures with higher diffusion). A quantitative analysis of water diffusion can be performed by calculating the so-called “apparent diffusion coefficient” (ADC). Diffusion in the extracellular-extravascular space, cellular diffusion and intravascular perfusion all contribute to ADC. Significantly lower ADC value of pancreatic cancer compared with that of normal pancreas has been reported (Matsuki et al. 2007).

In the evaluation of chronic pancreatitis, DWI may help to detect mass-forming pancreatitis, to assess exocrine function and to monitor effects of steroid treatment in autoimmune pancreatitis.

The employment of image fusion technique to help evaluate diffusion-weighted images has been recently suggested (Tsushima et al. 2007). This post-processing procedure consists in the combination of T2-weighted images and diffusion-weighted images, in order to create fusion images in which the former are used as morphological reference and the latter give the functional information. Conspicuity of diffusion-positive lesions is greatly improved when this technique is applied (Fig. 11.20a,b).

11.4.1 Differential Diagnosis Between Mass-Forming Pancreatitis and Pancreatic Carcinoma

In a recent report, it was demonstrated that analysis of ADC, pure diffusion coefficient (D) and perfusion fraction (f) leads to an overall diagnostic performance in differentiating mass-forming pancreatitis from pancreatic carcinoma similar or slightly inferior to those of various diagnostic examinations (CT, MRI, serum CA 19-9). Significantly lower ADCs were noted for mass-forming pancreatitis compared with those for pancreatic carcinoma (Lee et al. 2008).

11.4.2 Exocrine Function Assessment

DWI obtained before and after intravenous administration of secretin could provide clinically useful information about physiopathologic alterations in chronic pancreatitis. In normal pancreas, in response to secretin an increase in water osmosis towards the pancreatic ducts and an increase in pancreatic perfusion occur, leading to signal loss on DWI and increased ADC values.

Erturk et al. (2006) measured ADC values of pancreatic parenchyma on a series of DW images obtained at different times after secretin injection. In subjects without demonstrable pancreatic disease, an early ADC peak occurred within the first 4 min after secretin injection. In a group of subjects at risk for alcoholic chronic pancreatitis and in patients with chronic pancreatitis that peak was delayed, mainly between 4 and 8 min in the former group and after more than 10 min in the latter. Decrease in secretin binding to its receptors on pancreatic duct cells and reduction of blood vessel density may explain these slower ADC peak values in chronic pancreatitis.

11.4.3 Monitoring of Autoimmune Pancreatitis Treatment

In autoimmune pancreatitis, steroid treatment usually leads to a rapid improvement in clinical symptoms, laboratory and morphological findings. It has been suggested that, during the first 2–4 weeks of therapy, CT or MRI/MRCP could be used to monitor the response (Song et al. 2008). A poor response to steroid treatment should raise the suspicion of pancreatic cancer or other forms of chronic pancreatitis. Dense lymphoplasmacytic infiltration and large amount of fibrosis are typical histological features of autoimmune pancreatitis. These features may cause a restriction in water diffusion and be responsible

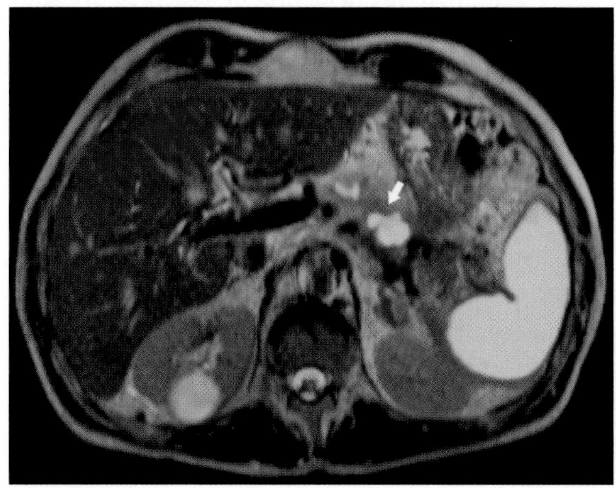

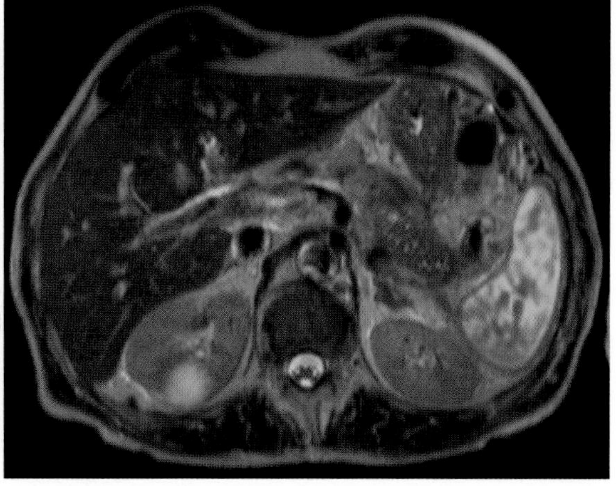

Fig. 11.20a,b. Chronic pancreatitis with an acute inflammatory mass in the tail. Combined T2-weighted TSE and diffusion-weighted images display an area of abnormal signal intensity within the pancreatic body (*arrow* in **a**), that resolved spontaneously after 2 months (**b**)

for high-signal intensity in DWI before treatment. Decrease of signal intensity in diffusion-weighted images might therefore mirror a reduction of cell infiltration and inflammation, supporting evidence of response to treatment (Fig. 11.21a,b).

11.5 Appendix

Pratical Setup for an MR Study of Chronic Pancreatitis

Basic Protocol

1. Locator
   - **Technique:** Fast GRE T1-weighted axial, coronal and sagittal sections obtained during the same respiratory-gated acquisition
   - **Information Provided:** identification of correct positioning of the phased-array coil
2. Cross-sectional T2-weighted sequences
   - **Technique:** respiratory gating; coronal and axial planes; scans through liver and pancreas
   - **Information Provided:** depiction of bile and pancreatic ducts in cross-section; useful guide for MRCP acquisition
3. Cross-sectional T1-weighted sequence
   - **Technique:** breath-hold three-dimensional sequence with fat-saturation; axial plane; scan through liver and pancreas
   - **Information Provided:** visualization of pancreatic parenchyma and borders and of focal masses
4. Magnetic resonance cholangiopancreatography (MRCP)
   - **Technique:** breath-hold; projective technique with acquisition in coronal and axial planes according to the pancreatic angulation
   - **Information Provided:** visualization of the main pancreatic duct, pancreatic branch ducts, bile ducts and gallbladder

Optional Steps

1. Oral T2-negative contrast agent administration before performing MRCP
   - **Indication:** to avoid overlap of the pancreatic ducts and other fluid-containing organs due to residual fluid in the bowel
   - **Technique:** oral administration of 1–2 ml of water-diluted gadolinium
2. Intravenous gadolinium injection
   - **Indications:**
     - To detect pancreatic focal masses when chronic pancreatitis determines diffuse abnormal signal of the gland
     - To rule out vascular complications before endoscopic treatment
   - **Technique:** axial, breath-hold, three-dimensional gadolinium-enhanced sequences with fat-saturation; scans through liver and pancreas; dynamic acquisition in arterial, portal venous and late phase
3. Intravenous secretin administration
   - **Indications:**
     - To detect subtle duct changes when chronic pancreatitis at early stage is suspected and to improve the detection of pancreas divisum

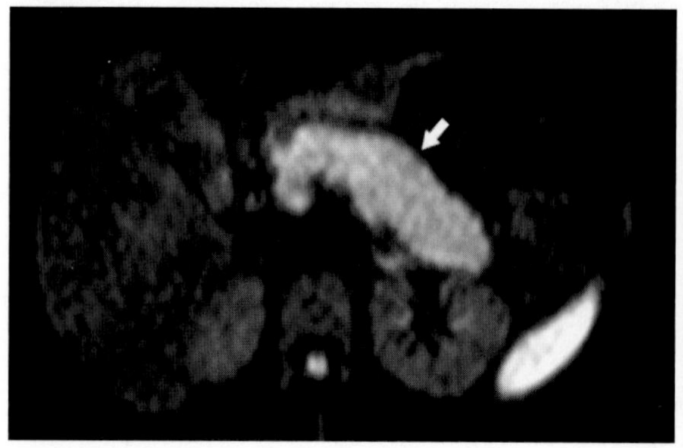
a

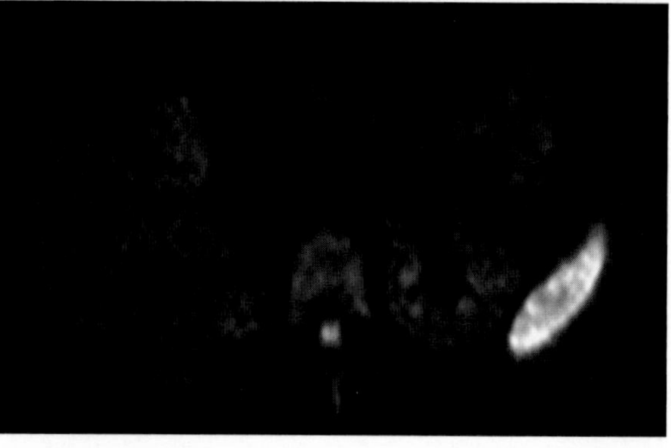
b

Fig. 11.21a,b. Autoimmune pancreatitis and diffusion-weighted imaging. Baseline axial diffusion-weighted image (**a**) displays a diffuse hyperintense pancreas related to an extensive restriction of water diffusion (*arrow*). Control after 7 months (**b**) displays normal signal intensity of the pancreas related to a complete recovery

- To detect mechanical obstruction in a normal pancreas
- To rule out duct disruption when the main pancreatic duct is not completely visible
- To help in differentiating focal inflammatory mass and pancreatic carcinoma ("duct penetrating" sign)
- To estimate pancreatic fluid output

- **Technique**: repeat the appropriate projection (usually coronal) every 30 s for 10–15 min, starting immediately after intravenous administration of 0.5–1 ml of secretin/10kg of body weight

4. More heavily T2-weighted sequences
   - **Indication**: to gain a better evaluation of peripancreatic exudate
   - **Technique**: acquire a more heavily T2-weighted sequence in axial plane
5. Three-dimensional MRCP
   - **Indication**: to provide better delineation of pancreatobiliary anatomy
   - **Technique**: acquire a three-dimensional, respiratory-gated, MRCP sequence covering the pancreatobiliary region
6. Diffusion-weighted images (Work In Progress)
   - **Indications:**
     - Differentiate between mass-forming pancreatitis and pancreatic carcinoma
     - Monitor the treatment of autoimmune pancreatitis
     - Diagnose acute pancreatitis superimposed to chronic pancreatitis
   - **Technique**: acquire respiratory triggered axial diffusion-weighted images with b values of 0 and 1000 s/mm^2; scan through pancreas and liver with the same geometry as T2-weighted scans (FOV, slice thickness); ADC measurements available

References

Ahualli J (2007) The double duct sign. Radiology 244:314–315

Axon ATR, Classen M, Cotton P, et al. (1984) Pancreatography in chronic pancreatitis: international definition. Gut 25:1107–1112

Ammann RW, Heitz PU, Klöppel G (1996) Course of alcoholic chronic pancreatitis: a prospective clinicomorphological long-term study. Gastroenterology 111:224–23

Baker ME (1991) Pancreatic adenocarcinoma: are there pathognomonic changes in the fat surrounding the superior mesenteric artery? Radiology 180:613–614

Balakrishnan V, Unnikrishnan AG, Thomas V, et al. (2008) Chronic pancreatitis: a prospective nationwide study of 1,086 Subjects from India. JOP. J Pancreas (Online) 9:593–600

Bali MA, Sztantics A, Metens T, et al. (2005) Quantification of pancreatic exocrine function with secretin-enhanced magnetic resonance cholangiopancreatography: normal values and short-term effects of pancreatic duct drainage procedures in chronic pancreatitis. Initial results. Eur Radiol 15:2110–2121

Balthazar EJ (2005) Pancreatitis associated with pancreatic carcinoma. Preoperative diagnosis: role of CT imaging in detection and evaluation. Pancreatology 5:330–344

Blasbalg R, Baroni RH, Costa DN, et al. (2007) MRI features of groove pancreatitis. AJR 189:73–80

Braganza JM, Hunt LP, Warwick F (1982) Relationship between pancreatic exocrine function and ductal morphology in chronic pancreatitis. Gastroenterology 82:1341–1347

Cappeliez O, Delhaye M, Deviere J, et al. (2000) Chronic pancreatitis: evaluation of pancreatic exocrine function with MR pancreatography after secretin stimulation. Radiology 215:358–364

Chatelain D, Vibert E, Yzet T, et al. (2005) Groove pancreatitis and pancreatic heterotopia in the minor duodenal papilla. Pancreas 30:e92–95

Coenegrachts K, Van Steenbergen W, De Keyzer F, et al. (2004) Dynamic contrast-enhanced MRI of the pancreas: initial results in healthy volunteers and patients with chronic pancreatitis. J Magn Reson Imaging 20:990–997

Colagrande S, Carbone SF, Carusi LM, et al. (2006) Magnetic resonance diffusion-weighted imaging: extraneurological applications. Radiol Med 111:392–419

Cremer M, Toussaint J, Hermanus A, et al. (1976) Les pancréatites primitives: classification sur base de la pancréatographie endoscopique. Acta Gastroenterol Belg 39:522–546

Czakó L (2007) Diagnosis of early-stage chronic pancreatitis by secretin-enhanced magnetic resonance cholangiopancreatography. J Gastroenterol 42:113–117

Delhaye M, Matos C, Devière J (2003) Endoscopic management of chronic pancreatitis. Gastrointest Endoscopy Clin N Am 13:717–742

Dumonceau JM, Costamagna G, Tringali A, et al. (2007) Treatment for painful calcified chronic pancreatitis: extracorporeal shock wave lithotripsy versus endoscopic treatment a randomised controlled trial. Gut 56:545–552

Ebbehoj N, Borly L, Bulow J, et al. (1990) Evaluation of pancreatic tissue fluid pressure and pain in chronic pancreatitis. A longitudinal study. Scand J Gastroenterol 25:462–466

Elmas N (2001) The role of diagnostic radiology in pancreatitis. Eur J Radiol 38:120–32

Erturk SM, Ichikawa T, Motosugi U, et al. (2006) Diffusion-weighted MR imaging in the evaluation of pancreatic exocrine function before and after secretin stimulation. Am J Gastroenterol 101:133–136

Fulcher AS, Turner MA (1999) MR pancreatography: a useful tool for evaluating pancreatic disorders. Radiographics 19:5–24

Garg PK, Tandon RK (2004) Survey on chronic pancreatitis in the Asia-Pacific region. J Gastroenterol Hepatol 19:998–1004

Gillams AR, Lees WR (2007) Quantitative secretin MRCP (MRCPQ): results in 215 patients with known or suspected pancreatic pathology. Eur Radiol 17:2984–2990

Gillams A, Pereira S, Webster G, et al. (2008) Correlation of MRCP quantification (MRCPQ) with conventional non-invasive pancreatic exocrine function tests. Abdom Imaging 33:469–473

Graziani R, Tapparelli M, Malagò R (2005) The various imaging aspects of chronic pancreatitis. JOP. J Pancreas (Online) 6:73–88

Hellerhoff KJ, Helmberger H, Rösch T, et al. (2002) Dynamic MR pancreatography after secretin administration: image quality and diagnostic accuracy. AJR Am J Roentgenol 179:121–129

Heverhagen JT, Muller D, Battmann A, et al. (2001) MR hydrometry to assess exocrine function of the pancreas: initial results of noninvasive quantification of secretion. Radiology 218:61–67

Hirohashi S, Hirohashi R, Uchida H, et al. (1997) Pancreatitis: evaluation with MR cholangiopancreatography in children. Radiology 203:411–415

Howell DA, Elton E, Parsons WG (1998) Endoscopic management of pseudocysts of the pancreas. Gastrointenst Endosc Clin N Am 8:143–162

Howes N, Lerch MM, Greenhalf W, et al. (2004) European Registry of Hereditary Pancreatitis and Pancreatic Cancer (EUROPAC). Clinical and genetic characteristic of hereditary pancreatitis in Europe. Clin Gastroenterol Hepatol 2:252–261

Ichikawa T, Sou H, Araki T, et al. (2001) Duct-penetrating sign at MRCP: usefulness for differentiating inflammatory pancreatic mass from pancreatic carcinomas. Radiology 221:107–116

Irie H, Honda H, Baba S, et al. (1998a) Autoimmune pancreatitis: CT and MR characteristics. AJR Am J Roentgenol 170:1323–1327

Irie H, Honda H, Kuroiwa T, et al. (1998b) MRI of groove pancreatitis. J Comput Assist Tomogr 22:651–655

Johnson PT, Outwater EK (1999) Pancreatic carcinoma versus chronic pancreatitis: dynamic MR imaging. Radiology 212:213–218

Kim DH, Pickhardt PJ (2007) Radiologic assessment of acute and chronic pancreatitis. Surg Clin N Am 87:1341–1358

Kim JH, Kim MJ, Chung JJ, et al. (2002) Differential diagnosis of periampullary carcinomas at MR imaging. RadioGraphics 22:1335–1352

Kim JK, Altun E, Elias J Jr, et al. (2007) Focal pancreatic mass: distinction of pancreatic cancer from chronic pancreatitis using gadolinium-enhanced 3D-gradient-echo MRI. J Magn Reson Imaging 26:313–322

Klöppel G (2008) Chronic pancreatitis: consequences of recurrent acute episodes. In: Berger H, Warshaw A, Büchler M, Kozarek R, Lerch M, Neoptolemos J, Shiratori K, Whitcomb D (eds) The pancreas: an integrated textbook of basic science, medicine and surgery. Blackwell Publishing, Oxford, pp 375–382

Klöppel G, Maillet B (1991) Pseudocysts in chronic pancreatitis: a morphological analysis of 57 resection specimens and 9 autopsy pancreata. Pancreas 6:266–274

Klöppel G, Maillet B (1992) The morphological basis for the evolution of acute pancreatitis into chronic pancreatitis. Virchows Arch 420:1–4

Klöppel G, Maillet B (1993) Pathology of acute and chronic pancreatitis. Pancreas 8:659–670

Klöppel G, Luttges J, Lohr M, et al. (2003) Autoimmune pancreatitis: pathological, clinical, and immunological features. Pancreas 27:14–19

Klöppel G, Detlefsen S, Feyerabend B (2004) Fibrosis of the pancreas: the initial tissue damage and the resulting pattern Virchows Arch 445:1–8

Koga Y, Yamaguchi K, Sugitani A, et al. (2002) Autoimmune pancreatitis starting as a localized form. J Gastroenterol 37:133–137

Koh DM, Collins DJ (2007) Diffusion-weighted MRI in the body: applications and challenges in oncology. AJR Am J Roentgenol 188:1622–1635

Koinuma M, Ohashi I, Hanafusa K, et al. (2005) Apparent diffusion coefficient measurements with diffusion-weighted magnetic resonance imaging for evaluation of hepatic fibrosis. J Magn Reson Imaging 22:80–85

Laugier R (1994) Dynamic endoscopic manometry of the response to secretin in patients with chronic pancreatitis. Endoscopy 26:222–227

Le Bihan D, Breton E, Lallemand D, et al. (1988) Separation of diffusion and perfusion in intravoxel incoherent motion MR imaging. Radiology 168:497–505

Lee SS, Byun JH, Park BJ, et al. (2008) Quantitative analysis of diffusion-weighted magnetic resonance imaging of the pancreas: usefulness in characterizing solid pancreatic masses. J Magn Reson Imaging 28:928–936

Lowenfels AB, Maisonneuve P, Cavallini G, et al. (1993) Pancreatitis and the risk of pancreatic cancer. N Engl J Med 328:1433–1437

Lowenfels AB, Maisonneuve P, DiMagno EP, et al. (1997) Hereditary pancreatitis and the risk of pancreatic cancer. International Hereditary Pancreatitis Study Group. J Natl Cancer Inst 89:442–446

Malfertheiner P, Büchler M, Stanescu A, et al. (1986) Exocrine pancreatic function in correlation to ductal and parenchymal morphology in chronic pancreatitis. Hepatogastroenterology 33:110–114

Manfredi R, Costamagna G, Brizi MG, et al. (2000) Severe chronic pancreatitis versus suspected pancreatic disease: dynamic MR cholangiopancreatography after secretin stimulation. Radiology 214:849–855

Manfredi R, Graziani R, Cicero C, et al.(2008) Autoimmune pancreatitis: CT patterns and their changes after steroid treatment. Radiology 247:435–443

Matos C, Metens T, Devière J, et al. (1997) Pancreatic duct: morphology and functional evaluation with dynamic MR pancreatography after secretin stimulation. Radiology 203:435–441

Matos C, Devière J, Cremer M (1998) Acinar filling during secretin-stimulated MR pancreatography. AJR Am J Roentgeonol 171:165–169

Matos C, Metens T, Devière J, et al. (2001) Pancreas divisum: evaluation with secretin-enhanced magnetic resonance cholangiopancreatography. Gastrointest Endosc 53:728–733

Matos C, Cappeliez O, Winant C, et al. (2002) MR imaging of the pancreas: a pictorial tour. Radiographics 22(1):e2 (online only)

Matos C, Bali MA, Delhaye M, et al. (2006) Magnetic resonance imaging in the detection of pancreatitis and pancreas neoplasms. Best Pract Res Clin Gastroenterol 20:157–178

Matsuki M, Inada Y, Nakai G, et al. (2007) Diffusion-weighted MR imaging of pancreatic carcinoma. Abdom Imaging 32:481–483

Miller FH, Keppke AL, Wadhwa A, et al. (2004) MRI of pancreatitis and its complications: part 2, chronic pancreatitis. AJR Am J Roentgenol 183:1645–1652

Mitchell DG, Winston CB, Outwater EK, et al. (1995) Delineation of pancreas with MR imaging: multiobserver comparison of five pulse sequences. J Magn Reson Imaging 5:193–199

Okazaki K (2008) Autoimmune pancreatitis. In: Berger H, Warshaw A, Büchler M, Kozarek R, Lerch M, Neoptolemos J, Shiratori K, Whitcomb D (eds) The pancreas: an integrated textbook of basic science, medicine and surgery. Blackwell Publishing, Oxford, pp 420–425

Okazaki K, Kawa S, Kamisawa T, et al. (2006) Research Committee of Intractable Diseases of the Pancreas. Clinical diagnostic criteria of autoimmune pancreatitis revised proposal. J Gastroenterol 41:626–631

Otte M (1979) Pankreasfunktionsdiagnostik. Internist 20:331–340

Pezzilli R, Lioce A, Frulloni L (2008) Chronic pancreatitis: a changing etiology? JOP J Pancreas (Online) 9:588–592

Procacci C, Graziani R, Zamboni G, et al. (1997) Cystic dystrophy of the duodenal wall: radiologic findings. Radiology 205:741–747

Punwani S, Gillams AR, Lees WR (2003) Non-invasive quantification of pancreatic exocrine function using secretin-stimulated MRCP. Eur Radiol 13:273–276

Ryu JK, Lee JK, Kim YT, et al. (2005) Korean Multicenter Study Group on Chronic Pancreatitis. Clinical features of chronic pancreatitis in Korea: a multicenter nationwide study. Digestion 72:207–211

Sahani DV, Kalva SP, Farrell J, et al. (2004) Autoimmune pancreatitis: imaging features. Radiology 233:345–352

Sai JK, Suyama M, Kubokawa Y, et al. (2008) Diagnosis of mild chronic pancreatitis (Cambridge classification): Comparative study using secretin injection-magnetic resonance cholangiopancreatography and endoscopic retrograde pancreatography. World J Gastroenterol 14:1218–1221

Schlaudraff E, Wagner HJ, Klose KJ, et al. (2008) Prospective evaluation of the diagnostic accuracy of secretin-enhanced magnetic resonance cholangiopancreticography in suspected chronic pancreatitis. Magn Reson Imaging (Epub ahead of print)

Schneider ARJ, Hammerstingl R, Heller M, et al. (2006) Does secretin-stimulated MRCP predict exocrine pancreatic insufficiency? A comparison with noninvasive exocrine pancreatic function tests. J Clin Gastroenterol 40:851–855

Semelka RC, Kroeker MA, Shoenut JP, et al. (1991) Pancreatic disease: prospective comparison of CT, ERCP, and 1.5-T MR imaging with dynamic gadolinium enhancement and fat suppression. Radiology 181:785–791

Semelka RC, Shoenut JP, Kroeker MA, et al. (1993) Chronic pancreatitis: MR imaging features before and after administration of gadopentetate dimeglumine. J Magn Reson Imaging 3:79–82

Siddiqi AJ, Miller F (2007) Chronic pancreatitis: ultrasound, computed tomography, and magnetic resonance imaging features. Semin Ultrasound CT MRI 28:384–394

Song Y, Liu QD, Zhou NX, et al. (2008) Diagnosis and management of autoimmune pancreatitis. Experience from China. World J Gastroenterol 14:601–606

Steer ML, Waxman I, Freedman S (1995) Chronic pancreatitis. N Engl J Med 332:1482–1490

Stolte M, Weiss W, Volkholz H, et al. (1982) A special form of segmental pancreatitis: „groove pancreatitis." Hepatogastroenterology 29:198–208

Talukdar R, Saikia N, Singal DK, et al. (2006) Chronic pancreatitis: evolving paradigms. Pancreatology 6:440–449

Tajima Y, Kuroki T, Tsutsumi R, et al. (2007) Pancreatic carcinoma coexisting with chronic pancreatitis versus tumor-forming pancreatitis: diagnostic utility of the time-signal intensity curve form dynamic contrast-enhanced MR imaging. World J Gastroenterol 13:858–865

Takayama M, Hamano H, Ochi Y, et al. (2004) Recurrent attacks of autoimmune pancreatitis result in pancreatic stone formation. Am J Gastroenterol 99:932–937

Tsushima Y, Takano A, Taketomi-Takahashi A, et al. (2007) Body diffusion-weighted MR imaging using high b-value for malignant tumor screening: usefulness and necessity of referring to T2-weighted images and creating fusion images. Acad Radiol 14:643–650

Van Hoe L, Vanbeckevoort D, Mermuys K et al. (2006) MR cholangiopancreatography. Atlas with cross-sectional imaging correlation, 2nd edn. Springer, Berlin Heidelberg New York, p 338

Yang DH, Kim KW, Kim TK, et al. (2006) Autoimmune pancreatitis: radiologic findings in 20 patients. Abdom Imaging 31:94–102

Zhang J, Israel GM, Hecht EM, et al. (2006) Isotropic 3D T2-weighted MR cholangiopancreatography with parallel imaging: feasibility study. AJR Am J Roentgenol 187:1564–1570

Zhang XM, Shi HS, Parker L, et al. (2003) Suspected early or mild chronic pancreatitis: enhancement patterns on gadolinium chelate dynamic MRI. J Magn Reson Imaging 17:86–94

The Role of Endoscopic Retrograde Cholangiopancreatography (ERCP)

12

Myriam Delhaye

CONTENTS

12.1 **Introduction** *209*

12.2 **Technical Principles of ERCP** *210*
12.2.1 Technical Success *211*
12.2.2 Complications *212*

12.3 **ERCP for the Diagnosis of CP** *215*
12.3.1 Indications for Diagnostic ERCP *215*
12.3.1.1 Diagnosis of Early CP *216*
12.3.1.2 ERCP for CP Severity Assessment *218*
12.3.1.3 ERCP for Complications Assessment *218*
12.3.2 New Diagnostic Applications of ERCP *218*
12.3.2.1 ERCP Tissue Sampling *218*
12.3.2.2 Intraductal Optical Coherence Tomography *219*

12.4 **ERCP for the Treatment of CP** *219*
12.4.1 Pancreatic Ductal Stones *219*
12.4.1.1 Selection of Patients *219*
12.4.1.2 Pre-Procedural Evaluation *220*
12.4.1.3 Techniques and Timing of ERCP *220*
12.4.1.4 Results *220*
12.4.2 Pancreatic Ductal Strictures *221*
12.4.2.1 Selection of Patients *222*
12.4.2.2 Techniques of Pancreatic Ductal Stenting *222*
12.4.2.3 Results of Pancreatic Ductal Stenting *223*
12.4.2.4 Timing of ERCP for Stent Exchange *223*
12.4.2.5 Timing of ERCP for Stent Removal *224*
12.4.2.6 Endoscopy or Surgery as the Best First-line Treatment for Symptomatic CP? *224*

12.5 **Conclusions** *225*

References *225*

M. Delhaye, MD, PhD
Department of Gastroenterology, Hospital Erasme, Université Libre de Bruxelles Route de Lennik 808, 1070 Brussels, Belgium

Abstract/Summary

Since its introduction, 40 years ago, the diagnostic workload of ERCP has been dramatically reduced in benefit of non- or less invasive imaging procedures such as magnetic resonance imaging or endoscopic ultrasonography.

A few additional pieces of diagnostic information can be obtained through ERCP such as cytology and biopsy tissue sampling, visual inspection of the ducts through pancreatoscopy and thanks to new development of intraductal imaging.

However, ERCP is an operator-dependent procedure requiring training, experience and associated with low failure and complications rates.

The major field of ERCP consists in the therapeutic options provided by this procedure, including relief of pancreatic ductal obstruction related to stone(s) and/or stricture(s) in the setting of painful chronic pancreatitis.

ERCP should therefore be applied to patients with chronic pancreatitis who may benefit from endoscopic treatment or for whom tissue sampling would be required.

12.1 Introduction

Chronic pancreatitis (CP) is a progressive, destructive inflammatory process, characterized by recurrent attacks of abdominal pain, leading to irreversible pancreatic ductal and parenchymal changes, and results in a decrease in exocrine and endocrine functions late in the disease (Steer et al. 1995; Etemad and Whitcomb 2001).

The reported incidence (5–7/100,000 inhabitants per year) and prevalence (10–15/100,000 inhabitants) of CP in Western countries underestimate the true spectrum of this disorder because its diagnosis is often problematic, particularly in the early stage of the disease (Steer et al. 1995; Levy et al. 2006).

The origin of CP is mixed, with about 70% of the cases being attributed to alcohol abuse. The remaining cases are classified as idiopathic CP (20%), tropical pancreatitis or unusual causes including hereditary pancreatitis and CP-associated metabolic and congenital factors. Recent studies reveal that subjects with CP usually have multiple risk factors including a number of underlying genetic susceptibility gene mutations (Etemad and Whitcomb 2001).

Once CP is initiated, it appears to progress unrelentingly toward inflammatory destruction of the total organ.

The diagnosis of CP can be based on the presence of the three following criteria: ductal abnormalities, presence of pancreatic calcifications, or fibrosis in histological specimen (Alazmi et al. 2006). The first two signs are late indicators and generally appear several years after the onset of symptoms. Moreover, an histological specimen obtained after surgical resection or pancreatic biopsy is rarely available, especially in the early stages of the disease (Varadarajulu et al. 2007). The formal diagnosis of CP is therefore often delayed, the average length of time to diagnosis of CP being approximately 5 years (Levy et al. 2006).

Traditionally, ERCP has been considered as the gold standard study for diagnosing the subtle and overt ductal abnormalities in cases of CP (Catalano et al. 1998). However, since its introduction in 1968 (McCune et al. 1968), 40 years ago, ERCP has evolved from a purely diagnostic procedure to a therapeutic modality when the first sphincterotomy was carried out in 1974 (Kawai et al. 1974).

As a diagnostic test of CP, the role of ERCP has been dramatically decreased as access to competing non- or less-invasive imaging techniques such as magnetic resonance imaging (MRI) and endoscopic ultrasonography (EUS) is becoming widely available (Adler et al. 2005). Actually, the vast majority of patients undergoing ERCP have evidence of structural disease on pre-ERCP imaging and 9 out of 10 patients are scheduled with therapeutic intent.

In patients who have CP, the aims of the endoscopic therapy are to alleviate outflow obstruction of the pancreatic duct to decrease ductal hypertension and relieve pain. Available endoscopic modalities include ERCP which is used to treat pancreatic ductal strictures, pancreatic ductal stones, bile duct strictures and some pseudocysts (Delhaye et al. 2003).

12.2 Technical Principles of ERCP

ERCP is a technically challenging procedure in CP patients and requires intravenous sedation and analgesia or most often general anesthesia of the patient (Ong et al. 2007).

Cannulation of the pancreatic duct with injection of contrast medium at the major and/or the minor papilla allows for complete evaluation of the pancreatic ducts in a single radiograph.

Indeed, ERCP is a dynamic, operator-dependent procedure that requires immediate interpretation of cholangiograms and pancreatograms to make diagnostic and therapeutic decisions. Radiologists are not provided formal training in post-ERCP film interpretation. So, currently, the endoscopist would selectively consult with other advanced ERCP endoscopists about the findings noted on a cholangiogram or a pancreatogram instead of relying on radiologists for interpretation of post-procedure ERCP films (Kucera et al. 2007).

However, a sufficient experience and competency can be acknowledged to expert radiologists in the field of magnetic resonance cholangiopancreatography (MRCP) (Matos et al. 1997).

Appropriate selection of patients for ERCP is of utmost importance. ERCP should be almost exclusively therapeutic with avoidance of diagnostic ERCP by using a combination of clinical assessment and prior imaging so that limiting ERCP to patients with a near-certain probability of requiring therapy (Williams et al. 2007). ERCP is therefore not indicated for patients with abdominal pain without objective evidence of pancreatico-biliary disease by laboratory or noninvasive imaging studies (Baron et al. 2006).

Standard ERCP cannulas typically are 5F-catheters (Fig. 12.1a,b) that can accept a 0.035-inch guidewire (Fig. 12.1b). Guidewires often are used in conjunction with cannulas or sphincterotomes (Fig. 12.1c) to obtain and to secure deep cannulation, and to perform wire-guided sphincterotomy, stent placement, stone extraction, and other therapeutic techniques (Delhaye et al. 2003).

The overall outcome of a procedure like ERCP is a balance between technical success, complications, and clinical efficacy (Freeman and Guda 2005) (Table 12.1).

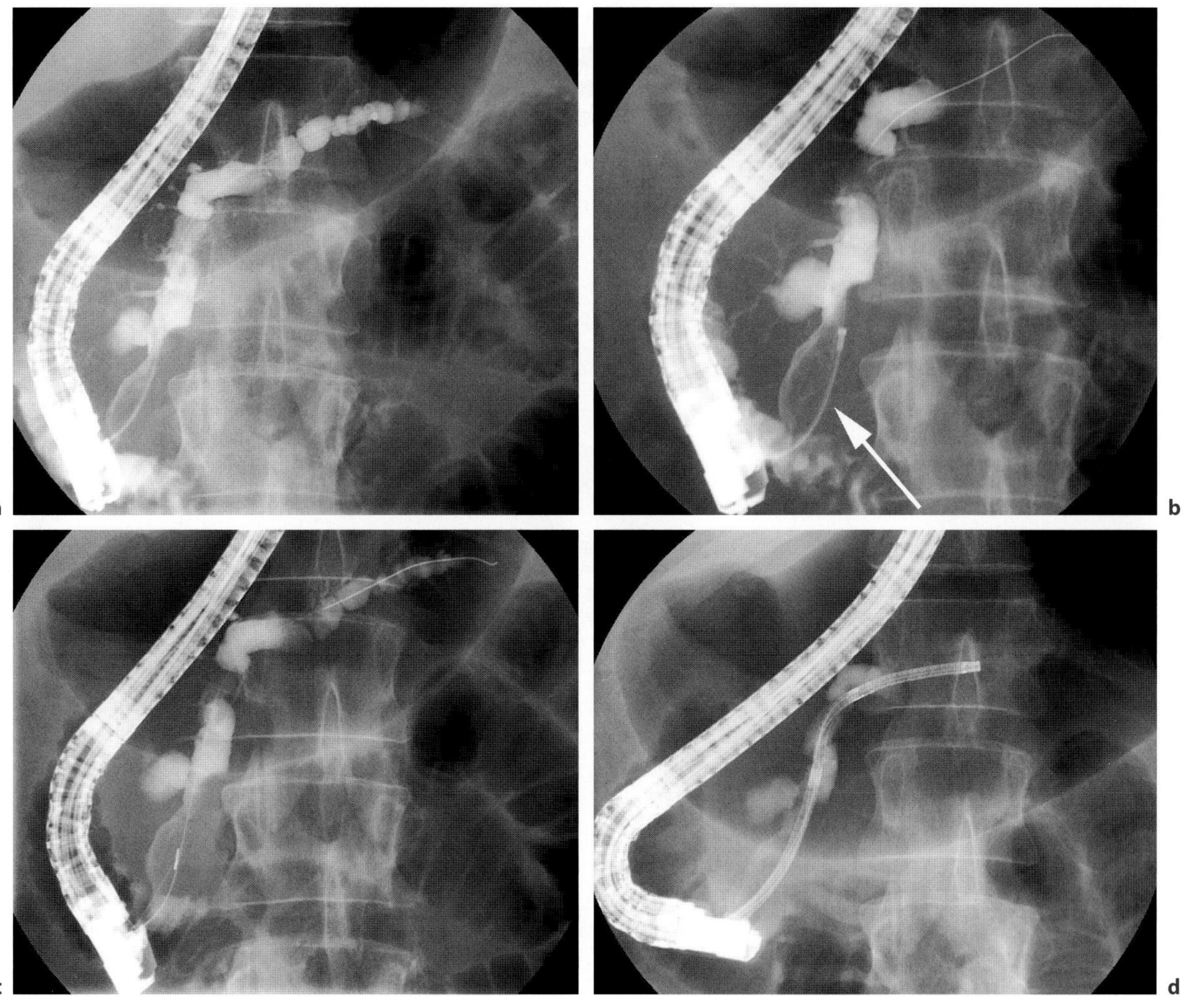

Fig. 12.1a–d. A 51-year-old man presented with epigastric pain radiating through the back over 2 years, with acute exacerbation of pain one week before ERCP. There was a history of slight alcohol consumption (1–2 units/week) and heavy smoking (20–40 cigarettes/day). CT had shown a huge dilatation of the main pancreatic duct (9–10 mm) but no calcifications. Cannulation of the major papilla using a 5F-catheter allowed the deep opacification of the main pancreatic duct which was dilated (**a**). At higher magnification (**b**), a radiolucent filling defect was suspected in the distal part of the main pancreatic duct (*arrow* in **b**), suggesting an intraductal mucus-secreting lesion. Endoscopic pancreatic sphincterotomy was performed with a standard pull-type sphincterotome (**c**) and subsequently a pancreatoscope was inserted to delineate the extension of the intraductal papillary mucinous tumor. (**d**) Three weeks later, the patient underwent a pylorus-preserving duodenopancreatectomy. Pathology revealed a malignant T2N0 intraductal papillary mucinous tumor

12.2.1 Technical Success

ERCP is one of the most technically demanding and highest-risk procedure perfomed by gastrointestinal endoscopists. A five-point difficulty scale has been described for ERCP (Schutz and Abbott 2000) and it was shown that technical success was dependent on ERCP degree of difficulty, but complications were not. Interestingly, all pancreatic therapeutic procedures were included in grade 5 procedures.

Successful deep cannulation of the desired duct is achieved at or above 95%, consistently, by experienced endoscopists (Calvo et al. 2002; Freeman and Guda 2005; Baron et al. 2006).

However, some confounding anatomical variables such as location of the papilla adjacent to or within a diverticulum, or altered surgical anatomy such as Billroth II gastrectomy or bariatric surgery, are some of the limitations of successful access and cannulation of the papilla.

Table 12.1. Advantages and limitations of ERCP in CP patients

Advantages	Limitations
• Ductal anatomic mapping most precise and reliable	• Expensive
• High level of spatial resolution	• Invasive (complication rate ~ 5%–10%)
• Precise assessment of: - Ductal stricture(s) - Filling defect(s) - Ductal communication of cyst(s) - Anatomical variations	• Operator-dependent (failure rate ~ 3%–10%)
• Additional diagnostic information (tissue and secretion sampling, OCT, pancreatoscopy,...)	• Incomplete examination: - Of extraductal structures - Above the site of complete ductal obstruction or disruption - In failed access to the papilla
• Interventional procedures concurrent with imaging (relief of pancreatic ductal obstruction)	• False increase in MPD diameter
	• Radiation exposure

ERCP: endoscopic retrograde cholangiopancreatography; CP: chronic pancreatitis; OCT: optical coherence tomography; MPD: main pancreatic duct

Technical success of ERCP in CP patients is not only dependent on successful cannulation. In fact, once cannulation is achieved, other maneuvers are required to achieve complete technical success, including traversing of a stricture, extraction of stones, and successful stent placement.

12.2.2 Complications

ERCP complications are heavily dependent on patient-related factors and, on technique and operator characteristics (Freeman et al. 2001; Vandervoort et al. 2002). For example, the risk of overall complication is more than doubled in patients with suspected sphincter of Oddi dysfunction.

Overall complication rate is around 10%, the most common complication being a procedure-related acute pancreatitis (2%–7%) which is mild in the majority of patients (Freeman 2002). The frequency of post-ERCP pancreatitis is similar for both diagnostic and therapeutic procedures.

Many studies have identified the risk factors for the development of post-ERCP pancreatitis (Freeman et al. 2001; Vandervoort et al. 2002).

Temporary stent placement across the pancreatic duct orifice is a cost-effective method of prevention of post-ERCP pancreatitis in high-risk groups.

Indeed, in a meta-analysis of controlled trials involving 481 patients, the non-stented group had a threefold higher risk of developing pancreatitis than the group with prophylactic stent insertion (Singh et al. 2004).

Endoscopic pancreatic sphincterotomy (Figs. 12.1c, 12.2b and 12.3f) is often the first step in accessing the pancreatic duct for therapeutic maneuvers, such as pancreatic duct stricture dilatation (Figs. 12.2c and 12.3g), pancreatic duct stone removal (Fig. 12.3h), and pancreatic duct stent placement (Fig. 12.2d) in CP patients.

The complications of pancreatic sphincterotomy in CP patients have been specifically studied by our group (Hookey et al. 2006). In a large series of 572 endoscopic pancreatic sphincterotomies performed for the management of CP patients in 70% of the cases, post-ERCP pancreatitis occurred in 9% among the patients with CP, and was severe in 1%. Multivariate analysis identified female sex as the single factor being associated with a higher risk of pancreatitis, while pancreatic ductal stones, sphincterotomy at only the major papilla, and pancreatic duct drainage with a nasopancreatic catheter or a stent were associated with a lower risk.

Nasopancreatic catheters were placed more frequently than stents in this series (50.7% vs 18.7% of cases). Advantages of nasopancreatic catheter in comparison with stent included the ability to remove them after 24–48 h without an additional endoscopy, and to assess of the need for therapeutic stent placement in patients with CP (Fig. 12.3j). Indeed, pain during perfusion of the nasopancreatic catheter with saline and little or no drainage under fluoroscopic control after contrast injection represented criteria for more permanent stenting.

CP was also found to provide some protection against ERCP-induced pancreatitis in other studies (Freeman et al. 2001). This could be explained by atrophy and decreased enzymatic activity in severe CP.

Other complications, excluding pancreatitis, occurred in 3%–5% of the cases and included significant post-sphincterotomy bleeding (0%–3%), sepsis or cholangitis (1%–2%) and retroperitoneal perforation (<1%) (Papachristou and Baron 2007). Therefore coagulopathy should be corrected if sphincterotomy is anticipated and antibiotic prophylaxis is indicated in the setting of suspected biliary obstruction, known pancreatic pseudocyst, or ductal leaks (Adler et al. 2005). Mortality was reported in 1 patient out of 398 with CP (0.25%) (Hookey et al. 2006).

The complications of pancreatic duct stenting in CP patients are similar to those of pancreatic sphincterotomy for the early complications, and included, as late complications, proximal migration into the main pancreatic duct (MPD) (1%–5%) or distal migration into the duodenum (7%–9%), and occlusion which can be associated with recurrent pain, pancreatitis or infection in 10%–20% of the cases (Adler et al. 2006; Somogyi et al. 2006). Digestive tract perforation and pancreatic duct disruption secondary to stent impaction were rarely reported.

Finally, stent-induced ductal changes were observed mainly in patients with normal pancreatic ducts prior to stent placement and were not clinically significant in patients with severe CP (Kozarek 1990).

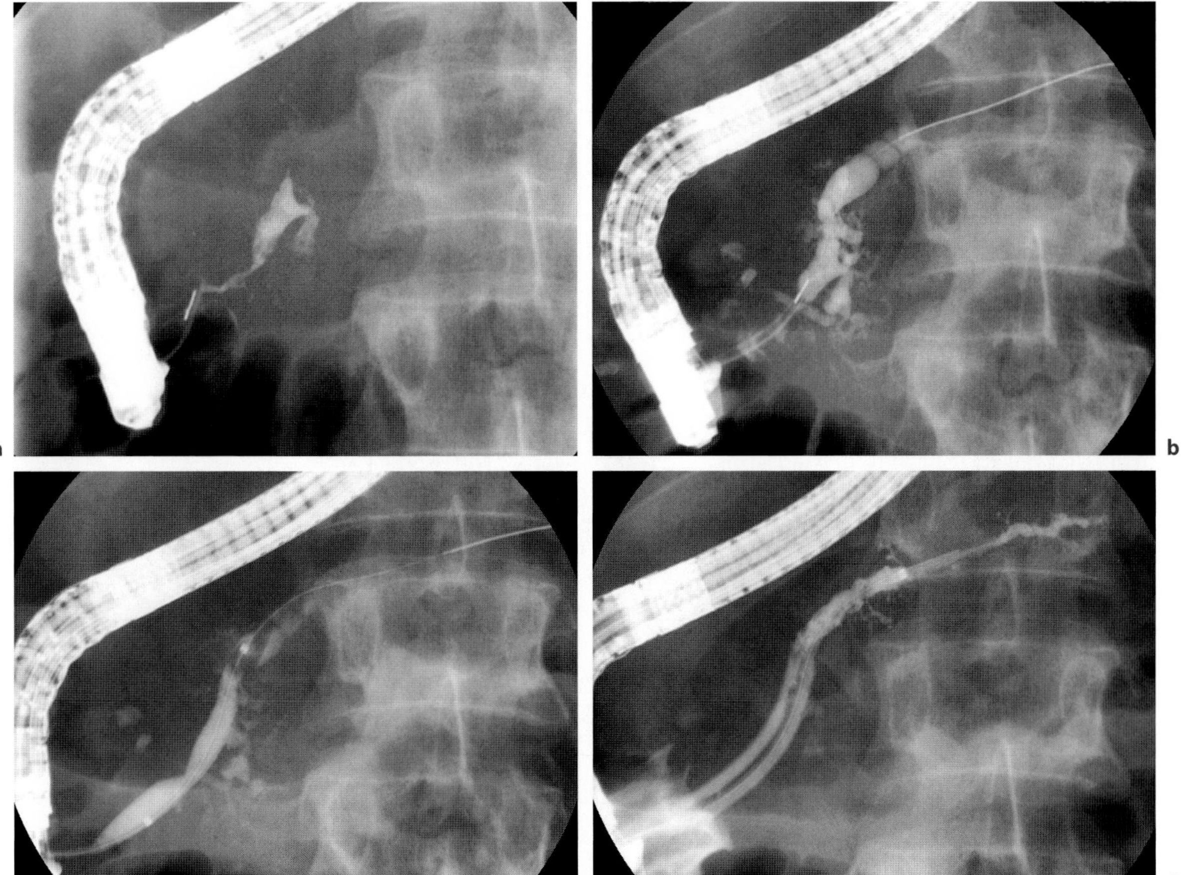

Fig. 12.2a–d. A 51-year-old man with chronic alcoholic pancreatitis presented with epigastric pain relapse radiating through the back. ERCP demonstrated a main pancreatic duct distal stricture (**a**). Endoscopic pancreatic sphincterotomy was performed using a wire-guided sphincterotome (**b**). Dilatation of the distal stricture was performed by means of a 6 mm/4 cm hydrostatic balloon catheter threaded over a guide-wire (**c**). Subsequently two straight 3 cm-10-F stents were implanted in the main pancreatic duct to allow adequate drainage of pancreatic secretions (**d**). A significant decrease in the main pancreatic duct diameter was obtained (compare pictures **b** and **d**)

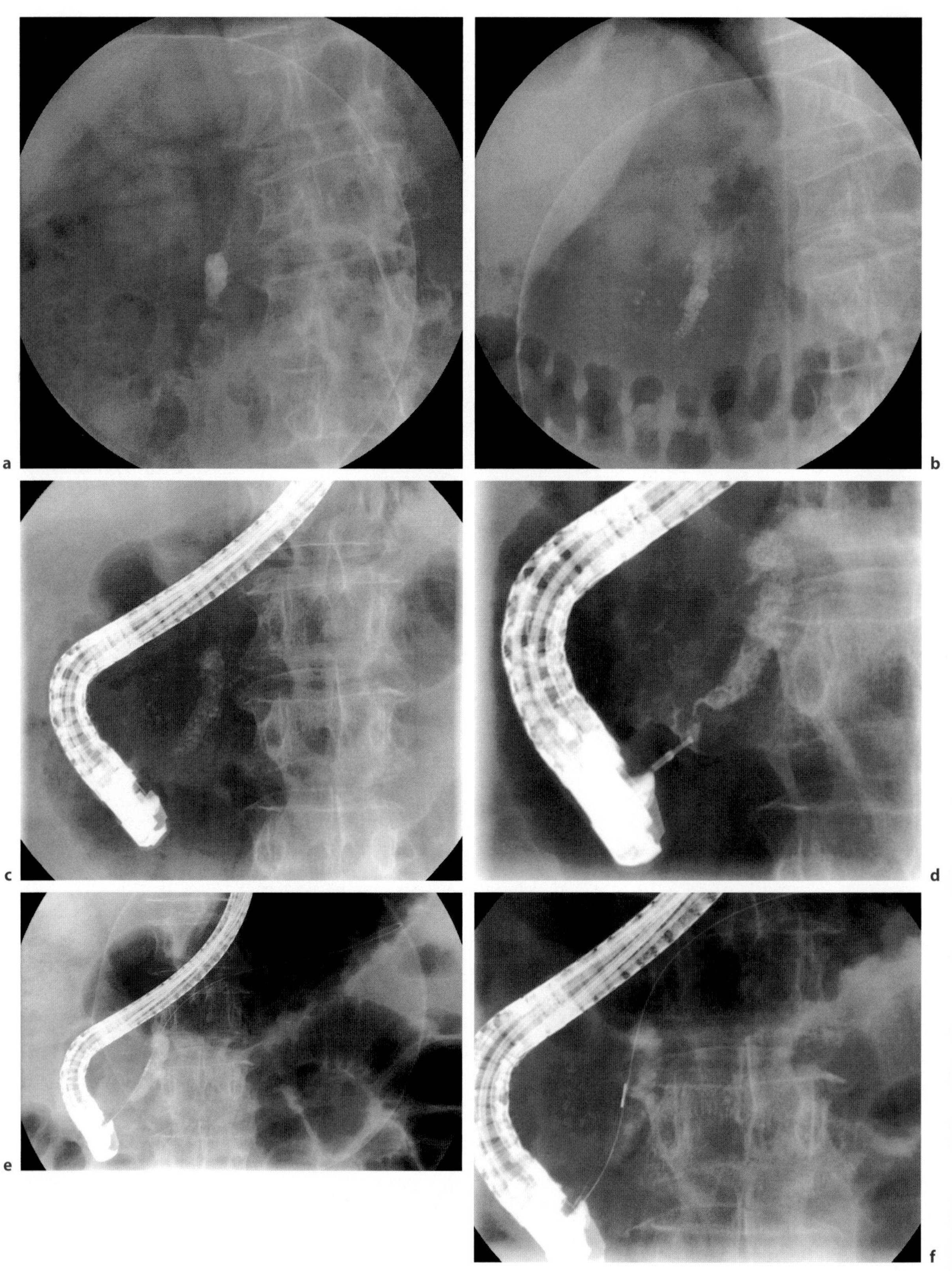
a
b
c
d
e
f

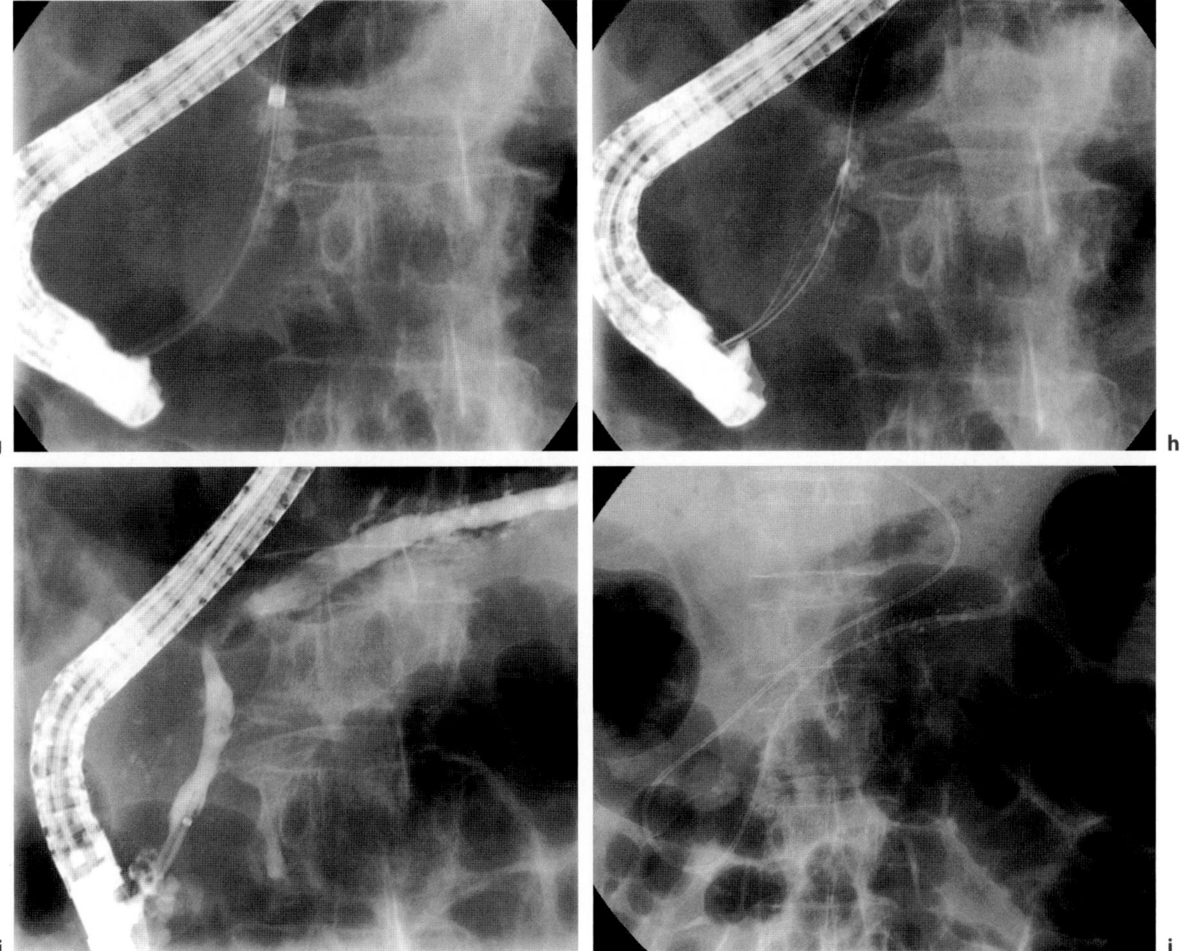

Fig. 12.3a–j. A 66-year-old woman presented with intermittent pain in the left upper quadrant increasing after meals. Previous alcohol abuse. Plain film centered on the head of the pancreas showing a big calcification before extracorporeal shock wave lithotripsy (**a**). Plain film immediately after one session (**b**) and after two sessions of lithotripsy (**c**), just before ERCP with the duodenoscope in front of the major papilla. ERCP demonstrated intraductal fragment stones and dilatation of the main pancreatic duct (**d**,**e**). Endoscopic pancreatic sphincterotomy was performed (**f**) followed by dilatation of the distal part of the main pancreatic duct using bougienage (**g**), just before extraction of fragment stones with a Dormia basket (**h**). After complete ductal clearance was obtained, contrast medium flowed freely alongside the catheter into the duodenum (**i**). Subsequently, a 6-F nasopancreatic catheter was inserted for lavage with saline for 24 h (**j**)

12.3 ERCP for the Diagnosis of CP

In clinical practice, the diagnosis of CP is based on a combination of clinical, laboratory and imaging findings (Fry et al. 2007). The challenge is to diagnose patients correctly with CP in earlier stages of the disease.

12.3.1 Indications for Diagnostic ERCP

The indications for diagnostic ERCP will diminish as alternative imaging modalities achieve better visualization of the biliary and pancreatic ducts without the procedural risks of ERCP.

ERCP will retain a portion of its traditional diagnostic role in clarifying areas that are poorly visualized by the other imaging procedures, such as the side-branches of the pancreatic duct, in differentiating CP from pancreatic neoplasm (by means of intraductal tissue sampling) in cases when adenocarcinoma (Fig. 12.4) or intraductal papillary mucinous neoplasm (Fig. 12.1) are in the differential diagnosis, in evaluating precisely location, size and aspect of strictures, ductal communication of cysts, pancreatic duct stones and ductal leaks (Devereaux and Binmoeller 2000; Lehman 2002; Attasaranya et al. 2007).

However, CT better depicts the parenchyma changes, including atrophy and the presence of calcifications. MRI has the advantage of evaluating both the ductal anatomy and the parenchyma, allowing a more global assessment, but calcifications are poorly seen at MRI and side branches may remain difficult to visualize at MRCP (Kim and Pickhardt 2007).

12.3.1.1 Diagnosis of Early CP

There is controversy regarding the gold standard for the early diagnosis of CP. Indeed, most diagnostic tests are not sensitive enough, costly, risky or not widely available and there is no single test able to make the diagnosis of CP in all patients (Forsmark 2000). So, in patients referred for evaluation of abdominal pain in whom there are few clinical grounds for suspecting CP, or in presence of risk factors, particularly alcohol use, the first step is to search for pancreatic calcifications and/or dilatation of the MPD using the test which is the least costly and risky.

In the absence of calcifications/dilatation of the MPD, the test with the maximum sensitivity has to be chosen.

In earlier reports, sensitivity and specificity of ERCP for the diagnosis of CP ranged from 71% to 94% and from 89% to 100% respectively (Etemad and Whitcomb 2001; Adler et al. 2006; Attasaranya et al. 2007).

So, in most studies evaluating the role of a new diagnostic test for CP, ERCP is chosen as the gold standard. However, CP can exist in the presence of a normal pancreatogram, the interpretation of ERCP is subjective with substantial interobserver and intraobserver variability, and finally acute pancreatitis, pancreatic cancer and aging can all produce changes in the pancreatic ducts similar to any or all of the features of CP (Forsmark and Toskes 1995).

In subgroups of patients with early disease (no calcifications, majority of patients with normal ducts or mild to moderate ductal changes), the sensitivity of EUS seems to be better than ERCP (on an average 87% vs 71%) (Wiersema et al. 1993; Catalano et al. 1998; Sahai et al. 1998).

However, what remains unknown is the clinical implication of mild abnormalities on ERCP (or EUS), because actually there is no criteria to predict the disease outcome, to formulate therapeutic guidelines or to plan the management strategy in such patients.

Another way to establish the diagnosis of CP could be through the detection of an abnormal function of the diseased pancreas. The intraductal secretin test performed at the time of ERCP consists in the collection of pure pancreatic juice after deep cannulation of the MPD and secretin intravenous administration. The highest bicarbonate concentration (105 mEq/L as the cut-off criteria for CP diagnosis) measured on pure pancreatic juice collected over 15 min showed, however, poor overall accuracy against the results of the standard secretin test or against the results of ERCP (Draganov et al. 2005). Therefore, the intraductal secretin test does not measure pancreatic function accurately, is an inadequate method to diagnose CP and should therefore no longer be performed in this setting.

Fig. 12.4a–f. A 69-year-old woman presented acute abdominal pain radiating through the back associated with increase of serum amylase and lipase, one week before ERCP. Magnetic resonance imaging showed a huge dilatation of the main pancreatic duct above a stricture. No mass was identified around the stricture, even after gadolinium administration. Cannulation of the major papilla allowed opacification of an irregular main pancreatic duct (**a**) without associated stricture of the common bile duct (**b**). However, an irregular long stricture was noted on the distal part of the duct of Santorini (*arrow* in **c**) with upstream dilatation of the main pancreatic duct (*asterisk* in **c**). Selective cannulation of the dorsal duct was obtained by the "rendez-vous" technique using a hydrophilic guide-wire passing from the major papilla (*black arrow*) to the minor papilla (*white arrow*) (**d**). Brush cytology of the stricture displayed rare malignant glandular cells. The ductal stricture was dilated using a 6 mm/4 cm hydrostatic balloon catheter (**e**) and subsequently one straight 5 cm–10-F stent was inserted in the Santorini duct (**f**). One month later the patient underwent a pylorus-preserving duodenopancreatectomy. Pathology revealed a 3-cm ductal adenocarcinoma at the stage T3N0

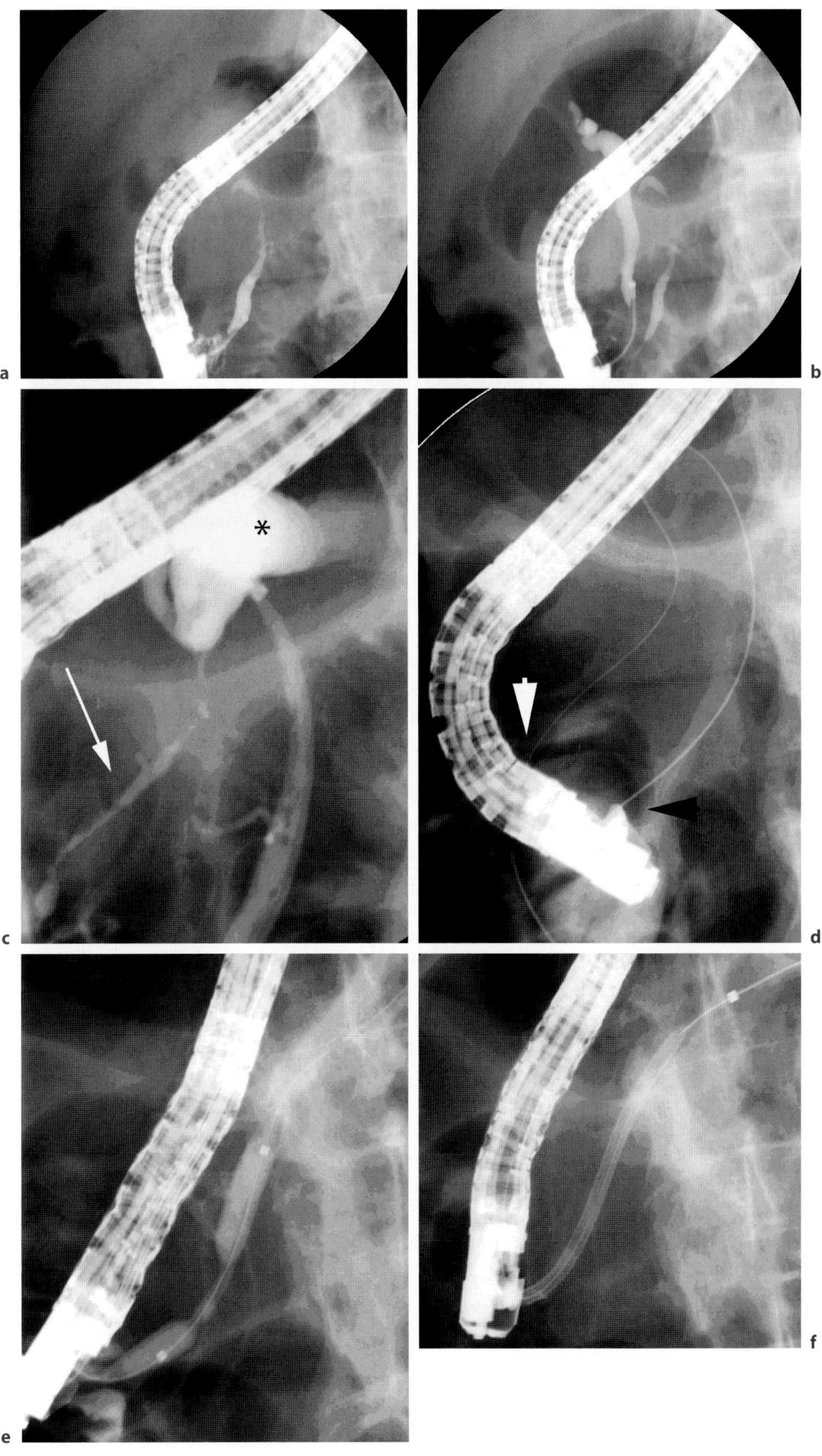
a
b
*
c
d
e
f

12.3.1.2
ERCP for CP Severity Assessment

The Cambridge classification is the most commonly used method for defining and grading the severity of CP and was initially based on the ductal changes evaluated by ERCP (Axon et al. 1984).

Severity was divided into normal, mild, moderate or severe changes of CP.

Abnormalities (dilatation and irregularity) in three or more side branches with a normal MPD were considered to indicate mild or early CP. When the MPD was also abnormal, moderate changes were considered to be present. Severe CP was considered to be present when one or more of the following features were seen: severe dilatation or irregularity of the MPD, a large cavity, filling defects or obstruction of the MPD. Dilatation of the MPD was defined according to the reported normal parameters for MPD diameter (3–4 mm in the head, decreasing to 2–3 mm in the body, and 1–2 mm in the tail) (Gabbrielli et al. 2005). Changes were also classified as focal (head, body or tail) or diffuse.

In a recent study (Tamura et al. 2006), the pancreas was examined both by MRCP and ERCP according to the criteria in the Cambridge classification of CP, with ERCP considered as the accepted reference standard.

The accuracy of MRCP for irregularity in the MPD was 88%, for dilatation of branch ducts was 92%, for irregularity in branch ducts was 79%, for cystic lesions was 100%, for stenosis or obstruction of the MPD was 92% and for pancreatic stones was 94%.

MRCP was found to have the lowest sensitivity (76%) for irregularity of branch ducts and the lowest specificity (94%) for pancreatic stone.

Moreover, the measured MPD diameter at ERCP was 1.5 times larger, on average, than that of MRCP, probably because of injection of contrast medium during ERCP may have distended the duct.

In the particular form of autoimmune CP, pancreatography is showing diffuse or segmental irregularities of the MPD, or some narrowing of the MPD together with bile duct strictures. Both features improved after therapy with corticosteroids (Horiuchi et al. 2002).

12.3.1.3
ERCP for Complications Assessment

Complications seen in CP included pseudocyst that can be a source of pain (see Chap. 15), gastrointestinal or biliary obstruction (see Chap. 16), pseudoaneurysms of the visceral arteries or splenic vein thrombosis, pancreatic ductal leaks (see Chap. 15), and ductal adenocarcinoma with an overall lifetime risk of 4% (Lowenfels et al. 1993).

The imaging appearances of focal CP and ductal adenocarcinoma demonstrate significant overlap, making differential diagnosis difficult. Indeed, both may present as focal masses with obstruction of the pancreatic or biliary ducts. This aspect will be treated in Chapter 15.

12.3.2
New Diagnostic Applications of ERCP

12.3.2.1
ERCP Tissue Sampling

A tissue diagnosis can be obtained via ERCP biopsy and brush cytology (Papachristou et al. 2007).

This technique is straightforward, requires little time and has a good safety profile. The brush and catheter sheaths are inserted into the duct of interest under fluoroscopy over a guidewire. The brush is then advanced from the sheath to a point proximal to the stricture, withdrawn slightly, and moved across the stricture approximately 10 times. The brush is then withdrawn into the catheter and both are subsequently withdrawn from the endoscope as a single unit.

The sensitivity rate for ERCP-directed brush cytology or biopsy is 30%–50%, with a combination achieving sensitivity rates of 65%–70% (Pugliese et al. 2001). These procedures are however highly specific for the diagnosis of malignancy. Techniques to enhance the accuracy of brush cytology are in progress, namely using additional biological molecular markers including p53, telomerase activity and detection of K-ras mutations especially for patients without pancreatic calcifications (Arvanitakis et al. 2004).

The use of pancreatography as a means of obtaining tissue has been marginalized by the development of EUS in conjunction with fine-needle aspiration, a procedure that has a significantly higher cytologic yield than ERCP and brush cytology (Kozarek 2006).

Visually guided tissue sampling during pancreatoscopy (Fig. 12.1d) has also been described with the aim to increase the ability to differentiate pancreatic neoplasm from CP in cases with local stenosis or elevated lesions of the MPD (Devereaux and Binmoeller 2000). However, these techniques are not widely available.

12.3.2.2
Intraductal Optical Coherence Tomography

Optical coherence tomography (OCT) is an optical imaging technique that uses infrared light reflectance and produces high-resolution cross-sectional images of tissues in vivo. The depth of penetration of the light wave into the tissues is limited to 1–2 mm, so only mucosal and submucosal structures can be investigated. Testoni et al. (2007) reported preliminary results with insertion of the OCT catheter into the MPD during an ECRP procedure in 12 patients (7 cases of neoplastic lesion, 3 cases of CP with a segmental MPD stricture, 1 case of neuroendocrine tumor and 1 case of normal tissue). OCT imaging showed a recognizable three-layer structure in the cases with normal MPD or CP, but the layer structure was totally unrecognizable in all cases with ductal adenocarcinoma. However, OCT seems unable to discriminate between a normal MPD structure and other benign lesions of the MPD.

12.4
ERCP for the Treatment of CP

Ideally, ERCP should be reserved for treatment of abnormalities found by less invasive imaging techniques (Adler et al. 2005). Indeed, CT and MRI/MRCP allow pancreatic and biliary anatomy to be defined non-invasively, without risk of complications.

Obstruction of the MPD results in impaired pancreatic drainage and may be the principal cause of symptoms in some patients with CP. When ductal obstruction is present, drainage of the pancreatic duct may improve symptoms or prevent recurrent episodes of pancreatitis.

ERCP provides direct access to the pancreatic duct for evaluation and treatment of symptomatic ductal stones and strictures.

The aim of endoscopic treatment is to decompress the MPD and to obtain good ductal drainage with reduction of the MPD diameter. All these strategies are palliative. So, they should only be considered for symptomatic patients.

The application of a variety of techniques depends on the causes of ductal obstruction, such as stones (Fig. 12.3a), strictures (Fig. 12.2a), or their combinations and on the presence of complications amenable to endoscopic treatment like pseudocysts or biliary stricture.

In spite of its limited evidence, endotherapy has been frequently performed over the past 25 years, as a first-line procedure in selected patients with CP (Delhaye et al. 2005).

12.4.1
Pancreatic Ductal Stones

Irrespective of the etiology of CP, pancreatic ductal stones are a relatively common finding in advanced CP. Stones can cause ductal obstruction that leads to ductal hypertension, increased interstitial pressure, and abdominal pain or recurrent attacks of pancreatitis (Devière et al. 1998).

Endoscopic removal of pancreatic stones is difficult, mainly because pancreatic stones tend to be multiple, hard, and spiculed, and because they are usually stuck to the ductal epithelium or impacted behind fibrotic or angulated strictures. Some form of lithotripsy is therefore usually required before stone removal (Adler et al. 2005). Extracorporeal shock wave lithotripsy (ESWL) seems to be the best technique for disintegrating pancreatic stones (Devereaux and Binmoeller 2000).

12.4.1.1
Selection of Patients

The best candidates for endoscopic treatment of pancreatic stones are those patients having single or multiple stones located in a dilated MPD and who do not have any associated tight ductal stricture (Maydeo et al. 2007) (Fig. 12.3).

The worse candidates are those patients having stones located throughout the MPD or side branches, stones impacted behind tight strictures, stones located predominantly in the pancreatic tail, stones associated with proximal strictures, complex parenchymal/ductal disease, or multiple strictures. In these patients, the number of ESWL and ERCP sessions required is much higher, with higher rate of associated complications together with a limited technical and clinical success rates.

12.4.1.2
Pre-Procedural Evaluation

Adequate assessment of the bilio-pancreatic ductal morphology and of the pancreatic and surrounding anatomy is essential prior to ESWL to ascertain the patient's suitability for endotherapy. This is accomplished by obtaining good quality plain films of the pancreatic area in left and right oblique positions and MRCP. CT is not required routinely unless an inflammatory mass or a complex parenchymal pathology are suspected.

If the MPD is well visualized on the MRCP, ESWL is begun without doing an ERCP or a pancreatic sphincterotomy, except in patients who have radiolucent stones. In these patients, ERCP with a pancreatic sphincterotomy and the placement of a nasopancreatic catheter are required for allowing radiological focusing on the stones during ESWL (Delhaye et al. 1992).

12.4.1.3
Techniques and Timing of ERCP

The end point of ESWL should be complete stone disintegration (Fig. 12.3b,c) as evidenced by a decrease in the radiographic density of the stone, an increase in the stone surface area and heterogeneity of the stone which appears as powder-like material filling the pancreatic and the surrounding secondary ducts (Delhaye et al. 1992).

ERCP is then performed with the aim of achieving complete ductal clearance.

First, the pancreatic duct is opacified (Fig. 12.3d), then a hydrophilic guidewire is negotiated across the disintegrated stones as far as the pancreatic tail (Fig. 12.3e). A wire-guided sphincterotome is used for the pancreatic sphincterotomy (Fig. 12.3f) with a pure cutting current up to the limit of the ampullary bulge. Stone fragments are usually removed with stone extraction balloon or small basket alongside the previously placed guidewire (Fig. 12.3h), starting from the pancreatic head (Dumonceau et al. 1996; Delhaye et al. 2003).

In case of multiple pancreatic stones, 2–3 sessions of ESWL and 3–4 sessions of ERCP may be required in order to achieve the end-point of endotherapy which should be complete ductal clearance (Fig. 12.3i).

12.4.1.4
Results

Several observational, retrospective studies have reported benefit from removal of pancreatic stones in terms of improvement or relieving of abdominal pain and pancreatitis exacerbation in 54%–91% of the patients, in the largest series, during a mean follow-up ranging from 7 to 44 months (Delhaye et al. 1992; Dumonceau et al. 1996; Smits et al. 1996; Costamagna et al. 1997; Brand et al. 2000; Kozarek et al. 2002; Inui et al. 2005).

Moreover, about two-thirds of these patients have a sustained relief of pain at long-term follow-up (Rosch et al. 2002; Delhaye et al. 2004; Tadenuma et al. 2005).

Accordingly, a meta-analysis including a total of 588 patients found that ESWL was effective in relieving MPD obstruction and alleviating pain in chronic calcifying pancreatitis, most often in combination with endoscopic therapy (Guda et al. 2005).

Factors associated with immediate relief or improvement of pain were successful decompression of the MPD as evidenced by a decrease in its diameter and stone clearance (Delhaye et al. 1992; Dumonceau et al. 1996; Brand et al. 2000).

In a long-term study (Tadenuma et al. 2005), pain relapse occurred significantly more frequently in patients with incomplete removal of stones after the initial therapy (hazard ratio, 3.7) and in those with a MPD stricture (hazard ratio, 3.4). Both factors were significant risk factors for pain relapse by multivariate analysis.

As expected, complete removal of stones was attained more frequently in patients with a single stone and without a MPD stricture.

At long-term follow-up, 10%–20% of the patients were still receiving endotherapy (Rosch et al. 2002; Delhaye et al. 2004), while surgery became necessary for about 20% of these CP patients initially treated with endotherapy, either for pancreatic ductal drainage when repetitive endoscopic treatment is considered too frequent in these young patients, or in case of technical or clinical failure after endotherapy (Rosch et al. 2002; Delhaye et al. 2005; Farnbacher et al. 2006a) (Table 12.2).

From the functional point of view, the exocrine function of the pancreas deteriorated more significantly in the incomplete removal group (Tadenuma

Table 12.2. Results of endoscopic pancreatic ductal drainage in CP patients (selected retrospective series including more than 50 patients followed for a mean period of more than 3 years)

Authors (y)	Number of patients (n)	Clinical improvement (%)	Conversion to surgery (%)	Ongoing endoscopic therapy (%)
CREMER et al. (1991)	76	84	15	NA
BINMOELLER et al. (1995)	93	65	26	13
ADAMEK et al. (1999)	80	76	10	NA
ROSCH et al. (2002)	996	65	24	16
DELHAYE et al. (2004)	56	66	21	18
TADENUMA et al. (2005)	70	70	1	20
FARNBACHER et al. (2006a)	96	67	23	18

CP: chronic pancreatitis; y: year; NA: not available

et al. 2005), in patients with a long duration of symptomatic ductal obstruction (DELHAYE et al. 2004) and in the alcohol abuse group (DELHAYE et al. 2004; TADENUMA et al. 2005).

However, the pancreatic endocrine function of the patients treated for pancreatic stones deteriorated after long-term follow-up evaluation independently of the successful removal of ductal stones (DELHAYE et al. 2004; TADENUMA et al. 2005).

Besides these previous retrospective studies, a bicenter prospective randomized controlled trial recently reported the results of ESWL alone vs ESWL in conjunction with endotherapy in highly selected patients with painful uncomplicated calcified CP (DUMONCEAU et al. 2007). These investigators randomized 55 patients, 26 to ESWL alone and 29 to ESWL combined with endotherapy (Table 12.3). A total of 38% of the patients treated with lithotripsy alone and 45% of those treated with combination therapy had relapse of pain 2 years after treatment. No significant differences in the outcome of pancreatic pain were reported in both groups; however, costs of treatment were about three times higher in the combination group compared with the ESWL alone group.

On the basis of this trial, ESWL might be the best initial option in selected patients with calcifications confined to the head of the pancreas, because it is non-invasive, is less expensive, and does not preclude further endoscopic or surgical therapy.

However, patients who would not be eligible for ESWL alone are those with a concomitant fluid collection, a symptomatic biliary obstruction or with a huge stone burden or multiple side branch calcifications.

Specific complications related to ESWL are rarely severe and include petechiae on the skin at the area of shock waves penetration and erosions in the gastric antrum or the duodenum, sometimes hemorrhagic that have been observed when ERCP has been performed immediately following ESWL, but without clinical consequences.

12.4.2 Pancreatic Ductal Strictures

Approximately half of the patients with severe CP presented with obstruction of the MPD caused by a dominant stricture usually located in the pancreatic head (ELEFTHERIADIS et al. 2005).

A stricture was defined as a main-duct narrowing (Fig. 12.2a and Fig. 12.4c) with partial or complete obstruction to contrast flow with or without associated stone or pseudocyst (COSTAMAGNA et al. 2006).

Benign strictures of the MPD are generally due to inflammation or fibrosis around the MPD (ADLER et al. 2006). Ductal obstruction may lead to pain or acute pancreatitis superimposed on CP.

Numerous studies have described symptomatic benefit of pancreatic duct stenting for painful CP (Cremer et al. 1991; Ponchon et al. 1995; Vitale et al. 2004; Eleftheriadis et al. 2005).

12.4.2.1 Selection of Patients

The best candidates for pancreatic stenting are those patients with one dominant stricture in the pancreatic head with upstream ductal dilatation combined with typical pain (Type IV according to Cremer's classification; Cremer et al. 1976).

The worse candidates are those with multiple strictures on the MPD, resulting in a picture sometimes described as a "chain of lakes" or Type III according to Cremer's classification (Cremer et al. 1976).

12.4.2.2 Techniques of Pancreatic Ductal Stenting

Pancreatic duct strictures are best demonstrated at ERCP at which time attempts at excluding malignancy must always be pursued, namely by appropriate tissue sampling of the stricture (Fig. 12.4c).

In most patients, pancreatic sphincterotomy (with or without biliary sphincterotomy) by way of the major or minor papilla is performed to facilitate access to the MPD. A hydrophilic guidewire is maneuvered upstream to the narrowing (Fig. 12.2b). High-grade strictures require dilatation before stent insertion. This may be performed with graduated bougienage (Fig. 12.3g) or hydrostatic balloon dilatation (Figs. 12.2c and 12.4e) (Delhaye et al. 2005).

Occasionally the pancreatic duct strictures are extremely tight or angulated and may not be traversable with conventional dilators. Therefore, new devices have been applied to improve the technical success rate of passing difficult ductal strictures. The Soehendra stent retriever has been used to core a path through high grade strictures (Binmoeller et al. 1998). "Dissection" or "stricturoplasty" of refractory strictures on the MPD using a sphincterotome or a pre-cutting needle-knife (Kawamoto et al. 2006) was recently described.

Thereafter, one or more polyethylene pancreatic duct stents are placed through the strictures (Fig. 12.2d), as described previously (Delhaye et al. 2003), to expand the narrowing adequately such that it allows good flow long after the stent is removed (Attasaranya et al. 2007).

In case of multiple stenting, it is recommended to begin with the stent of the largest diameter and maximal length in order to reduce the risk of migration of the first stent into the pancreatic duct during insertion of the next stent (Costamagna et al. 2006).

The technical success rate of pancreatic duct stenting is reported at or above 95% by experienced endoscopists (Farnbacher et al. 2006a).

Table 12.3. Randomized controlled trials related to the treatment of CP

Authors (y)	Dite et al. (2003)		Cahen et al. (2007)		Dumonceau et al. (2007)	
Design of the RCT	Endotherapy vs Surgery		Endotherapy vs Surgery		ESWL vs ESWL + endotherapy	
Number of randomized patients	36	36	19	20	26	29
Mean follow-up	5 years		2 years		4 years	
Complete pain relief (%)	15	34*	16	40*	58	55[a]
Partial pain relief (%)	46	52[a]	16	35*	ND	ND
Total group (n)	64	76	19	20	26	29
Technical success (%)	97	100[a]	53	100*	100	100[a]
Morbidity (%)	8	8	58	35[a]	0	3[a]
Mortality (%)	0	0	5	0[a]	0	0[a]
Need for surgery (%)	0	3	21	5	4	10[a]

CP: chronic pancreatitis; y: year; RCT: randomized controlled trial; ESWL: extracorporeal shockwave lithotripsy; [a] not significant; * $p<0.05$

Pancreatic stricture resolved if a free flow of contrast medium was seen alongside a 6-F nasopancreatic catheter and no pain was recorded during forced injection (Delhaye et al. 2003; Costamagna et al. 2006).

12.4.2.3 Results of Pancreatic Ductal Stenting

Observational retrospective studies have shown that pancreatic ductal stenting resulted in initial pain relief in 75%–95% of patients while long-term results were less promising (Cremer et al. 1991; Binmoeller et al. 1995, 1998; Ponchon et al. 1995; Smits et al. 1995; Adler et al. 2005; Farnbacher et al. 2006a).

Indeed, 25%–50% of patients presented pain relapse after stent removal requiring re-intervention in the follow-up period.

There are at least two drawbacks of pancreatic stenting: the first is the high relapse rate for symptomatic MPD stricture after stent removal (for example, 38% of patients required re-stenting after a supposedly definitive stent removal (Eleftheriadis et al. 2005) and the second is the occurrence of early stent clogging leading to frequent ERCPs for stent exchanges. In a recent study, a mean of 4.6 ERCPs/patient were required for stent exchanges (Farnbacher et al. 2006a).

Accordingly, we had shown that a significant predictive factor for completion of endotherapy in patients with severe CP, followed during a mean period of 14 years, was the absence of pancreatic duct stenting (Delhaye et al. 2004).

As definitive stent removal seems to be impracticable in a subset of patients due to recurrent pain caused by persisting stricture of the MPD, self-expandable metal stents have also been tested, but with unsatisfactory results because of frequent stent dysfunction secondary to tissue ingrowth through the mesh of these stents (Eisendrath and Devière 1999).

More recently, the insertion of multiple stents into the MPD has been proposed as a new strategy in order to obtain a greater stricture dilatation, a lower frequency of simultaneous stent occlusion, a possible drainage of pancreatic secretions alongside the stents even if all stents occlude, and maybe a longer interval between sent replacements and a higher rate of stricture calibration. Costamagna et al. (2006) recently performed a prospective non-randomized trial in 19 patients with symptomatic dominant MPD stricture located in the head of the pancreas, that persisted at ERCP after at least two placements of a single stent. Resolution of the dominant stricture at the time of removal was noted in 18/19 (95%) patients after a mean duration of stenting of 7 months (5–11) and a median number of simultaneous stents of 3 (2–4). During a mean follow-up period of 38 months after stent removal, pain recurred in 3/19 (16%) patients and repeat MPD stenting was resumed in 2 of them. The symptom-free period after removal of multiple stents was significantly longer when compared with the previous symptom-free period achieved with placement of a single stent in the same patients.

12.4.2.4 Timing of ERCP for Stent Exchange

At some centers, stents are exchanged on a regular basis (every 2–3 months) to avoid complications related to stent clogging (Ponchon et al. 1995; Smits et al. 1995; Vitale et al. 2004), whereas other endoscopists carry out stent exchange "on demand", i.e., in patients with recurrence of pain and recurrent dilatation of the MPD (Cremer et al. 1991; Binmoeller et al. 1995; Eleftheriadis et al. 2005).

This strategy means that stent replacement is required after a mean period of 8–12 months. Comparable clinical results were reported with both strategies.

In fact, there are no reliable clinical or laboratory parameters that indicate clogging of pancreatic stents. Stent clogging occurs very early and frequently (Ikenberry et al. 1994) but does not seem to be clinically relevant. So, in most of the cases with CP, the need for a scheduled stent exchange is not obvious. A symptom-oriented approach seems to be an attractive and potentially cost-effective alternative.

In an attempt to predict the optimal time interval for exchanging pancreatic stents, Farnbacher et al. (2006b) have reported that a stent diameter >8.5 F, a stent length >8 cm, the female gender and the need for regular enzyme supplementation were independent risk factors for stent occlusion. From these findings, the authors established a score significantly associated with a higher risk of occlusion within 90 days, suggesting that stent exchange or removal should be performed after 3 months at the latest when the score is high. They suggested also that multiple, 8.5 F, as short as possible stents should be inserted to reduce the advent of early stent occlusion. However, these recommendations should be prospectively validated in independent studies.

12.4.2.5 Timing of ERCP for Stent Removal

Clinical success includes symptom relief while the stent is in place and more importantly after stent removal.

Stents were removed and not replaced if the stricture could be easily passed with a 6-F catheter and if there was a prompt drainage of the contrast after ductal filling on ECRP (BINMOELLER et al. 1995).

Resolution of the stricture is not a pre-requisite for long-term symptomatic improvement. Indeed, symptomatic improvement may persist after pancreatic stent removal despite persistence of the stricture (PONCHON et al. 1995; SMITS et al. 1995).

Three large studies evaluated the long-term outcome of patients after definitive removal of the pancreatic stent (BINMOELLER et al. 1995; ELEFTHERIADIS et al. 2005; FARNBACHER et al. 2006a) (Table 12.4).

In one study, stents could be removed from 49 patients out of a total of 93 (53%) after a mean stenting period of 15.7 months, and 73% of these patients remained pain-free without a stent during a mean follow-up of 46 months (BINMOELLER et al. 1995). In the second study, after a median total duration of stenting of 23 months before stent removal, 62% of the patients maintained satisfactory pain control without pancreatic stent replacement during a median time of 27 months (ELEFTHERIADIS et al. 2005).

In the last retrospective study, after a total stenting duration of 10 months for 96 patients with symptomatic CP, 57 did not need secondary intervention, 22 underwent surgical treatment (9 patients for persistent pain despite endotherapy) and 17 resumed endotherapy following a pain-free interval after stent removal. Therefore, temporary pancreatic stenting may be considered as a definitive treatment for 55% (48/87) of these patients (FARNBACHER et al. 2006a).

12.4.2.6 Endoscopy or Surgery as the Best First-line Treatment for Symptomatic CP?

Pain relief following surgical pancreatico-jejunostomy was observed in 80% of the cases in the short-term follow-up period and in 40%–50% of the cases in the long-term follow-up period (WARSHAW et al. 1998).

There are few randomized controlled trials related to the treatment of CP (Table 12.3).

The first prospective randomized trial comparing endoscopic and surgical therapy for CP included 72 patients (36 in the endotherapy group and 36 in the surgery group) (DITE et al. 2003). Surgery consisted of resection (80%) and drainage (20%) procedures, while endotherapy included sphincterotomy and stenting (52%) and/or stone removal (23%). The initial success rates were similar for surgery and endoscopic treatment (92.1% vs 92.2% of complete or partial pain relief at 1-year follow-up). At 5-year follow-up, the complete absence of pain was more frequent among the surgically treated patients (34% vs 15% among the endoscopically treated patients) while the rates of partial relief were similar (52% and 46%). However, in this study, treatment was tailored to the patient, so that surgery involved resection in the majority of patients, which is difficult to compare with endoscopic ductal drainage. Moreover, endoscopic-drainage techniques were not optimally applied, in that they did not include ESWL, cumulative stenting, or repeated treatment after recurrence of symptoms, all factors which may have contributed to the reduced success rate for patients randomized in the endoscopic treatment group.

A second recent randomized trial compared the endoscopic drainage of the MPD with surgical pancreatico-jejunostomy (CAHEN et al. 2007). A total of 39 symptomatic patients having CP with distal obstruction of the MPD and without an inflamma-

Table 12.4. Clinical results after removal of pancreatic ductal stent

Authors (y)	Design of the study	Number of patients (n)	Mean duration of stenting (m)	Long-term pain relief after stent removal (%)	FU (m)
BINMOELLER et al. (1995)	Single stent exchange on demand	49	16	73	46
ELEFTHERIADIS et al. (2005)	Single stent exchange on demand	100	23	62	27
FARNBACHER et al. (2006a)	Single stent exchange every 3 m	96	10	55	46

y: year; m: month; FU: follow-up after stent removal

tory mass were randomized: 19 in the endotherapy group with 16 of them undergoing pancreatic ductal stent placement after ESWL, and 20 in the surgical pancreatic duct decompression group. Complete or partial pain relief was achieved in only 32% of patients assigned to endoscopic drainage as compared with 75% of patients assigned to surgical drainage (p=0.007), at the end of a 2-year follow-up period.

Rates of complications, length of hospital stay and changes in pancreatic function were similar in the two treatment groups, but patients receiving endoscopic treatment required more procedures than did the patients in the surgical group.

The conclusion of this trial was that surgical drainage of the pancreatic duct is more effective than endoscopic treatment in patients with pain from obstruction of the MPD attributable to CP.

However, the very high incidence of pancreatic ductal strictures (84%) in the endoscopically treated patients, who were treated by a short-term not optimal stenting duration (median, 27 weeks) could explained, at least partly, the disappointing rate of pain relief in the endoscopy group.

Moreover, the rate of common bile duct strictures and pseudocysts are not reported, which could also have allowed the inclusion of more refractory patients into the endoscopy group.

Despite these randomized trials showing a superiority of the surgical approach to CP patients, the conclusion of the accompanying editorial (Elta, 2007) was that endotherapy could be preferable as the first therapeutic option in patients with amenable ductal lesions, given its low degree of invasiveness, while surgery might be considered as the second-line therapy for patients in whom endoscopic therapy fails or is ineffective.

12.5 Conclusions

A multidisciplinary diagnostic and therapeutic approach of CP patients is actually required between radiologists, endoscopists, pathologists and surgeons.

As imaging modalities such as MRCP/MRI, CT and EUS progress, diagnostic ERCP should be reserved for the few patients in whom the diagnosis is still unclear after these non-invasive or less invasive imaging studies have been performed.

A refined selection of patients with CP for endoscopic treatment should take into account the heterogeneity of patient characteristics, the multiple anatomical changes to be treated, the goals of therapy and the prophylactic measures to prevent unplanned outcomes, so that an individual treatment strategy could be optimally applied to each patient.

Because of its low invasiveness and safety, endotherapy may be preferred as a first-line approach to the relief of MPD obstruction by stones and/or strictures, reserving surgery in cases of failure and/or recurrence of symptoms.

Therefore, ERCP has yet major roles to play in the management of CP and its complications. These roles will yet increase in parallel with technologic development and refinement of endoscopes and their accessories.

References

Adamek HE, Jakobs R, Buttmann A et al (1999) Long term follow up of patients with chronic pancreatitis and pancreatic stones treated with extracorporeal shock wave lithotripsy. Gut 45:402–405

Adler DG, Baron TH, Davila RE et al (2005) ASGE guideline: the role of ERCP in diseases of the biliary tract and the pancreas. Gastrointest Endosc 62:1–8

Adler DG, Lichtenstein D, Baron TH et al (2006) The role of endoscopy in patients with chronic pancreatitis. Gastrointest Endosc 63:933–937

Alazmi WM, Fogel EL, Schmidt S et al (2006) ERCP findings in idiopathic pancreatitis: patients who are cystic fibrosis gene positive and negative. Gastrointest Endosc 63:234–239

Arvanitakis M, Van Laethem J-L, Parma J et al (2004) Predictive factors for pancreatic cancer in patients with chronic pancreatitis in association with K-ras gene mutation. Endoscopy 36:535–542

Attasaranya S, Aziz AMA, Lehman GA (2007) Endoscopic management of acute and chronic pancreatitis. Surg Clin N Am 87:1379–1402

Axon ATR, Classen M, Cotton PB et al (1984) Pancreatography in chronic pancreatitis: international definitions. Gut 25:1107–1112

Baron TH, Petersen BT, Mergener K et al (2006) Quality indicators for endoscopic retrograde cholangiopancreatography. Gastrointest Endosc 63:S29–S34

Binmoeller KF, Jue P, Seifert H et al (1995) Endoscopic pancreatic stent drainage in chronic pancreatitis and a dominant stricture: long-term results. Endoscopy 27:638–644

Binmoeller KF, Rathod VD, Soehendra N (1998) Endoscopic therapy of pancreatic strictures. Gastrointest Endosc Clin N Am 8:125–142

Brand B, Kahl M, Sidhu S et al (2000) Prospective evaluation of morphology, function and quality of life after extracorporeal shockwave lithotripsy and endoscopic treatment of chronic calcific pancreatitis. Am J Gastroenterol 95:3428–3438

Cahen DL, Gouma DJ, Nio Y et al (2007) Endoscopic versus surgical drainage of the pancreatic duct in chronic pancreatitis. N Engl J Med 356:676–684

Calvo MM, Bujanda L, Calderon A et al (2002) Comparison between magnetic resonance cholangiopancreatography and ERCP for evaluation of the pancreatic duct. Am J Gastroenterol 97:347–353

Catalano MF, Lahoti S, Geenen JE et al (1998) Prospective evaluation of endoscopic ultrasonography, endoscopic retrograde pancreatography, and secretin test in the diagnosis of chronic pancreatitis. Gastrointest Endosc 48:11–17

Costamagna G, Gabbrielli A, Multignani M et al (1997) Extracorporeal shockwave lithotripsy of pancreatic stones in chronic pancreatitis: immediate and medium-term results. Gastrointest Endosc 46:231–236

Costamagna G, Bulajic M, Tringali A et al (2006) Multiple stenting of refractory pancreatic duct strictures in severe chronic pancreatitis: long-term results. Endoscopy 38:254–259

Cremer M, Toussaint J, Hermanus A et al (1976) Les pancréatites chroniques primitives; classification sur base de la pancréatographie endoscopique. Acta Gastroent Belg 39:522–546

Cremer M, Devière J, Delhaye M et al (1991) Stenting in severe chronic pancreatitis: results of medium-term follow-up in seventy-six patients. Endoscopy 23:171–176

Delhaye M, Vandermeeren A, Baize M et al (1992) Extracorporeal shock wave lithotripsy of pancreatic calculi. Gastroenterology 102:610–620

Delhaye M, Matos C, Devière J (2003) Endoscopic management of chronic pancreatitis. Gastrointest Endosc Clin N Am 13:717–742

Delhaye M, Arvanitakis M, Verset G et al (2004) Long-term clinical outcome after endoscopic pancreatic ductal drainage for patients with painful chronic pancreatitis. Clin Gastroenterol Hepatol 2:1096–1106

Delhaye M, Arvanitakis M, Bali M et al (2005) Endoscopic therapy for chronic pancreatitis. Scand J Surg 94:143–153

Devereaux CE, Binmoeller KF (2000) Endoscopic retrograde cholangiopancreatography in the next millennium. Gastrointest Endosc Clin N Am 10:117–133

Devière J, Delhaye M, Cremer M (1998) Pancreatic duct stones management. Gastrointest Clin N Am 8:163–179

Dite P, Ruzicka M, Zboril V et al (2003) A prospective, randomized trial comparing endoscopic and surgical therapy for chronic pancreatitis. Endoscopy 35:553–558

Draganov P, Patel A, Fazel A et al (2005) Prospective evaluation of the accuracy of the intraductal secretin stimulation test in the diagnosis of chronic pancreatitis. Clin Gastroenterol Hepatol 3:695–699

Dumonceau J-M, Devière J, Le Moine O et al (1996) Endoscopic drainage in chronic pancreatitis associated with ductal stones: long-term results. Gastrointest Endosc 43:547–555

Dumonceau J-M, Costamagna G, Tringali A et al (2007) Treatment for painful calcified chronic pancreatitis: extracorporeal shockwave lithotripsy versus endoscopic treatment: a randomised controlled trial. Gut 56:545–552

Eisendrath P, Devière J (1999) Expandable metal stents for benign pancreatic duct obstruction. Gastrointest Endosc Clin N Am 9:547–554

Eleftheriadis N, Dinu F, Delhaye M et al (2005) Long-term outcome after pancreatic stenting in severe chronic pancreatitis. Endoscopy 37:223–230

Elta GH (2007) Is there a role for the endoscopic treatment of pain from chronic pancreatitis? N Engl J Med 356:727–729

Etemad B, Whitcomb DC (2001) Chronic pancreatitis: diagnosis, classification and new genetic developments. Gastroenterology 120:682–707

Farnbacher MJ, Mühldorfer S, Wehler M et al (2006a) Interventional endoscopic therapy in chronic pancreatitis including temporary stenting: a definitive treatment? Scand J Gastroenterol 41:111–117

Farnbacher MJ, Radespiel-Tröger M, König MD et al (2006b) Pancreatic endoprostheses in chronic pancreatitis: criteria to predict stent occlusion. Gastrointest Endosc 63:60–66

Forsmark CE (2000) The diagnosis of chronic pancreatitis. Gastrointest Endosc 52:293–298

Forsmark CE, Toskes PP (1995) What does an abnormal pancreatogram mean? Gastrointest Endosc Clin N Am 5:105–123

Freeman ML (2002) Adverse outcomes of ERCP. Gastrointest Endosc 56(suppl):S273–S282

Freeman ML, Guda NM (2005) ERCP cannulation: a review of reported techniques. Gastrointest Endosc 61:112–125

Freeman ML, DiSario JA, Nelson DB et al (2001) Risk factors for post-ERCP pancreatitis: a prospective, multicenter study. Gastrointest Endosc 54:425–434

Fry LC, Mönkemüller K, Malfertheiner P (2007) Diagnosis of chronic pancreatitis. Am J Surg 194:S45–S52

Gabbrielli A, Pandolfi M, Mutignani M et al (2005) Efficacy of main pancreatic-duct endoscopic drainage in patients with chronic pancreatitis, continuous pain, and dilated duct. Gastrointest Endosc 61:576–581

Guda NM, Partington S, Freeman ML (2005) Extracorporeal shockwave lithotripsy in the management of chronic calcific pancreatitis: a meta-analysis. JOP 6:6–12

Hookey LC, RioTinto R, Delhaye M et al (2006) Risk factors for pancreatitis after pancreatic sphincterotomy: a review of 572 cases. Endoscopy 38:670–676

Horiuchi A, Kawa S, Hamano H et al (2002) ERCP features in 27 patients with autoimmune pancreatitis. Gastrointest Endosc 55:494–499

Ikenberry SO, Sherman S, Smith M (1994) The occlusion rate of pancreatic stents. Gastrointest Endosc 40:611–613

Inui K, Tazuma S, Yamaguchi T et al (2005) Treatment of pancreatic stones with extracorporeal shockwave lithotripsy: results of a multicenter survey. Pancreas 30:26–30

Kawai K, Akasaka Y, Murakami K et al (1974) Endoscopic sphincterotomy of the ampulla of Vater. Gastrointest Endosc 20:148–151

Kawamoto H, Ishida E, Ogawa T et al (2006) Dissection of a refractory pancreatic-duct stricture by using a pre-cutting needle-knife. Gastrointest Endosc 63:190–192

Kim DH, Pickhardt PJ (2007) Radiologic assessment of acute and chronic pancreatitis. Surg Clin North Am 87:1341–1358

Kozarek RA (1990) Pancreatic stents can induce ductal changes consistent with chronic pancreatitis. Gastrointest Endosc 36:93–95

Kozarek RA (2006) Pancreatic ERCP. Endoscopy 38:110–115

Kozarek RA, Brandabur JJ, Ball TJ et al (2002) Clinical outcomes in patients who undergo extracorporeal shockwave lithotripsy for chronic calcific pancreatitis. Gastrointest Endosc 56:496–500

Kucera S, Isenberg G, Chak A et al (2007) Postprocedure radiologist's interpretation of ERCP X-ray films: a prospective outcomes study. Gastrointest Endosc 66:79–83

Lehman GA (2002) Role of ERCP and other endoscopic modalities in chronic pancreatitis. Gastrointest Endosc 56:S237–S240

Lévy P, Barthet M, Mollard BR et al (2006) Estimation of the prevalence and incidence of chronic pancreatitis and its complications. Gastroenterol Clin Biol 30:838–844

Lowenfels AB, Maisonneuve P, Cavallini G et al (1993) Pancreatitis and the risk of pancreatic cancer. N Engl J Med 328:1433–1437

Matos C, Metens T, Devière J et al (1997) Pancreatic duct: morphologic and functional evaluation with dynamic MR pancreatography after secretin stimulation. Radiology 203:435–441

Maydeo A, Soehendra N, Reddy N et al (2007) Endotherapy for chronic pancreatitis with intracanalar stones. Endoscopy 39:653–658

McCune WS, Shorb PE, Moscovitz H (1968) Endoscopic cannulation of the ampulla of Vater: a preliminary report. Ann Surg 167:752–756

Ong WC, Santosh D, Lakhtakia S et al (2007) A randomized controlled trial on use of propofol alone versus propofol with midazolam, ketamine, and pentazocine «sedato-analgesic cocktail» for sedation during ERCP. Endoscopy 39:807–812

Papachristou GI, Baron TH (2007) Complications of therapeutic endoscopic retrograde cholangiopancreatography. Gut 56:854–868

Papachristou GI, Smyrk TC, Baron TH (2007) Endoscopic retrograde cholangiopancreatography tissue sampling: when and how? Clin Gastroenterol Hepatol 5:783–790

Ponchon T, Bory RM, Hedelius F et al (1995) Endoscopic stenting for pain relief in chronic pancreatitis: results of a standardized protocol. Gastrointest Endosc 42:452–456

Pugliese V, Pujic N, Saccomanno S et al (2001) Pancreatic intraductal sampling during ERCP in patients with chronic pancreatitis and pancreatic cancer: cytologic studies and k-ras-2 codon 12 molecular analysis in 47 cases. Gastrointest Endosc 54:595–599

Rosch T, Daniel S, Scholz M et al (2002) Endoscopic treatment of chronic pancreatitis: a multicenter study of 1000 patients with long-term follow-up. Endoscopy 34:765–771

Sahai AV, Zimmerman M, Aabakken L et al (1998) Prospective assessment of the ability of endoscopic ultrasound to diagnose, exclude, or establish the severity of chronic pancreatitis found by endoscopic retrograde cholangiopancreatography. Gastrointest Endosc 48:18–25

Schutz SM, Abbott RM (2000) Grading ERCPs by degree of difficulty: a new concept to produce more meaningful outcome data. Gastrointest Endosc 51:535–539

Singh P, Das A, Isenberg G et al (2004) Does prophylactic pancreatic stent placement reduce the risk of post-ERCP acute pancreatitis? A meta-analysis of controlled trials. Gastrointest Endosc 60:544–560

Smits ME, Badiga SM, Rauws EAJ et al (1995) Long-term results of pancreatic stents in chronic pancreatitis. Gastrointest Endosc 42:461–467

Smits ME, Rauws EAJ, Tytgat GNJ et al (1996) Endoscopic treatment of pancreatic stones in patients with chronic pancreatitis. Gastrointest Endosc 43:556–560

Somogyi L, Chuttani R, Croffie J et al (2006) Biliary and pancreatic stents. Gastrointest Endosc 63:910–919

Steer ML, Waxman I, Freedman S (1995) Chronic pancreatitis. N Engl J Med 332:1482–1490

Tadenuma H, Ishihara T, Yamaguchi T et al (2005) Long-term results of extracorporeal shockwave lithotripsy and endoscopic therapy for pancreatic stones. Clin Gastroenterol Hepatol 3:1128–1135

Tamura R, Ishibashi T, Takahashi S (2006) Chronic pancreatitis: MRCP versus ERCP for quantitative caliber measurement and qualitative evaluation. Radiology 238:920–928

Testoni PA, Mariani A, Mangiavillano B et al (2007) Intraductal optical coherence tomography for investigating main pancreatic duct strictures. Am J Gastroenterol 102:269–274

Vandervoort J, Soetikno RM, Tham TCK et al (2002) Risk factors for complications after performance of ERCP. Gastrointest Endosc 56:652–656

Varadarajulu S, Eltoum I, Tamhane A et al (2007) Histopathologic correlates of non-calcific chronic pancreatitis by EUS: a prospective tissue characterization study. Gastrointest Endosc 66:501–509

Vitale GC, Cothron K, Vitale EA et al (2004) Role of pancreatic duct stenting in the treatment of chronic pancreatitis. Surg Endosc 18:1431–1434

Warshaw AL, Banks PA, Fernandez-Del Castillo C (1998) AGA technical review: treatment of pain in chronic pancreatitis. Gastroenterology 115:765–776

Wiersema MJ, Hawes RH, Lehman GA et al (1993) Prospective evaluation of endoscopic ultrasonography and endoscopic retrograde cholangiopancreatography in patients with chronic abdominal pain of suspected pancreatic origin. Endoscopy 25:555–564

Williams EJ, Taylor S, Fairclough P et al (2007) Are we meeting the standards set for endoscopy? Results of a large-scale prospective survey of endoscopic retrograde cholangio-pancreatograph practice. Gut 56:821–829

Complications of Acute and Chronic Pancreatitis

Pathology of Chronic Pancreatitis

13

Giuseppe Zamboni, Paola Capelli, and Günter Klöppel

CONTENTS

13.1 **Introduction** *231*

13.2 **Alcoholic Chronic Pancreatitis** *232*
13.2.1 Macroscopy *232*
13.2.2 Microscopy *232*
13.2.3 Pathogenesis *236*

13.3 **Hereditary Pancreatitis** *237*
13.3.1 Pathology *238*

13.4 **Autoimmune Pancreatitis** *240*
13.4.1 Macroscopy *242*
13.4.2 Microscopy *242*
13.4.3 Extrapancreatic Involvement *245*
13.4.4 Relationship to Inflammatory Pseudotumor *246*
13.4.5 Differential Diagnosis *246*

13.5 **Paraduodenal Pancreatitis and Cysts of the Duodenal Wall** *247*
13.5.1 Macroscopy *248*
13.5.2 Microscopy *248*
13.5.3 Differential Diagnosis *250*

13.6 **Obstructive Chronic Pancreatitis** *250*

13.7 **Idiopathic Chronic Pancreatitis** *251*

13.8 **Metabolic Chronic Pancreatitis** *252*

13.9 **Tropical Chronic Pancreatitis** *252*

13.1 **Pancreatic Fibrosis Not Associated with Symptoms of Chronic Pancreatitis** *252*

13.1 **Complications of Chronic Pancreatitis** *252*
13.11.1 Biliary Stricture *252*
13.11.2 Duodenal Stenosis *253*
13.11.3 Pseudocysts *253*
13.11.4 Retention Cysts *253*
13.11.5 Internal Pancreatic Fistulas *254*
13.11.6 Splenic Vein Thrombosis *254*
13.11.7 Concomitant Pancreatic Cancer *254*

References *254*

G. Zamboni, MD
Department of Pathology University of Verona, Ospedale S. Cuore-Don Calabria, Via don Sempreboni 5, 37024 Negrar-Verona, Italy
P. Capelli, MD
Department of Pathology University of Verona, Strada le Grazie 8, 37134 Verona, Italy
G. Klöppel, MD
Professor and Head, Department of Pathology, University of Kiel, Michaelisstrasse 11, 24105 Kiel, Germany

Supported by European Community Grant FP6, MolDiagPaca

13.1 Introduction

Chronic pancreatitis (CP) is a benign, progressive fibroinflammatory process which leads to irreversible damage to both exocrine and endocrine components of the pancreas, resulting in gland atrophy. The reported incidence in industrialized countries ranges from 3.5–10 persons/100,000 per year (Witt et al. 2007). The reported increased incidence likely represents increased recognition in its earlier stage due to improved radiological imaging.

The aetiological factors associated with CP are summarized using the TIGAR-O classification: *T*oxic-metabolic (alcohol, tobacco), *I*diopathic, *G*enetic, *A*utoimmune, *R*ecurrent and *O*bstructive (Etemad and Whitcomb 2001). In Western countries alcohol abuse is the leading cause of CP, accounting for approximately 80% of cases. Alcoholic pancreatitis and most of the other aetiological forms clinically present in adulthood. Exceptions are hereditary pancreatitis, which may already occur in childhood, and tropical pancreatitis, which often affects adolescents.

The crucial lesions of CP are chronic inflammation, pancreatic fibrosis, acinar atrophy and duct dilatation and obstruction. Some morphological features, such as the composition of the inflammatory infiltrate and the fibrosis pattern, may be a clue to a specific aetiology (Adsay et al. 2004; Klöppel et al. 2004). For instance, the pattern of fibrosis, i.e. inter(peri)lobular or intralobular, depends very much on the site of the initial injury in the pancreas and this is related to the aetiological factor. These observations have been included in a new classification that also considers clinical and immunological features (Klöppel 2007b) So far, it is possible to distinguish alcoholic chronic pancreatitis, hereditary pancreatitis, autoimmune pancreatitis, obstructive chronic pancreatitis and paraduodenal pancreatitis ("groove pancreatitis") (Adsay and Zamboni 2004; Etemad and Whitcomb 2001; Klöppel 2007a; Stolte et al. 1982; Witt et al. 2007). Table 13.1 shows the classification that we use.

Table 13.1. Aetiological classification of chronic pancreatitis and pancreatic fibrosis

Chronic pancreatitis
• Alcoholic
• Hereditary
• Autoimmune
• Metabolic (hypercalcaemia, hyperlipidaemia)
• Tropical
• Idiopathic
Obstructive chronic pancreatitis
• Paraduodenal pancreatitis
• Chronic pancreatitis associated with anatomic abnormalities
• Other types (Oddi disorders, tumor obstruction)
Pancreatic fibrosis not associated with symptoms of chronic pancreatitis
• Pancreatic fibrosis in the elderly
• Cystic fibrosis
• Pancreatic fibrosis in long-term insulin-dependent diabetes mellitus
• Haemochromatosis

13.2 Alcoholic Chronic Pancreatitis

Although alcoholic chronic pancreatitis (ACP) accounts for up to 80%–90% of cases of CP many aspects of the disease remain unexplained; it is far from clear where to set the limit of alcohol consumption and why clinical CP develops only in about 10% of heavy drinkers. Moreover, the differential diagnosis between acute and chronic alcoholic pancreatitis is difficult (there is a continuum of disease manifestations). In the early stage of ACP patients experience relapsing episodes of acute pancreatitis, particularly with severe recurrent pain, whereas in advanced stages pain, steatorrhea and diabetes predominate. The patients are usually young to middle-aged men (25–50 years), who develop the disease after approximately 10 years of alcohol abuse. ACP has been proven to be a risk factor for the development of pancreatic cancer (Lowenfels et al. 1993; Talamini et al. 2000).

13.2.1 Macroscopy

Alcoholic chronic pancreatitis may present as a predominantly focal disease involving only a portion of the gland as a mass-like lesion, or it may show extensive involvement, resulting in global atrophy of the gland.

In the early stages the gland shows irregularly distributed fibrosis. The involved parts of the gland, either small foci or large areas, appear indurated and may be enlarged, showing coarse lobulation and/or nodular scarring on the cut surface. Only those ducts that are embedded in fibrotic tissue show irregularities and occasionally may contain calculi (calcified protein plugs). In 30%–50% of cases there may be pseudocysts associated with necrotic foci (Klöppel and Maillet 1991).

In the advanced stages the pancreas is extensively involved, atrophic and shrunken with an irregular contour and loss of the normal lobulation. The fibrotic process occasionally leaves the lobular pattern of the organ preserved in some areas. The pancreatic ducts are generally dilated and distorted. The severity and multifocality of the duct involvement and the calculi formation depend on the extent of the periductal fibrosis. The calculi, which consist of calcium carbonate, vary in size from less than 1 mm to many centimetres in diameter (Ammann et al. 1996; Klöppel and Maillet 1992) (Fig. 13.1).

13.2.2 Microscopy

In most of the cases microscopic examination reveals a variable degree of parenchymal involvement, with spared glandular lobules alternating

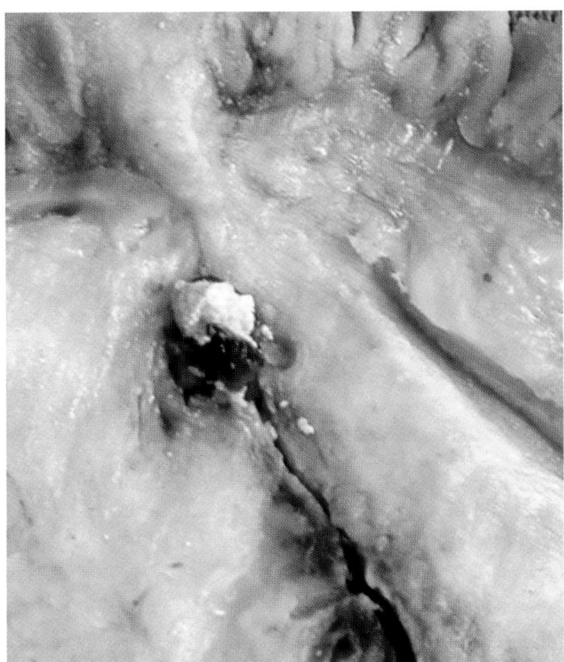

Fig. 13.1. Alcoholic chronic pancreatitis: head of the pancreas with extensive fibrosis and loss of the normal lobulation. Calculi are present within the main pancreatic duct which shows upstream dilatation. The terminal bile duct shows intrapancreatic and intraduodenal stenosis and moderate dilatation of the proximal part

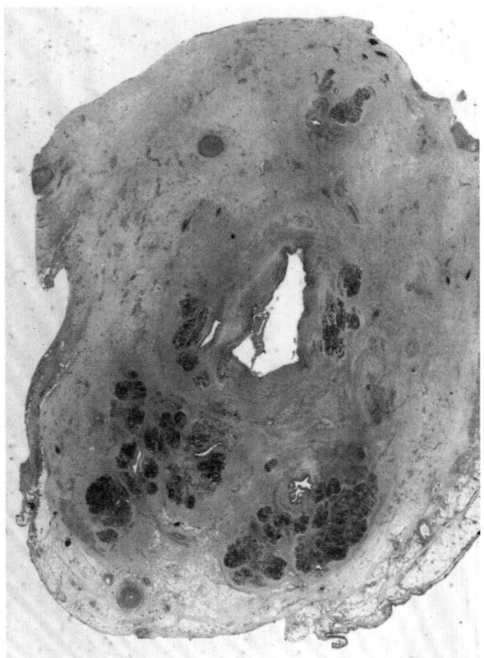

Fig. 13.2. Severe atrophic pancreatitis with main duct dilatation, diffuse fibrosis; despite the extensive fibrosis focally spared glandular lobules can be recognized

with mild to severe atrophic areas, embedded in fibrotic tissue (Fig. 13.2). Except for extremely advanced cases, the pancreatic lobular architecture is retained (Fig. 13.3). This is an extremely important key diagnostic feature in the differential diagnosis versus pancreatic carcinoma.

In the early stages the pancreas reveals interlobular (perilobular) cell-rich fibrosis (Ammann et al. 1996; Detlefsen et al. 2006). The distorted intralobular ducts, frequently lined by mucinous metaplastic and hyperplastic epithelium, may contain eosinophilic secretions, so-called protein plugs (Fig. 13.4). Chronic inflammatory infiltration, characterized by lymphocytes, plasma cells, and macrophages are present, either focally around nerve trunks (Fig. 13.5) or scattered diffusely throughout the fibrous tissue. In the perilobular tissue there may be foci of resolving fat necrosis with large numbers of vacuolated macrophages in the immediate vicinity and cell-rich fibrosis in the surrounding area.

In advanced stages, fibrosis affects most of the parenchyma, though still sparing some areas. Perilobular fibrosis causes duct distortions and dilatations with frequent deposition of protein plugs and

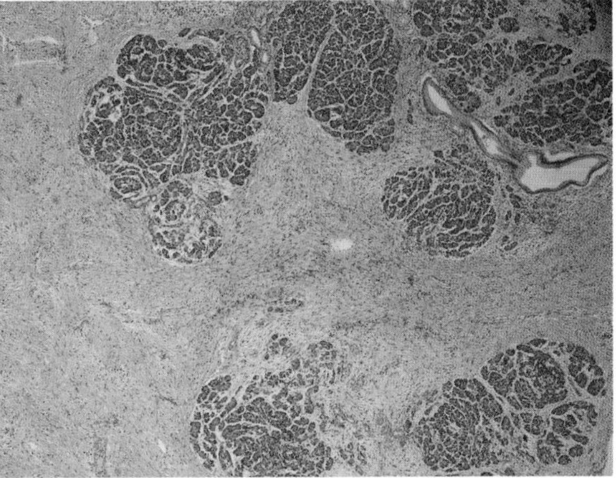

Fig. 13.3. Preserved lobular architecture of the gland with the presence of perilobular and intralobular fibrosis, duct distortion with periductal inflammatory infiltration and mucinous metaplastic change of the duct epithelium

calculi (Fig. 13.6), which are responsible for the atrophic changes in the epithelium and eventually for its denudation with complete replacement by inflammatory granulation tissue. With the progressive loss of the acinar cell component, the pancreatic lobule, which still retains its lobular architec-

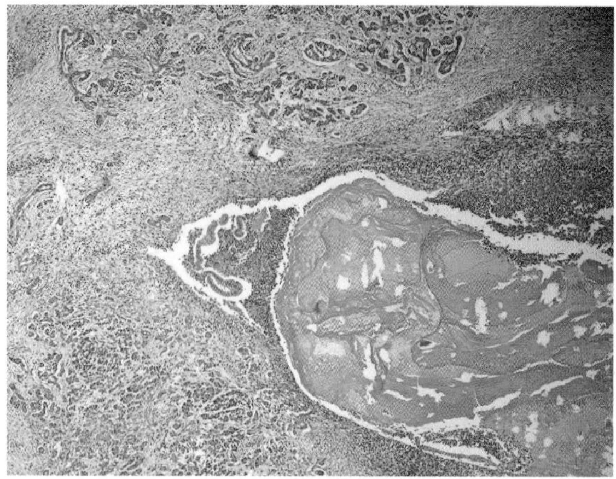

Fig. 13.4. Intralobular fibrosis with dilated duct with protein plug, intense inflammatory infiltration with epithelial destruction and focal epithelial denudation

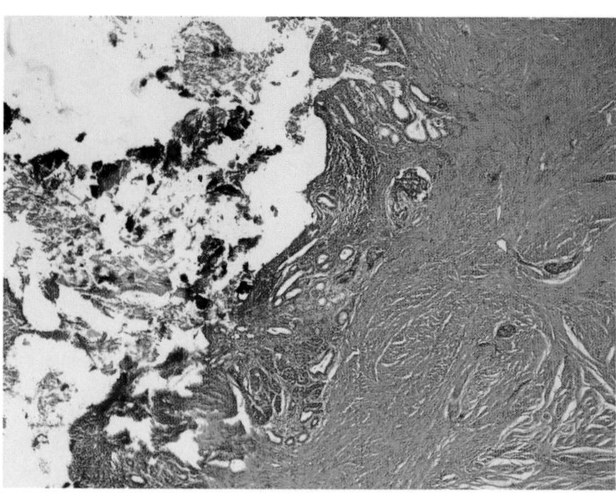

Fig. 13.6. Calcified protein plug with disruption of the ductal lining epithelium, replaced by granulation tissue, and severe periductal fibrosis

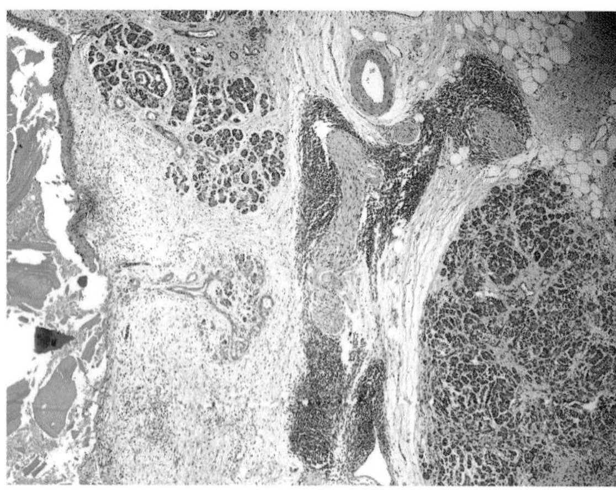

Fig. 13.5. Intense perineural lymphocytic infiltration. The duct, containing a protein plug, presents with focal squamous metaplasia

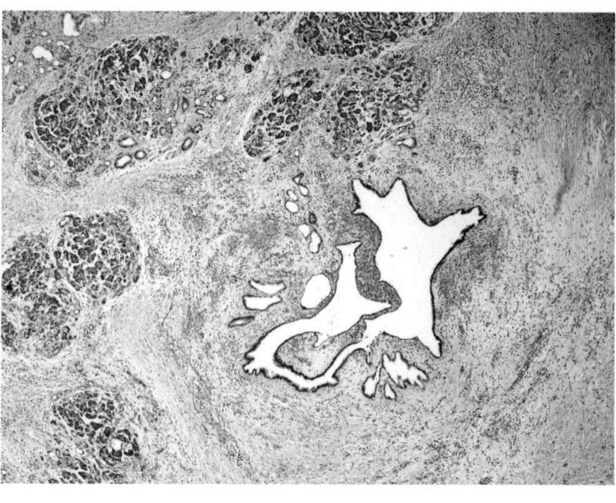

Fig. 13.7. Pancreatic lobule with partially conserved lobular architecture and markedly distorted central duct surrounded by fibrous tissue

ture, is characterized by central ducts surrounded by remnants of acinar cells (Fig. 13.7) undergoing apoptosis and forming so-called tubular complexes (Bockman et al. 1982). With more pronounced atrophy, the lobules are constituted exclusively of clusters of ductules separated by fibrous tissue (Fig. 13.8a,b). In areas with intralobular fibrosis the elements that remain are islets. They usually aggregate together in pseudonodular formations, resulting in an apparent increase in mass or adenomatoid changes (Fig. 13.9). Frequently, the endocrine cell component forms ductulo-insular complexes (Fig. 13.10). In a few instances benign perineural invasion of endocrine cell clusters can be observed, as well as their presence within the adipose tissue. The latter phenomenon does not reflect true proliferation and adipose tissue infiltration, but rather the result of a marked fibro-adipose transformation of the pancreatic parenchyma simulating adipose tissue infiltration.

In pancreatic atrophy the only recognizable structures embedded in the fibrous tissue are thick-walled blood vessels (Fig. 13.11) and prominent, hypertrophic nerves damaged by the inflammatory process (Bockman et al. 1988).

Immunohistochemistry can be useful for demonstrating the preservation of the lobular architecture of the pancreas and for demonstrating the endocrine nature of the round cell clusters in perineu-

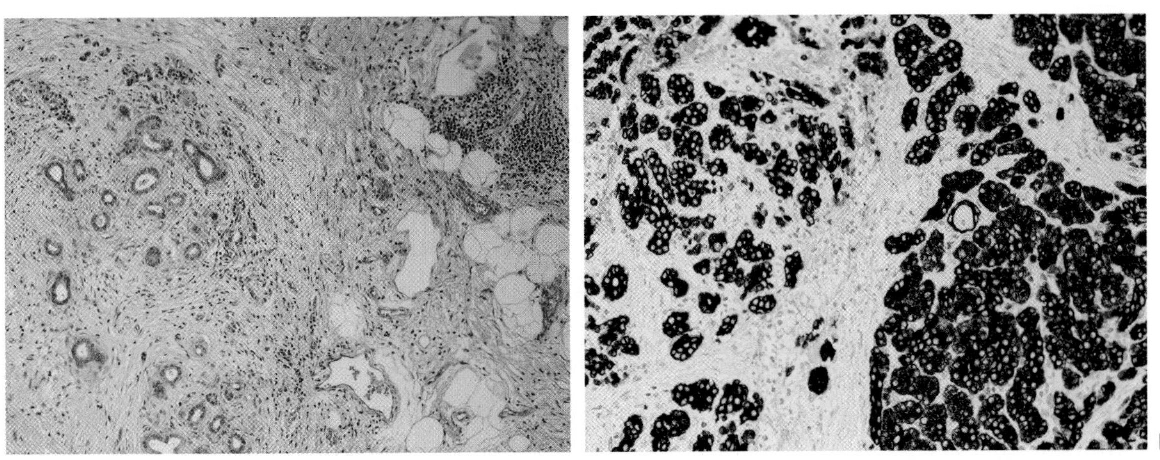

Fig. 13.8a,b. Tubular complexes constituted by ductules, separated by fibrous tissue but still retaining their lobular architecture, intermingled with endocrine cell component (**a**). Immunohistochemical staining for Keratin highlights the progressive lobular atrophy (*right*) and tubular complexes formation (*left*) (**b**)

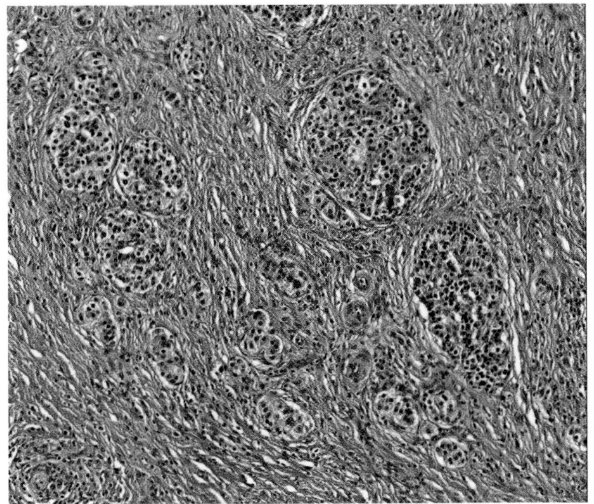

Fig. 13.9. Diffuse atrophy with the only presence of islets, with apparent increase of mass

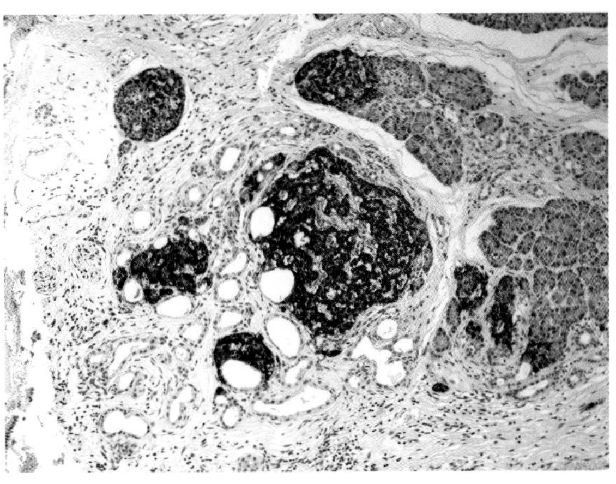

Fig. 13.10. Immunohistochemical staining with Chromogranin showing a ductulo-insular complex, with insulae budding from ductular structures

ral spaces or in apparently inappropriate locations within the adipose tissue. Immunohistochemically, the duct epithelium commonly expresses HLA-DR and cytokines such as transforming growth factors alpha and beta (TGFα, TGFβ1) and fibroblast growth factor (FGF) (Bedossa et al. 1990; Bovo et al. 1987; van Laethem et al. 1995). TGFβ1 and platelet derived growth factor (PDGF) are also found in fibroblasts, macrophages and/or platelets (Ebert et al. 1998). Fibroblasts are vimentin-positive, whereas positivity for α-smooth muscle actin (SMA) and desmin are the markers for the identification of the activated stellate pancreatic cells (SPCs) (Bachem et al. 2006) (Fig. 13.12a,b). The majority of the inflam-

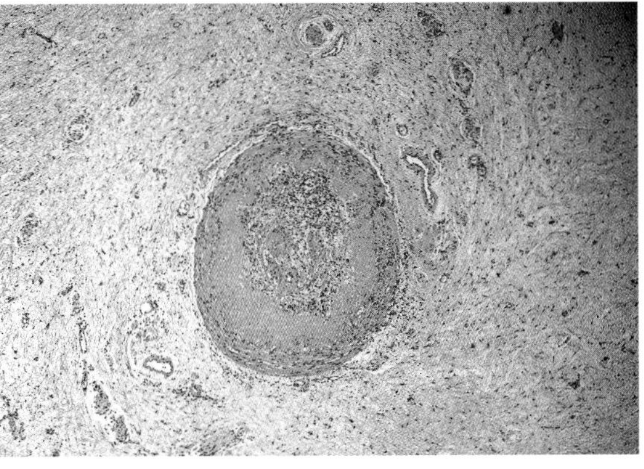

Fig. 13.11. Thick walled blood vessel with intimal proliferation and occlusion of the lumen

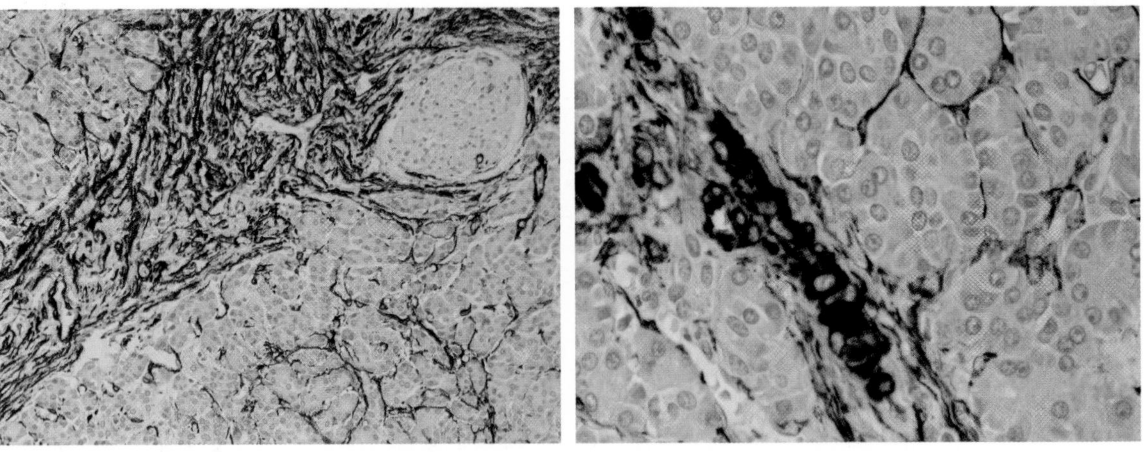

Fig. 13.12a,b. Perilobular and intralobular fibrosis characterized by the presence of smooth muscle actin (SMA)-positive myofibroblast, both with spindle shape (**a**) and oval shape (activated stellate cells) (**b**)

matory cells in ACP tissue are macrophages and T lymphocytes, with a minority of B lymphocytes and plasma cells (Farkas et al. 2007). Although IgG4 – positive plasma cells – can be found in 63% of the cases of alcoholic pancreatitis, they are not clustered around periductal areas, nor do they exceed the cut-off of 20 cells per high power field (HPF). In terms of specificity, this implies that IgG4 expression in more than 20 cells/HPF is 100% specific for the diagnosis of autoimmune pancreatitis and rules out alcoholic chronic pancreatitis (Kojima et al. 2007). The hypertrophic nerves express calcitonin-gene related peptide and substance P (Buchler et al. 1992). Both the endothelial cells and endocrine beta and alpha cells show strong endothelin-1 expression in chronic pancreatitis (Kakugawa et al. 1996).

13.2.3 Pathogenesis

Significant advances have been made in the comprehension of the pathogenetic mechanisms of ACP. This refers particularly to the direct toxic effects of alcohol and its metabolites on the pancreatic acinar cells, which may predispose to relapsing necrotizing pancreatitis episodes, but also to the molecular mechanisms responsible for pancreatic recruitment and activation of inflammatory cells, the activation of PSCs, fibrin deposition and scarring.

The traditional view of ACP was that it is chronic from the start and only punctuated during its course by acute exacerbation. However, this concept has been challenged and the prevalent current opinion is that the necrosis-fibrosis hypothesis (Klöppel and Maillet 1993) can better explain the progression of tissue damage from an early acute process that progresses to chronic irreversible damage as a result of repeated relapsing severe attacks of acute pancreatitis (Ammann and Muellhaupt 1994).

Ethanol derived toxic metabolites induce reactive oxygen species (ROS) and oxidative stress induces necrosis of acinar cells through alterations in cell calcium metabolism. The pancreatic acinar cells respond to the noxious stimuli by upregulating signalling systems that mediate the proinflammatory cytokines and chemokines and other inflammatory molecules. These signalling pathways include the activation of the transcription factors nuclear factor-kB (NF-kB) and activator protein-1 (AP-1) and the p38-MAP kinase, which mediate the production of proinflammatory cytokines TNFα, IL-6 and chemokines (Pandon and Raraty 2007).

Significant progress in the understanding of the fibrosis process has been made as the result of the identification and characterization of PSCs. PSCs are similar morphologically to the hepatic stellate cells, the principal effector of hepatic fibrosis. Activated PSCs play a key role in the fibrinogenic process, both in pancreatitis and pancreatic carcinoma, regulating the synthesis, deposition and degradation of the extracellular matrix protein of the fibrous tissue (Apte et al. 1998, 2004; Apte and Wilson 2003; Vonlaufen et al. 2008). In the activation process, the PSCs lose their ability to store vitamin A, express the cytoskeletal protein SMA and produce and secrete large amounts of extracellular matrix protein. PSC activation is mediated by the proinflammatory cytokines TNFα, IL-1, IL-6 and the chemokines transforming growth factors-β (TGF-β) and platelet-derived growth factors (PDGF) produced and secreted by acinar cells, inflammatory cells and by PSCs themselves. TGF-β stimulates the production and secretion of type-1 collagen, fibronectin, laminin and MMPs, whereas PDGF induces proliferation and migration of PSCs. In vitro studies have established that PSCs show alcohol dehydrogenase activity, indicating that ethanol can also be metabolized by non-parenchymal cells in the pancreas. During alcohol abuse PSCs are potentially exposed not only to cytokines and growth factors, but also to alcohol. Ethanol and its metabolites may stimulate PSC activation through the production of ROS. PSCs can be activated early during chronic alcohol intake, even in the absence of necro-inflammation, by ethanol and its metabolite, acetaldehyde, with the subsequent generation of oxidative stress. Persistent activation of PSCs leads to an imbalance between fibrin protein synthesis and degradation, resulting in irreversible pancreatic fibrosis (Jaster et al. 2008).

The fibrosis develops primarily in the perilobular space, where fat necrosis and most of the hemorrhagic necrosis occur (Adsay et al. 2004; Detlefsen et al. 2006). Perilobular fibrosis, in turn, affects the structure of the interlobular ducts, creating duct dilatations and strictures. In these altered ducts the flow of secretions is presumably impaired, a situation that may trigger the spontaneous precipitation of proteins with subsequent calcification. In addition, the impaired and eventually interrupted flow of pancreatic secretions leads to fibrotic replacement of the acinar cells upstream from the occluded duct and finally results in intralobular fibrosis. Although the necrosis-fibrosis sequence explains the perilobular fibrosis pattern, the patchy distribution of fibrosis and the late occurrence of calcifications in the pancreas of patients with alcoholic chronic pancreatitis, it does not explain why only a small proportion of heavy drinkers develop acute or chronic pancreatitis. A possible explanation is that ethanol alone is not enough to develop the disease. Alcohol may sensitize an individual to pancreatitis, but a second hit is necessary to precipitate a clinical attack of pancreatitis. Hypothetical triggers or additional cofactors include smoking, a high-fat diet, gallstones, obstruction and a genetic predisposition (Haber et al. 1995; Witt et al. 2007).

13.3 Hereditary Pancreatitis

Hereditary pancreatitis (HP) is an autosomal dominant condition with 70%–80% penetrance characterized by recurrent attacks of acute pancreatitis and progressing to CP over a variable period of time. Symptoms usually start already in childhood or adolescence and are characterized by recurring, suddenly appearing epigastric pain (Whitcomb 1999). Clinically, it resembles alcoholic pancreatitis, although the progression toward pancreatic insufficiency, with steatorrhoea and diabetes normally occurs later. Only 4% of patients develop severe CP, whereas 50% of the mutation carriers have few or no complications (Teich and Mossner 2008). The condition was considered very rare, accounting for no more than 1%–2% of all patients. However, recent research indicates that a significant percentage of 25% of patients with so-called idiopathic chronic pancreatitis may also have a genetic basis for their condition (Treiber et al. 2008).

Genetic alterations in chronic pancreatitis involve the cationic trypsinogen gene (PRSS1) (Whitcombe et al. 1996), the serine protease inhibitor Kazal type 1 (SPINK1) gene (Witt et al. 2000), the cystic fibrosis transmembrane conductance regulator gene (CFTR) (Cohn et al. 1998; Durie 1998; Sharer et al. 1998), Chymotrypsin C (CTRC) (Rosendahl et al. 2008), the anionic trypsinogen (PRSS2) (Witt et al. 2006), and mutation of keratin 8 gene (Cavestro et al. 2003).

The majority of patients with HP express one of two gain-of-function mutations (R 122H and N291) in the cationic trypsinogen gene (PRSS1 gene) (Antonarakis 1998). These mutations increase autocatalytic conversion of trypsinogen to active trypsin, causing premature intrapancreatic trypsinogen activation, which in turn disturbs the intrapancreatic balance of proteases and their inhibitors with subsequent autodigestive necrosis and inflammation. A transgenic animal model, R122H, which reveales histological lesions similar to those typically seen in human CP underlines the significance of PRSS1 mutations (Archer et al. 2006). In contrast, A16V-PRSS1 mutation is associated with idiopathic pancreatitis.

If one considers intrapancreatic trypsin activation to be the beginning of pancreatitis (see Chapter 1), SPINK1 was an obvious candidate gene. SPINK1 is a strong antiprotease capable of temporarily hampering intrapancreatic trypsin activity. SPINK1 mutations could lead to a loss-of-function thereby resulting in elevated trypsin levels within the pancreas (Witt et al. 2007). However, since in the normal pancreas the trypsin inhibition by SPINK1 is only temporary and results in rapid degradation of SPINK1 by trypsin itself with restoration of normal trypsin activity, the pathogenetic role of SPINK1 mutations remains enigmatic (Kiraly et al. 2007).

The aetiological link between CP and cystic fibrosis was supported by several observations: 1.24% of patients developed CP with exocrine and endocrine insufficiency, and both diseases may be accompanied by abnormal sweat chloride concentration and pancreatic duct obstruction. At least one CFTR mutation has been found in 20%–25% of patients with idiopathic CP. CFTR is an integral membrane protein found in the apical membrane of chloride secretory epithelial cells that, within the pancreas, are localized to centroacinar and proximal duct and regulate ductal bicarbonate secretion (Denning et al. 1992). To date, the role of the CFTR mutations in the pathogenesis of chronic pancreatitis is unclear. Although initial reports suggested that idiopathic CP was associated with a single allelic mutation of CFTR, recent evidence suggests that patients with CP are mixed heterozygous for CFTR mutations or transheterozygous (CFTR and SPINK1 mutation), emphasizing the importance of mutation combinations or the association with other cofactors, like alcohol or autoimmunity (Audrezet et al. 2002; Teich and Mossner 2008). More than 1500 mutations of the CFTR gene have been described, yet of these only 1%–2% of patients with cystic fibrosis develop CP.

Recently, two chymotrypsin C (CTRC) variants have been associated not only with hereditary and idiopathic but also with alcoholic and tropical pancreatitis. The detected mutations are loss-of-function mutations leading to reduced trypsin-degrading activity (Rosendahl et al. 2008). Although PRSS2 mutations were thought to enhance the risk of CP, a recent study indicated that G191R PRSS2 variants may be a protective factor against CP, mitigating intrapancreatic trypsin activity (Witt et al. 2006). Mutations of keratin 8 interfering with normal filament reorganization and the related regulation of pancreatic exocrine homeostasis have been reported in patients with CP from Italy (Cavestro et al. 2003). However, the same mutations were not confirmed in a population from the United States (Schneider et al. 2006).

13.3.1 Pathology

The pathological features of HP are considered to be similar to those of alcoholic CP, with frequent presence of complications such as pseudocysts (Konzen et al. 1993). However, the distinct pathological findings have not been reported in adequate detail. Most of the resected cases displayed advanced chronic pancreatitis with massively dilated ducts containing protein plugs and calculi (personal observation) (Figs. 13.13 and 13.14). The fibrosis showed a periductal and interlobular pattern. In one case there was ductal necrosis in some of the medium-sized interlobular ducts that destroyed the duct epithelium and led to an intense chronic inflammatory reaction in the periductal area. This finding suggests that the autodigestive process in hereditary chronic pancreatitis may occur in the duct lumen, resulting initially in necrosis of the duct-lining cells and subsequently affecting the surrounding interstitial tissue. A possible hypothesis is that the relapsing autodigestive necrosis occurs particularly in the large ducts and gradually induces scarring of the surrounding interstitial tissue with subsequent dilatation of the involved duct segments. In addition, there may also be necrotic events in the interlobular areas resulting in interlobular fibrosis. The calculi found in the dilated ducts are probably a result of the obstructed flow of pancreatic secretions, which promotes the precipitation of calcium from the pancreatic juice.

Cystic fibrosis was initially considered a primary disease of the pancreas characterized by cysts filled with viscid mucous and fibrous atrophy of the exocrine pancreas (Fig. 13.15a,b). The term mucoviscidosis indicated that the disease is systemic and characterized by abnormal mucous secretion. Subsequently, the sweat electrolyte abnormalities were discovered. The disease is now recognized as resulting from mutations of CFTR, and the pathogenesis has been clarified. The early histological lesion is recognized in the acinar tissue and is essentially characterized by increased luminal volume of the acinar and intralobular ducts (Fig. 13.16). The intraluminal eosinophilic secretion was considered for a long time to be a mucous substance because of its PAS positivity (intraluminal mucous plugging). This led to the conclusion that hypersecretion of viscid mucus leads to duct obstruction with subsequent cystic dilatation and eventually surrounding parenchymal atrophy. Ultrastructural and immu-

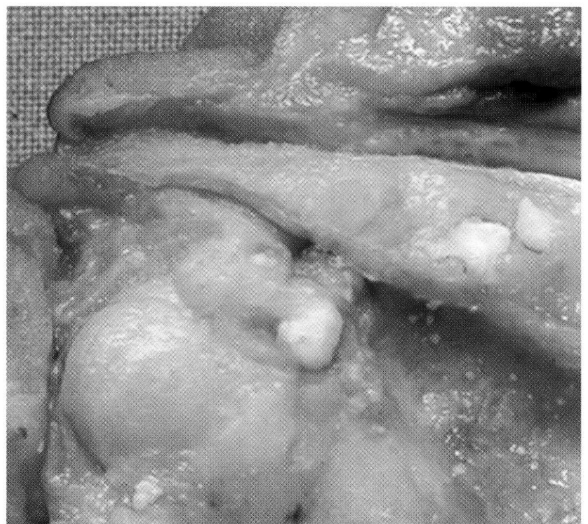

Fig. 13.13. Hereditary chronic pancreatitis (SPINK1-mutation): severe fibrosis of the head of the pancreas with multiple calculi and marked dilatation of the main pancreatic duct

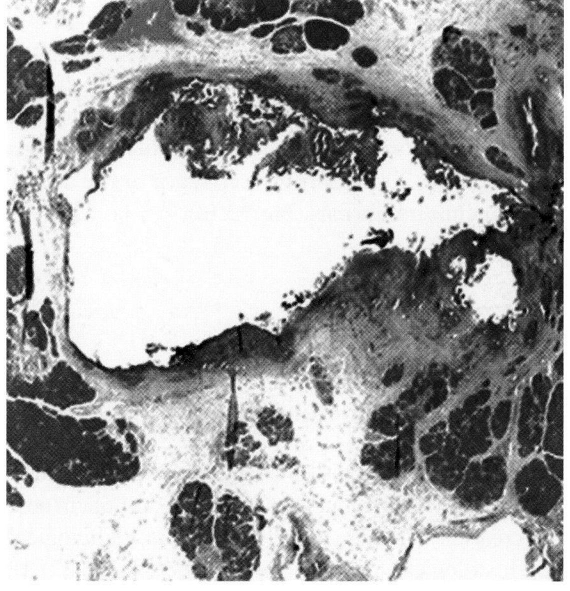

Fig. 13.14. Hereditary chronic pancreatitis (SPINK1-mutation): histological macrosection showing a dilated main pancreatic duct containing a calcified calculus with epithelial denudation and severe parenchymal fibrosis and widely separated acinar lobuli

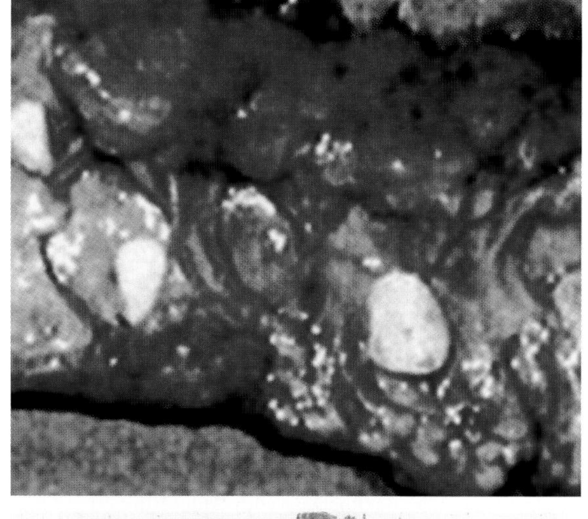

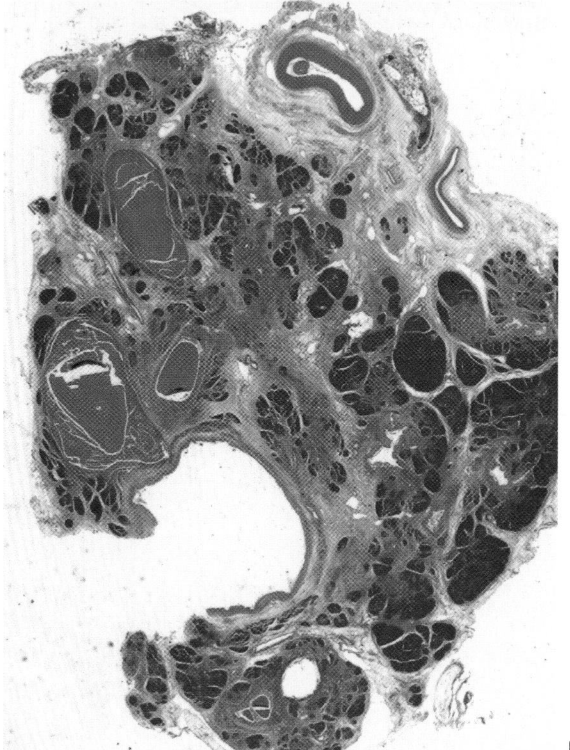

Fig. 13.15a,b. Hereditary chronic pancreatitis (CFTR-mutation): marked dilated main pancreatic duct containing multiple white calculi (**a**). Histological macrosection showing multiple dilated ducts with eosinophilic bodies, moderate fibrosis with partial conservation of the lobular architecture (**b**)

nohistochemical studies demonstrated that early intraluminal plugs are composed of zymogen material rather than mucus, and that the intracystic concretions have the same staining pattern as the zymogen secretions. Ultrastructurally, they have a concentric fibrillar structure similar to acinar plugs and correspond to the eosinophilic, laminated, PAS-negative or only weakly positive deposits seen on light microscopy (Fig. 13.17a). These findings fit the molecular pathology of cystic fibrosis: CFTR appears to be expressed in the apical plasma membrane of chloride-secreting centroacinar cells and

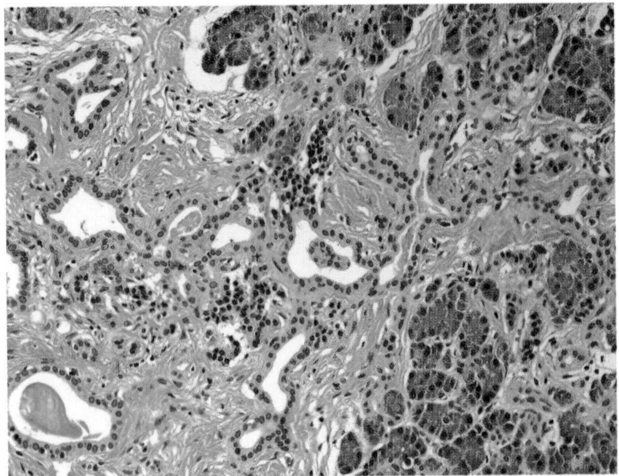

Fig. 13.16. Hereditary chronic pancreatitis (CFTR-mutation): intralobular duct ectasia with "ductulinization" and intraluminal precipitation of eosinophilic material

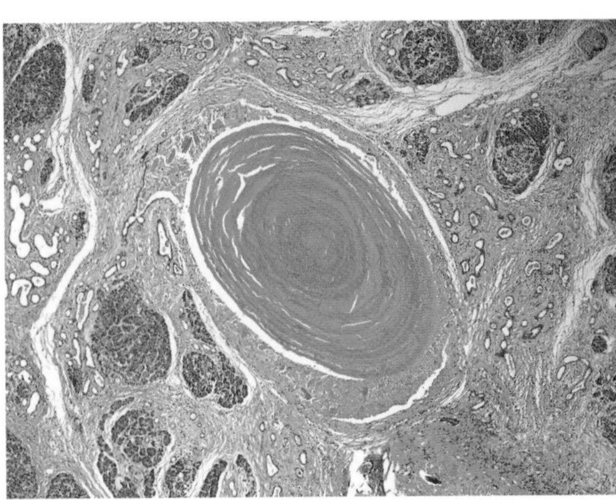

Fig. 13.18. Hereditary chronic pancreatitis (CFTR-mutation): intraductal eosinophilic plug with concentric laminated structure, periductal and intralobular fibrosis, acinar atrophy, and ductular ectasia with multiple eosinophilic precipitates

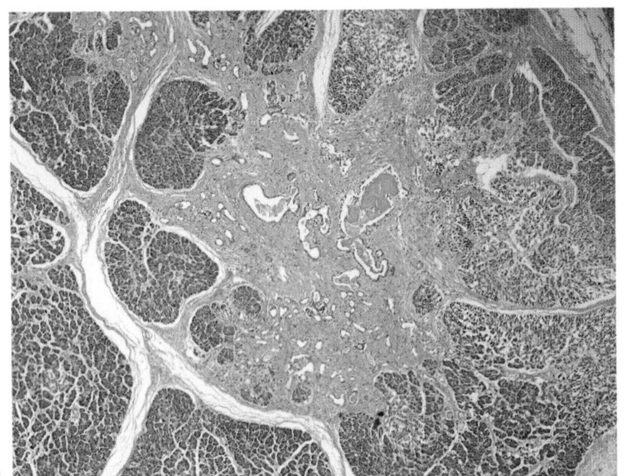

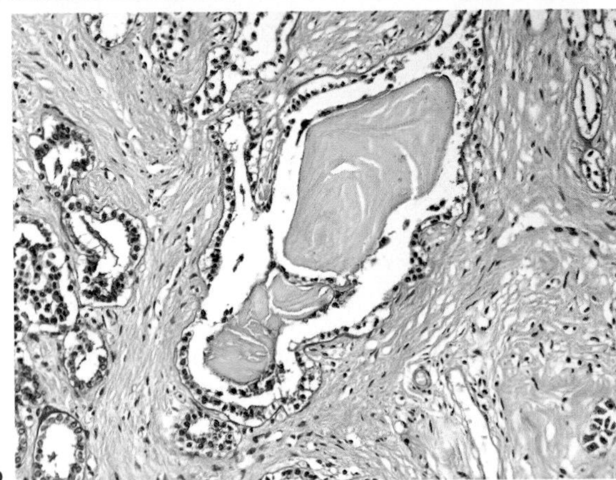

Fig. 13.17a,b. Hereditary chronic pancreatitis (CFTR-mutation): moderate intralobular fibrosis with increasingly dilated ductules with multiple globular intraluminal eosinophilic material (**a**). The intralobular ductules show PAS-positive cells (focal mucinous metaplasia), whereas, the PAS-negative intraluminal precipitate in the central duct shows a peripheral rim of PAS-positive mucoid material (**b**)

intralobular duct cells. The alteration of CFTR results in a chloride-secretion defect with inadequate hydration and inspissation of zymogen secretions. Mucinous metaplasia of centroacinar and ductular cells follows (Fig. 13.17b) leading to progressive duct obstruction and destruction (Iwasa et al. 2001; Tucker et al. 2003), atrophic changes in the acinar component and fibrosis (Fig. 13.18).

13.4 Autoimmune Pancreatitis

Autoimmune pancreatitis (AIP) represents a distinct and increasingly frequently detected form of chronic pancreatitis with characteristic clinical, radiological and histological features (Zamboni et al. 2004). AIP is now considered the pancreatic manifestation of a systemic fibroinflammatory disease in which affected extrapancreatic organs also demonstrate a lymphoplasmacytic infiltration with abundant IgG4-positive plasma cells (Kamisawa et al. 2003b). The first cases of AIP were probably observed by Ball and Sarles, who described them using the terms chronic interstitial pancreatitis and primary inflammatory sclerosis, associated respectively with ulcerative colitis (Ball et al. 1950) and hypergammaglobulinemia (Sarles et al. 1961). The disease was later referred to by various names, depending on whether it was studied by pathologists, clinicians, or radiologists. The most widely used names are chronic sclerosing pancreatitis (Sood et al. 1995), lymphoplasmacytic sclerosing pancreatitis (Kawaguchi et al. 1991), duct-destructive chronic pancreatitis (Ectors et al. 1997), tumor-forming pancreatitis (Takase and Suda 2001) and mass-forming pancreatitis (Yamaguchi et al. 1996). The name autoimmune pancreatitis has the advantage of being simple and suggestive of the aetiology (Yoshida et al. 1995), although it is apparent that autoimmune pancreatitis is a heterogeneous disease (Deshpande et al. 2006; Zamboni et al. 2004).

Clinically, it can present with either the classical symptoms of acute or severe pancreatitis or can produce a mass-like lesion that frequently simulates a carcinoma clinically and radiologically (Cavallini and Frulloni 2001; Pearson et al. 2003). Pathologically, it is characterized by a mixed inflammatory cell infiltrate centered on the pancreatic ducts and small periductal veins.

In around 40% of patients a peculiar granulocytic infiltration of the epithelial duct has been reported that was termed "granulocytic epithelial lesion" (GEL) (Zamboni et al. 2004). Two main subtypes with differing clinicopathological features can be distinguished: one called lymphoplasmacytic sclerosing pancreatitis (Notohara et al. 2003), lobulocentric (Deshpande et al. 2005a), or GEL-negative pancreatitis (Zamboni et al. 2004), the other ductocentric (Notohara et al. 2003; Deshpande et al. 2005a) or GEL-positive pancreatitis (Zamboni et al. 2004). GEL-positive patients had a mean age of 40.5 years, an almost equal male-female ratio and a high coincidence of ulcerative colitis or Crohn's disease, whereas patients without GELs were older (mean age 64 years), showed a male preponderance, commonly had Sjögren's syndrome and often developed recurrent bile-duct stenosis (Zamboni et al. 2004).

Although many reported immunological and genetic anomalies suggest that autoimmune mechanisms may be involved, the pathogenesis remain largely unknown. Typical immunological abnormalities are increased levels of serum γ-globulin, IgG, IgG4 and the presence of autoantibodies (antinuclear, antilactoferrin, anticarbonic anhydrase-II). In patients with a high level of IgG4 serum concentration and/or dense IgG4-positive lymphoplasmacytic infiltration, IgG4 has been suggested to play a major role in the pathogenesis. The presence of granular deposits containing IgG4 in renal tubular basal membranes in patients with AIP might suggest an immune complex-mediated disease (Deshpande et al. 2006).

So far, several risk factors have been implicated, including the HLA DRB1*0405-DQB1*0401 haplotype (Kawa et al. 2002) and polymorphisms of the Fc receptor-like gene 3 (FCRL3), which lies outside the major histocompatibility complex region (Kawa et al. 2002). The lymphocytic infiltration includes predominantly CD4 or CD8 T lymphocytes. Th1-type CD4+ T cells have been reported to be increased in the peripheral blood of AIP patients in Japan (Okazaki et al. 2000). Recently, great interest has focused on factors regulating T-cell function as well as the switching of B cells to IgG4-producing plasma cells in the development of AIP. A possible candidate associated with an increased risk for various autoimmune diseases is the inhibitory molecule cytotoxic T-lymphocyte antigen 4 (CTLA4; CD152) expressed on the cell surface of activated memory T cells and on CD4+CD25+ regulatory T cells, which acts largely as a negative regulator of the T-cell response (Gough et al. 2005). Although CTLA4+6230SNP polymorphism may be functionally linked to AIP, it has been reported to play a role in both susceptibility to and protection from AIP (Chang et al. 2007; Umemura et al. 2008). Circulating CD4+CD25+ T lymphocytes have been reported to be increased in the peripheral blood of patients with AIP in comparison with both healthy people and other types of CP (Miyoshi et al. 2008). There is no direct evidence of increased pancreatic infiltration of these CD4+CD25+ T lymphocytes, but there is agreement that in many autoimmune diseases there is an increased recruitment at inflammatory sites. Therefore, the increased circulating CD4+CD25+ T lymphocytes may correlate with IL-10 at the local sites of the pancreas and extrapancreatic lesions (Zen et al. 2007), which might influence the switching of B cells to IgG4-producing plasma cells and the production of serum IgG4 (Miyoshi et al. 2008). Interestingly, in Mikulicz's disease, another IgG4-related disease characterized by bilateral lacrimal and salivary gland swelling, some clonally related IgG4 positive cells exist between lacrimal glands and the peripheral blood. This may be important for the understanding of the multiple organ involvement of an IgG4-related disease (Yamada et al. 2008). The disease-specific antigen resulting in activation of both Th-1-type lymphocytes and CD4+CD25+ suppressing Th-2 type immune cells remains to be clarified. Pancreatic secretory trypsin inhibitor (PSTI), lactoferrin (LF) and carbonic anhydrase-II (CA) could be candidates for target antigens in AIP, because they are demonstrated in the commonly involved organs, such as the pancreas, biliary tree, salivary glands, gastrointestinal tract and distal renal tubules. Anti-CA-II and anti- PSTI autoantibodies are frequently detected in patients with AIP (Asada et al. 2006; Frulloni et al. 2000).

13.4.1 Macroscopy

Macroscopically, AIP may appear either focal or diffuse; in a few cases the lesions can be multifocal. In most cases the focal type involves the head of the pancreas and resemble pancreatic or terminal bile duct carcinoma. In both cases, the lesions are typically ill-defined and narrow the pancreatic duct, which, contrary to the usual situation in ACP, is neither dilated nor contains calculi. If duct dilatation or calculi occur, they do so late in the course of the disease (Hamano et al. 2001). Stenosis and narrowing of the terminal bile duct are frequently seen. In a minority of cases the inflammatory process is concentrated in the body or tail of the pancreas or can diffusely involve the entire pancreas, mimicking a pancreatic lymphoma. In contrast to other types of chronic pancreatitis, such as ACP, hereditary pancreatitis and tropical pancreatitis, there are no pseudocysts. Both the reduced vascularization of the involved pancreatic area and its increase in size give it a neoplastic appearance (Procacci et al. 2001).

13.4.2 Microscopy

The microscopic features of AIP are dominated by an intense inflammatory cell infiltration consisting mainly of lymphocytes, plasma cells and macrophages, which characteristically show a periductal distribution, causing periductal fibrosis, ductal distortion and obstruction (Fig. 13.19). In many case, intermingled with the lymphocytes there is an acute inflammatory component, which constitutes the "granulocytic-epithelial" lesions (GELs) (Zamboni et al. 2004) (Fig. 13.20). Characteristic of the GELs is invasion of the ductal structures by neutrophilic granulocytes, with detachment, disruption and destruction of the duct epithelium. Sometimes the eosinophilic component is conspicuous (Abraham et al. 2003b). The process affects the main and secondary pancreatic ducts and frequently the distal bile duct.

The extension and severity of the chronic and acute changes in AIP vary from case to case and even from one area to another within a single case. Four grade of severity have been proposed that take into account the distribution and intensity of inflammatory infiltration, fibrosis, duct distortion and destruction, the presence of lymphoid follicles and vasculitis (Table 13.2) (Zamboni et al. 2004).

In the early stages, grade 1 and grade 2, when the pancreatic parenchyma is only slightly affected, the inflammatory infiltration focuses almost entirely on the ducts, which show mild periductal fibrosis and duct obliteration, whereas the acinar cells are only focally affected (Fig. 13.21). Grade 1–2 AIP may only rarely cause clinical symptoms (e.g. pain and jaundice) of such intensity that they become an indication for resection. In advanced stages (grade 3 and grade 4), the diffuse periductal lymphoplasmacytic infiltrates are associated with severe periductal fibrosis, duct obstruction and eventually duct destruction. The fibroinflammatory process extends to the interlobular and intralobular ducts as well as to the acinar component which progressively atrophy and are replaced by fibrosis (Fig. 13.22). At this stage, venulitis is always found (Fig. 13.23), and the lymphoid follicles may be diffusely scattered throughout the lesion (Fig. 13.24). Grade 3–4 is present in 90% of resected cases of AIP. Another characteristic finding is the patchy distribution of the fibroinflammatory process, with variable involvement of lobules.

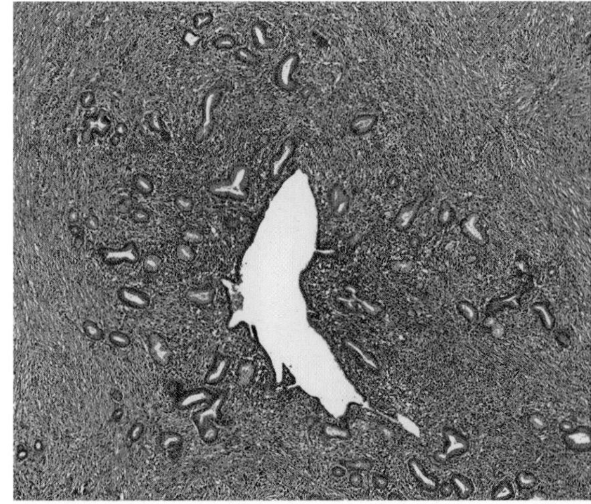

Fig. 13.19. Autoimmune pancreatitis (AIP): Periductal fibrosis and inflammatory cell infiltration, characterized by lymphocytes, plasma cells and macrophages, causing ductal distortion

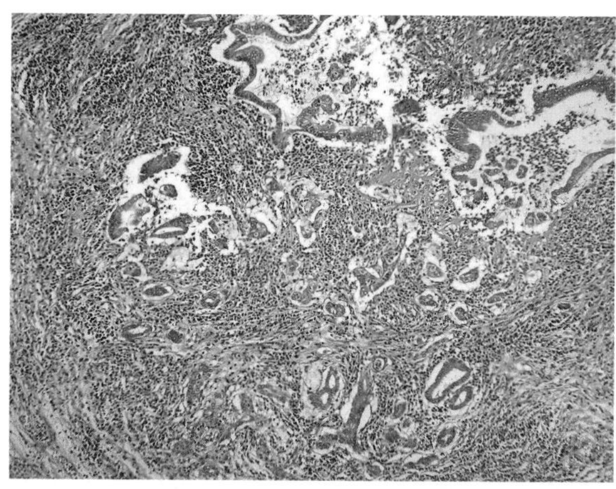

Fig. 13.20. Autoimmune pancreatitis (AIP): granulocytic-epithelial lesion (GEL), characterized by the invasion of the ductal structures by neutrophilic granulocytes, with detachment, disruption and destruction of the duct epithelium

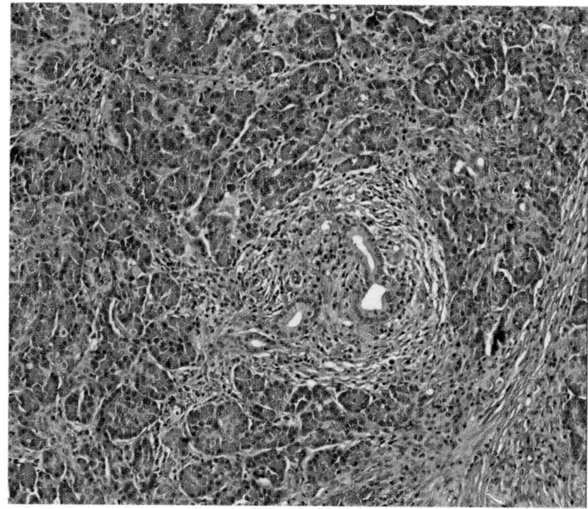

Fig. 13.21. Autoimmune pancreatitis (AIP): grade 1–2, with mild periductal inflammatory infiltration and fibrosis, whereas the acinar component is well preserved

Table 13.2. Grades of severity of AIP

Grade 1	Scattered periductal lymphoplasmacytic infiltrates; mild duct obliteration; almost no interlobular and acinar involvement
Grade 2	Multiple periductal lymphoplasmacytic infiltrates; mild periductal fibrosis and duct obliteration; mild interlobular and acinar involvement; focal inflammatory storiform fibrosis; occasional, mild venulitis
Grade 3	Diffuse periductal lymphoplasmacytic infiltrates; marked periductal fibrosis and duct obstruction; moderate interlobular and acinar involvement; moderate focal inflammatory storiform fibrosis; frequent venulitis; scattered lymphoid follicles
Grade 4	Diffuse periductal lymphoplasmacytic infiltrates; severe periductal fibrosis and duct obstruction/disappearance; severe interlobular and acinar involvement; severe inflammatory storiform fibrosis and diffuse sclerosis; frequent venulitis and occasional arteritis; scattered and occasionally prominent lymphoid follicles

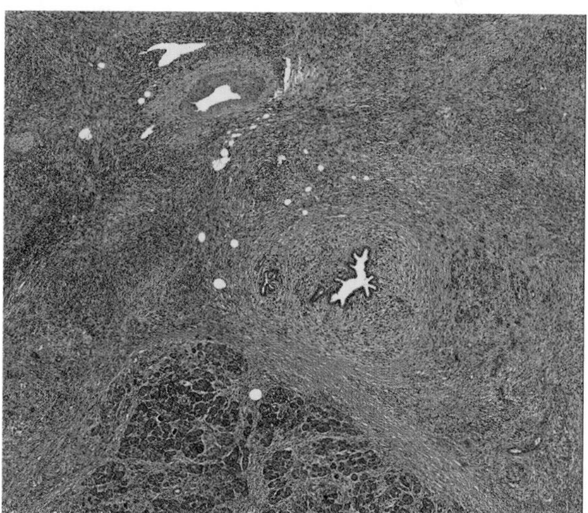

Fig. 13.22. Autoimmune pancreatitis (AIP): grade 3, with marked periductal lymphoplasmacytic infiltrates, associated to severe periductal fibrosis, duct obstruction and extension to the interlobular and intralobular ducts as well as to the acinar component. Presence of venulitis

A special type of fibrosis with storiform pattern, present in about half of the patients, is characterized by the presence of inflammatory cells and plump myofibroblasts (PSCs) intermingled with collagen bundles (Fig. 13.25). Less frequently, the storiform fibrosis occupies a large area, mimicking a fibroinflammatory pseudotumor. The stellate cells express smooth muscle actin (activated SPCs) (Fig. 13.26), whereas most of the intermingled mononuclear cells are CD68+ macrophages, T lymphocytes and plasma cells do not. Scattered HLA-DR expression is seen in duct cells, endothelial cells, inflammatory cells and myofibroblastic cells. The inflammatory process is usually well demarcated from the surrounding peripancreatic fatty tissue and only occasionally shows some small tongue-like extensions.

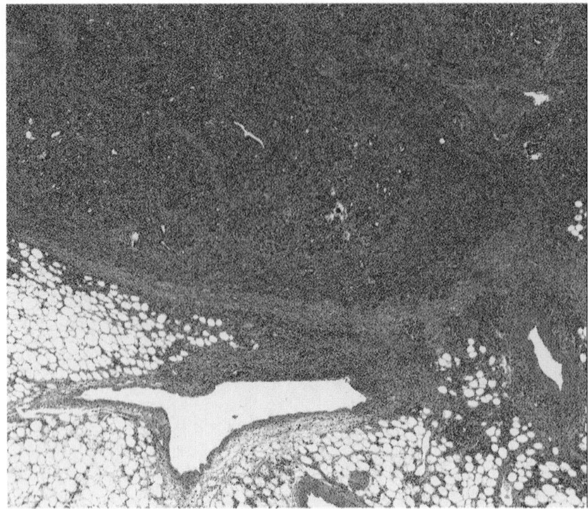

Fig. 13.23. Autoimmune pancreatitis (AIP): grade 3, extensive intralobular inflammatory infiltration sub sub-total acinar atrophy and presence of venulitis

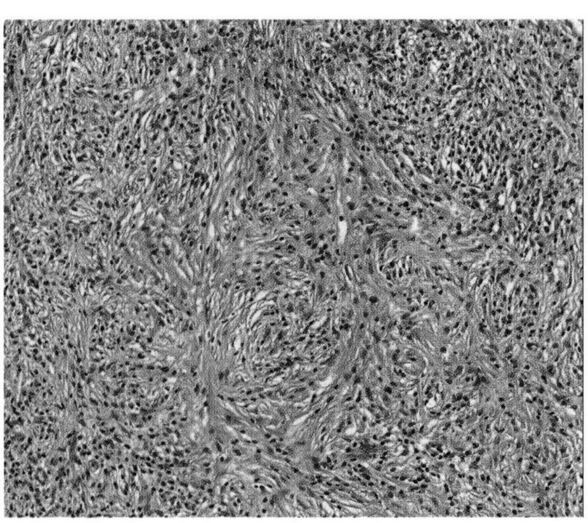

Fig. 13.25. Autoimmune pancreatitis (AIP): grade 4, severe atrophy with storiform fibrosis, characterized by myofibroblast mixed with inflammatory cells

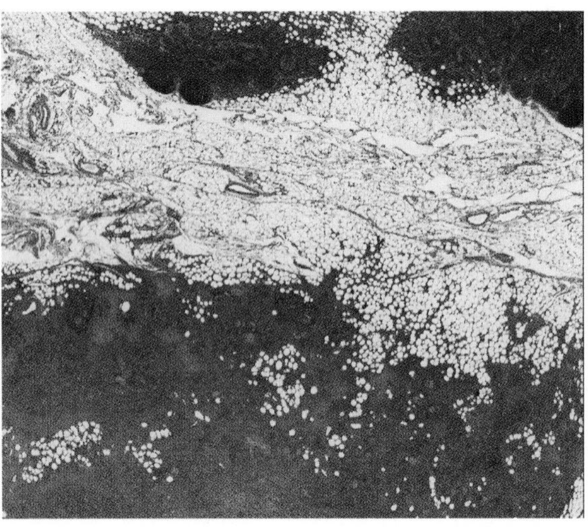

Fig. 13.24. Autoimmune pancreatitis (AIP): grade 4, severe lobular atrophy with fibrosis and diffuse presence of lymphoid follicles, within and outside the pancreatic parenchyma

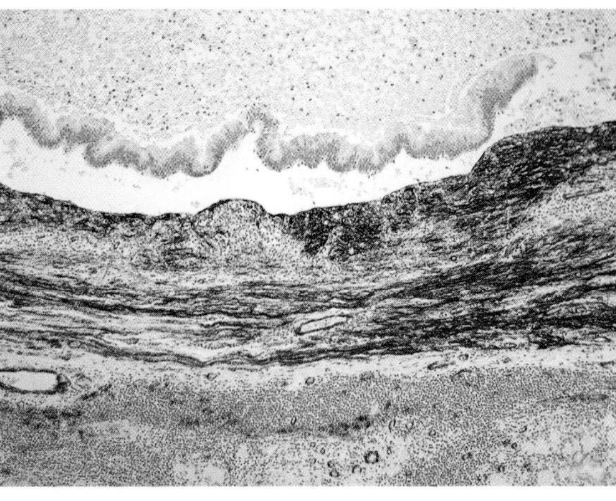

Fig. 13.26. Autoimmune pancreatitis (AIP): periductal myofibroblastic proliferation (activated stellate cells), smooth muscle actin-positive

The peripancreatic lymph nodes are enlarged and show follicular hyperplasia. If the inflammatory process affects the head of the gland (as in approximately 80% of the cases), it usually also involves the distal common bile duct, where it leads to a marked thickening of the bile duct wall due to a diffuse lymphoplasmacytic infiltration combined with fibrosis (Zen et al. 2004). In about 25% of cases the inflammation also extends to the gallbladder and biliary tree (Abraham et al. 2003a).

Immunohistochemical typing of the lymphocytes reveals a predominance of CD3+, CD4+ and CD8+ T lymphocytes in the inflammatory infiltrates surrounding the medium-sized and large interlobular ducts, with occasional invasion of the duct epithelium. The CD2O+ B lymphocytes are sparse or aggregate to form lymphoid follicles, which are found either scattered in sclerotic tissue or around ducts.

The most relevant and important feature is the increased number of IgG4-positive plasma cells

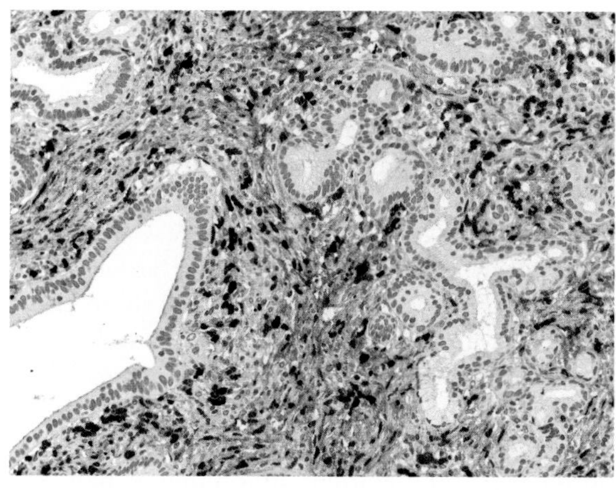

Fig. 13.27. Autoimmune pancreatitis (AIP): dense, periductal and intralobular infiltration of IgG4-positive plasma cells

reported in the majority of cases (Fig. 13.27). IgG4 levels have been proposed as a useful tool in the differential diagnosis of pancreatic masses; IgG4 levels are low in pancreatic carcinoma and chronic obstructive or biliary pancreatitis and high in AIP (Hirano et al. 2004, 2006). The diagnostic significance of IgG4 positivity depends mainly on the cut-off level used. Kojima et al. reported a sensitivity of 43% and specificity of 100% for more than 20 IgG4-positive cells at a magnification of ×40 (Kojima et al. 2007). With a cut-off of more than 10 IgG4-positive cells per HPF the sensitivity was 72% and the specificity 88% (Zhang et al. 2007), whereas Deshpande reported 76% sensitivity and 70% specificity for more than 10 IgG4-positive cells at a magnification of ×20 (Deshpande et al. 2006).

13.4.3 Extrapancreatic Involvement

Autoimmune pancreatitis is part of a systemic disease that may involve many organs. All of these manifestations show similar lymphoplasmacytic infiltration, fibrosclerosis and frequently dense IgG4-positive cell infiltration. For this reason Kamisawa suggested the term IgG4-related systemic disease (Kamisawa et al. 2003b). The recognition of this extrapancreatic involvement is of great importance in the diagnosis of so called "mass-forming pancreatitis" (Yamaguchi et al. 1996). The biliary tree is involved in about 70% of cases, with intra- or extrahepatic sclerosing cholangitis mimicking a cholangiocarcinoma or primary sclerosing cholangitis (Fig. 13.28). The number of associated conditions recognized has increased immensely and includes ulcerative colitis, Crohn's disease, primary sclerosing cholangitis (Kamisawa et al. 2006; Kawamura et al. 2007; Mendes et al. 2006; Okazaki 2007; Prasad et al. 2004), lymphoplasmacytic cholecystitis (Abraham et al. 2003a), primary biliary cirrhosis (Hastier et al. 1998), Sjogren's syndrome (Etemad and Whitcomb 2001; Kamisawa et al. 2003a), chronic sclerosing sialoadenitis resembling Mikulicz's disease (Dooreck et al. 2004; Yamada et al. 2008), thyroiditis (Merino et al. 2004), the family of tumor-like lesions known as multifocal idiopathic fibrosclerosis, including mediastinal and retroperitoneal fibrosis, Riedel's thyroiditis, and inflammatory pseudotumor of the orbit (Bartholomew et al. 1963; Chutaputti et al. 1995; Comings et al. 1967; Levey and Mathai 1998; Renner et al. 1980; Uchida et al. 2003), tubulointerstitial nephritis (Nishi et al. 2007;Takeda et al. 2004; Uchiyma-Tanaka et al. 2004), interstitial pneumonia (Taniguchi et al. 2004), lymphadenopathy (Cheuk et al. 2008), prostatitis (Yoshimura et al. 2006) and inflammatory abdominal aortic aneurysm (Sakata et al. 2008).

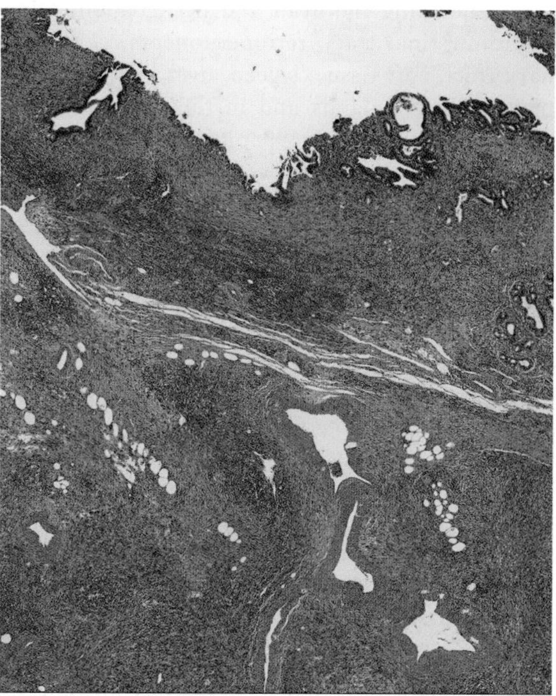

Fig. 13.28. Autoimmune pancreatitis (AIP): extrapancreatic bile duct involvement. The fibroinflammatory infiltrate is similar to that present in the pancreatic tissue (*lower part*)

Steroid therapy not only improves the pancreatic lesions but also significantly decreases the IgG4 levels (Aoki et al. 2005; Hamano et al. 2001).

13.4.4 Relationship to Inflammatory Pseudotumor

Inflammatory pseudotumor (IP) usually presents as a mass-forming lesion characterized by spindle cell proliferation with a characteristic fibroinflammatory appearance. It has not yet been resolved whether IP is an excessive reactive process (infection-associated inflammatory pseudotumor) or a true neoplasm (neoplastic inflammatory myofibroblastic tumor) (Dehner 2000). The pseudotumoral nature of the lesions can be supported by their clinical, radiological and pathological findings. Clinically, the lesions mimic a neoplastic process, the sign and symptoms depending on the particular site or organ involved, and on the production of cytokines by inflammatory cells. Radiologically, the various procedures, US, CT and MRI, reveal the presence of a suspicious mass indistinguishable from carcinoma or sarcoma. Inflammatory pseudotumor, originally described in the lung, has been subsequently described in many extrapulmonary locations, including the head and neck region, orbit, gastrointestinal tract, retroperitoneum, genitourinary tract, soft tissue, spleen, liver, lymph nodes, major salivary glands and in the submandibular glands (Dehner et al. 1998; Rasanen et al. 1972; Williams et al. 1992). There have been a number of reports of IP of the pancreas using different designations: inflammatory pseudotumors (Casadei et al. 2004; DeRubertis et al. 2004; Esposito et al. 2004; Kroft et al. 1995; Palazzo and Chang 1993; Wreesmann et al. 2001; Zen et al. 2005), fibrous pseudotumor (Zhao et al. 2004), plasma cell granuloma (Abrebanel et al. 1984), inflammatory myofibroblastic tumor (Walsh et al. 1998), localized lymphoplasmacellular pancreatitis (Petter et al. 1998), or lymphoplasmacytic sclerosing pancreatitis (Kawaguchi et al. 1991). All of these cases are characterized, like AIP, by a triad of characteristic histological features: diffuse infiltration by lymphocytes and plasma cells and myofibroblastic proliferation.

Macroscopically, most of the reported cases were solid lesions with diffuse or indistinct mass. They were frequently localized in the head of the pancreas, fibrous in appearance and involved the distal bile duct.

Microscopically, the pancreatic parenchyma is replaced by a proliferation of myofibroblasts with spindle-shaped nuclei and eosinophilic cytoplasm and inflammatory cells consisting mainly of lymphocytes and plasma cells. In some areas fibrosis and atrophy of the parenchyma predominate, in others the inflammatory reaction. Vasculitis and particularly venulitis are frequently present. The fibroinflammatory areas found in AIP share histological features with those described in inflammatory pseudotumors of the pancreas (Palazzo and Chang 1993; Uchida et al. 2003; Walsh et al. 1998; Wreesmann et al. 2001), including the myofibroblastic proliferation. Autoimmune pancreatitis might be regarded as the initiating event in the evolution of IP, in which the fibroinflammatory storiform fibrosis has acquired a tumorlike appearance (Zamboni et al. 2004; Kawaguchi et al. 1991; Petter et al. 1998). Evidence supporting an autoimmune aetiology includes the association of IP with other autoimmune diseases such as Sjogren's syndrome (Eckstein et al. 1995) and sclerosing cholangitis (Jafri et al. 1983), retroperitoneal fibrosis (Chutaputti et al. 1995; Renner et al. 1980; Uchida et al. 2003) and the regression seen in some cases after treatment with corticosteroids (Chutaputti et al. 1995). The finding of an oligoclonal pattern of T cell receptor δ-gene rearrangements suggests that the pathogenesis of both IP and AIP could be related to the development of an intense and self-maintaining immune response, with the emergence of clonal populations of T-lymphocytes (Esposito et al. 2004). The frequent association of AIP with inflammatory pseudotumors involving the common bile duct and liver (Chutaputti et al. 1995; Fukushima et al. 1997; Nonomura et al. 1997) induced some authors to consider all of these lesions to belong to the spectrum of AIP. More recently, a massive infiltration of IgG4-positive plasma cells in IP of many sites, such as the breast, lung and kidney, has been reported (Diakowska et al. 2005; Takeda et al. 2004; Taniguchi et al. 2004; Zen et al. 2004).

13.4.5 Differential Diagnosis

Clinically, radiographically and grossly the disease most commonly mimics pancreatic carcinoma, because it produces a mass predominantly affecting the pancreatic head and the bile duct (Abraham et al. 2003a; HARDACRE et al. 2003; NOTOHARA et al. 2003; WEBER et al. 2003). Histologically, however, it is not difficult to distinguish from ductal adenocarcinoma of the pancreas or other pancreatic malignancies. Fine needle aspiration cytology and core biopsy may confirm the clinically and radiologically suspected diagnosis (ZAMBONI et al. 2004; BANG et al. 2008; DESHPANDE et al. 2005b; PEARSON et al. 2003). It is therefore essential to increase our ability to recognize AIP features in cytological smears and in small tissue fragments. Unfortunately, mainly due to the patchy distribution of the lesions, biopsy specimens were diagnostic or suggestive of AIP in only about half of the patients. The biopsy diagnosis of AIP relies on its specific features, i.e. lymphoplasmacellular infiltration, especially around ducts, granulocytic infiltration with GELs and venulitis. However, the presence of highly cellular stroma characterized by myofibroblastic proliferation and lymphoplasmacellular infiltration, in the appropriate clinical context, can help establish a preoperative diagnosis of AIP. In addition, the presence of abundant IgG4-positive cells has to be considered together with the other morphological features of AIP present in the core biopsy specimen and coupled with a high IgG4 serum level (BANG et al. 2008; KAMISAWA et al. 2003b).

The association between AIP and pancreatic cancer is still largely unknown. To date only a few cases have been reported. Long-term studies on large cohorts of AIP patients are needed to determine whether AIP predisposes to the subsequent development of pancreatic carcinoma. This may be difficult to prove, because cancer typically occurs decades after the onset of chronic pancreatitis and AIP occurs in older men who are likely to die of comorbid conditions before such a complication develops (YAMADA et al. 2008; FUKUI et al. 2008; GHAZALE and CHARI 2007).

AIP has to be distinguished from alcoholic chronic pancreatitis. Autoimmune pancreatitis almost consistently lacks the features that are common in alcoholic chronic pancreatitis: calculi, dilated and tortuous ducts, pseudocyst formation and areas of fat necrosis. Histologically, alcoholic chronic pancreatitis lacks the dense periductal lymphoplasmacytic infiltration, the obliterative venulitis, the often diffuse fibrosis and the common inflammatory involvement of the bile duct. The immunohistochemical evidence of dense, periductal IgG4-positive plasma cells can rule out alcoholic chronic pancreatitis (KOJIMA et al. 2007).

13.5 Paraduodenal Pancreatitis and Cysts of the Duodenal Wall

Duodenal involvement is frequently observed in the typical long clinical course of chronic pancreatitis, and duodenal stenosis is a well known complication in a proportion of cases ranging from 19.6% (STOLTE et al. 1982) to 31% (BECKER and MISCHKE 1991). Much less well known is the occurrence of pancreatitis related cysts within the duodenal wall.

Duodenal wall cysts may arise in various situations: enterogenous duplication, retention cysts in Brunner's glands or as the result of pancreatitis in duodenal heterotopic pancreas. The latter possibility, described either as a pure lesion or associated with chronic pancreatitis, has been reported under many different names. In the World Health Organization classification of tumours and tumour-like lesions of the pancreas it was referred as to "para-ampullary duodenal wall cyst" (KLÖPPEL et al. 1996), while POTET and DUCLERT (1970) suggested the term cystic dystrophy of the duodenal wall (CDDW). They described the presence of cysts lined by pancreatic duct-like epithelium or surrounded by inflammatory granulation tissue in ectopic pancreas in the duodenal wall though the histology of the pancreas proper was normal. Subsequently, a frequent association of chronic alcoholic pancreatitis with CDDW was reported (ELOIT et al. 1987; LÉGER et al. 1974; PALAZZOET al. 1992). Thus, two clinicopathological forms of CDDW may be envisaged: a "pure" type, in which only the intraduodenal pancreatic tissue shows pancreatitic changes and the pancreas proper is normal (FEKETE et al. 1996), and a more common type associated with chronic calcific pancreatitis (COLARDELLE et al. 1994). Cystic dystrophy in duodenal heterotopic pancreas was found in 26 of 96 cases reported by MARTIN (1977) and in 17 of 50 cases studied by VANKEMMEL et al. (1975). BECKER (1973) described segmental pancreatitis involving the dorsocranial portion of the pancreas with extension to the region between the C-loop of the duodenum and the head of the pancreas. He used the term "groove" to describe that plane interfacing the two organs that serves as a "bed" for the large vessels, lymph nodes and the common bile duct. All those cases in which the inflammatory and fibrous process involved the "groove" he then called "groove pancreatitis". In "pure" groove pancreatitis the scarring is restricted to the groove without any pancreatic head involvement. In "segmental" groove pancreatitis the scarring involves the dorsocranial portion of the head of the pancreas without any involvement of the main pancreatic duct. In advanced cases more diffuse pancreatic involvement with duct dilatation is present (Becker and Mischke 1991). Although groove pancreatitis represents a heterogeneous group of lesions, i.e. the extension of biliary, gastric or duodenal lesions to the groove, it has many clinical and pathological aspects in common with CDDW, including the extremely high prevalence of duodenal wall cysts (49%) in cases with groove scarring (Becker and Mischke 1991). In the large majority of reported cases, the clinical presentation (pain, vomiting and jaundice), imaging and pathological features overlap in so many important aspects that they may be considered variants of the same disease (Fekete et al. 1996). For these reasons the unifying name "paraduodenal pancreatitis" has been proposed (Adsay and Zamboni 2004).

The knowledge of the clinical and pathological features of this disease allows a preoperative diagnosis that in most cases correctly differentiates it from pancreatic and periampullary neoplasms and may prevent unnecessary surgical resections.

Although sporadic cases have been reported in women (Abraham et al. 2002; Shudo et al. 1998) and in non-alcohol abusers (Colardelle et al. 1994; Fekete et al. 1996), it is important to stress that almost all cases are young or middle-aged men with a history of alcohol abuse.

In comparison to the long clinical course of the typical diffuse form of chronic pancreatitis, in which the symptoms are mainly related to the dilatation of the main duct and the loss of the acinar component, the symptoms of patients with paraduodenal pancreatitis are specifically related to the duodenal wall and groove involvement. Typically, the pain and vomiting have a waxing and waning character. In a proportion of patients the stenosis of the distal common bile duct may be associated with jaundice.

13.5.1 Macroscopy

The large majority of cases present with a stenosis of the second portion of the duodenum. The most characteristic and constant feature is the presence of multiple cysts within a thickened duodenal wall containing clear liquid or in some cases white concretions and stones (Fekete et al. 1996). These cysts, which occur in the submucosa and in the muscularis, may in some cases extend to the "groove" compressing the common bile duct. In the involved areas the duodenal mucosa usually shows nodular appearance, ulcerations and scar retractions.

Macroscopically, two types can be considered. The first is a "cystic" variant characterized by the presence of multiple cysts (Fig. 13.29) with a diameter varying between 1 and 10 cm protruding on the mucosal surface of the periampullary duodenum, which shows a dome-like appearance. The larger cysts might be confused with intestinal duplication. The second is a "solid" variant characterized by a marked thickening of the muscular layer of the duodenal wall, within which cysts less than 1 cm in diameter are found (Fig. 13.30). Both types share a more or less marked thickening of the duodenal wall, more evident at the pancreatic side of the periampullary duodenum, at the level of the papilla minor. The "groove" region (between the dorso-cranial portion of the pancreatic head, the duodenum and the common bile duct) is markedly expanded, either due to the presence of fibrotic tissue or to the extension of the cysts from the duodenal wall, with frequent stenosis of the common bile duct. The severity of the duodenal stenosis and bile duct stenosis depends on the degree of duodenal thickening, the presence and dimension of duodenal wall cysts and the degree of groove involvement. The presence of numerous enlarged peripancreatic lymph nodes is a constant feature of the disease.

The pancreatic parenchyma of the head is normal in the early stages of the disease, whereas at the time of surgery most cases usually show mild to moderate fibrosis. The involvement of the pancreatic parenchyma, in the early stage, affects the dorsocranial portion with obstruction and dilatation of Santorini's duct and spares the remaining pancreatic parenchyma of the head. As the disease progresses all the pancreatic parenchyma is involved.

13.5.2 Microscopy

Histologically, the cysts are localized in the submucosal and muscular layers of the duodenal wall

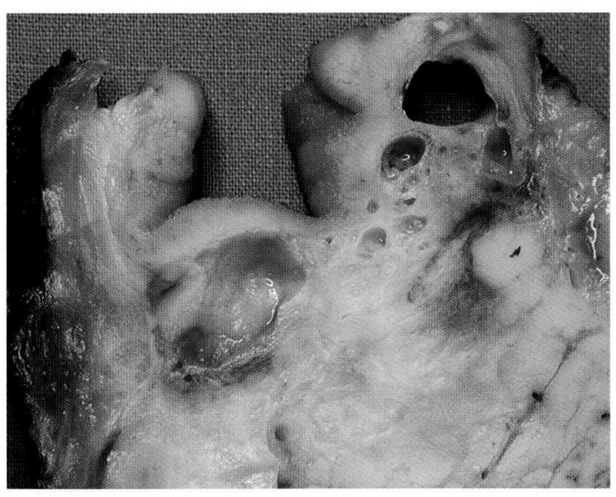

Fig. 13.29. Paraduodenal pancreatitis, cystic-type: multiple cysts in the submucosal layer of the duodenal wall, associated with fibrotic tissue focally extended to the pancreatic parenchyma

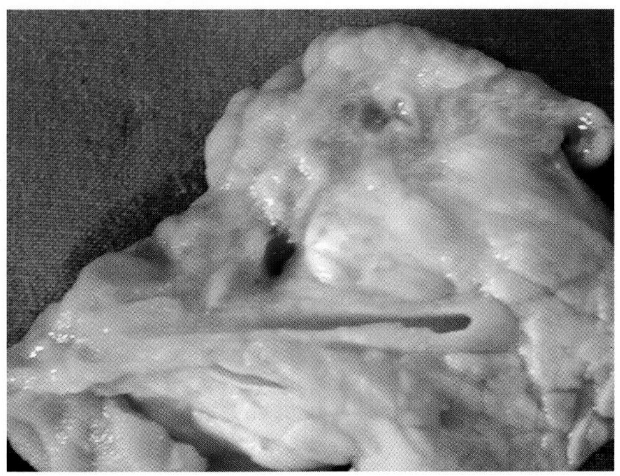

Fig. 13.30. Paraduodenal pancreatitis, solid-type: marked thickening of the muscular layer of the duodenal wall associated with small cysts of less than 1 cm of diameter; the white fibrotic tissue involves the groove region with fibrotic stricture of the terminal common bile duct

(Fig. 13.31), with frequent extension to the "groove" region. The internal surface is mainly lined by columnar pancreatic duct-like epithelium which may be lost and replaced by inflammatory granulation tissue. The duodenum shows Brunner's gland hyperplasia (Fig. 13.32) and variable thickening and disarray of the muscular layer, due to smooth muscle hyperplasia and fibrosis (Fig. 13.33). Heterotopic pancreatic tissue is intimately associated with the cysts either within the muscular layer or in the submucosa. In most cases the "groove" area shows marked fibrosis and chronic inflammation (Fig. 13.34a,b). The pancreatic parenchyma frequently shows fibrosis, an inflammatory reaction and ductal ectasia with calcifications.

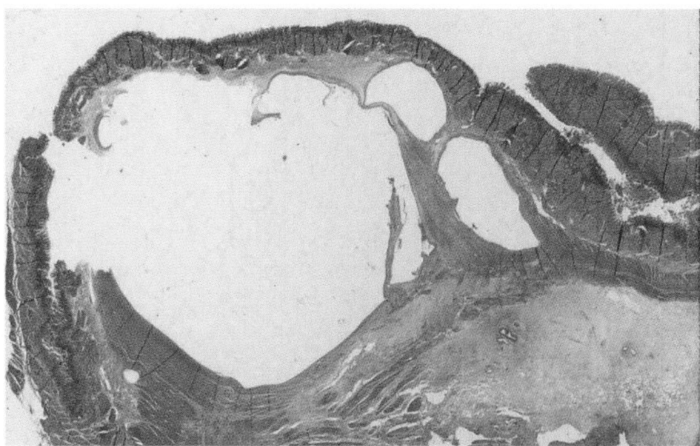

Fig. 13.31. Paraduodenal pancreatitis, cystic-type: multiple submucosal and intramuscular cysts in duodenal wall, associated with fibrotic enlargement of the groove region

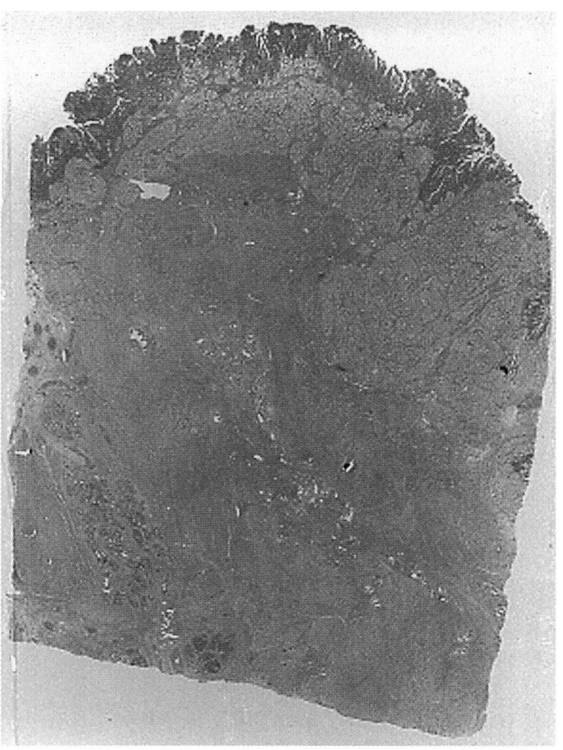

Fig. 13.32. Paraduodenal pancreatitis: histological section showing Brunner's gland hyperplasia with thickening of duodenal wall

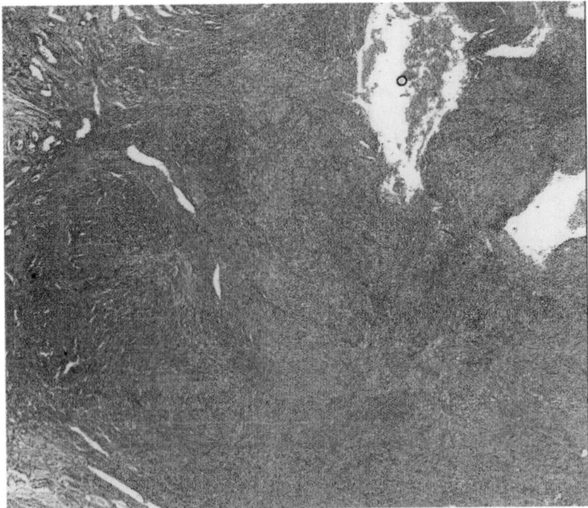

Fig. 13.33. Paraduodenal pancreatitis, solid-type: small cysts lacking epithelial lining, associated with thickening and disarray of the muscular layer

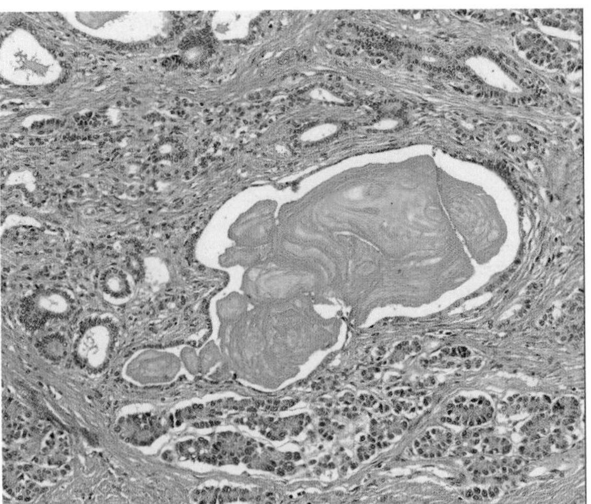

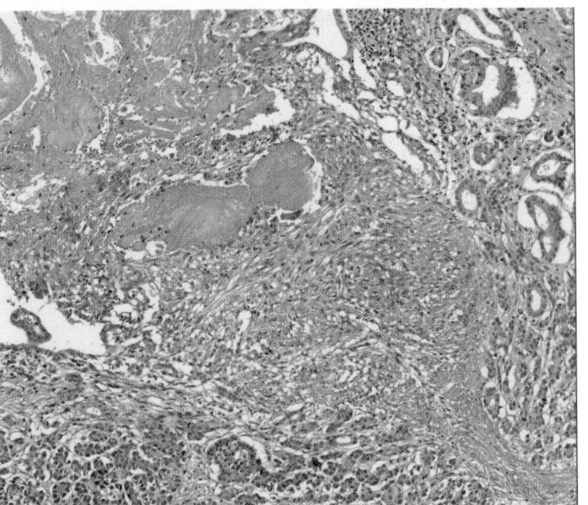

Fig. 13.34a,b. Paraduodenal pancreatitis: intraduodenal pancreas with fibrosis, duct ectasia and intraluminal inspissated eosinophilic secretions (**a**). The eosinophilic secretions, which fill the lumen, partially erode the epithelial lining (**b**)

13.5.3 Differential Diagnosis

The knowledge of the existence of these two variants, solid and cystic, is of practical importance, since only the cystic component is recognized by standard imaging procedures, and most of the solid cases might be misdiagnosed by imaging as ampullary or pancreatic head carcinoma (Procacci et al. 1997).

13.6 Obstructive Chronic Pancreatitis

Obstructive chronic pancreatitis develops upstream from an area in which there is obstruction of the main pancreatic duct or one of the secondary ducts, leading to ductal dilatation, atrophy of the acinar cells and replacement by fibrous tissue. Although it may occasionally present as clinically acute pancreatitis, it is often painless and usually does not present with intraductal and intraparenchymal calculi. There are various possible causes for a duct obstruction, but the most important and common cause is ductal carcinoma in the head of the pancreas occluding the main pancreatic duct (Fig. 13.35). This process leads to a generalized involvement of the gland with interlobular fibrosis, which in long-standing cases is increasingly accompanied by intralobular fibrosis (Fig. 13.36). Other causes include bile duct calculi, sphincter of Oddi dysfunction, tumours and tumour-like lesions of the papilla of Vater, intraductal papillary-mucinous neoplasms, some cystic and endocrine neoplasms, acquired fibrous strictures of the pancreatic ducts, ductal papillary hyperplasia narrowing the duct lumen and finally viscous mucin blocking the duct lumen. The effects of all of these duct obstructing mechanisms can be compared with those of duct ligation in the pancreas (Isaksson et al. 1983). In the early phase after duct ligation the acini are transformed into small ductal (tubular) complexes. In the next step the acinar cells disappear, probably due to apoptosis.

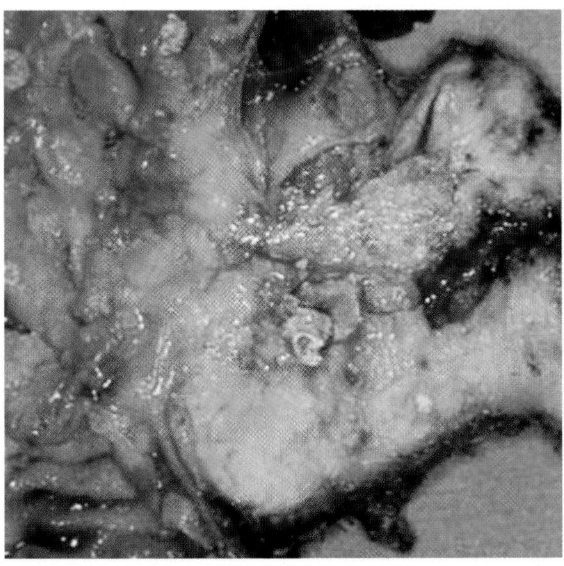

Fig. 13.35. Obstructive pancreatitis: pancreatic head carcinoma with obstruction of the main duct, which show a marked dilatation

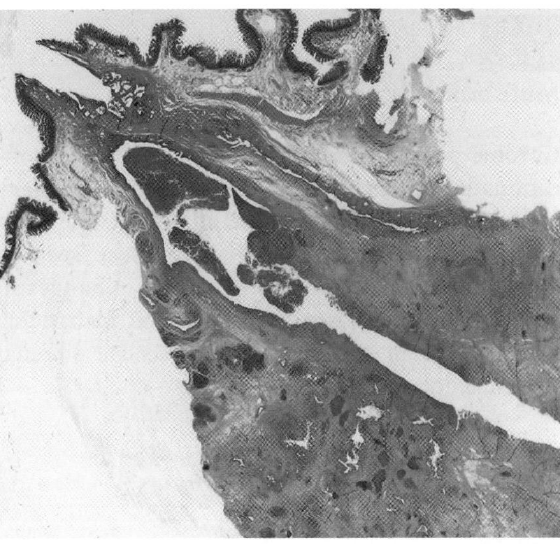

Fig. 13.36. Obstructive pancreatitis: whole mount histological macrosection, showing an intraductal tumor, with main duct and focally branch ducts dilatation, and extensive pancreatic atrophy

These changes are associated with an inflammatory and fibrotic reaction involving macrophages. The macrophages are the potential source of cytokines, which stimulate fibrogenesis by fibroblasts that acquire the properties of myofibroblasts (Klöppel et al. 2004). Because the inflammatory reaction takes place in all of the interlobular and intralobular areas of the pancreatic tissue that were once drained by the occluded duct, fibrosis develops in these regions at the same pace, producing interlobular and intralobular fibrosis in equal distribution.

13.7 Idiopathic Chronic Pancreatitis

The term idiopathic pancreatitis is applied to all those cases of CP in which it was possible to exclude the presence of recognized aetologies of CP occurring in up to 10%–25% of patients despite a careful diagnostic work-up. With the considerable progress made in the understanding the pathogenesis of alcoholic CP and in the hereditary and autoimmune mechanisms underlying the development of chronic pancreatitis, a specific aetiology can be determined in an increasing proportion of cases. The possibility of sharply distinguishing idiopathic CP from hereditary or autoimmune pancreatitis has been challenged by the discovery of several combinations of mutations in various genes. Patients may be transheterozygous for a CFTR alteration and PRSS1 or SPINK1 variants. Two loss-of-function mutations of chymotrypsin C (CTRC) variants leading to reduced trypsin-degrading activity have been associated not only with hereditary pancreatitis but also with idiopathic, alcoholic and tropical pancreatitis (Masson et al. 2008; Rosendahl et al. 2008). An enhanced susceptibility to exogenous noxious agents such as alcohol and smoking, an increased frequency of gene mutations affecting activation or inactivation of SPINK1, CFTR, PRSS1, CTRC function, and an increased disposition to autoimmune reactions may all have a role in the development of idiopathic CP (Keller and Layer 2008).

Two types of idiopathic pancreatitis have been reported, one occurring in young patients and the other in elderly patients (Layer and Keller 2006). Patients with early-onset idiopathic chronic pancreatitis usually have severe pain, but slowly develop morphological and functional pancreatic damage. By contrast, patients with late-onset idiopathic chronic pancreatitis have a milder and often painless course.

Morphologically, there are no systematic studies on this type of pancreatitis; however, calcifications seem to be less frequent than in alcoholic chronic pancreatitis (Ammann and Mullhaupt 2007).

13.8 Metabolic Chronic Pancreatitis

Chronic pancreatitis may be associated with conditions producing hypercalcemia such as primary hyperparathyroidism (Cope et al. 1957). The morphological changes are similar to those seen in alcoholic chronic pancreatitis. Fibrotic changes in the pancreas have also been observed in patients who underwent chronic dialysis because of renal insufficiency.

13.9 Tropical Chronic Pancreatitis

Tropical pancreatitis may be referred to as a type of idiopathic chronic pancreatitis occurring in tropical regions in central Africa, Brazil and southern Asia, especially India. This disease has also been referred to as tropical calculous pancreatitis and, if diabetes is the prevailing symptom, as fibrocalculous pancreatic diabetes. The disease is associated with malnutrition in childhood and usually occurs in adolescents. Recently, it was found that PRSS1, R122H and SPINK1 mutations are associated with tropical pancreatitis and therefore seem to be involved in its aetiopathogenesis (Rossi et al. 2004). Morphologically, tropical pancreatitis has been compared to alcoholic chronic pancreatitis. In its late stages it shows intense inter- and partly also intralobular fibrosis and contains numerous small and larger calculi. Nothing is known so far about the early stages of the disease.

13.10 Pancreatic Fibrosis Not Associated with Symptoms of Chronic Pancreatitis

A special type of duct fibrosis is encountered in cystic fibrosis of the pancreas and in pancreatic lobular fibrosis, which is frequently observed in elderly persons. Whereas the first condition causes duct obstruction due to clogging with viscous mucin, the second condition leads to narrowing of the duct lumen by papillary hyperplasia of the duct epithelium. In cystic fibrosis complete or almost complete (inter- and intralobular) fibrosis develops slowly after birth, which, after many years, is replaced by fatty tissue, a process that is not understood so far, but is of great interest for the resolution of fibrosis (Lack 2003).

In elderly persons the pancreas may contain ducts narrowed by ductal papillary hyperplasia, a lesion that has now been termed pancreatic intraepithelial neoplasia type 1B (PanIN-1B) (Hruban et al. 2004). In association with this lesion there may be patchy lobular fibrosis in the periphery of the pancreas. The fibrosis affects the lobes that are drained by ducts showing PanIN-1B lesions. The extent of this lobular fibrosis varies from person to person; the most severe form and the highest incidence (up to 50%) are found in persons older than 60 years (Detlefsen et al. 2005).

13.11 Complications of Chronic Pancreatitis

In addition to pain, malabsorption and diabetes, as a consequence of parenchymal atrophy (Ammann et al. 1996), in the course of the disease chronic pancreatitis can be associated with a number of local complications, including biliary stricture, duodenal obstruction, formation of pseudocysts and retention cysts, splenic vein thrombosis with spleen infarction, internal pancreatic fistulas, and pancreatic ascites. Chronic pancreatitis has also been reported to be an independent risk factor for the development of pancreatic cancer.

13.11.1 Biliary Stricture

Persistent stenosis of the bile duct develops in approximately 10% of the cases (Cunha et al. 2004; Warshaw 1985). This complication is either due to direct extension of the fibroinflammatory process into the wall of the bile duct, causing permanent obstruction, which can lead to cholangitis and in exceptional cases to biliary cirrhosis, or to the development of a pseudocyst in the head of the pancreas.

13.11.2 Duodenal Stenosis

Although some degree of duodenal stenosis is commonly found in chronic pancreatitis during radiological examination, consistent obstruction is only seen in a minority of cases (CHAUDHARY et al. 2004). The patients have a "head-predominant" type of pancreatitis or in the majority of cases they reveal the characteristics of paraduodenal pancreatitis (ADSAY and ZAMBONI 2004), groove pancreatitis (STOLTE et al. 1982), or cystic dystrophy of duodenal wall (POTET and DUCLERT 1970). Less frequently, stomach and colon obstruction might be observed, as the result of diffusion of necrotic material through the mesocolon.

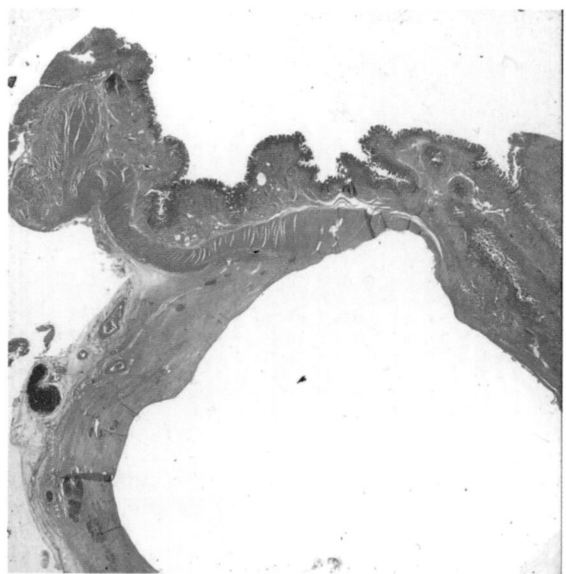

Fig. 13.37. Extra pancreatic pseudocyst

13.11.3 Pseudocysts

Pseudocysts are found in 30%–50% of patients with chronic pancreatitis (AMMANN et al. 1996; KLÖPPEL and MAILLET 1991). The wall is composed of granulation and fibrous tissue and lacks an epithelial lining, and the lumen contains fibrin, necrotic debris and hemorrhagic material (KLÖPPEL and MAILLET 1991). Identical features are observed in pseudocysts associated with acute pancreatitis. Pseudocysts are usually connected with the duct system and therefore rich in pancreatic enzymes. They may expand and exert pressure on the surrounding organs. Inflammatory pseudocysts present as extrapancreatic (usually large) (Fig. 13.37) or intrapancreatic cavities, which may have a thick fibrous capsule lined by inflammatory tissue (Fig. 13.38) and filled with necrotic and haemorrhagic material (KLÖPPEL and MAILLET 1993). The cysts have no internal septations. Calcification in the fibrous capsule is rare but can be preesent.

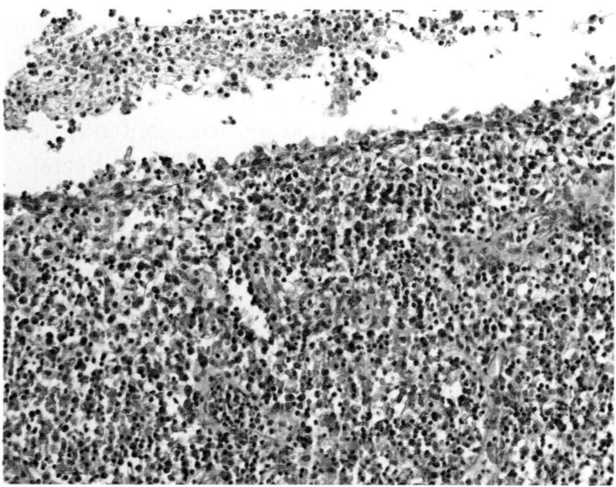

Fig. 13.38. Pseudocyst: a fibrous capsule with dilated blood vessels, lined by inflammatory tissue

13.11.4 Retention Cysts

Retention cysts may occur as single or multiple intrapancreatic lesions completely or partially lined by ductal epithelium. They represent a cystically dilated pancreatic duct (Fig. 13.39) resulting from mechanical obstruction. Occasionally they become so large that they are radiologically detectable. In such cases they have to be differentiated from cystic neoplasms. The most important differential diagnosis of pseudocysts is that vs mucinous neoplasms of both types: (1) mucinous cystic neoplasms (MCNs) characterized by strict female prevalence and composed of uni- or multilocular cysts with no connection to the main pancreatic duct that are lined by mucin secreting epithelium supported by an ovarian type stroma (ZAMBONI et al. 1999); (2) intraductal papillary-mucinous neoplasms (IPMNs) characterized by dilatation of the main and/or branch ducts, mucinous epithelium with mucus hyperproduction and intraductal growth (KLÖPPEL et al. 1996). The preoperative diagnosis of cystic lesions is of para-

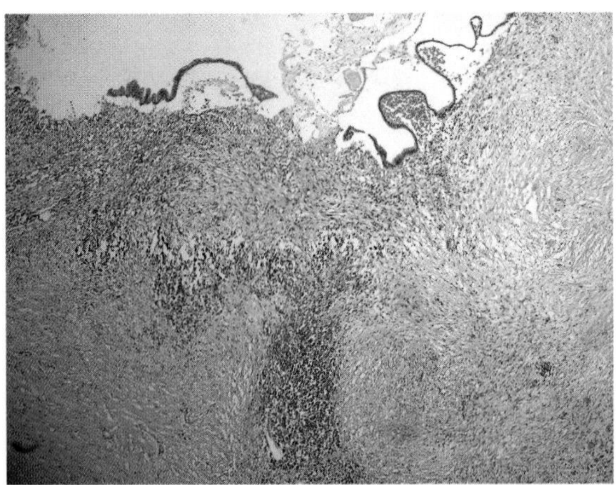

Fig. 13.39. Retention cyst: a thick fibrous capsule with inflammatory infiltration, lined by epithelial lining, with focal epithelial disruption and denudation

mount importance in planning the appropriate surgical treatment. Differentiating a pseudocyst from a mucinous neoplasm may be not only a clinical problem but also a morphological one. Especially in MCN, due to degenerative processes the tumour epithelium may be denuded and the content exclusively characterized by cellular debris and haemorrhagic material. The necessity of appropriate sampling for the correct diagnosis must be emphasized (Warshaw and Rutledge 1987; Zamboni et al. 1994, 1999). Clinical and radiological criteria may be of some value in the differential diagnosis, but they may be not reliable in an individual case. Fine needle aspiration biopsy (Warshaw et al. 1990) and cyst fluid analysis (Lewandrowski et al. 1993) have been reported to improve the preoperative diagnosis. Intraoperative frozen sections is useful, but may fail due to the lack of the epithelial layer in the biopsy specimen (Warshaw and Rutledge 1987). In some cases, the definite diagnosis is reached only after histopathological examination of the resected specimen.

13.11.5 Internal Pancreatic Fistulas

Internal pancreatic fistulas are characterized by pancreatic ascites and/or pleural effusion caused by leakage of pancreatic juice into the peritoneal cavity from pseudocysts or by disruption of the main pancreatic duct. In rare cases, disseminated fat necrosis with subcutaneous nodular panniculitis, polyarthritis and necrotic bone marrow lesions may be observed (Klöppel 2000).

13.11.6 Splenic Vein Thrombosis

Pancreatic fistulas occasionally may erode the splenic artery, causing splenic infarct and secondary left-sided portal hypertension (Bradley 1987).

13.11.7 Concomitant Pancreatic Cancer

Patients with chronic pancreatitis have an increased risk of developing pancreatic carcinoma in relation to the general population. The cumulative risk varies from 2.3% to 26.7% (Lowenfels et al. 1993), especially in smokers (Falconi et al. 2000; Talamini et al. 2000). In hereditary pancreatitis the cumulative risk is about 40% and reaches almost 75% for patients with a paternal hereditary pattern (Lowenfels et al. 1997).

The differential diagnosis between CP and pancreatic carcinoma is of the utmost importance, but may sometimes be problematic. However, FNA-Cytology, FNA-Biopsy and intraoperative frozen sections combined with the knowledge of the pertinent clinical and radiological features may establish a correct diagnosis in most cases.

It is interesting that the pancreatic intraepithelial lesions, PanIN-1 and PanIN-2, which are associated with pancreatic carcinoma, as well as K-ras mutations, which are very common in ductal adenocarcinoma, may also occur in patients with chronic pancreatitis (Hruban et al. 2004; Lohr et al. 2005).

Another important differential diagnosis is vs the intraductal papillary mucinous neoplasms, which frequently present with symptoms similar to chronic pancreatitis (Talamini et al. 2006).

References

Abraham SC, Lee JH, Boitnott JK et al (2002) Microsatellite instability in intraductal papillary neoplasms of the biliary tract. Mod Pathol 15:1309–1317

Abraham SC, Cruz-Correa M, Argani P et al (2003a) Diffuse lymphoplasmacytic chronic cholecystitis is highly specific for extrahepatic biliary tract disease but does not distinguish between primary and secondary sclerosing cholangiopathy. Am J Surg Pathol 27:1313–1320

Abraham SC, Leach S, Yeo CJ et al (2003b) Eosinophilic pancreatitis and increased eosinophils in the pancreas. Am J Surg Pathol 27:334–342

Abrebanel P, Sarfaty S, Gal R et al (1984) Plasma cell granuloma of the pancreas. Arch Pathol Lab Med 108:531–532

Adsay NV, Zamboni G (2004) Paraduodenal pancreatitis: a clinico-pathologically distinct entity unifying "cystic dystrophy of heterotopic pancreas", "para-duodenal wall cyst", and "groove pancreatitis". Semin Diagn Pathol 21:247–254

Adsay NV, Bandyopadhyay S, Basturk O et al (2004) Chronic pancreatitis or pancreatic ductal adenocarcinoma? Semin Diagn Pathol 21:268–276

Ammann RW, Muellhaupt B (1994) Progression of alcoholic acute to chronic pancreatitis. Gut 35:552–556

Ammann RW, Mullhaupt B (2007) Do the diagnostic criteria differ between alcoholic and nonalcoholic chronic pancreatitis? J Gastroenterol 42(Suppl 17):118–126

Ammann RW, Heitz PU, Klöppel G (1996) Course of alcoholic chronic pancreatitis: a prospective clinicomorphological long-term study. Gastroenterology 111:224–231

Antonarakis SE (1998) Recommendations for a nomenclature system for human gene mutations. Nomenclature Working Group. Hum Mutat 11:1–3

Aoki S, Nakazawa T, Ohara H et al (2005) Immunohistochemical study of autoimmune pancreatitis using anti-IgG4 antibody and patients' sera. Histopathology 47:147–158

Apte MV, Wilson JS (2003) Stellate cell activation in alcoholic pancreatitis. Pancreas 27:316–320

Apte MV, Haber PS, Applegate TL et al (1998) Periacinar stellate shaped cells in rat pancreas: identification, isolation, and culture. Gut 43:128–133

Apte MV, Park S, Phillips PA et al (2004) Desmoplastic reaction in pancreatic cancer: role of pancreatic stellate cells. Pancreas 29:179–187

Archer H, Jura N, Keller J et al (2006) A mouse model of hereditary pancreatitis generated by transgenic expression of R122H trypsinogen. Gastroenterology 131:1844–1855

Asada M, Nishio A, Uchida K et al (2006) Identification of a novel autoantibody against pancreatic secretory trypsin inhibitor in patients with autoimmune pancreatitis. Pancreas 33:20–26

Audrezet MP, Chen JM, Le Marechal C et al (2002) Determination of the relative contribution of three genes-the cystic fibrosis transmembrane conductance regulator gene, the cationic trypsinogen gene, and the pancreatic secretory trypsin inhibitor gene-to the etiology of idiopathic chronic pancreatitis. Eur J Hum Genet 10:100–106

Bachem MG, Zhou Z, Zhou S et al (2006) Role of stellate cells in pancreatic fibrogenesis associated with acute and chronic pancreatitis. J Gastroenterol Hepatol 21(Suppl 3):S92–96

Ball WP, Baggenstoss AH, Bargen JA (1950) Pancreatic lesions associated with chronic ulcerative colitis. Arch Pathol (Chic) 50:347–358

Bang SJ, Kim MH, Kim do H et al (2008) Is pancreatic core biopsy sufficient to diagnose autoimmune chronic pancreatitis? Pancreas 36:84–89

Bartholomew LG, Cain JC, Woolner LB et al (1963) Sclerosing cholangitis: its possible association with Riedel's struma and fibrous retroperitonitis. Report of two cases. N Engl J Med 269:8–12

Becker V (1973) Bauchspeicheldrüse. Spezielle pathologische Anatomie, Bd. VI. Doerr W, Ühlinger E (eds). Springer, Berlin Heidelberg New York

Becker V, Mischke U (1991) Groove pancreatitis. Int J Pancreatol 10:173–182

Bedossa P, Bacci J, Lemaigre G et al (1990) Lymphocyte subsets and HLA-DR expression in normal pancreas and chronic pancreatitis. Pancreas 5:415–420

Bockman DE, Boydston WR, Anderson MC (1982) Origin of tubular complexes in human chronic pancreatitis. Am J Surg 144:243–249

Bockman DE, Buchler M, Malfertheiner P et al (1988) Analysis of nerves in chronic pancreatitis. Gastroenterology 94:1459–1469

Bovo P, Mirakian R, Merigo F et al (1987) HLA molecule expression on chronic pancreatitis specimens: is there a role for autoimmunity? A preliminary study. Pancreas 2:350–356

Bradley EL III (1987) Management of infected pancreatic necrosis by open drainage. Ann Surg 206:542–550

Buchler M, Weihe E, Friess H et al (1992) Changes in peptidergic innervation in chronic pancreatitis. Pancreas 7:183–192

Casadei R, Piccoli L, Valeri B et al (2004) Inflammatory pseudotumor of the pancreas resembling pancreatic cancer: clinical, diagnostic and therapeutic considerations. Chir Ital 56:849–858

Cavallini G, Frulloni L (2001) Autoimmunity and chronic pancreatitis: a concealed relationship. JOPp 2:61–68

Cavestro GM, Frulloni L, Nouvenne A et al (2003) Association of keratin 8 gene mutation with chronic pancreatitis. Dig Liver Dis 35:416–420

Chang MC, Chang YT, Tien YW et al (2007) T-cell regulatory gene CTLA-4 polymorphism/haplotype association with autoimmune pancreatitis. Clin Chem 53:1700–1705

Chaudhary A, Negi SS, Masood S et al (2004) Complications after Frey's procedure for chronic pancreatitis. Am J Surg 188:277–281

Cheuk W, Yuen HK, Chu SY et al (2008) Lymphadenopathy of IgG4-related sclerosing disease. Am J Surg Pathol 32:671–681

Chutaputti A, Burrell MI, Boyer JL (1995) Pseudotumor of the pancreas associated with retroperitoneal fibrosis: a dramatic response to corticosteroid therapy. Am J Gastroenterol 90:1155–1158

Cohn JA, Friedman KJ, Noone PG et al (1998) Relation between mutations of the cystic fibrosis gene and idiopathic pancreatitis. N Engl J Med 339:653–658

Colardelle P, Chochon M, Larvon L et al (1994) Dystrophie kystique sur pancreas aberrant antro-bulbaire. Gastroenterol Clin Biol 18:277–280

Comings DE, Skubi KB, Van Eyes J et al (1967) Familial multifocal fibrosclerosis. Findings suggesting that retroperitoneal fibrosis, mediastinal fibrosis, sclerosing cholangitis, Riedel's thyroiditis, and pseudotumor of the orbit may be different manifestations of a single disease. Ann Intern Med 66:884–892

Cope O, Culver PJ, Mixter CG Jr et al (1957) Pancreatitis, a diagnostic clue to hyperparathyroidism. Ann Surg 145:857–863

Cunha JE, Penteado S, Jukemura J et al (2004) Surgical and interventional treatment of chronic pancreatitis. Pancreatology 4:540–550

Dehner LP (2000) The enigmatic inflammatory pseudotumours: the current state of our understanding, or misunderstanding. J Pathol 192:277–279

Dehner LP, Coffin CM (1998) Idiopathic fibrosclerotic disorders and other inflammatory pseudotumors. Semin Diagn Pathol 15:161–173

Denning GM, Anderson MP, Amara JF et al (1992) Processing of mutant cystic fibrosis transmembrane conductance regulator is temperature-sensitive. Nature 358:761–764

DeRubertis BG, McGinty J, Rivera M et al (2004) Laparoscopic distal pancreatectomy for inflammatory pseudotumor of the pancreas. Surg Endosc 18:1001

Deshpande V, Mino-Kenudson M, Brugge W et al (2005a) Autoimmune pancreatitis: more than just a pancreatic disease? A contemporary review of its pathology. Arch Pathol Lab Med 129:1148–1154

Deshpande V, Mino-Kenudson M, Brugge WR et al (2005b) Endoscopic ultrasound guided fine needle aspiration biopsy of autoimmune pancreatitis: diagnostic criteria and pitfalls. Am J Surg Pathol 29:1464–1471

Deshpande V, Chicano S, Finkelberg D et al (2006) Autoimmune pancreatitis: a systemic immune complex mediated disease. Am J Surg Pathol 30:1537–1545

Detlefsen S, Sipos B, Feyerabend B et al (2005) Pancreatic fibrosis associated with age and ductal papillary hyperplasia. Virchows Arch 447:800–805

Detlefsen S, Sipos B, Feyerabend B et al (2006) Fibrogenesis in alcoholic chronic pancreatitis: the role of tissue necrosis, macrophages, myofibroblasts and cytokines. Mod Pathol 19:1019–1026

Diakowska D, Knast W, Diakowski W et al (2005) [Abnormal metabolism of triglycerides fractions in chronic pancreatitis and results after the operation treatment]. Pol Merkur Lekarski 18:629–633

Dooreck BS, Katz P, Barkin JS (2004) Autoimmune pancreatitis in the spectrum of autoimmune exocrinopathy associated with sialoadenitis and anosmia. Pancreas 28:105–107

Durie PR (1998) Pancreatitis and mutations of the cystic fibrosis gene. N Engl J Med 339:687–688

Ebert M, Kasper HU, Hernberg S et al (1998) Overexpression of platelet-derived growth factor (PDGF) B chain and type beta PDGF receptor in human chronic pancreatitis. Dig Dis Sci 43:567–574

Eckstein RP, Hollings RM, Martin PA et al (1995) Pancreatic pseudotumor arising in association with Sjogren's syndrome. Pathology 27:284–288

Ectors N, Maillet B, Aerts R et al (1997) Non-alcoholic duct destructive chronic pancreatitis. Gut 41:263–268

Eloit S, Charles JF, L'Heveder G et al (1987) Dystrophie kystique sur pancréas aberrant. Sem Hop Paris 63:2545–2549

Esposito I, Bergmann F, Penzel R et al (2004) Oligoclonal T-cell populations in an inflammatory pseudotumor of the pancreas possibly related to autoimmune pancreatitis: an immunohistochemical and molecular analysis. Virchows Arch 444:119–126

Etemad B, Whitcomb DC (2001) Chronic pancreatitis: diagnosis, classification, and new genetic developments. Gastroenterology 120:682–707

Falconi M, Valerio A, Caldiron E et al (2000) Changes in pancreatic resection for chronic pancreatitis over 28 years in a single institution. Br J Surg 87:428–433

Farkas G Jr, Hofner P, Balog A et al (2007) Relevance of transforming growth factor-beta1, interleukin-8, and tumor necrosis factor-alpha polymorphisms in patients with chronic pancreatitis. Eur Cytokine Netw 18:31–37

Fekete F, Noun R, Sauvanet A et al (1996) Pseudotumor developing in heterotopic pancreas. World J Surg 20:295–298

Frulloni L, Bovo P, Brunelli S et al (2000) Elevated serum levels of antibodies to carbonic anhydrase I and II in patients with chronic pancreatitis. Pancreas 20:382–388

Fukui T, Mitsuyama T, Takaoka M et al (2008) Pancreatic cancer associated with autoimmune pancreatitis in remission. Intern Med 47:151–155

Fukushima N, Suzuki M, Abe T et al (1997) A case of inflammatory pseudotumour of the common bile duct. Virchows Arch 431:219–224

Ghazale A, Chari S (2007) Is autoimmune pancreatitis a risk factor for pancreatic cancer? Pancreas 35:376

Gough SC, Walker LS, Sansom DM (2005) CTLA4 gene polymorphism and autoimmunity. Immunol Rev 204:102–115

Haber P, Wilson J, Apte M et al (1995) Individual susceptibility to alcoholic pancreatitis: still an enigma. J Lab Clin Med 125:305–312

Hamano H, Kawa S, Horiuchi A et al (2001) High serum IgG4 concentrations in patients with sclerosing pancreatitis. N Engl J Med 344:732–738

Hardacre JM, Iacobuzio-Donahue CA, Sohn TA et al (2003) Results of pancreatico-duodenectomy for lymphoplasmacytic sclerosing pancreatitis. Ann Surg 237:853–858; discussion 858–859

Hastier P, Buckley MJ, Le Gall P et al (1998) First report of association of chronic pancreatitis, primary biliary cirrhosis, and systemic sclerosis. Dig Dis Sci 43:2426–2428

Hirano K, Komatsu Y, Yamamoto N et al (2004) Pancreatic mass lesions associated with raised concentration of IgG4. Am J Gastroenterol 99:2038–2040

Hirano K, Kawabe T, Komatsu Y et al (2006) High-rate pulmonary involvement in autoimmune pancreatitis. Intern Med J 36:58–61

Hruban RH, Takaori K, Klimstra DS et al (2004) An illustrated consensus on the classification of pancreatic intraepithelial neoplasia and intraductal papillary mucinous neoplasms. Am J Surg Pathol 28:977–987

Isaksson G, Ihse I, Lundquist I (1983) Influence of pancreatic duct ligation on endocrine and exocrine rat pancreas. Acta Physiol Scand 117:281–286

Iwasa S, Fujiwara M, Nagata M et al (2001) Three autopsied cases of cystic fibrosis in Japan. Pathol Int 51:467–472

Jafri SZ, Bree RL, Agha FP et al (1983) Inflammatory pseudotumor from sclerosing cholangitis. J Comput Assist Tomogr 7:902–904

Jaster M, Horstkotte D, Willich T et al (2008) The amount of fibrinogen-positive platelets predicts the occurrence of in-stent restenosis. Atherosclerosis 197:190–196

Kakugawa Y, Giaid A, Yanagisawa M et al (1996) Expression of endothelin-1 in pancreatic tissue of patients with chronic pancreatitis. J Pathol 178:78–83

Kamisawa T, Egawa N, Inokuma S et al (2003a) Pancreatic endocrine and exocrine function and salivary gland function in autoimmune pancreatitis before and after steroid therapy. Pancreas 27:235–238

Kamisawa T, Egawa N, Nakajima H (2003b) Autoimmune pancreatitis is a systemic autoimmune disease. Am J Gastroenterol 98:2811–2812

Kamisawa T, Nakajima H, Egawa N et al (2006) IgG4-related sclerosing disease incorporating sclerosing pancreatitis, cholangitis, sialadenitis and retroperitoneal fibrosis with lymphadenopathy. Pancreatology 6:132–137

Kawa S, Ota M, Yoshizawa K et al (2002) HLA DRB10405-DQB10401 haplotype is associated with autoimmune pancreatitis in the Japanese population. Gastroenterology 122:1264–1269

Kawaguchi K, Koike M, Tsuruta K et al (1991) Lymphoplasmacytic sclerosing pancreatitis with cholangitis: a variant of primary sclerosing cholangitis extensively involving pancreas. Hum Pathol 22:387–395

Kawamura E, Habu D, Higashiyama S et al (2007) A case of sclerosing cholangitis with autoimmune pancreatitis evaluated by FDG-PET. Ann Nucl Med 21:223–228

Keller J, Layer P (2008) Idiopathic chronic pancreatitis. Best Pract Res Clin Gastroenterol 22:105–113

Kiraly O, Wartmann T, Sahin-Toth M (2007) Missense mutations in pancreatic secretory trypsin inhibitor (SPINK1) cause intracellular retention and degradation. Gut 56:1433–1438

Klöppel G (2000) Pseudocysts and other non-neoplastic cysts of the pancreas. Semin Diagn Pathol 17:7–15

Klöppel G (2007a) Chronic pancreatitis, pseudotumors and other tumor-like lesions. Mod Pathol 20 (Suppl 1) S113–131

Klöppel G (2007b) Toward a new classification of chronic pancreatitis. J Gastroenterol 42(Suppl 17):55–57

Klöppel G, Maillet AB (1991) Pseudocyst in chronic pancreatitis: a morphological analysis of 57 resection specimens and 9 autopsy pancreata. Pancreas 6:266–274

Klöppel G, Maillet B (1992) The morphological basis for the evolution of acute pancreatitis into chronic pancreatitis. Virchows Arch A Pathol Anat Histopathol 420:1–4

Klöppel G, Maillet B (1993) Pathology of acute and chronic pancreatitis. Pancreas 8:659–670

Klöppel G, Solcia E, Longnecker D et al (1996) WHO. Histological typing of tumours of the exocrine pancreas, 2nd edn. Springer, Berlin Heidelberg New York, p 23

Klöppel G, Detlefsen S, Feyerabend B (2004) Fibrosis of the pancreas: the initial tissue damage and the resulting pattern. Virchows Arch 445:1–8

Kojima M, Sipos B, Klapper W et al (2007) Autoimmune pancreatitis: frequency, IgG4 expression, and clonality of T and B cells. Am J Surg Pathol 31:521–528

Konzen KM, Perrault J, Moir C et al (1993) Long-term follow-up of young patients with chronic hereditary or idiopathic pancreatitis. Mayo Clin Proc 68:449–453

Kroft SH, Stryker SJ, Winter JN et al (1995) Inflammatory pseudotumor of the pancreas. Int J Pancreatol 18:277–283

Lack E (2003) Cystic fibrosis and selected disorders with pancreatic insufficiency. Oxford University Press, Oxford

Layer P, Keller J (2006) Chronic pancreatitis: faces, facets, and facts. Swiss Med Wkly 136:163–165

Léger L, Lemaigre G, Lenriot J (1974) Kystes sur hétérotopies pancréatiques de la paroi duodénale. Nouv Press Med 3:2309–2314

Levey JM, Mathai J (1998) Diffuse pancreatic fibrosis: an uncommon feature of multifocal idiopathic fibrosclerosis. Am J Gastroenterol 93:640–642

Lewandrowski KB, Southern JF, Pins MR et al (1993) Cyst fluid analysis in the differential diagnosis of pancreatic cysts. A comparison of pseudocysts, serous cystadenomas, mucinous cystic neoplasms, and mucinous cystadenocarcinoma. Ann Surg 217:41–47

Lohr M, Klöppel G, Maisonneuve P et al (2005) Frequency of K-ras mutations in pancreatic intraductal neoplasias associated with pancreatic ductal adenocarcinoma and chronic pancreatitis: a meta-analysis. Neoplasia 7:17–23

Lowenfels AB, Maisonneuve P, Cavallini G et al (1993) Pancreatitis and the risk of pancreatic cancer. International Pancreatitis Study Group. N Engl J Med 328:1433–1437

Lowenfels AB, Maisonneuve P, DiMagno EP et al (1997) Hereditary pancreatitis and the risk of pancreatic cancer. International Hereditary Pancreatitis Study Group. J Natl Cancer Inst 89:442–446

Martin E (1977) Paraampullary duodenal cysts: their relationship with chronic pancreatitis. The sphincter of Oddi. Karger, Basel, pp 156–162

Masson E, Chen JM, Scotet V et al (2008) Association of rare chymotrypsinogen C (CTRC) gene variations in patients with idiopathic chronic pancreatitis. Hum Genet 123:83–91

Mendes FD, Jorgensen R, Keach J et al (2006) Elevated serum IgG4 concentration in patients with primary sclerosing cholangitis. Am J Gastroenterol 101:2070–2075

Merino JL, Fernandez Lucas M, Teruel JL et al (2004) [Membranous nephropathy associated to autoimmune thyroiditis, chronic pancreatitis and suprarrenal insufficiency]. Nefrologia 24:376–379

Miyoshi H, Uchida K, Taniguchi T et al (2008) Circulating naive and CD4+CD25high regulatory T cells in patients with autoimmune pancreatitis. Pancreas 36:133–140

Nishi H, Tojo A, Onozato ML et al (2007) Anti-carbonic anhydrase II antibody in autoimmune pancreatitis and tubulointerstitial nephritis. Nephrol Dial Transplant 22:1273–1275

Nonomura A, Minato H, Shimizu K et al (1997) Hepatic hilar inflammatory pseudotumor mimicking cholangiocarcinoma with cholangitis and phlebitis – a variant of primary sclerosing cholangitis? Pathol Res Pract 193:519–525; discussion 526

Notohara K, Burgart LJ, Yadav D et al (2003) Idiopathic chronic pancreatitis with periductal lymphoplasmacytic infiltration: clinicopathologic features of 35 cases. Am J Surg Pathol 27:1119–1127

Okazaki K (2007) Is primary sclerosing cholangitis different from sclerosing cholangitis with autoimmune pancreatitis? J Gastroenterol 42:600–601

Okazaki K, Uchida K, Ohana M et al (2000) Autoimmune-related pancreatitis is associated with autoantibodies and a Th1/Th2-type cellular immune response. Gastroenterology 118:573–581

Palazzo JP, Chang CD (1993) Inflammatory pseudotumour of the pancreas. Histopathology 23:475–477

Palazzo L, Roseau G, Chaussade S et al (1992) Dystrophie kystique sur pancreas aberrant de la paroi duodenale (DKPA) associée à la pancreatite chronique calcificante alcoolique (PCCA): une affection frequente et meconnue (resumé). Gastroenterol Clin Biol 16(suppl. 2 bis):A141

Pandol SJ, Raraty M (2007) Pathobiology of alcoholic pancreatitis. Pancreatology 7:105–114

Pearson RK, Longnecker DS, Chari ST et al (2003) Controversies in clinical pancreatology: autoimmune pancreatitis: does it exist? Pancreas 27:1–13

Petter LM, Martin JK Jr, Menke DM (1998) Localized lymphoplasmacellular pancreatitis forming a pancreatic inflammatory pseudotumor. Mayo Clin Proc 73:447–450

Potet F, Duclert N (1970) [Cystic dystrophy on aberrant pancreas of the duodenal wall]. Arch Fr Mal App Dig 59:223–238

Prasad P, Salem RR, Mangla R et al (2004) Lymphoplasmacytic sclerosing pancreato-cholangitis: a case report and review of the literature. Yale J Biol Med 77:143–148

Procacci C, Graziani R, Zamboni G et al (1997) Cystic dystrophy of the duodenal wall: radiologic findings. Radiology 205:741–747

Procacci C, Carbognin G, Biasiutti C et al (2001) Autoimmune pancreatitis: possibilities of CT characterization. Pancreatology 1:246–253

Rasanen O, Jokinen K, Dammert K (1972) Sclerosing inflammation of the submandibular salivary gland (Kuttner tumour). A progressive plasmacellular ductitis. Acta Otolaryngol 74:297–301

Renner IG, Ponto GC, Savage WT III et al (1980) Idiopathic retroperitoneal fibrosis producing common bile duct and pancreatic duct obstruction. Gastroenterology 79:348–351

Rosendahl J, Witt H, Szmola R et al (2008) Chymotrypsin C (CTRC) variants that diminish activity or secretion are associated with chronic pancreatitis. Nat Genet 40:78–82

Rossi L, Parvin S, Hassan Z et al (2004) Diabetes mellitus in tropical chronic pancreatitis is not just a secondary type of diabetes. Pancreatology 4:461–467

Sakata N, Tashiro T, Uesugi N et al (2008) 0IgG4-positive plasma cells in inflammatory abdominal aortic aneurysm: the possibility of an aortic manifestation of IgG4-related sclerosing disease. Am J Surg Pathol 32:553–559

Sarles H, Sarles JC, Muratore R et al (1961) Chronic inflammatory sclerosis of the pancreas – an autonomous pancreatic disease? Am J Dig Dis 6:688–698

Schneider A, Lamb J, Barmada MM et al (2006) Keratin 8 mutations are not associated with familial, sporadic and alcoholic pancreatitis in a population from the United States. Pancreatology 6:103–108

Sharer N, Schwarz M, Malone G et al (1998) Mutations of the cystic fibrosis gene in patients with chronic pancreatitis. N Engl J Med 339:645–652

Shudo R, Obara T, Tanno S et al (1998) Segmental groove pancreatitis accompanied by protein plugs in Santorini's duct. J Gastroenterol 33:289–294

Sood S, Fossard DP, Shorrock K (1995) Chronic sclerosing pancreatitis in Sjogren's syndrome: a case report. Pancreas 10:419–421

Stolte M, Weiss W, Volkholz H et al (1982) A special form of segmental pancreatitis. "Groove pancreatitis". Hepatogastroenterology 29:198–208

Takase M, Suda K (2001) Histopathological study on mechanism and background of tumor-forming pancreatitis. Pathol Int 51:349–354

Takeda S, Haratake J, Kasai T et al (2004) IgG4-associated idiopathic tubulointerstitial nephritis complicating autoimmune pancreatitis. Nephrol Dial Transplant 19:474–476

Talamini G, Butturini G, Bassi C et al (2000) [Clinical evolution of chronic pancreatitis and quality of life]. Chir Ital 52:647–53

Talamini G, Zamboni G, Salvia R et al (2006) Intraductal papillary mucinous neoplasms and chronic pancreatitis. Pancreatology 6:626–634

Taniguchi T, Ko M, Seko S et al (2004) Interstitial pneumonia associated with autoimmune pancreatitis. Gut 53:770; author reply 771

Teich N, Mossner J (2008) Hereditary chronic pancreatitis. Best Pract Res Clin Gastroenterol 22:115–130

Treiber M, Schlag C, Schmid RM (2008) Genetics of pancreatitis: a guide for clinicians. Curr Gastroenterol Rep 10:122–127

Tucker JA, Spock A, Spicer SS et al (2003) Inspissation of pancreatic zymogen material in cystic fibrosis. Ultrastruct Pathol 27:323–335

Uchida K, Okazaki K, Asada M et al (2003) Case of chronic pancreatitis involving an autoimmune mechanism that extended to retroperitoneal fibrosis. Pancreas 26:92–94

Uchiyama-Tanaka Y, Mori Y, Kimura T et al (2004) Acute tubulointerstitial nephritis associated with autoimmune-related pancreatitis. Am J Kidney Dis 43:e18–25

Umemura T, Ota M, Hamano H et al (2006) Genetic association of Fc receptor-like 3 polymorphisms with autoimmune pancreatitis in Japanese patients. Gut 55:1367–1368

Umemura T, Ota M, Yoshizawa K et al (2008) Association of cytotoxic T-lymphocyte antigen 4 gene polymorphisms with type 1 autoimmune hepatitis in Japanese. Hepatol Res 38:689–695

Vankemmel M, Paris JC, Houcke M et al (1975) [Paraduodenal cysts near Vater's ampulla and chronic pancreatitis]. Med Chir Dig 4:181–185

van Laethem JL, Deviere J, Resibois A et al (1995) Localization of transforming growth factor beta 1 and its latent binding protein in human chronic pancreatitis. Gastroenterology 108:1873–1881

Vonlaufen A, Joshi S, Qu C et al (2008) Pancreatic stellate cells: partners in crime with pancreatic cancer cells. Cancer Res 68:2085–2093

Walsh SV, Evangelista F, Khettry U (1998) Inflammatory myofibroblastic tumor of the pancreatico-biliary region: morphologic and immunocytochemical study of three cases. Am J Surg Pathol 22:412–418

Warshaw AL (1985) Surgical treatment of pancreatitis. Ala J Med Sci 22:36–39

Warshaw AL, Rutledge PL (1987) Cystic tumors mistaken for pancreatic pseudocysts. Ann Surg 205:393–398

Warshaw AL, Compton CC, Lewandrowski K et al (1990) Cystic tumors of the pancreas. New clinical, radiologic, and pathologic observations in 67 patients. Ann Surg 212:432–443; discussion 444–445

Weber SM, Cubukcu-Dimopulo O, Palesty JA et al (2003) Lymphoplasmacytic sclerosing pancreatitis: inflammatory mimic of pancreatic carcinoma. J Gastrointest Surg 7:129–137; discussion 137–139

Whitcomb DC (1999) New insights into hereditary pancreatitis. Curr Gastroenterol Rep 1:154–160

Whitcomb DC, Gorry MC, Preston RA et al (1996) Hereditary pancreatitis is caused by a mutation in the cationic trypsinogen gene. Nat Genet 14:141–145

Williams SB, Foss RD, Ellis GL (1992) Inflammatory pseudotumors of the major salivary glands. Clinicopathologic and immunohistochemical analysis of six cases. Am J Surg Pathol 16:896–902

Witt H, Luck W, Hennies HC et al (2000) Mutations in the gene encoding the serine protease inhibitor, Kazal type 1 are associated with chronic pancreatitis. Nat Genet 25:213–216

Witt H, Sahin-Toth M, Landt O et al (2006) A degradation-sensitive anionic trypsinogen (PRSS2) variant protects against chronic pancreatitis. Nat Genet 38:668–673

Witt H, Apte MV, Keim V et al (2007) Chronic pancreatitis: challenges and advances in pathogenesis, genetics, diagnosis, and therapy. Gastroenterology 132:1557–1573

Wreesmann V, van Eijck CH, Naus DC et al (2001) Inflammatory pseudotumour (inflammatory myofibroblastic tumour) of the pancreas: a report of six cases associated with obliterative phlebitis. Histopathology 38:105–110

Yamada K, Kawano M, Inoue R et al (2008) Clonal relationship between infiltrating immunoglobulin G4 (IgG4)-positive plasma cells in lacrimal glands and circulating IgG4-positive lymphocytes in Mikulicz's disease. Clin Exp Immunol 152:432–439

Yamaguchi K, Chijiiwa K, Saiki S et al (1996) "Mass-forming"pancreatitis masquerades as pancreatic carcinoma. Int J Pancreatol 20:27–35

Yoshida K, Toki F, Takeuchi T et al (1995) Chronic pancreatitis caused by an autoimmune abnormality. Proposal of the concept of autoimmune pancreatitis. Dig Dis Sci 40:1561–1568

Yoshimura Y, Takeda S, Ieki Y et al (2006) IgG4-associated prostatitis complicating autoimmune pancreatitis. Intern Med 45:897–901

Zamboni G, Bonetti F, Castelli P et al (1994) Mucinous cystic tumor of the pancreas recurring after 11 years as cystadenocarcinoma with foci of choriocarcinoma and osteoclast-like giant cell tumor. Surgical Pathology 5:253–262

Zamboni G, Scarpa A, Bogina G et al (1999) Mucinous cystic tumors of the pancreas: clinicopathological features, prognosis, and relationship to other mucinous cystic tumors. Am J Surg Pathol 23:410–422

Zamboni G, Luttges J, Capelli P et al (2004) Histopathological features of diagnostic and clinical relevance in autoimmune pancreatitis: a study on 53 resection specimens and 9 biopsy specimens. Virchows Arch 445:552–563

Zen Y, Harada K, Sasaki M et al (2004) IgG4-related sclerosing cholangitis with and without hepatic inflammatory pseudotumor, and sclerosing pancreatitis-associated sclerosing cholangitis: do they belong to a spectrum of sclerosing pancreatitis? Am J Surg Pathol 28:1193–1203

Zen Y, Kasahara Y, Horita K et al (2005) Inflammatory pseudotumor of the breast in a patient with a high serum IgG4 level: histologic similarity to sclerosing pancreatitis. Am J Surg Pathol 29:275–278

Zen Y, Fujii T, Harada K et al (2007) Th2 and regulatory immune reactions are increased in immunoglobin G4-related sclerosing pancreatitis and cholangitis. Hepatology 45:1538–1546

Zhang L, Notohara K, Levy MJ et al (2007) IgG4-positive plasma cell infiltration in the diagnosis of autoimmune pancreatitis. Mod Pathol 20:23–28

Zhao MF, Tian Y, Guo KJ et al (2004) Common bile duct obstruction due to fibrous pseudotumor of pancreas associated with retroperitoneal fibrosis: a case report. World J Gastroenterol 10:3078–3079

Clinical Aspect of Complications: Features and Prognoses

14

Claudio Bassi, Giovanni Butturini, Nora Sartori, Massimo Falconi, and Paolo Pederzoli

CONTENTS

14.1 **Introduction** *261*
14.2 **Acute Pancreatitis** *261*
14.3 **Complications** *261*
14.3.1 Systemic Complications: Multi-organ Failure *261*
14.3.2 Local Complications *262*
14.3.2.1 Pancreatic Necrosis *262*
14.3.2.2 Fluid Collections *262*
14.3.2.3 Pseudocyst *263*
14.3.2.4 Infected Necrosis *263*
14.3.2.5 Abscess *264*
14.3.2.6 Fistulas *264*
14.3.2.7 Fibrosis *264*
14.4 **Chronic Pancreatitis** *264*
14.4.1 Malabsorption *265*
14.4.2 Diabetes *265*
14.4.3 Ductal Carcinoma *265*
14.5 **Local Complications** *265*
References *266*

C. Bassi, MD; G. Butturini, MD; N. Sartori, MD
M. Falconi, MD; P. Pederzoli, MD
Surgical and Gastroenterological Department, Hospital "GB Rossi", Piazzale LA Scuro 10, University of Verona, 37134 Verona, Italy

14.1 Introduction

The development of complications in inflammatory pancreopathies is often the main factor responsible for the presence and severity of the clinical syndrome. A comprehensive short evaluation of clinical features and their significance is difficult since various manifestations, clinical developments, treatments and prognoses differ wildly.

14.2 Acute Pancreatitis

As previously described in Chaps. 1 and 2, acute pancreatitis can be divided clinically into a mild, self-limiting form (interstitial or edematous pancreatitis) which accounts for 75% – 80% of cases and into a severe form (necrotizing pancreatitis) which is seen in about 20% – 25% of patients with acute pancreatitis (Banks 1994; Bradley 1993a; Bassi 1994; D'Egidio and Schein 1991).

14.3 Complications

14.3.1 Systemic Complications: Multi-organ Failure

The extravasation of pancreatic enzymes causes a systemic response in all forms of acute pancreatitis, which in most cases is mild and transitory without serious clinical consequences (Bradley 1993a; Pederzoli et al. 1994).

The triggering mechanism of acute pancreatitis is not fully understood but it starts at the intracellular level. Apparently there is a loss in the normal control of the intracytoplasmic traffic with accumulation of zymogen granules full of enzymes. Secretion of zymogen is deviated towards the interstices rather than excreted into the ductal system causing mild edematous changes seen in interstitial pancreatitis. If the activation of the extravasated pancreatic enzymes is not blocked, a chemical chain reaction ensues that induces tissue necrosis, leading to the development of severe necrotizing pancreatitis (Bassi 1994; Beger et al. 1998; Howard et al. 1998). The initial chemical and inflammatory events draw immuno-competent cells such as polymorphonuclear cells and mastocytes into the pancreas and releases vaso-active substances and activated cytokines responsible for the systemic inflammatory response. Severe manifestation of this clinical syndrome, called systemic inflammatory response syndrome (SIRS) can lead to organ or multi-organ impairment or failure (MOF) responsible for the early mortality in severe pancreatitis, even when the necrotic pancreas is sterile.

The target organs of SIRS are:

- The lungs where the abnormalities may range from pleural effusions usually on the left side, to respiratory distress syndrome due to the enzymatic destruction of the pulmonary surfactant;
- The cardio-vascular system with hypotension and even hypovolemic-toxic shock;
- The kidneys with hypoperfusion and subsequent oliguria and even anuria with acute renal failure necessitating dialysis;
- The liver and gastro-intestinal system causing acute hepatic steatosis and alterations in in intestinal permeability;
- Lastly, less frequent, involvement of the nervous system with demyelination and the expected central type neurological symptoms (Bradley 1993a).

Hypercatabolic activity may cause hypoproteinemia, hypoalbuminemia and hypocalcemia. Additionally, hyperglycemia, hyperlipidemia, ketoacidosis and coagulation disorders that may progress into disseminated intravascular coagulopathy (DIC) with high mortality rates, are sometimes seen (Banks 1994; Beger et al. 1998; Bradley 1993a; Pederzoli et al. 1994).

14.3.2 Local Complications

14.3.2.1 Pancreatic Necrosis

Whether or not pancreatic necrosis should be considered a complication of acute pancreatitis is controversial and debatable. It has been well documented that glandular necrosis is present at the beginning of an acute attack of severe pancreatitis and it is associated with a high incidence of local complications such as infected necrosis, abscesses, fistulous tracts and acute pseudocysts. Furthermore, patchy foci of necrosis can be present in the gland or commonly in the peripancreatic retroperitoneal fatty tissue even in patients with interstitial mild pancreatitis. In fact severe complications, sometimes life-threatening, do occur in a minority of patients with interstitial (non-necrotizing) pancreatitis which have peripancreatic fluid collections. Since early discernable glandular necrosis occurs only in the minority of patients (20% – 25%) with acute pancreatitis, due to the enzymatic activity of pancreatic secretions and microvascular thrombosis, necrosis has been considered by some clinicians an infrequent complications forecasting a prolong and dire clinical course (Pederzoli et al. 1994).

14.3.2.2 Fluid Collections

The appearance of peripancreatic fluid collections is a common event in acute pancreatitis, which occurs even in milder forms of disease. In the past fluid collections were considered manifestations of severe necrotizing pancreatitis and the distinction between fluid collections and pseudocysts difficult to establish. With the advent of ultrasonography and CT imaging, fluid collections are easily detected and their frequency and eventual resolution readily established. The appearance and natural history of fluid collections explains the development of pseudocysts that require 4–5 weeks to form (Bradley 1993b). Peripancreatic fluid is composed of exudate and transudate with a variable amount of activated pancreatic enzymes. It is thought that the amount of fluid and extent of activated pancreatic enzymes explains the severity of pancreatic and peripancreatic tissue auto-digestion and determines the speed of reabsorption or in some cases the formation of pseudocysts (Banks 1994).

14.3.2.3
Pseudocyst

The enzymatic contents of fluid collections trigger an inflammatory reaction that leads to the formation of a pseudo-wall or a capsule that surrounds the collection thus forming a pseudocyst. Its wall is made up of fibrous tissue devoid of a lining epithelium, while the fluid content of the cyst is rich in amylase. The color of the liquid varies from clear to transparent in chronic pseudocysts to degrees of light to dark brown in acute cysts. Imaging studies and particularly CT examinations document the progressive formation of the capsule and evaluate its thickness and maturation, which takes at least 4 weeks to mature (Bradley 1993b). Pseudocysts vary greatly in size, are generally round, sharply defined with a low fluid density that exhibits no contrast enhancement.

Considerations for treatment are controversial but are related to size of the cyst usually over 4–5 cm, and particularly to symptomatic cysts or unusual complications. Since the natural history of an acute pseudocyst is unpredictable, with some cysts resolving spontaneously, aggressive interventional procedures or surgery is delayed until and unless patients become ill. Compression of the stomach or duodenum produces gastric outlet obstruction while compression of the common bile duct leads to cholestasis and jaundice. Other clinical complications include rupture of the pseudocyst, hemorrhage and secondary infection (Bradley 1993a; Beger et al. 1998; Howard et al. 1998; Pederzoli et al. 1994).

Cyst rupture occurs infrequently and it is more common with longstanding chronic cysts. Smaller amounts of leakage are usually reabsorbed while continuous leakage secondary to a pancreatic duct peritoneal cavity fistula results in pancreatic ascites. Peritoneal irritation due to enzymatic peritonitis is a less common complication. Pseudocysts can get adherent to and can rupture into adjacent hollow organs such as stomach, duodenum or colon leading to their collapse and spontaneous resolution of the cyst without serious clinical implications.

Hemorrhage due to the enzymatic erosion of a vessel or rupture of a pseudo-aneurysm can manifest as a life-threatening dramatic event. Obviously, arterial bleeding is more severe while venous bleeding or capillary oozing can manifest as encapsulated hemorrhagic cysts. Lesions that involve the splenic artery in the splenic hilum adjacent to the tail of the pancreas are particularly worrisome. In most of these cases the radiologist's angiographic contribution in diagnosis and selective arterial embolizations is required to control the bleeding and obviate risky surgical interventions.

Lastly, infection is defined as symptomatic proliferation of germs in the pseudocyst contents which essentially leads to the formation of a pancreatic abscess. The presence of a few bacteria in the cyst in asymptomatic individuals has limited clinical value. Hence the term "infected pseudocyst" has lost clinical significance and should be avoided (Bradley 1993b).

14.3.2.4
Infected Necrosis

Infected necrosis is the most feared local complication of severe pancreatitis. This is why prevention, early recognition and adequate therapy for infected necrosis are among the main considerations in septic patients.

In most cases infected necrosis appears 3–4 weeks after the acute onset of pancreatitis. The devitalised pancreatic tissue is the ideal habitat for the colonisation and increased virulence of gram-negative germs originating in the intestine. Alteration of permeability of intestinal and colonic mucosa during the acute phase of acute pancreatitis, known as "intestinal failure", allows gram-negative bacteria to migrate through the intestinal wall and reach the retroperitoneum, colonizing necrotic pancreatic and peripancreatic tissue. Germs originating in the biliary tract, gram-positive, fungi and antibiotic resistant hospital breeds can also occur and be responsible for the development of infected pancreatic necrosis.

To avoid and/or limit the onset of this complication, early administration of antibiotic therapy in patients with pancreatic necrosis and adequate parenteral nutrition has been advocated.

The diagnosis is suspected clinically in septic individuals (fever, increased WBC) and imaging guided aspiration biopsy, gram stain diagnosis and culture of the necrotic material provide confirmation. Once demonstrated, infected necrosis is drained surgically by retroperitoneal debridement (Beger et al. 1998; Bradley 1987). If not treated, sepsis will gradually worsen with subsequent unfolding of MOF and death. The mortality rate remains high even in cases that are treated early, highlighting this complication as one of the most common causes of death in patients with acute pancreatitis (Bassi 1994).

14.3.2.5
Abscess

The consensus of the international meeting on acute pancreatitis in Atlanta defined a pancreatic abscess as an encapsulated collection of pus that develops following an episode of acute pancreatitis. This entity should be differentiated from infected necrosis since it is mainly composed of liquefied purulent material with absent or very minimal necrotic debris. The factors that determine the formation of a pancreatic abscess are similar to those that lead to the development of an infected pancreatic pseudocyst. Compared to infected necrosis, abscesses have a less severe clinical course and since they are liquefied and do not contain solid necrotic material, are generally amenable to percutaneous or endoscopic drainage procedures (Bassi et al. 1990).

14.3.2.6
Fistulas

Fistulas that occur following an attack of severe pancreatitis can be internal pancreato-intestinal or external pancreato-cutaneous. Internal fistulas and sinus tracts involving loops of hollow organs (colon, small bowel) are the consequence of the enzymatic activity of the extravasated pancreatic juice. Percutaneous radiologically guided drainage procedures and often surgical drainage can lead to the formation of an external fistula. The establishment of an external pancreato-cutaneous fistula is a worrisome complication which if not corrected can lead to serious dysmetabolic and malnutrition consequences (Pederzoli et al. 1992). The introduction of alternative nutrition supplying enough calories and protein (total enteral-parenteral nutrition) has helped alleviate this complication. The treatment requires the removal by drainage of infected necrotic material that collects in the retroperitoneum. Additionally the use of drugs based on somatostatin and derivatives that are powerful inhibitors of pancreatic secretion are used with optimal results (Bassi et al. 1998a). This conservative approach is able to resolve the majority of acute pancreatic fistulas. Anatomic considerations play a significant role in the evaluation and prognosis of pancreatic fistulas in order to avoid failure. For instance, the complete disruption of the main pancreatic duct prevents excretion of pancreatic juice into the duodenum compelling pancreatic secretion to enter the fistulous tract and maintaining a chronic pancreatic-cutaneous communication (Bassi et al. 1998b). Internal enteric fistulas and sinus tracts are less common and generally of less clinical significance (Pederzoli et al. 1992).

14.3.2.7
Fibrosis

The pancreatic inflammatory process that involves the retroperitoneum and the peritoneal cavity may cause fibrotic reactions that can involve adjacent solid or hollow organs.

Fibrosis can involve the pancreatic gland with the development of chronic pancreatitis. This evolution is rare and probably correlated to the etiology of acute pancreatitis (Angelini et al. 1993). Biliary pancreatitis, the most common etiologic factor in most European countries, once resolved usually does not develop into chronic pancreatitis. Alternatively, repeated episodes of alcoholic pancreatitis often evolve into chronic calcific pancreatitis. Other less common incriminating etiologic factors are sclero-odditis, cystic dystrophy of the duodenum or even slow-growing neoplasms obstructing the main pancreatic duct.

Peripancreatic enzymatic collections can also involve adjacent solid and hollow organs. Duodenal and colonic strictures are the most common and may require surgical interventions to relief obstructions. Ureteral and common bile duct strictures are less common but reported in the literature. These complications are usually seen late in the chronic phases of illness (Beger et al. 1998; Howard et al. 1998).

14.4
Chronic Pancreatitis

Failure of the endocrine and exocrine function of the pancreas dominates the clinical picture in chronic pancreatitis. Diagnosis is suggested by history and presence of abdominal pain, dyspepsia, malabsorption with steatorrhea and diabetes in more severe cases (Scuro et al. 1990; Sales 1991; Prinz 1993). All these clinical manifestations as well as other local complications such as intestinal strictures, fistulas and pseudocysts tend to develop slowly. Abdominal pain may be absent (painless pancreatitis) or when initially present tends to diminish or burns out with time (Amman et al. 1984; Ihse 1990; Cavallini et al. 1998; Falconi et al. 2000). The above mentioned clinical alterations that are linked to the progressive breakdown of the gland's endocrine and exocrine functions are considered systemic complications (Cavallini et al. 1998). An increased incidence of pancreatic carcinoma in patients with chronic pancreatitis has been reported but its relationship to chronic pancreatitis is still debatable. Apparently other factors such as genetic disposition and way of life (chronic alcoholic intake) may contribute to its development (Talamini et al. 1999b).

14.4.1 Malabsorption

Malabsorption in chronic pancreatitis is the result of progressive fibrous replacement of glandular pancreatic tissue associated with multiple strictures of the pancreatic ductal system and the duct occlusion by protein plugs and /or calcified calculi. These morphologic alterations lead to a decrease production of pancreatic secretions on one hand and to a decrease excretion of pancreatic juice in the duodenum on the other hand. This phenomena explains the progressive clinical syndrome of malabsorption characterised by steatorrhea, weight loss and malnutrition which when severe requires substitutive pancreatic enzyme maintenance therapy. These symptoms usually manifests when fibrosis affects 80% – 90% of the pancreatic parenchyma (Scuro et al 1990a; Scuro and Cavallini 1990).

14.4.2 Diabetes

The progressive fibrotic replacement of the pancreatic gland eventually involves the islands of Langerhans and hence it affects the endocrine function. In about 40% of cases of chronic pancreatitis pre-clinical insulin dependent diabetes sets in. This systemic complication generally occurs late and often coincides with resolution of recurrent painful episodes (Amman et al. 1984; Scuro and Cavallini 1990).

14.4.3 Ductal Carcinoma

As previously mentioned the assumed increased risk of pancreatic carcinoma in all patients with chronic pancreatitis is still challenged. There is evidence however of a significant increased risk of carcinoma in the hereditary form of chronic pancreatitis. The contribution of smoking and/or drinking habits to pancreatic carcinogenesis is less clearly defined (Talamini et al. 1996a,b, 1999).

14.5 Local Complications

Complications occur secondary to the extensive chronic inflammatory fibrotic reaction and to the acute recurrent inflammatory episodes (acute exacerbation) that are common in patients with chronic pancreatitis. The most common and most relevant complications are:

- **Stenotic strictures of the biliary tract and duodenum**
  Fibrotic tissue replacement in the head of the pancreas or an enlarging pseudocyst can obstruct the main common biliary duct and/or the duodenum with an incidence of about 10% or 3%, respectively. Biliary obstruction is suspected with signs and symptoms of cholestasis or frank jaundice whereas symptoms of gastric outlet obstruction should be suspected with the appearance of nausea and postprandial vomiting (Stahl et al. 1988).

- **Left-sided postal hypertension and pseudoaneurysm**
  Vascular complications and bleeding due to chronic pancreatitis are not frequent but they may be life-threatening and need early diagnosis and adequate treatment. Chronic pancreatic inflammation and fibrosis or a pseudocyst adjacent to the splenic vein, which is located on the posterior surface of the gland, can lead to splenic vein thrombosis and left sided portal hypertension. Thrombosis of the splenic vein, portal vein or mesenteric veins is reported with an incidence of 30% – 40% in chronic pancreatitis. In clinical practice, however, bleeding from gastric or esophageal vein, in patients with left-sided portal hypertension is a rare occurrence. The development and leaking with acute bleeding of pseudoaneurysms of the splenic, hepatic or gastroduodenal arteries is more commonly seen. Pseudoaneurysms may develop in the wall of a pseudocyst or outside

it in the peripancreatic arteries, caused by the enzymatic action of the extravasated pancreatic secretions (Scuro et al. 1990a).

- **Pseudocysts**
Pseudocysts are found in 30%–50% of patients suffering from chronic pancreatitis. Like pseudocysts detected during an acute episode of pancreatitis called "acute pseudocysts", chronic cysts are fully encapsulated pancreatic secretions with a fibrous wall without an epithelial lining. They sometime are unresolved residual acute cysts or they may develop later as a consequence of strictures and/or calculi in the pancreatic ductal system leading to ductal ectasia and rupture. These chronic pseudo- cysts sometimes referred to as "retention cysts" more often tend to communicate with the main or secondary pancreatic ducts. This anatomic feature has significant clinical implications in the management of chronic pseudocysts. If communication with pancreatic duct is patent and pancreatic secretions can not drain into duodenum because of ductal strictures, percutaneous, endoscopic or surgical drainage of such cysts may result in the formation of pancreatic fistulas (Scuro and Cavallini 1990; Falconi et al. 2000). In these cases endoscopic attempts to reestablish patency of the pancreatic duct are made before cysts drainage is performed.
Similar to the acute pseudocysts, other complications may occur in patient with chronic cysts. Secondary infection with the formation of an abscess, cyst bleeding, migration of cyst into the pelvis or into mediastinum through the esophageal hiatus or cyst rupture with fluid leakage into the peritoneal cavity have been reported.

- **Pancreatic ascites**
Chronic pancreatic ascites occurs when there is a fistulous connection established between the pancreatic duct and peritoneal cavity, usually associated with rupture and leakage of a pancreatic pseudocyst. Blockage of the pancreatic duct diverts pancreatic secretion into the peritoneal cavity maintaining the pancreatic ascites. In chronic forms seen in patients with stigmata of chronic pancreatitis the pancreatic enzymes in the ascitic fluid are not activated, and acute peritonitis does not develop. The diagnosis is confirmed by peritoneal top with the detection of an exudate-transudate rich in protein and enzymes. Chronic pancreatic ascites is difficult to treat requiring decompression of the obstructed pancreatic duct by endoscopy or surgical means (Scuro and Cavallini 1990).

- **Fistulas**
Both internal or external fistulas can develop in the course of chronic pancreatitis. External, pancreatic-cutaneous fistulas, as mentioned before, are usually the result of surgical or percutaneous drainage attempts of pseudocysts or fluid collections that communicate with the pancreatic ductal system. Internal fistulas may follow endoscopic drainage procedures or they may be spontaneous following pseudocysts rupture into adjacent hollow viscera. The stomach, small bowel or transverse colon may be involved in these cases. Less common fistulas tracts may extend into the left pleural space with the development of pleural effusion rich in amylase or may invade the mediastinum causing mediastinitis with high mortality rates (Pederzoli et al. 1992).

References

Amman RW, Akovbiantz A, Largiader F, Schueler G (1984) Course and outcome of chronic pancreatitis. Longitudinal study of a mixed medical-surgical series of 254 patients. Gastroenterology 86:820–828

Angelini G, Cavallini G, Pederzoli P, Bovo P, Bassi C, Di Francesco V, Frulloni L, Sgarbi D, Talamini G, Castagnini A (1993) Long term outcome of acute pancreatitis. Digestion 54:143–147

Banks PA (1994) Acute Pancreatitis: medical and surgical management. Am J Gastroenterol 89:78–85

Bassi C (1994) Infected pancreatic necrosis. Int J Pancreatol 16:1–10

Bassi C, Vesentini S, Nifosì F et al (1990) Pancreatic abscess and other pus-harboring collections related to pancreatitis: a review of 108 cases. World J Surg 14:505–512

Bassi C, Falconi M, Pederzoli P (1998a) Pancreatic fistula. In: Howard J, Idezuki Y, Ihse I, Prinz R (eds) Surgical diseases of the pancreas. Williams and Wilkins, pp 827–834

Bassi C, Falconi M, Pederzoli P (1998b) Management of pancreatic fistulas. In: Beger HG, Warshaw AL, Büchler MW, Carr-Loke DL, Neoptolemos JP, Russel C, Sarr MG (eds) The pancreas. Blackwell Science, pp 632–649

Beger HG, Büchler MW, Bittner R et al (1988) Necrosectomy and postoperative lavage in necrotizing pancreatitis. Br J Surg 9:972–979

Beger HG, Warshaw AL, Büchler MW, Carr-Loke DL, Neoptolemos JP, Russel C, Sarr MG (1998) The pancreas. Blackwell Science

Bradley EL (1987) Management of infected pancreatic necrosis by open drainage. Ann Surg 206:542–550

Bradley EL (1993a) Acute pancreatitis. Raven Press, New York

Bradley EL (1993b) A clinically based classification system for acute pancreatitis: summary of the Atlanta Symposium. Arch Surg 128:586–590

Cavallini G, Frulloni L, Pederzoli P, Talamini G, Bovo P, Bassi C, Di Francesco V, Vaona B, Falconi M, Sartori N, Angelini GP, Brunori MP, Filippini M (1998) LongtTerm follow-up of patients with chronic pancreatitis in Italy. Scand J Gastroenterol 33:880–889

D'Egidio A, Schein M (1991) Surgical strategies in the treatment of pancreatic necrosis and infection. Br J Surg 78:133–137

Falconi M, Valerio A, Caldiron E, Salvia R, Sartori N, Talamini G, Bassi C, Pederzoli P (2000) Changes in pancreatic resection for chronic pancreatitis over 28 years in a single institution. Br J Surg 87:428–433

Howard J, Idezuki Y, Ihse I, Prinz R (1998) Surgical diseases of the pancreas. Williams and Wilkins

Ihse I (1990) Pancreatic pain – causes, diagnosis and treatment. Acta Chir Scand 156:257–258

Pederzoli P, Bassi C, Vesentini S (1992) Pancreatic fistulas. Springer, Berlin Heidelberg New York

Pederzoli P, Cavallini G, Bassi C, Falconi M (eds) (1994) Facing the pancreatic dilemma. Springer, Berlin Heidelberg New York

Prinz RA (1993) Surgical options in chronic pancreatitis. Int J Pancreatol 14:97–105

Sales H (1991) Definitions and classifications of pancreatitis. Pancreas 6:470–474

Scuro LA, Cavallini G (1990) La patologia infiammatoria del pancreas. Relazione 91°Congresso della Società Italiana di Medicina Interna. Luigi Pozzi Ed

Scuro LA, Cavallini G, Benini L, Brocco G, Bovo P, Riela A, Togni M, Cataudella G, Bassi C, Pederzoli P, Micciolo R (1990) Pancreatic calcifications in patients with chronic pancreatitis. Int J Pancreatol 6:139–150

Stahl TJ, O'Connors AM, Ansel HJ, Venes JA (1988) Partial biliary obstruction caused by chronic pancreatitis. Ann Surg 207:26–32

Talamini G, Bassi C, Falconi M, Frulloni L, Di Francesco V, Vaona B, Bovo P, Rigo L, Castagnini A, Angelini G, Pederzoli P, Cavallini G (1996a) Cigarette smoking: an independent risk factor in alcoholic pancreatitis. Pancreas 12:131–137

Talamini G, Bassi C, Falconi M, Sartori N, Salvia R, Di Francesco V, Frulloni L, Vaona B, Bovo P, Vantini I, Pederzoli P, Cavallini G (1996b) Pain relapses in the first 10 years of chronic pancreatitis. Am J Surg 171:565–569

Talamini G, Falconi M, Bassi C, Sartori N, Salvia R, Caldiron E, Frulloni L, Di Francesco V, Vaona B, Bovo P, Vantini I, Pederzoli P, Cavallini G (1999a) Incidence of cancer in the course of chronic pancreatitis. Am J Gastroenterol 94:1253–1260

Talamini G, Bassi C, Falconi M, Sartori N, Salvia R, Rigo L, Castagnini A, Di Francesco V, Frulloni L, Bovo P, Vaona B, Angelini GP, Vantini I, Cavallini G, Pederzoli P (1999b) Alcohol and smoking as risk factors in chronic pancreatitis and pancreatic cancer. Dig Dis Sci 44:1303–1311

Imaging of Pancreatic Pseudocyst

15

Giovanni Carbognin, Carlo Biasiutti, Chiara Calciolari, Giovanni Foti, and Roberto Pozzi Mucelli

CONTENTS

15.1 **Definition** *269*
15.1.1 Epidemiology *269*
15.1.2 Pathogenesis *270*
15.2 **Pathological Findings** *274*
15.2.1 Macroscopic Findings *274*
15.2.2 Microscopic Findings *276*
15.3 **Role of Imaging** *276*
15.4 **US Imaging** *276*
15.5 **CT Imaging** *276*
15.6 **MR Imaging** *278*
15.7 **Endoscopic Ultrasound Imaging (EUS)** *281*
15.8 **Differential Diagnosis** *281*
15.8.1 Cystic Dystrophy of Duodenum *282*
15.8.2 Mucinous Cystic Pancreatic Tumor *283*
15.8.3 Serous Cystadenoma *283*
15.8.4 Intraductal Papillary Mucinous Tumors of the Collateral Ducts (IPMT II Type) *284*
15.8.5 Solid and Papillary Tumor *285*
15.8.6 Other Cystic Tumors *285*
15.9 **Role of Needle-Aspiration Biopsy** *286*
15.1 **Pre-operative Assessment** *286*
15.1 **Pseudocyst Evolution** *286*
15.1 **Complications** *287*
15.12.1 Infection and Pancreatic Abscess *287*
15.12.2 Vascular Complications *288*
15.12.3 Jaundice *288*
15.12.4 Compression on Gastro-intestinal and Urinary Tracts *288*
15.12.5 Rupture and Fistulas *289*
15.12.6 Pleural Effusion *292*
References *292*

G. Carbognin, MD
C. Biasiutti, MD
C. Calciolari, MD
G. Foti, MD
R. Pozzi Mucelli, MD
Department of Radiology, Policlinico "GB Rossi", Piazzale LA Scuro 10, 37134 Verona, Italy

15.1 Definition

Pseudocysts are fluid filled masses with a wall made of inflammatory and fibrotic tissue rather than a true epithelial lining. They develop from a fluid collection following a pancreatic injury and are circumscribed by a pseudo-capsule (Fig. 15.1) (Hammond et al. 2002; Kim et al. 2005).

15.1.1 Epidemiology

Pseudocysts are the most common cystic lesions of the pancreas, representing about 85% of all pancreatic cysts (Hammond et al. 2002; Kim et al. 2005; Yeo and Sarr 1994; Singhal et al. 2006b). They do not present any risk of neoplastic degeneration. They will reabsorb spontaneously in about 40% of cases. They are clinically significant since they are a frequent

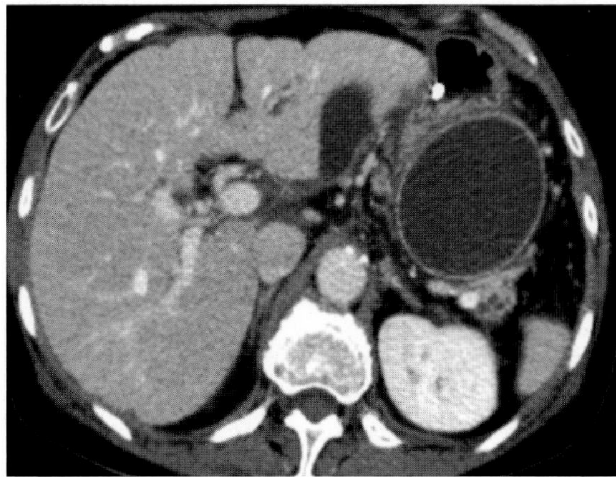

Fig. 15.1. Contrast enhanced CT (CECT), portal phase, axial plane: typical pseudocyst following acute pancreatitis. The lesion is characterized by homogenous fluid content and thin pseudocapsule

complication (30%–50% of cases) of acute pancreatitis (Soliani et al. 2004), abdominal trauma (10% in adults, 60% in children) and chronic pancreatitis (20%–40%) (Hammond et al 2002). Pseudocysts are usually located within the pancreatic parenchyma (85% in the region of the pancreatic body and tail, 15% in the head), or in the virtual spaces between the pancreas and the adjacent abdominal viscera.

15.1.2 Pathogenesis

Pancreatic pseudocysts are unabsorbed fluid collections that develop a fibrous pseudo-capsule over a period of 4–6 weeks.

The pathogenesis is based on the rupture of the pancreatic duct, with the subsequent release of pancreatic juice and activated enzymes, damaging the adjacent structures and forming the fluid collection (Yeo and Sarr 1994).

The following conditions can lead to the development of a pseudocyst:

1. *Severe acute pancreatitis* with parenchymal necrosis and hemorrhage: pancreatic duct rupture is an intrinsic characteristic of the autolysis process due to the release of pancreatic juice with a high concentration of pancreatic enzymes (Yeo and Sarr 1994; Soliani et al. 2004). Around 30%–50% of pseudocysts are due to severe acute pancreatitis; however, the majority resolve by spontaneous reabsorption (Yeo and Sarr 1994; Soliani et al. 2004).
2. *Blunt abdominal trauma* with pancreatic duct disruption is a relatively rare cause of pseudocyst in adults representing 10% of cases (Yeo and Sarr 1994; Procacci et al. 1997a). In contrast, post-traumatic lesions represent 60% of pseudocysts in children (Yeo and Sarr 1994; Soliani et al. 2004; Procacci et al. 1997b; Hall 1992). The most frequently involved regions are the pancreatic neck and body, closely located to the spine and indirectly damaged by the vertebrae (Fig. 15.2).
3. *Chronic pancreatitis* associated with stones obstructing the pancreatic duct, duct stenosis due to fibrous tissue and scarring or tumors invading the pancreatic duct causing an increase in intra-ductal pressure, duct dilation and their subsequent rupture and the release of pancreatic enzymes (Fig. 15.3) (Yeo and Sarr 1994; Bradley 1989; Klöppel 2000).

Pseudocysts following chronic pancreatitis will less frequently resorb spontaneously and often need to be drained (Yeo and Sarr 1994).

In all cases, fluid collections due to pancreatic injury develop a thin fibrous rim within 4 or 6 weeks after onset (Fig. 15.1) (Kim et al. 2005; Singhal et al. 2006b; Klöppel 2000). The lesion is either located within the pancreatic gland (Fig. 15.4) or adjacent to it (Fig. 15.5) (Yeo and Sarr 1994). The shape of the pseudocyst is frequently the same as the original fluid collection. At the beginning, the content is inhomogeneous because of the presence of blood clots and cellular debris (Fig. 15.5); a "mature" pseudocyst is characterized by a homogeneous, water-like content, resulting from the reabsorption of clots and debris (Fig. 15.6). A calcified wall can be found over a period of 5–6 months after onset (Yeo and Sarr 1994).

As regards extra-pancreatic pseudocysts, the typical locations are the lesser sac and the anterior para-renal spaces, most frequently on the left side (Klöppel 2000; Balthazar 2002).

Retrogastric pseudocysts can become large in size. They develop between the ventral border of the pancreas and the posterior parietal peritoneum, distending this potential space and protruding into the omental bursa (Fig. 15.7a). If the pseudocyst erodes into the posterior parietal peritoneum, a fluid collection can develop within the lesser sac or freely distribute within the peritoneal cavity as pancreatic ascites.

The anterior para-renal spaces are also the site of the origin and spread of a necrotic fluid collection coming from the pancreas (Fig. 15.7b). In the early phase, fluid collections are characterized by an inhomogeneous content due to the presence of blood clots, cellular debris, oxy-hemoglobin, deoxy-hemoglobin and methehemoglobin and adipose tissue (extracellular fat). The fluid collection tends to spread more frequently in the left anterior para-renal space because involvement of the body-tail region is more common in severe acute pancreatitis. The subsequent spread of the inflammatory process follows preferential paths: through the anterior para-renal space caudally, occupying the trough defined by the fusion of the renal fascia with the lateroconal fascia. More inferiorly, the collection dissects between the two layers of the posterior renal fascia and reaching the region of the quadratus lom-borum and psoas muscles.

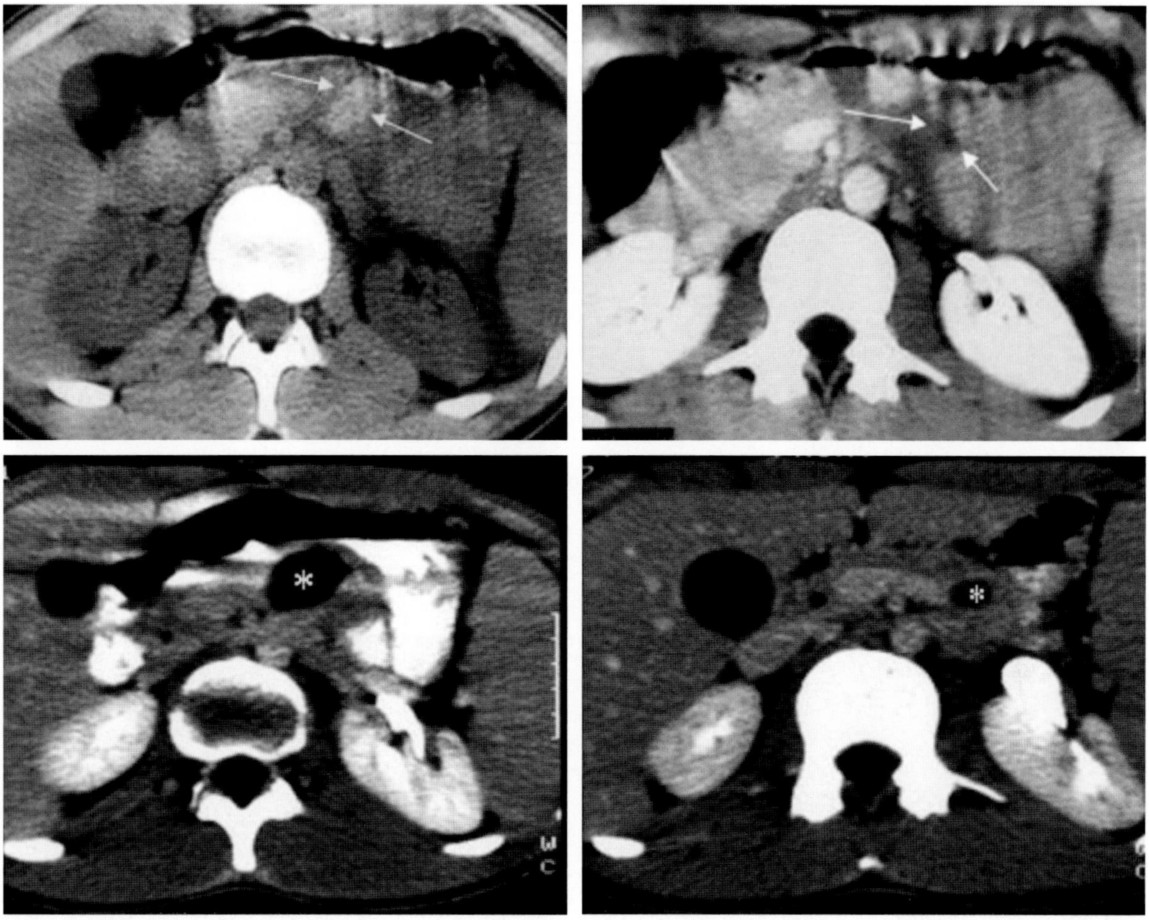

Fig. 15.2a–d. Post-traumatic pseudocyst. **a** Non-contrast-enhanced CT: non-homogenous hyperdense lesion located in the pancreatic neck (*arrows*). **b** CECT – Portal phase: hypodense non-enhancing lesion compared to pancreatic parenchyma (**c**) CT scan performed 3 months later: pseudocyst (*) in the region of pancreatic neck. **d** At 6 months later reduction in size of the pseudocyst (*) can be noted

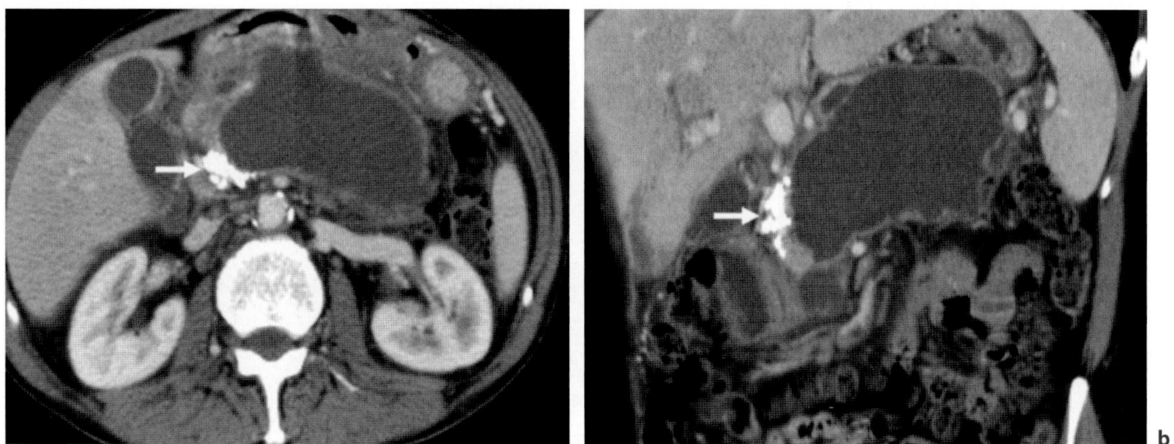

Fig. 15.3a,b. CECT – portal phase: axial (**a**) and coronal (**b**) CT show a large pseudocyst in a patient with chronic pancreatitis: multiple calcifications can be seen in pancreatic head (*arrows*)

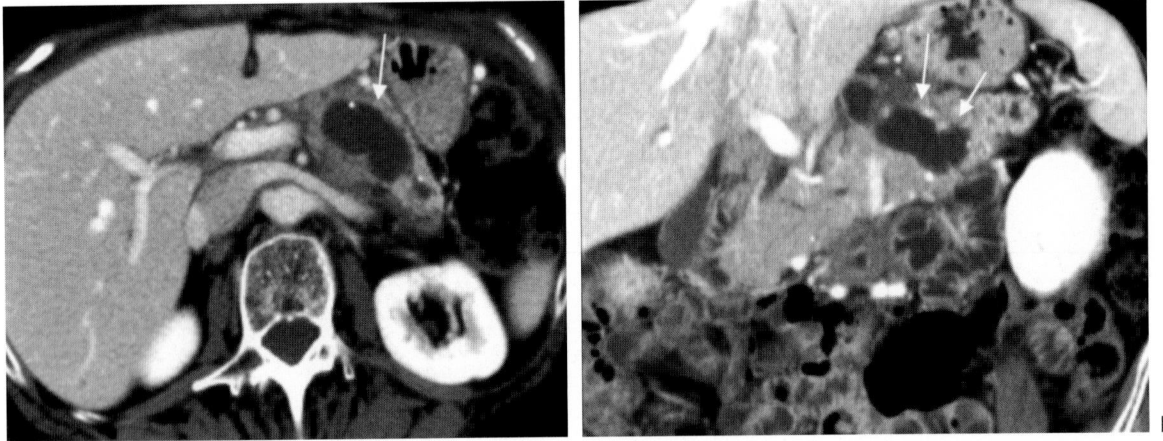

Fig. 15.4a,b. CECT – portal phase: axial (**a**) and coronal (**b**) planes show a intra-pancreatic pseudocyst involving the body and the tail of the pancreas (*arrows*)

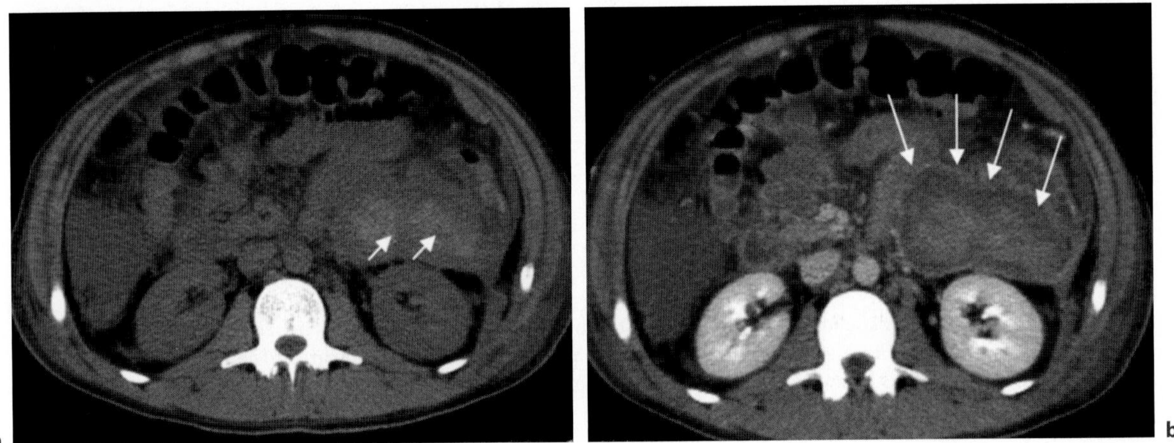

Fig. 15.5a,b. CT scan before (**a**) and after (**b**) the administration of iodinated contrast material: a large pseudocyst in the retroperitoneal left pararenal space. The pseudocyst is inhomogeneous due to the presence of clots and cellular debris (*short arrows*). Only the pseudocapsule enhances after contrast injection (*long arrows*)

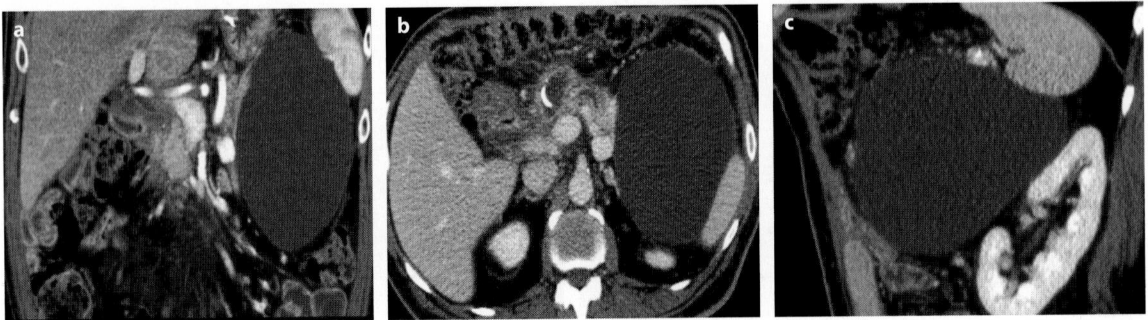

Fig. 15.6a–c. "Mature" pseudocyst. CECT during the portal phase in axial (**a**), coronal (**b**) and sagittal (**c**) planes shows a water-like homogenous mass encapsulated by a thin wall in the tail of pancreas

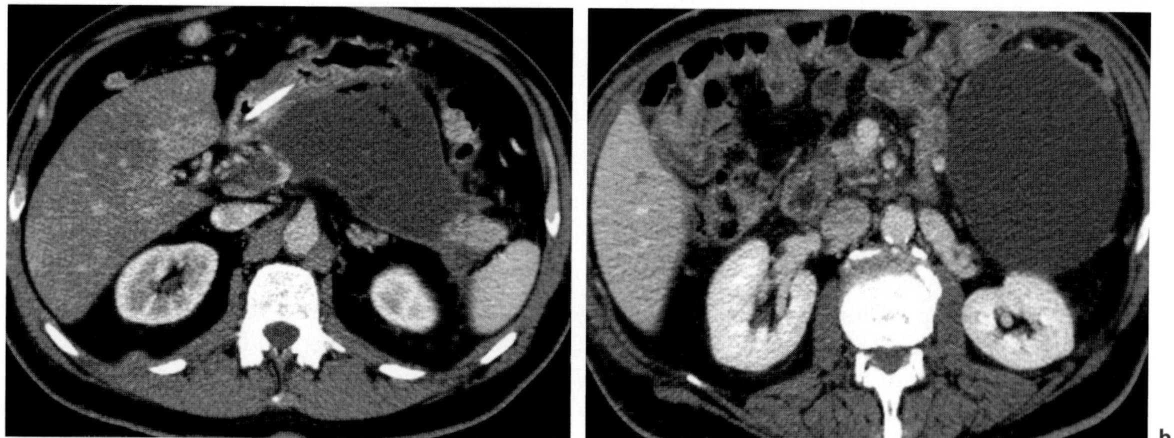

Fig. 15.7a,b. Large pseudocysts (two cases). **a** First case: large pseudocyst with predominant extension into the lesser sac. **b** Second case: large, round pseudocyst with extension to the left kidney, in the anterior pararenal space

Fig. 15.8a–c. Pseudocyst in the left pararenal space. CECT scan during the portal phase in axial (**a**), coronal (**b**) and sagittal (**c**) planes shows a pseudocyst in the tail of pancreas and a second pseudocyst in the left perirenal space, surrounding the upper pole of left kidney (*arrows*)

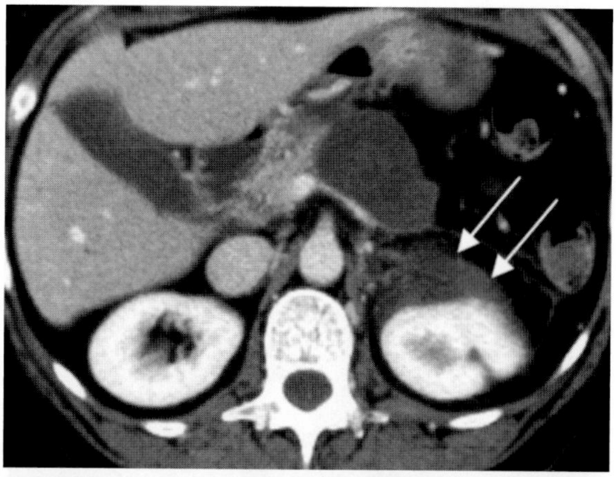

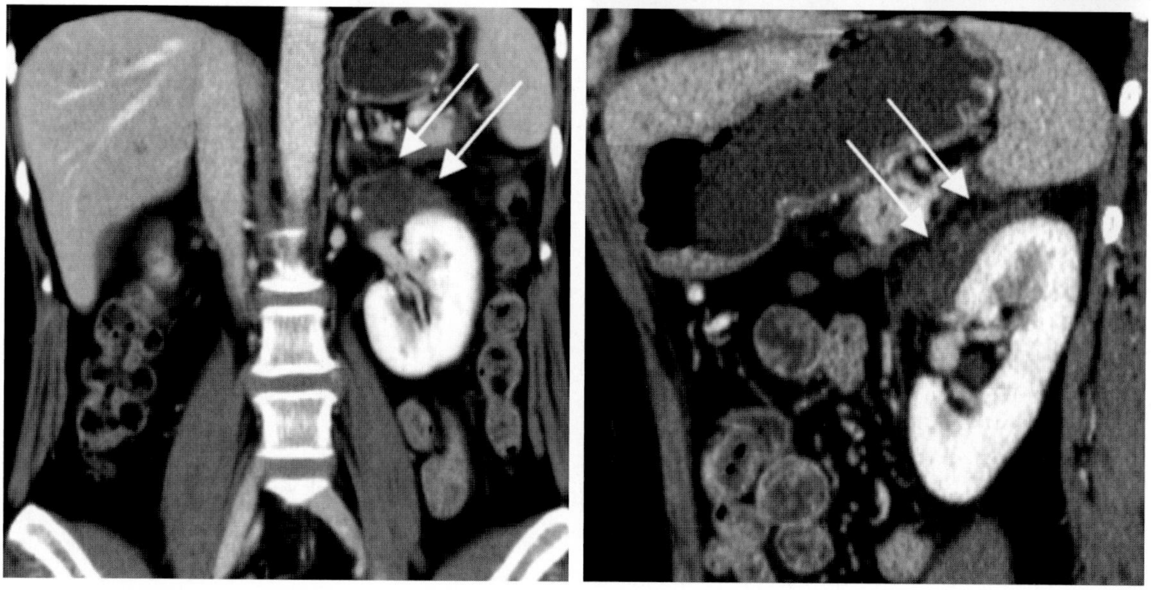

Larger fluid collections may involve the perirenal space (Fig. 15.8) and the posterior para-renal space either directly, due to erosion of the fascia or indirectly, in the case of large pelvic or iliac fluid collections spreading in a retrograde direction towards the upper regions of the retroperitoneal cavity (Fig. 15.9). From the pancreatic region, fluid collections can extend into the mesenteric layers, commonly the transverse mesocolon. Rarely pseudocysts can develop within the hepatoduodenal ligament occupying the hepatic hilum (Fig. 15.10). Lastly, pseudocysts can spread towards the diaphragm and the mediastinum or the pelvic extra-peritoneal space, following the psoas muscle (Fig. 15.11) and reaching, in extreme cases, the inguinal canal and scrotal bursa (Cooperman 2001; Sadat et al. 2007).

15.2 Pathological Findings

15.2.1 Macroscopic Findings

Small pseudocysts tend to be oval-shaped, whereas large ones are characterized by quite variable and irregular shapes. They often conform to the shape of the loculated fluid collection from which they arise. Intra-pancreatic pseudocysts are usually single and located in the body-tail region. Between 10%–20% of pseudocysts are multiple. The size range is wide, with lesions measuring about 10–15 cm or more, particularly those lesions located outside the pancreas (Kim et al. 2005; Klöppel 2000; Karantanus et al. 2003).

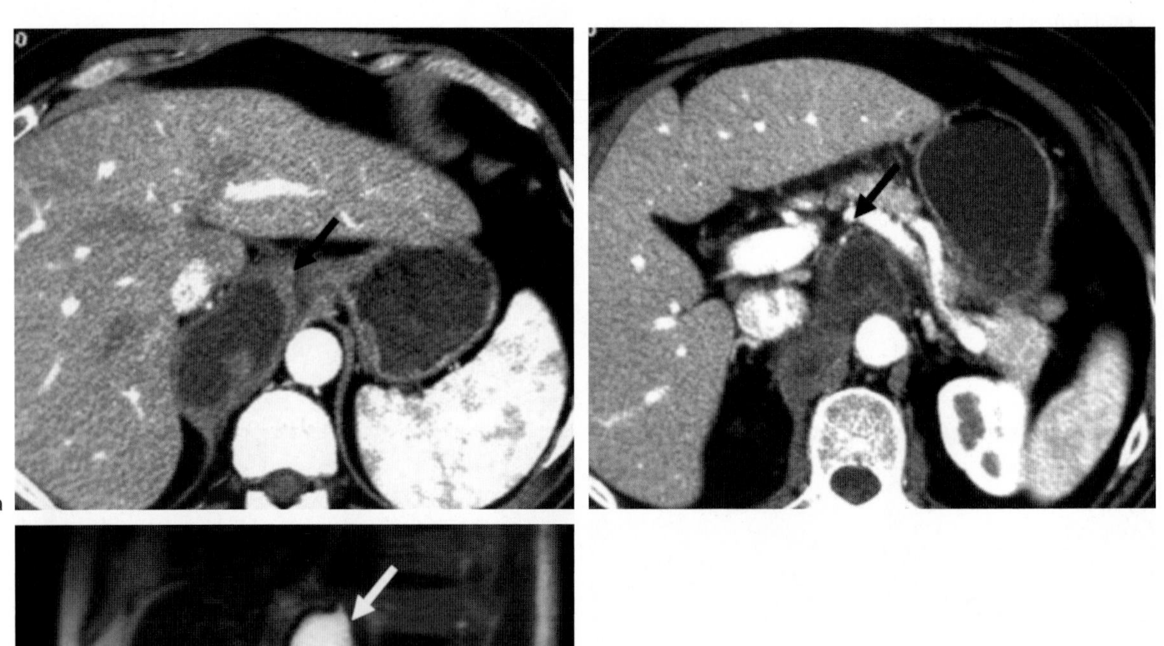

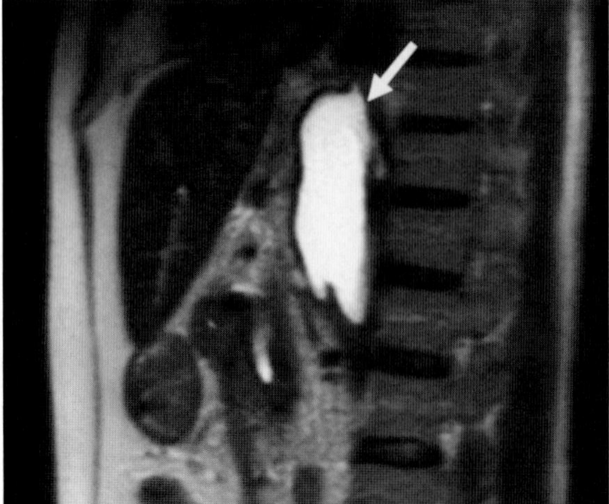

Fig. 15.9a–c. Pseudocyst with unusual location. Fluid collection (*arrows*) with thick wall involving the right crus of the diaphragm (**a**), and medial extension, anterior to the aorta is seen. **b** MR HASTE T2WI shows the same lesion in sagittal plane

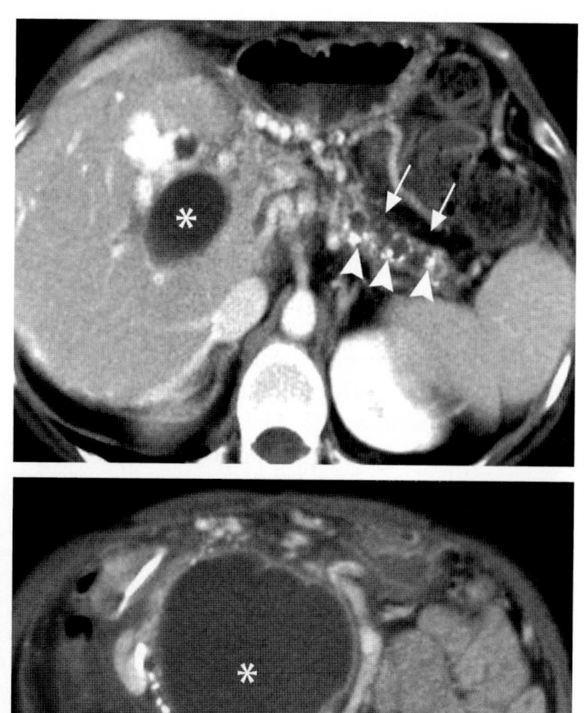

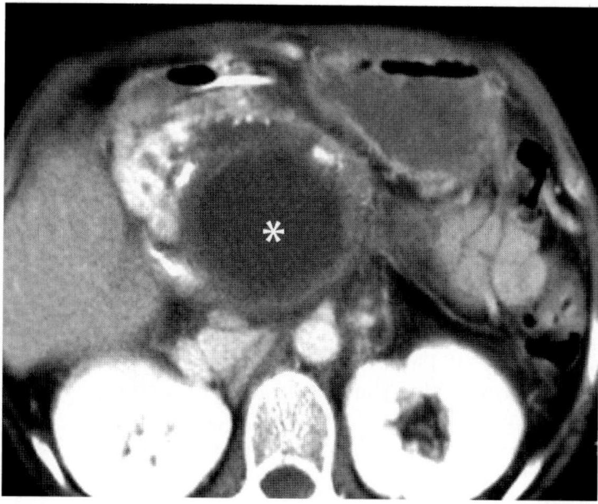

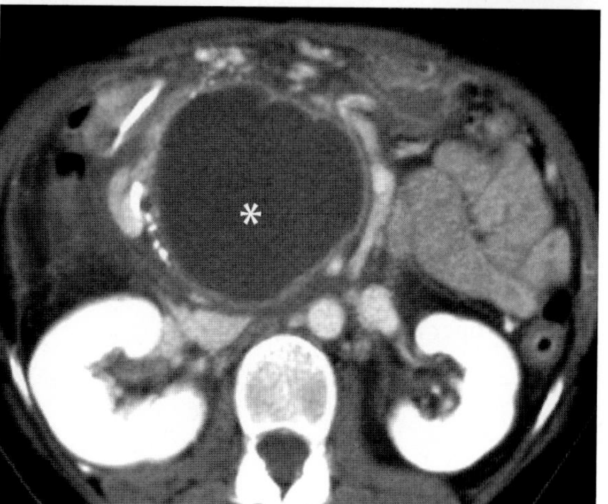

Fig. 15.10a–c. Large pseudocyst developing in the hepatic hilum (*). Pancreatic parenchyma is thin, main pancreatic duct is dilated (*arrows*) with a beaded tree pattern with multiple calcifications (*arrowheads*) (**a**). The portal vein is not visible but multiple venous collaterals are present (**b**,**c**)

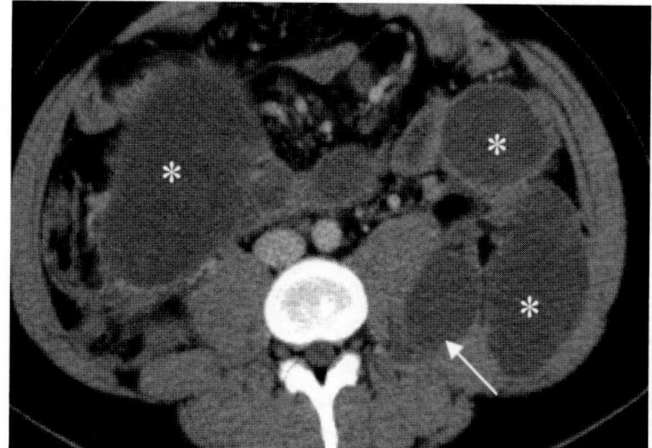

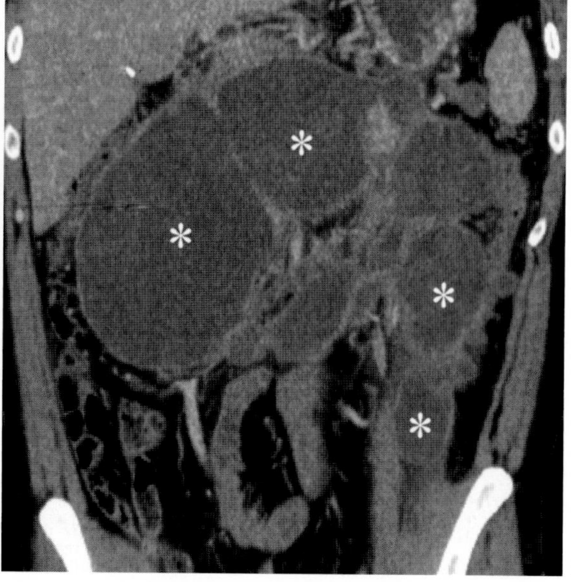

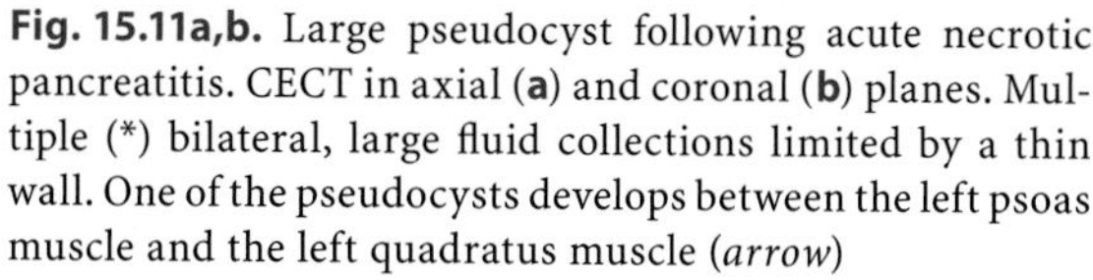

Fig. 15.11a,b. Large pseudocyst following acute necrotic pancreatitis. CECT in axial (**a**) and coronal (**b**) planes. Multiple (*) bilateral, large fluid collections limited by a thin wall. One of the pseudocysts develops between the left psoas muscle and the left quadratus muscle (*arrow*)

15.2.2 Microscopic Findings

The wall of the pseudocyst consists of necrotic, granulation and fibrous tissue, adipocytes, and collagen fibers, but no epithelial lining (Cooperman 2001). The pseudocapsule, developing over a period of 4–6 weeks after the onset of the fluid collection, has a variable thickness depending on the stage of evolution. The wall is characterized by inflammatory cells, hemoglobin pigments, hemorrhage and cholesterol. Wall calcifications can be found in "mature" pseudocysts. The content, inhomogeneous in the early stages due to the presence of necrotic debris, hemoglobin degradation products, pancreatic enzymes and adipose tissue, becomes more homogeneous as the cyst matures (Klöppel 2000; Karantanas et al. 2003). The presence of epithelial lining from the damaged pancreatic ducts incorporated into the pseudocyst wall causes some problems at histologic examination. However, the absence of atypical malignant cells together with typical clinical and radiological findings helps to lead to proper characterization.

15.3 Role of Imaging

The aims of imaging techniques are to detect the lesions, establishing the numbers, size and aspects of the pseudo-capsules, their internal architecture and content, as well as their precise location and the relationship with adjacent structures. Characterization and differential diagnosis from other pancreatic and peri-pancreatic cystic lesions should be carefully considered in order to choose the most appropriate therapy.

15.4 US Imaging

Typically, pseudocysts are solitary, unilocular cystic lesions characterized by a homogeneous anechoic content, encapsulated by a thin wall displaying acoustic enhancement of the posterior wall (Fig. 15.12). The presence of blood clots and cellular debris causes the inhomogeneity of the fluid content, producing internal echoes.The echoes are frequently stratified in the dependent regions and may demonstrate a fluid-debris level. Conversely, "mature" lesions are characterized by decreasing internal echoes due to autolysis, leaving a water-like anechoic content. The presence of internal septations is a rare finding and may suggest a complication such as infection or hemorrhage. In addition, US allows for the evaluation of the thickness of the pseudo-capsule and the presence of calcifications (Fig. 15.12). However, US imaging is limited in the evaluation of a pseudocyst with a markedly calcified wall, because of the mirror-effect that calcifications produce on the acoustic beam (Rickes and Wermke 2004).

Recently, thanks to the improvement of harmonic US imaging, with and without the administration of an ultrasonographic contrast agent, additional findings can be evaluated that could make differential diagnosis easier: young "immature" pseudocysts frequently show a moderate parietal enhancement, whereas "mature" ones are not usually associated with this finding (Rickes et al. 2006). US is the most appropriate technique in the follow-up of patients with known pseudocyst in order to evaluate any alteration in size that could lead to a change in the therapeutic approach (Yeo and Sarr 1994).

15.5 CT Imaging

CT is the imaging technique most frequently used in the assessment of cystic pancreatic lesions (Procacci et al. 1997a). The optimization of the contrast enhancement patterns of the pancreas and visualization of the peri-pancreatic vessels has made it possible to improve the sensitivity of CT in the detection of pseudocysts and their complications. The unenhanced CT examination aims at detecting any pancreatic calcifications (chronic pancreatitis) or hemorrhage. During this phase, pseudocysts appear as a near water-density mass, usually below 15 UH, encapsulated by a thin and homogeneous rim, isodense to the pancreatic parenchyma (Fig. 15.6) (Kim et al. 2005). Any inhomogeneity of the content is due to the presence of a large quantity of proteins, generally relatively high attenuating (> 40–50 UH), and frequently associated with the presence of fluid-fluid levels (Fig. 15.13) (Balthazar 2002; Morgan

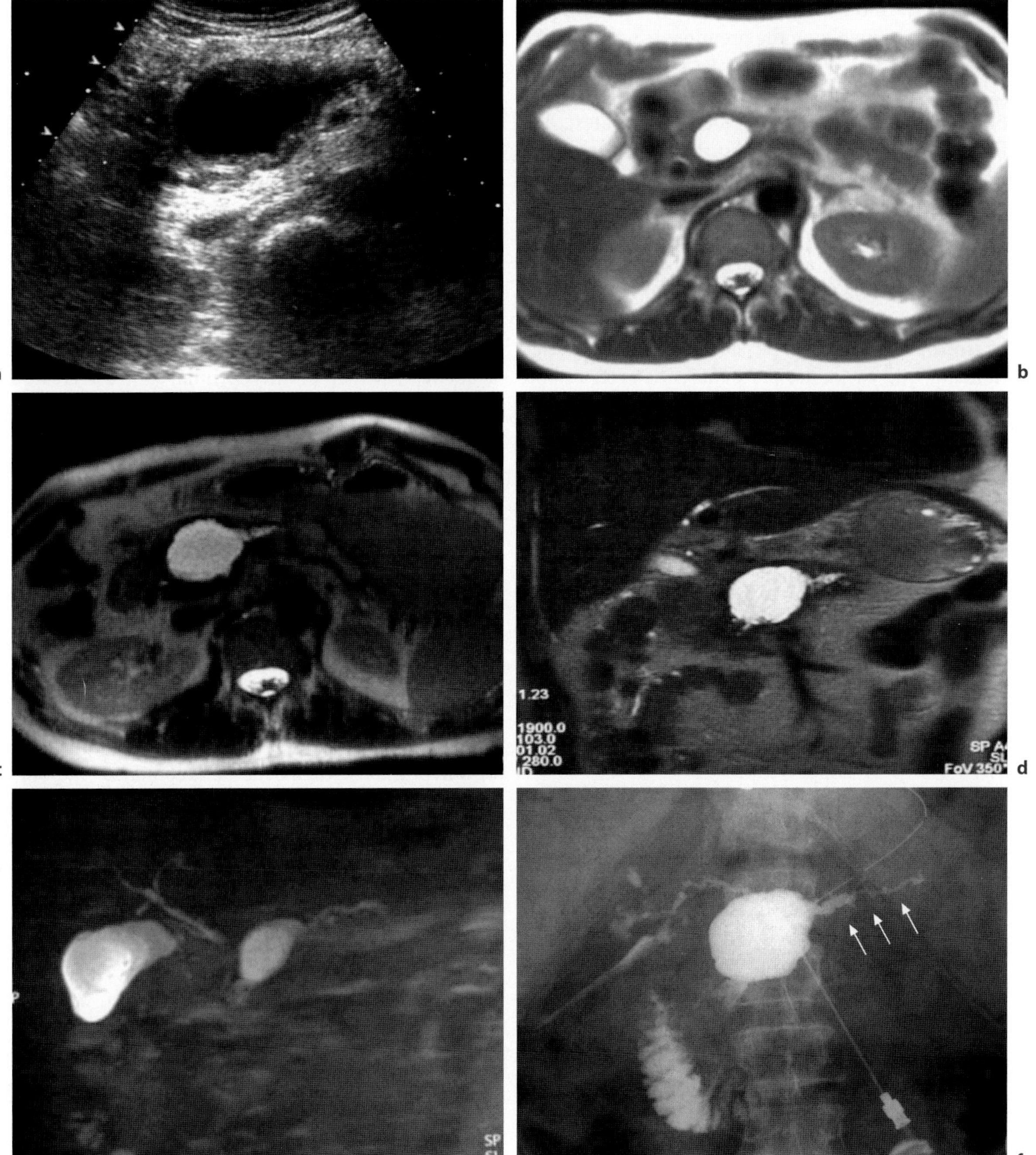

Fig. 15.12a–f. Abdominal ultrasound (**a**) shows the presence of a pseudocyst located in the region of pancreatic head characterized by thick wall and cellular debris in the dependent region. The MR HASTE sequences in axial (**b**,**c**) and coronal planes (**d**) and RARE sequences (**e**) show the communication of the cystic lesion with the main pancreatic duct. The communication is confirmed by the opacification of the tract through the percutaneous injection into the cyst (*arrows*) (**f**)

et al. 1997). In this phase it is possible to detect any calcifications involving the pseudocyst wall and the adjacent pancreatic parenchyma as well. The pancreatic arterial phase is optimal for the detection of pseudocysts since it provides the greatest difference of attenuation between the lesion, typically hypodense, and the normal pancreatic parenchyma (Klöppel 2000). Moreover, this phase helps in detecting and characterizing any possible neoplastic lesions (pseudocyst associated with pancreatic tumor) (Fig. 15.14). Thanks to the use of MDCT with the ability to rapidly acquire thin sections composed of isotropic voxels, it is possible to assess the relationship with the major peripancreatic arteries and veins.

The venous phase is used to assess the remainder of the abdominal cavity; with MDCT isotropic voxels can allow 3-D representations that can show the complex relationships that pseudocysts can develop with abdominal viscera. This information aids in assuring adequate drainage and surgical planning.

15.6 MR Imaging

Although CT is considered the primary imaging technique in the assessment of pseudocysts, MR imaging, thanks to its continuous technological advancement, can be considered as accurate as CT in the study of pancreatic pathologies and in particular of cystic lesions (Nishihara et al. 1996; Schima 2006).

On non-enhanced fat suppressed-gradient recalled echo T1 (FS-GRE T1)-weighted images, the pseudocyst appears as a homogeneous, encapsulated cystic lesion, usually oval-shaped and hypointense compared to the normally hyperintense pancreatic parenchyma (Fig. 15.15). The presence of hemorrhage or cellular debris within the cystic cavity is associated with an increase in the signal intensity of its content (Fig. 15.16). Extra-pancreatic lesions are well depicted with the breath-hold GRE sequence because of the optimal contrast created between the hypointense content of the pseudocyst and the typically hyperintense extra-cellular fat. Contrarily, these sequences are not able to show septations, which are usually hypointense like the pseudocyst content (Manfredi et al. 2001). The content is usually hyperintense on the TSE T2-weighted sequence. "Mature" and non-complicated pseudocysts are commonly homogeneously hyperintense, whereas "young" lesions and complicated ones are inhomogeneously hyperintense thanks to the presence of cellular debris, hemorrhage or infection (Fig. 15.17). A large quantity of proteins within the cyst is frequently associated with the presence of a hypointense meniscus or "geometric" hypointense material within the dependent portion of the cyst cavity. The use of a breath-hold FS-GRE 3-D T1-weighted sequence, during the i.v. administration of Gd-chelates, leads to the evaluation of imaging

a 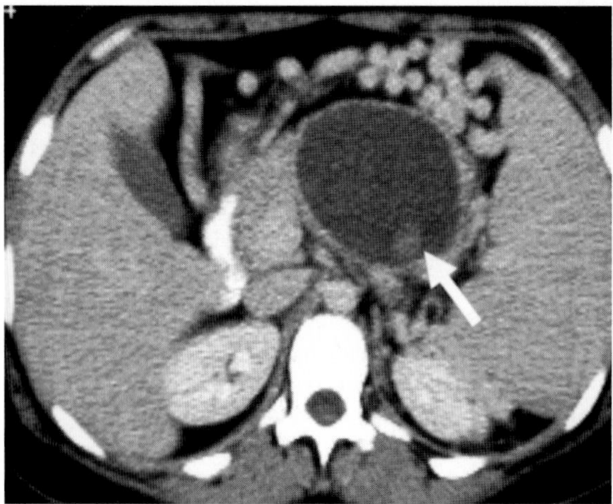

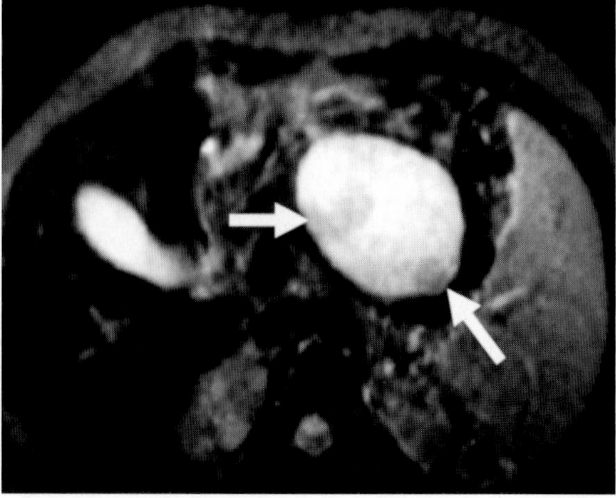 b

Fig. 15.13a,b. Clots and debris in a pseudocyst. Axial CECT scan during portal phase (**a**) and axial MR STIR sequence (**b**) show the presence of a pseudocyst following acute pancreatitis characterized by inhomogeneous content due to the presence of high density (**a**) (*arrow*), and low signal intensity areas (**b**) (*arrows*). Splenomegaly and multiple venous collaterals due to splenic vein thrombosis are also seen (**a**)

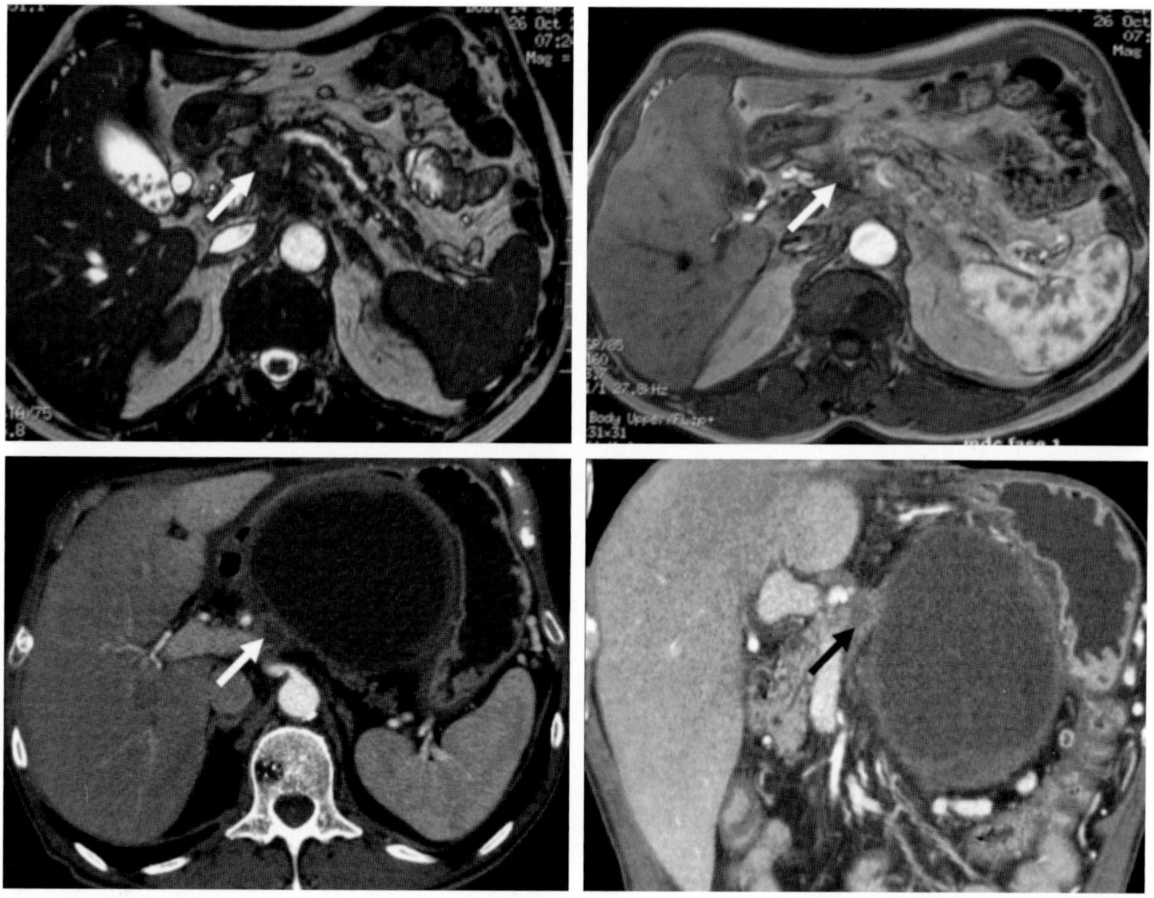

Fig. 15.14a–d. MR TRUE FISP (**a**) and VIBE (**b**) sequences in the arterial phase after the administration of intravenous gadolinium (**b**) show the presence of a small lesion (*arrow*) in the pancreatic head, slightly hyperintense on T2-weighted images and hypovascular following contrast injection when compared to pancreatic parenchyma (*arrow*). The lesion causes obstruction of main pancreatic duct, with upstream dilation. Three months later, a pseudocyst developed following an episode of acute pancreatitis. The CT scan in axial (**c**) and coronal (**d**) planes shows the cystic lesion and a hypodense lesion (*arrow*) in the region of the pancreatic neck. The biopsy of this lesion confirmed the diagnosis of pancreatic adenocarcinoma

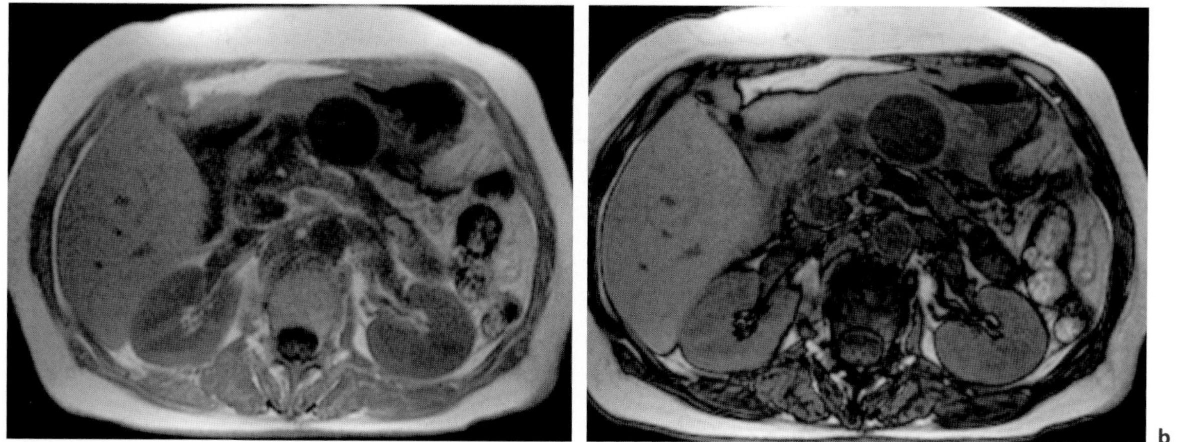

Fig. 15.15a,b. Typical pseudocyst. MR GRE T1-weighted in phase (**a**) and out of phase (**b**) images show the typical hypointense signal intensity of non-complicated pseudocyst

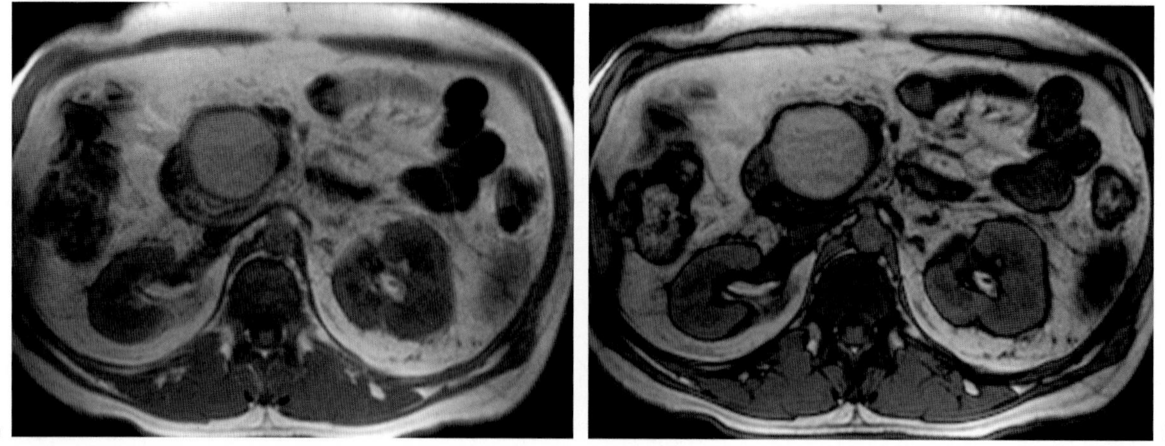

Fig. 15.16a,b. Hemorrhagic pseudocyst. MR GRE T1-weighted in phase (**a**) and out of phase (**b**) images show a hyperintense pseudocyst due to the presence of hemorrhagic content

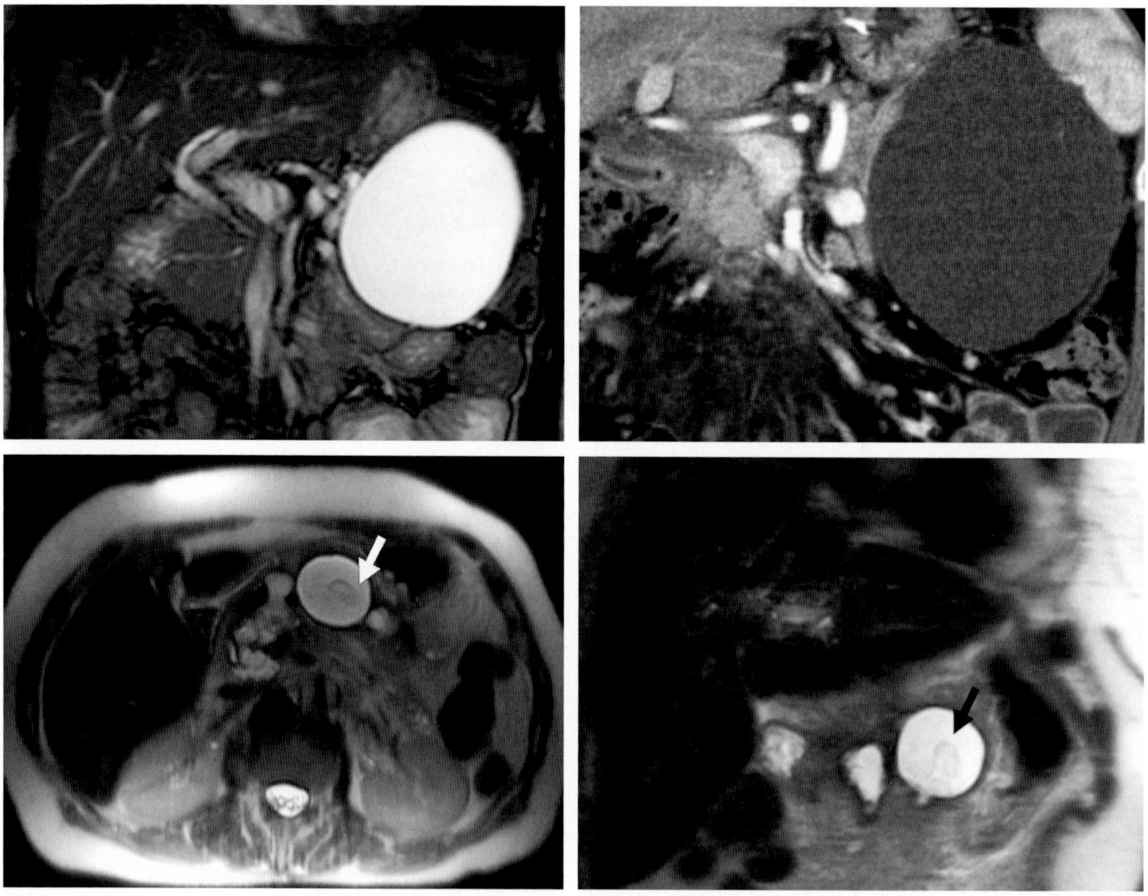

Fig. 15.17. a,b Imaging characterization of pseudocyst fluid. First case. T2-weighted MR images in the coronal plane adequately show the fluid homogeneous content of the pseudocyst (**a**). CT in the coronal plane (**b**) at the same level confirms the homogeneous water-like content of this mature pseudocyst. **c,d** Second case. MR HASTE sequences in axial (**c**) and coronal (**d**) planes show a cystic lesion characterized by inhomogeneous content due to clots and debris (*arrow*)

findings similar to that of contrast enhanced computed tomography (CECT) (Kim et al. 2005; Rickes et al. 2006; Morgan et al. 1997). Pancreatic and portal phases are obtained: the contrast enhancement makes it easier to depict septations and the pseudocapsule, which usually enhance during the portal phase (Fig. 15.18).

Because these sequences are obtained in 3-D, a precise assessment of the location and of the relationship of the lesion with adjacent organs and structures, particularly in respect to blood vessels is possible (Piironen et al. 2000).

MRCP, based on RARE single-shot and HASTE sequences, helps in the evaluation of the pancreatic ducts (Fig. 15.19). In particular, HASTE sequences, characterized by high spatial resolution (4 mm slice thickness), are able to show the presence of communication between the pseudocyst and the main pancreatic duct. To this purpose, 3-D sequences seem to be the most adequate, allowing for data to be reconstructed in order to obtain multiplanar images with different slice thickness, with the possibility of having 1.3 mm thick images reconstructed on any plane (Manfredi et al. 2001; Piironen et al. 2000; Calvo et al. 2002).

MR is preferred to CT in cases of patients with suspected allergy to iodinated contrast medium and in cases of pediatric patients that need several follow-up examinations. MR is indicated for characterizing highly inhomogeneous lesions in case of uncertain diagnosis after CT (Nisihara et al. 1996; Piironen et al. 2000).

15.7 Endoscopic Ultrasound Imaging (EUS)

EUS imaging can aid in the diagnosis of uncertain lesions, in particular if small and located close to the pancreatic area (Hammond et al. 2002; Yeo and Sarr 1994). EUS is more reliable and more precise than US in performing needle-aspiration biopsy in cases of undetermined lesions (Sahani et al. 2005; Giovannini et al. 2001).

EUS is able to facilitate the differential diagnosis between pseudocyst, mucinous cystic tumor (characterized by parietal nodules) and serous cystoadenoma. However, MR is still better than EUS in depicting any tiny communication between the cyst and the pancreatic duct.

15.8 Differential Diagnosis

The detection of a cystic pancreatic lesion generates the problem of distinguishing benign lesions from malignant ones, such as mucinous cystoadenoma, cystadenocarcinoma and intraductal papillary mucinous tumor (IPMT). Pre-operative diagnosis is based on US, CT, MR, EUS and needle-aspiration biopsy, completed by biochemical and cytological analysis of the lesion content (Kim et al. 2005;

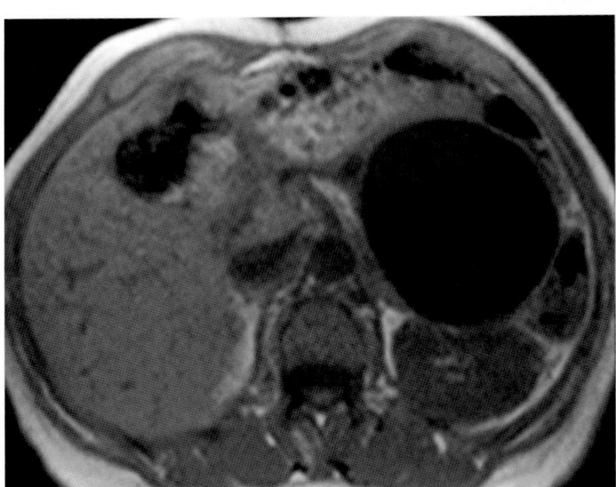

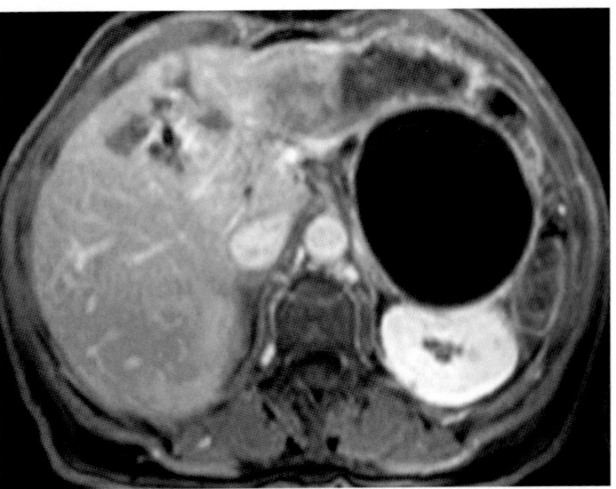

Fig. 15.18a,b. MR VIBE T1-weighted images before (**a**) and after the administration of contrast agent during portal phase (**b**) show the enhancement of pseudocyst wall. This post-contrast phase is the best to obtain the optimal contrast between the cystic lesion and the surrounding structures

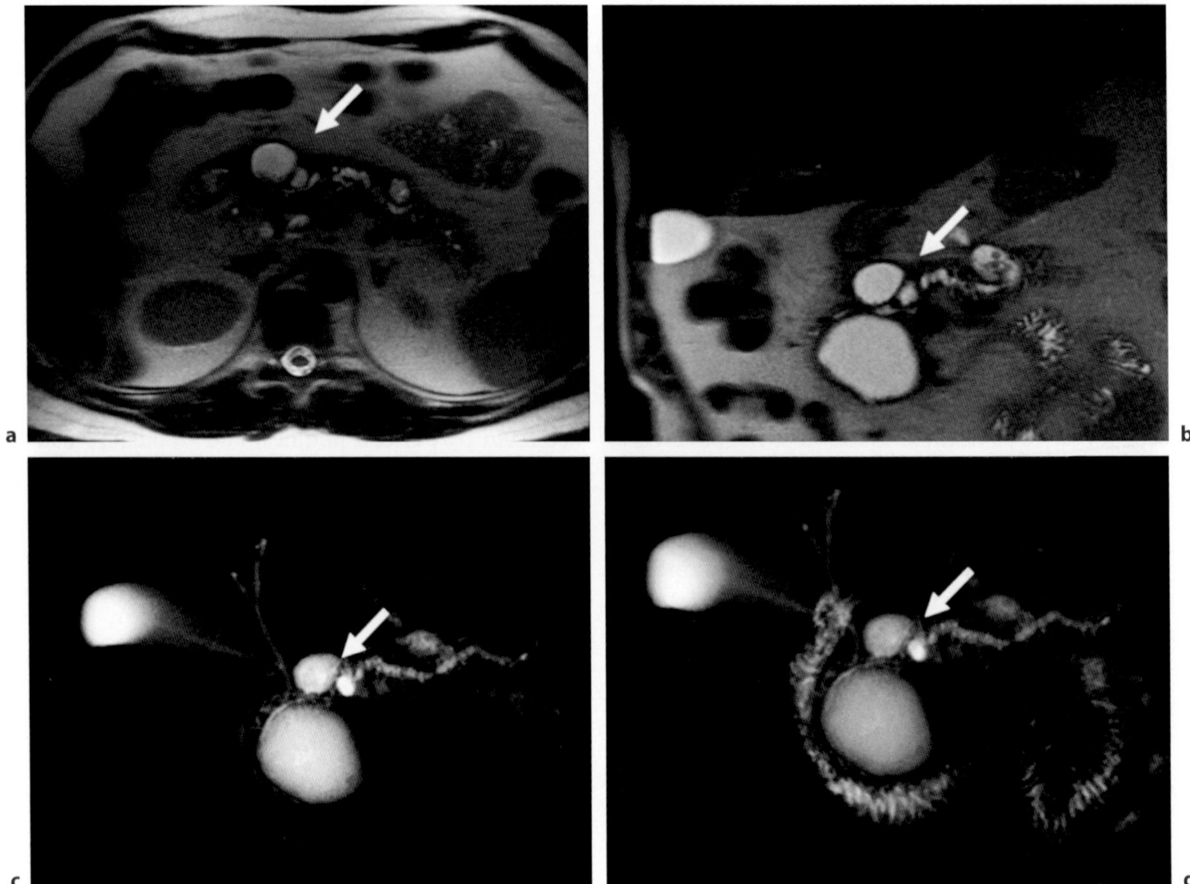

Fig. 15.19a–d. MR HASTE thin slice sequences (**a**,**b**) and RARE before (**c**) and after (**d**) the administration i.v. of secretin enables the evaluation of the relationship between the cystic lesion and the main pancreatic duct. In this patient, the absence of communication between the cysts (*arrow*) and the MPD in a clinical setting of chronic pancreatitis suggests the diagnosis of pancreatic pseudocysts (differential diagnosis with intraductal papillary mucinous tumour of the pancreas – IPMT)

Sahani et al. 2005; Giovannini et al. 2001; Brugge 2000; Breslin and Wallace 2002; Kalra et al. 2003; Fugazzola et al. 1991).

Clinical presentation often helps in the differential diagnosis. Usually pseudocysts develop in patients affected by severe acute pancreatitis, chronic pancreatitis, blunt abdominal trauma or surgical operations.

The differential diagnosis is much more difficult in cases of asymptomatic patients or atypical clinical presentation (Yeo and Sarr 1994).

Large size, liquid water-like content, scarce thin non-enhancing septations, a thin wall of homogeneous thickness and a demonstrable communication with the main pancreatic duct are features of a pseudocyst. The cytological examination of the liquid content after a CT- or US-guided needle-aspiration biopsy can confirm the diagnosis in the majority of cases (Yeo and Sarr 1994; Procacci et al. 2001). Although a wide variety of pancreatic cysts may have elevated amylase in the cyst fluid, extremely high levels favour pseudocyst.

An uncomplicated pseudocyst is usually followed by imaging to resolution. Interventional drainage is used if the pseudocyst increases in size or if it is not spontaneously reabsorbed. On the other hand, if infection or hemorrhage are present, surgical treatment becomes necessary (Singhal et al. 2006b; Spinelli et al. 2004).

15.8.1
Cystic Dystrophy of Duodenum

Duodenum cystic dystrophy (groove pancreatitis, DCD) is due to an inflammatory process, often associated with alcholism, arising within ectopic pancreatic tissue located in the duodenum wall. The inflammatory process causes the development of cystic lesions, with or without epithelial lining, circumscribed by inflammatory and fibrous tissue.

DCD is classified into two types: a solid and a cystic variant. The latter is the most frequent and must be distinguished from pancreatic pseudocysts. In addition, DCD may be associated with chronic pancreatitis and pseudocyst formation, determining obstruction of the main pancreatic duct (Chatelain et al. 2005).

CT and MR are able to show the presence of cystic lesions, resulting in an inhomogeneously thickened duodenum wall. Additional findings, useful in the differential diagnosis, are the dislocation of the common bile duct on the left and the dilation of the biliary and pancreatic ducts (Rebours et al. 2007). Stenosis of the terminal tract of the main pancreatic duct when it crosses the pancreatic head can be associated to chronic obstructing pancreatitis with parenchymal calcifications and pseudocysts.

15.8.2 Mucinous Cystic Pancreatic Tumor

Several clinical and epidemiological features help in the distinction between pseudocysts and mucinous cystic tumors of the pancreas. These tumors are typical in middle-aged women (mean age 50 years). They are generally located in the body and tail of the pancreas and usually detected incidentally in asymptomatic patients (Mulkeen et al. 2006). In contrast, patients affected by pseudocyst often suffer from acute or chronic pancreatitis, alcohol abuse, cholelithiasis or abdominal trauma. Furthermore, serum amylase levels are higher in 50%–75% of patients suffering from pseudocyst.

Some imaging findings are useful in the differential diagnosis: a mucinous cystic tumor is a thick-walled tumor frequently located in the body or tail of the pancreas. Very rarely it is connected to the main pancreatic duct (Sperti et al. 1996; Procacci et al. 2001; Spinelli et al. 2004). Usually round or oval shaped, it is characterized by a thick wall with smooth margins, with multiple internal septations, with or without septal and parietal nodules and calcifications (16%) (Kim et al. 2005).

At CT imaging it appears as a hypodense multilocular cystic lesion, consisting of a few large cysts (3 cm or more), with a thick wall and thin internal septations enhancing during the administration of contrast medium (Fig. 15.20) (Soliani et al. 2004; Kalra et al. 2003).

MR can further aid differentiation: "mature" pseudocysts are characterized by a homogeneous, hypointense signal intensity on T1-weighted images, whereas mucinous cystic tumors are often of variable signal intensity depending on the cyst content. Mucin, proteins and hemorrhage are typically hyperintense on T1-weighted images (short TR and TE) (Nishihara et al. 1996) as opposed to the low signal of uncomplicated pseudocyst content. MRCP and HASTE sequences are the most accurate in detecting the presence of a tiny communication with the main pancreatic duct in the presence of pseudocyst, whereas it usually results compressed, stenotic and dilated in the presence of mucinous tumor. This tumor is characterized by two different macroscopic patterns (Procacci et al. 2001): a micro-cystic one, similar to serous cystoadenoma, easily distinguished on the basis of the presence of a dilated main pancreatic duct and a macro-cystic pattern, much more common, characterized by a few thin internal septations separating wide cystic spaces and similar to a pseudocyst. Differential diagnosis is based on its inhomogeneous content (mucin and proteins) and on the presence of rare parietal nodules. Benign tumors are often characterized by thin and regular septations and capsule, whereas the malignant tumors usually have irregular septa and thick wall with mural nodules or vegetations.

15.8.3 Serous Cystadenoma

This is a benign tumor originating from acinar cells, frequently located in the pancreatic head. Females are most frequently affected in particular during their fifth decade. It is classified into two variants: the most common, defined as micro-cystic, consists of multiple tiny cysts with a mean diameter of 1–20 mm, configuring the typical "honeycomb" appearance and the macro-cystic form, less common, is characterized by one or a few large cysts encapsulated by a thin and homogeneous wall and divided by a few tiny septations. This form must be distinguished from pseudocyst and mucinous cystic tumor. Once more, clinical presentation is of fundamental importance in the differential diagnosis: patients affected by serous cystadenoma are usually asymptomatic, and rarely suffer from pancreatitis

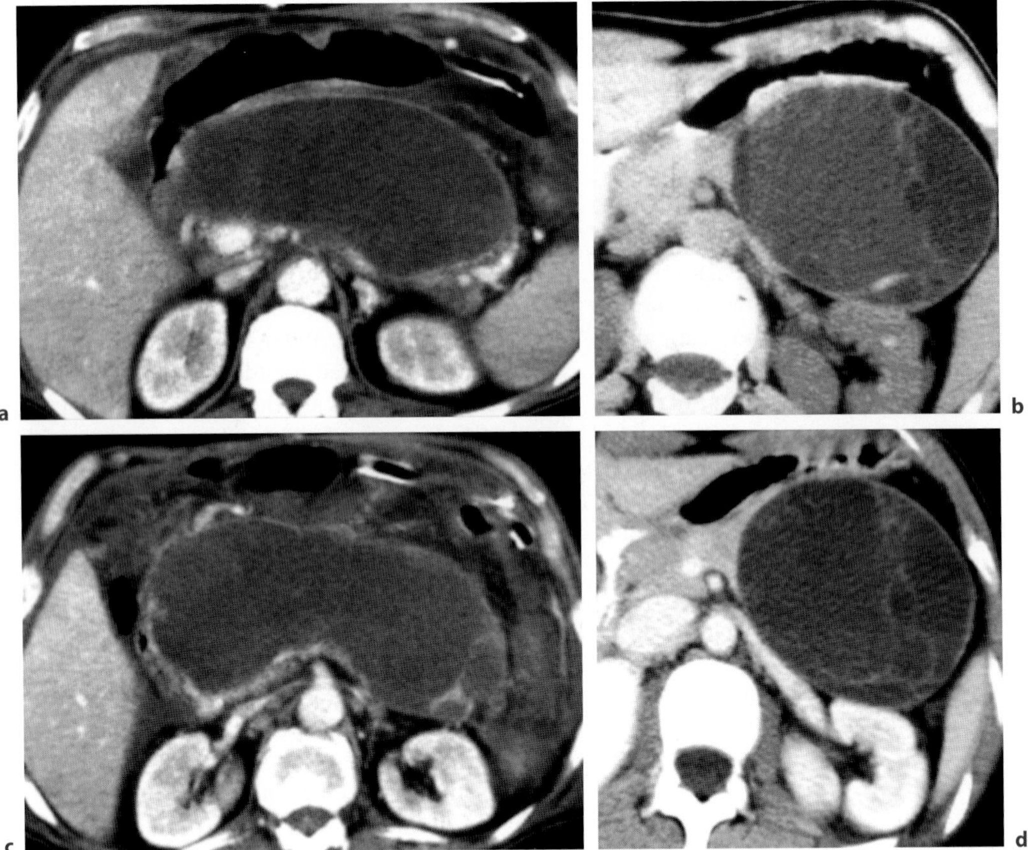

Fig. 15.20a–d. Pseudocyst: differential diagnosis. CECT in axial planes shows a pancreatic pseudocyst (**a,c**) and a mucinous cystoadenoma (**b,d**). Only the history of acute pancreatitis enables the differential diagnosis between these two cystic lesions

due to the compression of the main pancreatic duct by a large tumor located in the region of the head of the pancreas. On the other hand, imaging findings showing parietal nodules and communication with the main pancreatic duct are typically associated with mucinous tumor and pseudocyst respectively.

15.8.4 Intraductal Papillary Mucinous Tumors of the Collateral Ducts (IPMT II Type)

IPMT are intraductal mucin-producing pancreatic tumors developing from epithelial cells lining the main pancreatic duct (IPMT type I), branch pancreatic ducts (type II), or from both (combined IPMT or type III) (Lim et al. 2001; Prasad et al. 2003; Procacci et al. 1999; Sahani et al. 2006).

The branch pancreatic duct IPMT (type II) may appear similar to a pseudocyst. It usually consists of a multilocular cystic lesion of the pancreatic head or uncinate process associated with dilatation of the branch ducts. The mean age of onset is around the 5th decade with a slight prevalence in men. They are usually discovered incidentally, particularly if small in size; only rarely are they associated with acute or chronic obstructive pancreatitis (Fugazzola et al. 1991; Procacci et al. 2001).

These lesions are typically oval-shaped, with lobulated clustered cysts. Both external capsule and internal septations tend to enhance after the administration of contrast medium. Sometimes the cystic spaces may show a connection with a dilated duct. The characterization is easily achievable with MDCT and, above all, with MR, which shows the presence of a connection with the pancreatic duct.

In the late phase, additional findings are dilation of the main and collateral pancreatic ducts, atrophy of the gland and protrusion of the papilla of Vater into duodenum lumen (Procacci et al. 2001). However, these lesions grow slowly and, less frequently, they cause the obstruction of the duct and consequent acute pancreatitis. (Procacci et al. 2001).

MDCT has made it possible to create new reconstruction protocols (2-D curved reformations and volume rendered 3-D images) useful in the depiction of the relationship between the tumors, the pancreatic and the common bile ducts (Sahani et al. 2006). MRCP is considered as a gold standard in the study and follow-up of IPMT (Fig. 15.21). In addition, the use of secretin during MRCP improves the visualization of the internal structure of cystic lesions and of the communication of IPMT with the pancreatic duct (Carbognin et al. 2007).

15.8.5 Solid and Papillary Tumor

This tumor is distinguished from other cystic lesions of the pancreas by the presence of intra-lesional necrosis and cystic degeneration producing a lesion that simulates a unilocular cystic mass (Procacci et al. 2001). The lesional necrosisis is due to insufficient vascular supply, with thin, narrowed blood vessels (Procacci et al. 2001). Young women are usually affected by this tumor that is frequently characterized by a benign behaviour. However, it can be aggressive, with local invasion and distant hepatic and lymph node metastases (Procacci et al. 2001; Coleman et al. 2003). This tumor is usually discovered incidentally in asymptomatic patients. Large tumors may be associated with epigastric pain, palpable mass or peritoneal hemorrhage (Procacci et al. 2001). The cystic variant can show two different patterns: the first one, called mixed solid-liquid pattern, is typical of solid papillary tumors and enables the diagnosis. The second one, called macro-cystic, can simulate a pseudocyst (Procacci et al. 2001).

The MR findings of pseudo-papillary tumor are similar to that found on CT images. However, MR can facilitate the characterization of the lesion content, leading to the differential diagnosis: cystic areas are hypointense on T1 and hyperintense on T2, whereas solid tissue is iso-hypointense compared to the normal pancreatic parenchyma and show a moderate enhancement. Hemorrhage within the lesion is hyperintense on T1 (Yu et al. 2007).

T2-weighted images facilitate a differential diagnosis because they show the inhomogeneity due to the coexistence of strongly hyperintense cystic areas and mildly hyperintense or isointense solid tissue compared to the normal pancreas. Calcifications are rare (Procacci et al. 2001).

15.8.6 Other Cystic Tumors

Almost any of the multiple types of pancreatic neoplasms can appear as a cystic mass. Ductal adenocarcinoma may rarely undergo cystic degeneration due to insufficient blood supply in large and rapid growing tumors (Lumsden and Bradley 1989). Anaplastic carcinomas may also show a cystic pattern.

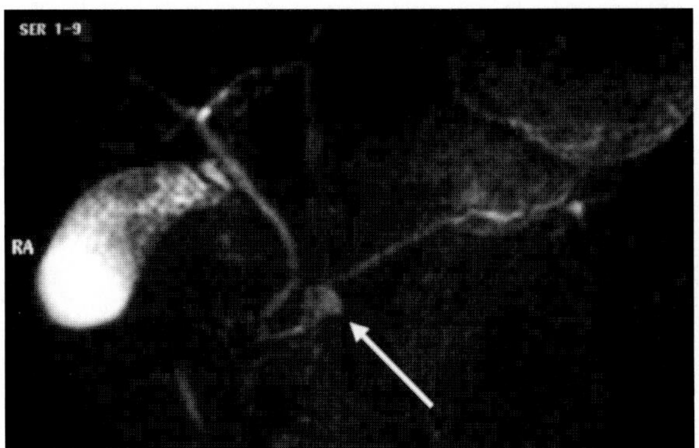

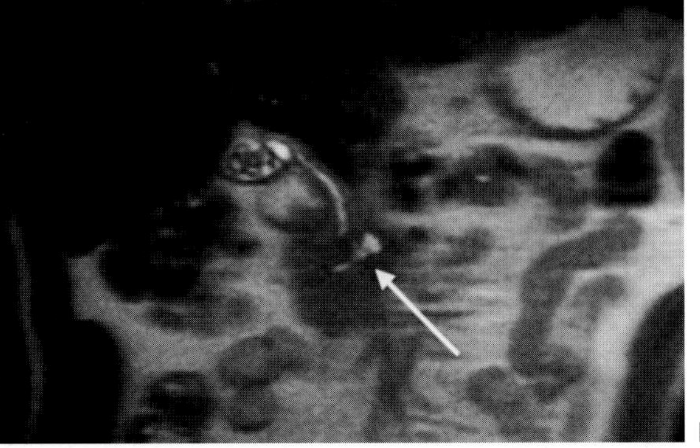

Fig. 15.21a,b. Intraductal papillary mucinous tumour of the pancreas (IPMT). MR RARE (**a**) and HASTE (**b**) sequences show a lobular cystic lesion (*arrow*) of pancreatic head communicating with pancreatic duct: the findings suggest the diagnosis of IPMT

Acinar carcinoma, in its multilocular cystic form, may be similar to other cystic lesions of the pancreas. On the contrary, its histologic diagnosis is easy (Lumsden and Bradley 1989; Horton and Fishman 2002; Warshaw and Rutledge 1986).

Neuroendocrine pancreatic tumors have a clearly cystic pattern in less than 10% of cases, usually due to central necrosis. Differential diagnosis is based on the hypervascularity of the solid component if present (Procacci et al. 2001).

The osteoclast-like giant cell tumor is a rare abdominal tumor involving the pancreas in the majority of cases, usually located in the head or body. This tumor consists of pleomorphic malignant cells and giant osteoclast-like cells. Generally it is diagnosed in a late phase, when large in size (mean diameter at diagnosis 6 cm) and inhomogeneous because of the coexistence of large cystic areas, necrosis and hemorrhage. It must be distinguished from cystic adenocarcinoma, neuroendocrine cystic tumors and particularly from pseudocysts (Oehler et al. 1997; Bauditz et al. 2006). The prognosis is usually poor because of frequent lymph node metastases and local recurrence after surgical resection.

15.9 Role of Needle-Aspiration Biopsy

Needle biopsy is of fundamental importance in diagnosing cystic pancreatic lesions. The biopsy can be performed under US or CT guidance and allows for the evaluation of cytologic, enzymatic and tumoral markers of the cyst content (Lewandrowski et al. 1995). Pancreatic pseudocysts are frequently characterized by their typical clinical presentation, absence of septations or solid enhancing tissue and by a high level of amylase. According to some authors (Ros et al. 2000; Frossard et al. 2003), this procedure is useful in the differential diagnosis between pseudocyst, lympho-epithelial cyst and cystic tumors (Yeo and Sarr 1994; Klöppel 2000; Ros et al. 2000; Frossard et al. 2003). In fact, a high level of CA 19-9, CEA and LDH, a low value of amylase, a low viscosity of the liquid content and the presence of malignant cells make it easier to diagnose a cystic tumor. Therefore, a well executed needle biopsy can avoid an unnecessary surgical resection of benign lesions (Yeo and Sarr 1994; Klöppel 2000).

Needle-biopsy does not have a high negative predictive value to exclude tumor. Moreover, there may be a high variability in the concentration of enzymes and tumoral markers within the same cystic lesions in different patients.

15.10 Pre-operative Assessment

CT and MR are the most widely used imaging techniques in the pre-operative assessment of pseudocysts for deciding on the proper treatment. With the use of i.v. contrast medium the wall and the septations can be studied. Furthermore, it is possible to perform the assessment of a normal, spared pancreatic parenchyma and evaluate the presence of other pathologies. The spared pancreas is characterized by regular thickness, normal density (at CT), and normal signal intensity (hyperintense on FS T1-weighted images at MR) with homogeneous enhancement in the arterial phase. MR imaging leads to a better study of pancreatic ducts: HASTE and MRCP sequences are the reference standard as regards non-invasive imaging techniques in the evaluation of stenosis, dilation, filling defects and communications with the cystic lesion.

Both CT and MR are able to create a precise vascular map, which is of fundamental importance for surgeons during treatment planning. The portal venous phase is able highlight venous thrombosis with or without imaging findings of portal hypertension. In contrast, rare lesions of the arteries (aneurysm, pseudoaneurysm) are well characterized during the arterial phase.

15.11 Pseudocyst Evolution

The presence of a pseudocyst requires planned imaging follow-up, and, if spontaneous reabsorption has not occurred, its drainage under US or CT guidance (Singhal et al. 2006b.

Pseudocyst evolution is strictly correlated to its size (Yeo and Sarr 1994; Demos et al. 2002). According to O'Malley et al. (1985), lesions of 4 cm spontaneously reabsorb in 55% of patients, and complications occur in 10% of cases. Furthermore, 67% of lesions measuring 6 cm need to be treated surgically, whereas smaller ones must be treated only in 40% of cases (YEO and SARR 1994; O'MALLEY et al. 1985).

In contrast, a pseudocyst can maintain a stable size and shape for a long time. These lesions are usually encapsulated by a thick pseudo-capsule. In such cases, watchful waiting is necessary in order to diagnose any complication in the early phase. Nowadays US- or CT-guided (Fig. 15.22) drainage of pseudocysts is the treatment of choice for lesions without complications that tend to increase in size.

15.12 Complications

Infections, hemorrhage, intestinal stenosis or obstruction, and rupture into adjacent organs or into the peritoneal/retroperitoneal cavity are considered the most frequent complications of pancreatic pseudocysts. Complications arise in 30%–50% of patients. In particular, 5%–20% of pancreatic pseudocysts are complicated by infections, and the majority are due to infected necrosis.

15.12.1 Infection and Pancreatic Abscess

Infection is one of the most feared complications of pancreatic pseudocysts and of any inflammatory pancreatic disease. The prompt diagnosis is of fundamental importance in order to rapidly deploy proper treatment. Gram-negative bacteria (*E. coli*), followed by anaerobes and fungi are the most likely offending organisms. The source of contamination is the colon. Imaging techniques can show the presence of inhomogeneous content and much more rarely the presence of gas within the cystic lesion (Fig. 15.23) (YEO and SARR 1994; O'MALLEY et al. 1985).

A pancreatic abscess consists of a well-circumscribed fluid-collection containing pus, localized within or in adjacent to the pancreas. It typically develops in cases of severe acute pancreatitis as result of infection of the original necrosis. The most important bacteria involved are *E. coli*, Klebsiella species, *S. aureus*. The prognosis is very poor, particularly when diagnosis and treatment are delayed: the rapid involvement of adjacent structures may cause acute bleeding or peritonitis, with consequent sepsis, shock and a high risk of death. CT imaging is the reference standard for the diagnosis of abscess: it usually appears as a round hypodense mass (0–45 UH), encapsulated, with or without the cluster sign (small abscesses tending to coalesce into a

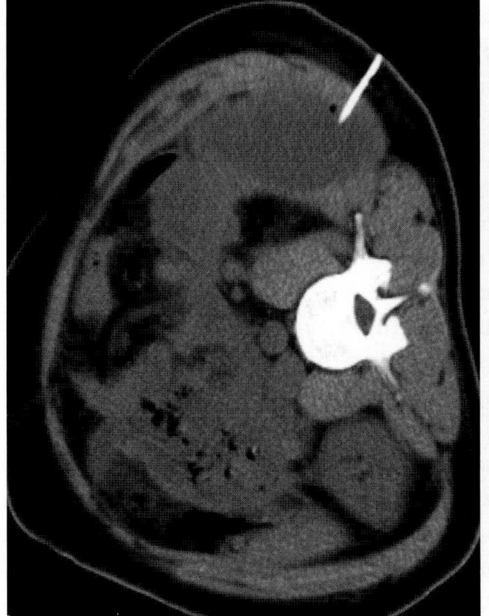

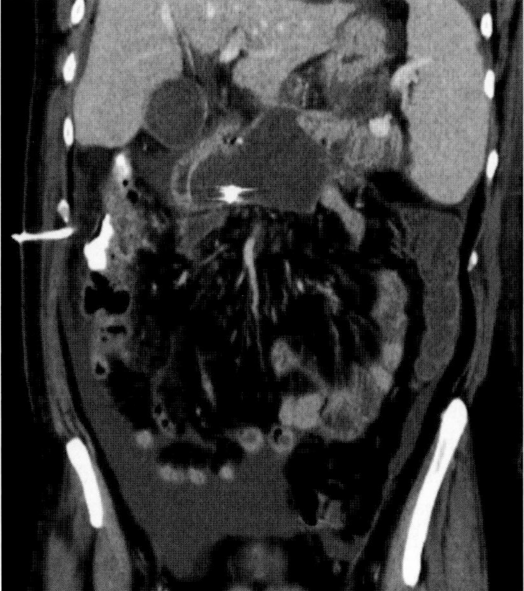

Fig. 15.22a,b. Pseudocyst drainage. Examples of percutaneous drainage approach under CT guidance

single septated cavity). The presence of gas (bubbles of air) or of an air-fluid level is a specific sign but occurs only in 20% of cases. In most cases, the imaging appearance will *not* be specific for the diagnosis of an abscess. Aspiration of cyst content in a febrile patient is necessary to establish an infected cyst.

15.12.2 Vascular Complications

Arterial complications include acute bleeding (arterial disruption) or the development of a pseudoaneurysm. The pseudocyst, increasing in size, may push on a vessel wall causing its necrosis with consequent arterial disruption and acute bleeding into the peritoneal cavity or within the pseudocyst. Depending on the size of the lesion and on the quantity of the bleeding, the cystic cavity can turn into a bleeding pseudocyst or into a pseudoaneurysm. A pseudoaneurysm develops in cases of small lesions (Fig. 15.24). In contrast, larger lesions turn into a bleeding pseudocyst, characterized by the emptying of an arterial vessel into the cyst and carrying a high risk of rupture into the peritoneum or retroperitoneum as a result of its rapid increase in size (Coleman et al. 2003; Yu et al. 2007). Small asymptomatic pseudoaneurysms can be an incidental finding during follow-up imaging examinations. The most frequently involved vessels are the splenic artery, gastro-duodenal artery, pancreatic-duodenal arteries and left gastric artery. The wall, consisting only of fibrous tissue, can rupture under constant arterial pressure. For this reason, a pseudoaneurysm must be promptly treated. Catheter based endovascular embolization techniques will be effective.

US-Doppler allows evaluation of the blood flow within the pseudoaneurysm. Sometimes the involved artery can be identified. These lesions usually show a good flow during the systole, with the exception of cases where the vessel is thrombosed. At CT imaging, pseudoaneurysms appear as round homogeneously and arterially enhancing foci located within or adjacent to a pancreatic pseudocyst. At MR imaging, pseudoaneurysms are characterized by signal void phenomenon due to the pure arterial flow and appear hypointense (Fig. 15.24). On T2-weighted sequences, alternate isointense and hypointense bands in the dependent region of the pseudoaneurysm, due to the presence of hemoglobin breakdown products, can be detected confirming the presence of thrombus. The i.v. administration of contrast medium helps to confirm the diagnosis. Recent advances in MDCT and MR 3-D reconstructions have made it possible to create maps of the arteries in the pancreatic area aiding in the identification of the involved artery. In cases of a bleeding pseudocyst, CT or US follow-up will highlight the rapid increase in size of the lesion (Fig. 15.25). The US-Doppler can confirm the presence of arterial flow.

A pseudocyst can be associated with thrombosis of the pancreatic veins, fistulas between the portal vein and the pancreatic duct, pylephlebitis and portal hypertension (Singhal et al. 2006a).

Thrombosis of the pancreatic veins is frequently associated with acute pancreatitis complicated by pseudocysts (McCormick et al. 1990). The pathogenesis is based on compression of veins and on the inflammatory process due to the release of pancreatic juice and enzymes, causing vasculitis. The splenic vein seems to be the most frequently involved vessel as a result of its contiguity to the pancreatic tail, above all in cases of chronic pancreatitis with formation of a calcified pseudocyst.

A fistula between the pancreatic duct and the portal system is due to the rupture of a pseudocyst in the portal vein. It is a rare complication and only a few cases are described in the literature (Ridell et al. 2005).

15.12.3 Jaundice

Compression of the common bile duct by a pseudocyst may cause the onset of obstructive jaundice, cholangitis and biliary dilatation (Warshaw and Rattner 1980). The pathogenesis is based on compression, fibrous tissue and scarring resulting from the original inflammatory and necrotic process.

15.12.4 Compression on Gastro-intestinal and Urinary Tracts

Any portion of the GI tract can become extrinsically narrowed secondary to the pressure of or, less commonly, due to fibrotic tissue developing during the primary inflammatory process. In such cases the colon is the most frequently involved segment as a result of a fluid collection commonly being located in the transverse mesocolon and in the para-renal spaces, followed by the duodenum. It is a rare but

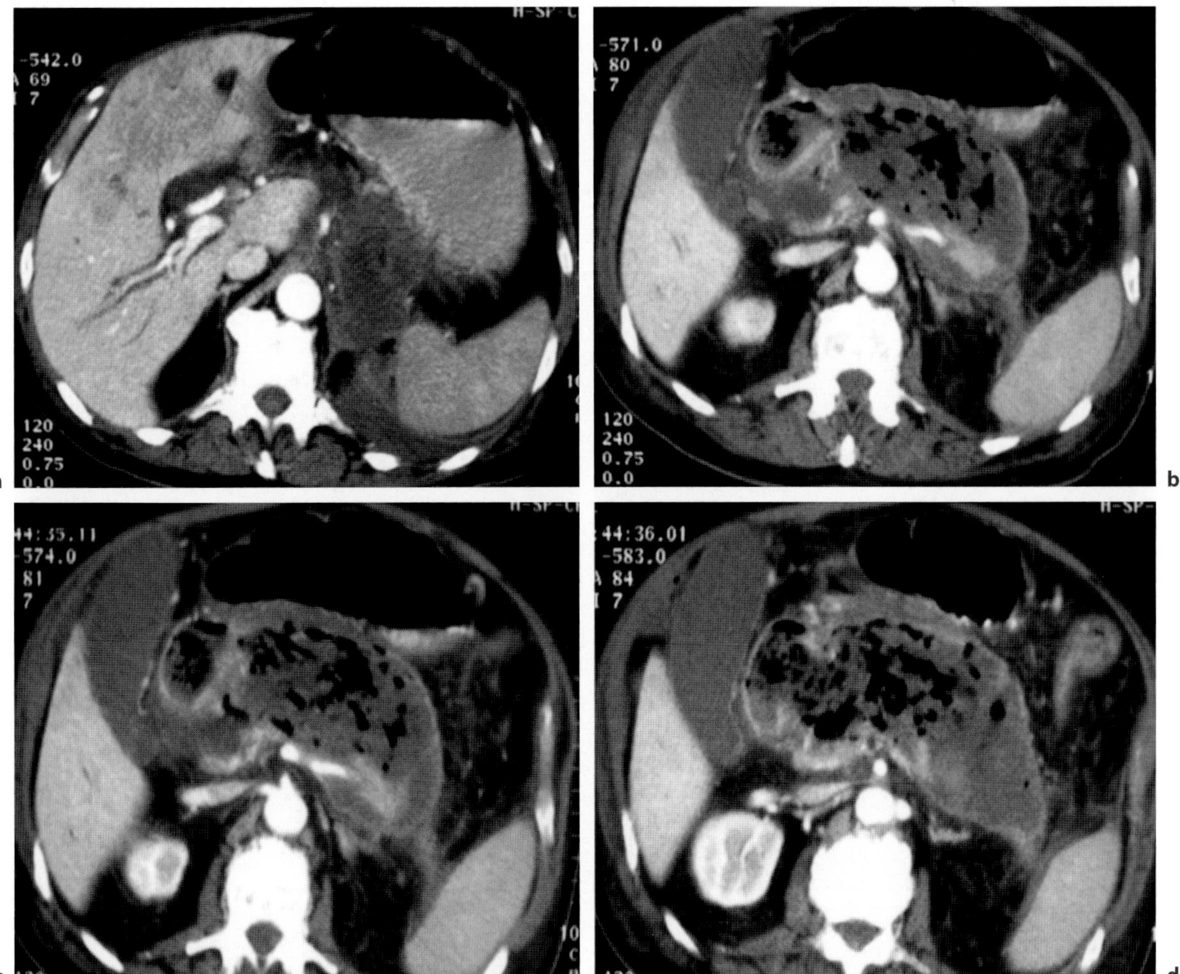

Fig. 15.23. Pseudocyst infection. CECT in axial planes at different levels show the presence of multiple air bubbles within the large pancreatic pseudocyst: the findings suggest the infection

hazardous complication that requires quick therapy. Percutaneous decompression of the cyst under US or CT guidance or a transgastric drainage under ERCP or EUS guidance can be performed (Fig. 15.26).

Large pseudocysts can produce urinary tract obstruction, with resulting hydronephrosis. Leg edema due to compression of the inferior vena cava (Demos et al. 2002; Bernades et al. 1992) can also be seen.

15.12.5 Rupture and Fistulas

Rupture occurs in less than 3% of pseudocysts. The clinical presentation can be either dramatic with severe abdominal pain or insidious with ascites or pleural effusion in the case of a slow emptying of the pseudocyst through a fistulous tract (O'Malley et al. 1985; Warshaw and Ratner 1980). If the pancreatic duct is involved, the subsequent release of pancreatic juice and enzyme will be followed by severe abdominal pain and pancreatic ascites. If the rupture occurs in the retroperitoneum, the fluid collection can spread to the pelvis and towards the thorax with subsequent pleural effusion (Yanagië et al. 1997).

The enteric fistula is the most common. The fistulas between the pancreas and colon have a high mortality rate (50%) as a result of the frequent association with infections and bleeding. CT may easily detect the presence of air bubbles in the absence of any sign of infection (Ros et al. 2000). MRCP with secretin administration confirms the diagnosis of fistula, demonstrating the duct rupture and involvement of the pseudocyst.

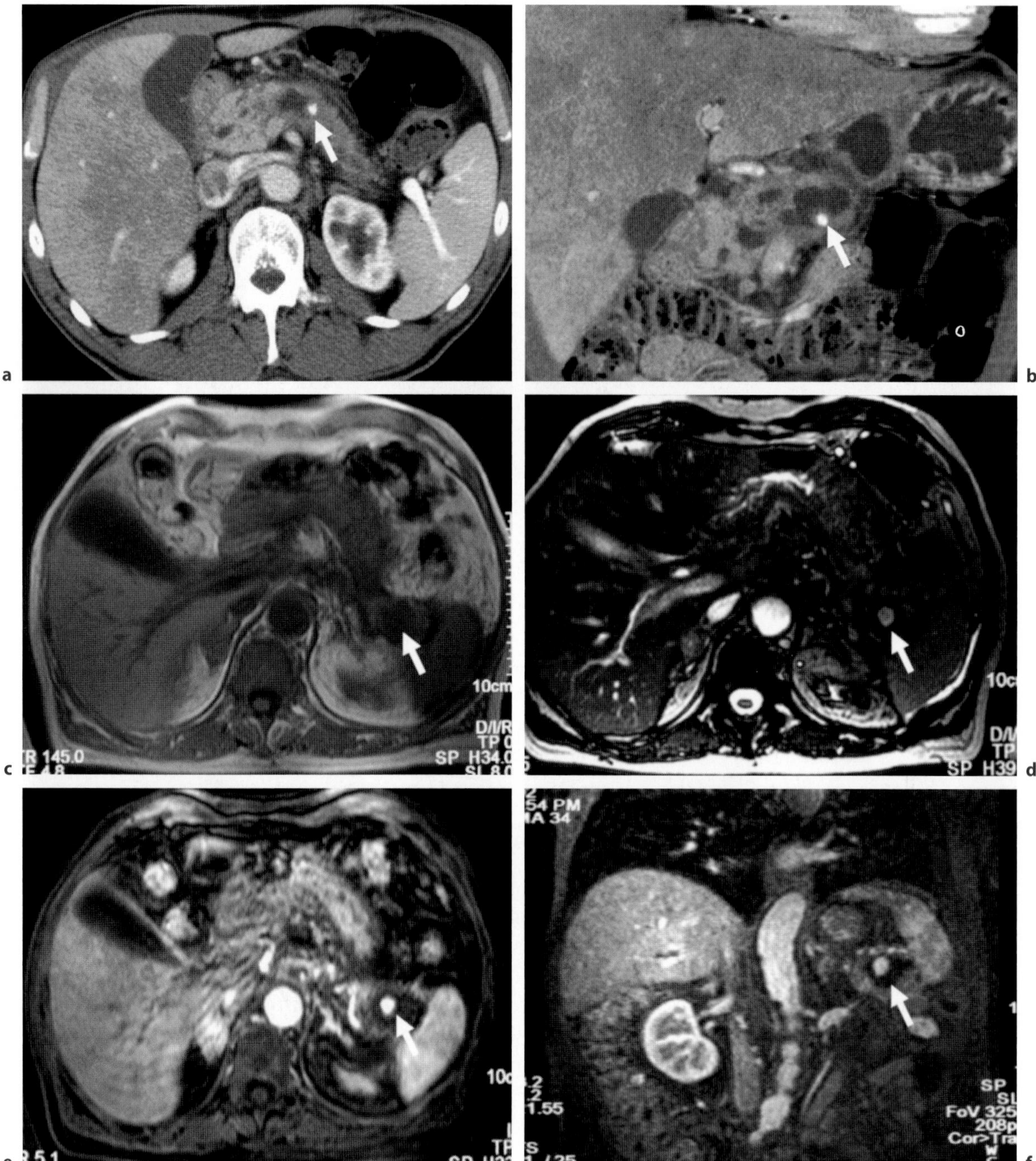

Fig. 15.24a–f. Pseudoaneurysm: CT scan in axial (**a**) and coronal curved reformation (**b**) show a focal hyperdense arterially enhancing focus inside a small pseudocyst, isodense with abdominal aorta. MR examination shows similar findings in a pseudocyst of splenic hilum. The lesion is nearly isointense (*arrow*) in the T1-weighted (**c**) image in which a faint hypointensity due to the "flow void" phenomenon is seen. The lesion is hyperintense in the T2-weighted image (**d**). The pseudoaneurysm is hyperintense similar to the abdominal aorta following the administration of gadolinium (**e**,**f**)

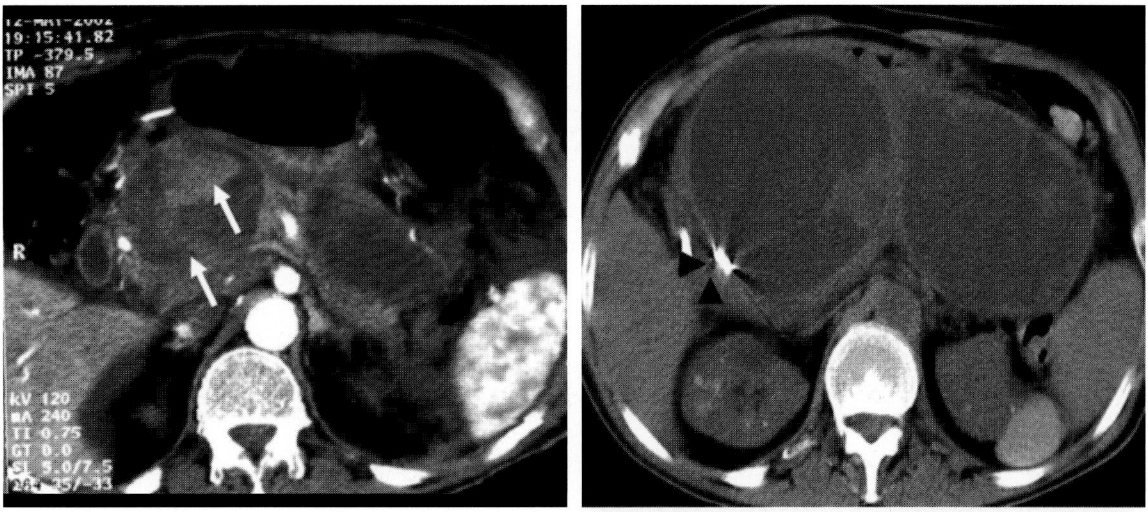

Fig. 15.25a–c. Bleeding pseudocyst. Contrast enhanced CT scan during the arterial phase (**a**) shows multiple hyperdense areas (*arrows*) within the pancreatic pseudocyst due to hemorrhagic content; after endovascular treatment of acute bleeding with two coils (*arrowhead*), the CT scan before (**b**) and after the administration of iodinated contrast agent shows the increase in size of the cystic lesion, but the absence of active bleeding (**c**)

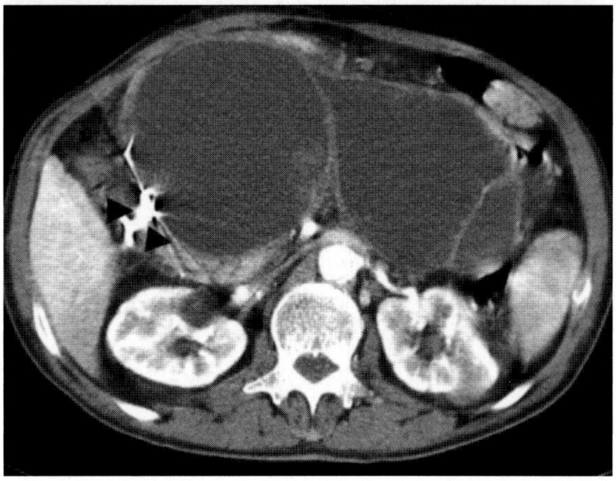

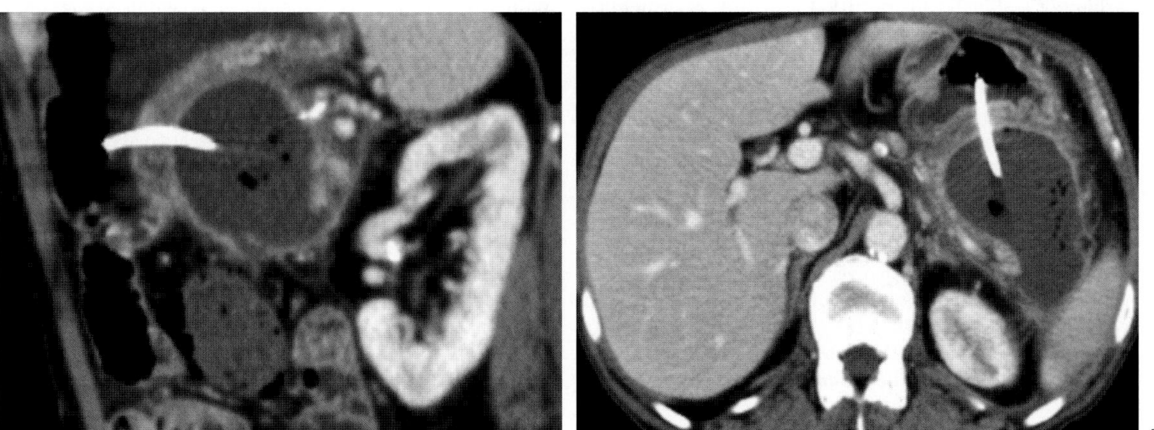

Fig. 15.26. Trans-gastric drainage of pseudocyst. Contrast-enhanced CT scan shows a large pseudocyst with air bubbles inside due to the presence of trans-gastric drainage positioned under ERCP-guidance

15.12.6 Pleural Effusion

Pleural effusion can be the consequence of various pathophysiologic mechanisms associated with pseudocyst. These include the spread of a retroperitoneal fluid collection through the diaphragmatic hiatus into the pleural cavity, a fistula between the pseudocyst and the pleural space and the rupture of a mediastinal pseudocyst.

References

Balthazar EJ (2002) Complications of acute pancreatitis Clinical and CT evaluation. Radiol Clin N Am 40:1211–1227

Bauditz J, Rudolph B, Wermke W (2006) Osteoclast-like giant cell tumors of the pancreas and liver. World J Gastroenterol 12(48):7878–7883

Bernades P, Baetz A, Lévy P, Belghiti J, Menu Y, Fékété F (1992) Splenic and portal venous obstruction in chronic pancreatitis. Digest Dis Sci 37(3):340–346

Bradley EL III (1989) Complications of chronic pancreatitis. Surg Clin North Am 69(3):481–497. Review

Breslin N, Wallace MB (2002) Diagnosis and fine needle aspiration of pancreatic pseudocysts: the role of endoscopic ultrasound. Gastrointest Endosc Clin N Am 12(4):781–790, viii. Review

Brugge W (2000) The role of EUS in the diagnosis of cystic lesion of the pancreas. Gastroint Radiol 52(6):s18–s22

Calvo MM, Bujanda L, Calderon A, Heras I, Cabriada JL, Bernal A, Orive V, Astigarraga E (2002) Comparison between magnetic resonance cholangiopancreatography and ERCP for evaluation of the pancreatic duct. Am J Gastroenterol 97:(2)347–353

Carbognin G, Pinali L, Girardi V, Casarin A, Mansueto G, Mucelli RP (2007) Collateral branches IPMTs: secretin-enhanced MRCP. Abdom Imaging 32(3):374–380

Chatelain D, Vibert E, Yzet T, Geslin G, Bartoli E, Manaouil D, Delcenserie R, Brevet M, Dupas JL, Regimbeau JM (2005) Groove pancreatitis and pancreatic heterotopia in the minor duodenal papilla. Pancreas 30(4):e92–95

Coleman KM, Doherty MC, Bigler SA (2003) Solid-pseudopapillary tumor of the pancreas. Radiographics 23(6):1644–1648

Cooperman AM (2001) An overview of pancreatic pseudocysts: the emperor's new clothes revisited. Surg Clin North Am 81(2):391–397, XII

Demos TC, Posniak HV, Harmat C, Olson MC, Aranha G (2002) Cystic lesion of the pancreas. AJR Am J Roentgenol 179:1375–1388

Frossard JL, Amouyal P, Palazzo L, Amaris J, Soldan M, Giostra E, Spahr L, Hadengue A, Fabre M (2003) Performance of endosonography-guided fine needle aspiration and biopsy in the diagnosis of pancreatic cystic lesions. Am J Gastroenterol 98(7):1516–1524

Fugazzola C, Procacci C, Bergamo Andreis IA, Iacono C, Portuese A, Dompieri P, Laveneziana S, Zampieri PG, Jannucci A, Serio G, Pistolesi GF (1991) Cystic tumors of the pancreas: evaluation by ultrasonography and computed tomography. Gastrointest Radiol 16:53–61

Giovannini M, Pesenti C, Rolland AL, Moutardier V, Delpero JR (2001) Endoscopic ultrasound-guided drainage of pancreatic pseudocysts or pancreatic abscesses using a therapeutic echo endoscope. Endoscopy 33(6):473–477

Hall KN (1992) Pediatric pancreatic pseudocyst: a case report and review of the literature. J Em Med 10:573–576

Hammond N, Miller FH, Sica GT, MPH, Gore RM (2002) Imaging of cystic disease of the pancreas. Radiol Clin N Am 40:1243–1262

Horton KM, Fishman EK (2002) Adenocarcinoma of the pancreas: CT imaging. Radiol Clin N Am 40:1263–1272

Kalra MK, Maher MM, Muller PR, Saini S (2003) State-of-the-art imaging of pancreatic neoplasms. Br J Radiol 76(912):857–865. Review

Karantanas AK, Sandris V, Tsikirika A, Karakousis K, Karaiscou E (2003) Extension of pancreatic pseudocysts into the neck: CT and RM imaging findings. AJR Am J Roentgenol 180(3):843–845

Kim YH, Saini S, Sahani D, Hahn PF, Muller PR, Auh YH (2005) Imaging diagnosis of cystic pancreatic lesions: pseudocyst versus nonpseudocyst. Radiographics 25:671–685

Klöppel G (2000) Pseudocysts and other non-neoplastic cysts of the pancreas. Semin Diagn Pathol 17(1):7–15

Lewandrowski K, Lee J, Southern J, Centeno B, Warshaw A (1995) Cyst fluid analysis in the differential diagnosis of pancreatic cysts: a new approach to the preoperative assessment of pancreatic cystic lesions. AJR Am J Roentgenol 164(4):815–819

Lim JH, Lee G, Oh YL (2001) Radiologic spectrum of intraductal papillary mucinous tumor of the pancreas. Radiographics 21(2):323–337; discussion 337–340. Review

Lumsden A, Bradley EL III (1989) Pseudocyst or cystic neoplasm? Differential diagnosis and initial management of cystic pancreatic lesions. Hepato-Gastroenterology 36:462–466

Manfredi R, Brizi M G, Tancioni V, Vecchioli A, Marano P (2001) Magnetic resonance pancreatography (MRP): morphology and function. RAYS 26(2):127–133

McCormick PA, Chronos N, Burroughs AK, McIntyre N, McLaughlin JE (1990) Pancreatic pseudocyst causing portal vein thrombosis and pancreatico-pleural fistula. Gut 31:561–563

Morgan DE, Baron TH, Smith JK, Robbin ML, Kenney PJ (1997) Pancreatic fluid collections prior to intervention: evaluation with MR imaging compared with CT and US. Radiology 203(3):773–778

Mulkeen AL, Yoo PS, Cha C (2006) Less common neoplasms of the pancreas. World J Gastroenterol 12(20):3180–3185. Review

Nishihara K, Kawabata A, Ueno T, Miyahara M, Hamanaka Y, Suzuki T (1996) The differential diagnosis of pancreatic cysts by MR imaging. Hepato-Gastroenterology 43:714–720

Oehler U, Jürs M, Klöppel G, Helpap B (1997) Osteoclast-like giant cell tumour of the pancreas presenting as a pseudocyst-like lesion. Wirch Arch 431(3):215–218

O'Malley VP, Cannon JP, Postier RG (1985) Pancreatic pseudocysts: cause, therapy, and results. Am J Surg 150(6):680–682

Piironen A, Kivisaari R, Kemppainen E, Laippala P, Koivisto AM, Poutamen VP, Kivisaari L (2000) Detection of severe acute pancreatitis by contrast-enhanced magnetic resonance imaging. Eur Radiol 10:354–361

Prasad SR, Sahani D, Nasser S, Farrell J, Fernandez-Del Castillo C, Hahn PF, Mueller PR, Saini S (2003) Intraductal papillary mucinous tumors of the pancreas. Abdom Imaging 28(3):357–365

Procacci C, Graziani R, Bicego E, Mainardi P, Bassi C, Bergamo Andreis IA, Valdo M, Guarise A, Girelli M (1997a) Blunt pancreatic trauma. Role of CT. Acta Radiol 38:543–549

Procacci C, Graziani R, Zamboni G, Cavallini G, Pederzoli P, Guarise A, Bogina G, Biasiutti C, Carbognin G, Bergamo Andreis IA, Pistolesi GF (1997b) Cystic dystrophy of the duodenal wall: radiologic findings. Radiology 205:741–747

Procacci C, Megibow AJ, Carbognin G, Guarise A, Spoto E, Biasiutti C, Pistolesi GF (1999) Intraductal papillary mucinous tumor of the pancreas: a pictorial essay. Radiographics 19(6):1447–1463

Procacci C, Biasiutti C, Carbognin G, Capelli P, El-Dalati G, Falconi M, Misiani G, Ghirardi C, Zamboni G (2001) Pancreatic neoplasm and tumor-like conditons. Eur Radiol 11(s2):S167–192

Rebours V, Lévy P, Vullierme MP, Couvelard A, O'Toole D, Aubert A, Palazzo L, Sauvanet A, Hammel P, Maire F, Ponsot P, Ruszniewski P (2007) Clinical and morphological features of duodenal cystic dystrophy in heterotopic pancreas. Am J Gastroent 102(4):871–879. E-pub Feb 23

Rickes S, Wermke W (2004) Differentiation of cystic pancreatic neoplasms and pseudocysts by conventional and echo-enhanced ultrasound. J Gastroenter Hepatol 19(7):761–766

Rickes S, Mönkemüller K, Malfertheiner P (2006) Echo-enhanced ultrasound with pulse inversion imaging: a new imaging modality for the differentiation of cystic pancreatic tumours. World J Gastroent 12(14):2205–2208

Riddell A, Jhaveri K, Haider M (2005) Pseudocyst rupture into portal vein diagnosed with MRI Br J Radiol 78(927):265–268

Ros LH, Helmberger T, Ros PR (2000) Cystic pancreatic lesions. Eur Radiol 10(Suppl 2):S209–S217

Sadat U, Jah A, Huguet E (2007) Mediastinal extension of a complicated pancreatic pseudocyst; a case report and literature review. J Med Case Rep 1:12

Sahani DV, Kadavigere R, Saokar A, Fernandez-del Castillo C, Brugge WR, Hahn PF (2005) Cystic pancreatic lesions: a simple imaging-based classification system for guiding management. Radiographics 25(6):1471–1484

Sahani DV, Kadavigere R, Blake M, Fernandez-Del Castillo C, Lauwers GY, Hahn PF (2006) Intraductal papillary mucinous neoplasm of pancreas: multi-detector row CT with 2D curved reformations – correlation with MRCP. Radiology 238(2):560–569

Schima W (2006) MRI of the pancreas: tumors and tumors-simulating processes. Cancer Imaging 6:199–203

Singhal D, Kakodkar R, Soin AS, Gupta S, Nundy S (2006a) Sinistral portal hypertension. A case report. JOP 7(6):670–673

Singhal D, Kakodkar R, Sud R, Chaudhary A (2006b) Issues in management of pancreatic pseudocyst. J of the Pancreas: 7(5)

Soliani P, Franzini C, Ziegler S, Del Rio P, Dell'Abate P, Piccolo D, Japichino GG, Cavestro GM, Di Mario F, Sianesi M (2004) Pancreatic pseudocysts following acute pancreatitis: risk factors influencing therapeutic outcomes. J of the Pancreas 5(5):338–347

Sperti C, Pasquali C, Guolo P, Polverosi R, Liessi G, Pedrazzoli S (1996) Serum tumor markers and cyst fluid analysis are useful for the diangosis of pancreatic cystic tumors. Cancer 15(2):237–243

Spinelli KS, Fromwiller TE, Daniel RA, Kiely JM, Nakeeb A, Komorowski RA, Wilson SD, Pitt HA (2004) Cystic pancreatic neoplasms: observe or operate. Ann Surg 239(5):651–657; discussion 657–9

Warshaw A, Rattner DW (1980) Facts and fallacies of common bile duct obstruction by pancreatic pseudocysts. Ann Surg 192(1):33–37

Warshaw A, Rutledge PL (1986) Cystic tumors mistaken for pancreatic pseudocysts. Ann Surg 393–398

Yanagië H, Tani T, Sairennji T, Ogata M, Eriguchi M (1997) A pancreatic pseudocyst with pancreatic pleural effusion: report of a case. Jpn J Surg 27:1064–1068

Yeo CJ, Sarr MG (1994) Cystic and pseudocystic diseases of the pancreas. Curr Prob Surg 31(3):169–243

Yu CC, Tseng JH, Yeh CN, Hwang TL, Jan YY (2007) Clinicopathological study of solid and pseudopapillary tumor of pancreas: emphasis on magnetic resonance imaging findings. World J Gastroenterol 13(12):1811–1815

Imaging of Biliary and Vascular Complications

16

Giancarlo Mansueto, Daniela Cenzi, Giulia Armatura, Riccardo Sante Murano and Alessia Tognolini

CONTENTS

16.1 **Introduction** *295*

16.2 **Vascular Complications** *295*
16.2.1 Arterial Complications *295*
16.2.1.1 Arterial Disruption *296*
16.2.1.2 Pseudoaneurysm and Bleeding Pseudocyst *297*
16.2.1.3 Haemosuccus Pancreaticus *300*
16.2.1.4 Acute Bleeding in Acute Pancreatitis *300*
16.2.2 Venous Complications *302*
16.2.2.1 Venous Thrombosis *302*
16.2.2.2 Pancreatic Duct/Portal Vein Fistula *302*
16.2.2.3 Thrombophlebitis of the Peripancreatic Tributaries of the Portal Vein *302*

16.3 **Biliary Complications** *302*
16.3.1 Biliary Tract Obstruction *306*
16.3.2 Pancreaticobiliary Fistula *306*

References *309*

16.1 Introduction

Multidetector CT (MDCT), magnetic resonance imaging (MRI) and color Doppler ultrasound (US), have significantly modified the role of diagnostic imaging in the study of splanchnic vessels and biliary tree in pancreatitis (Ito et al. 2001; Balthazar 2002a,b). Today, noninvasive imaging modalities can provide an immediate diagnosis, and catheter angiography has become the modality of choice in the treatment of vascular complications. Percutaneous transhepatic cholangiography (PTC) and its applications are useful in the treatment of biliary tract injuries (Gadacz et al. 1983).

This chapter describes the physiopathological mechanisms underlying vascular and biliary involvement in pancreatitis and the role of imaging in the diagnosis of these complications.

16.2 Vascular Complications

The erosive action of active pancreatic proteolytic enzymes in acute pancreatitis, mechanical pressure from the pseudocyst and drainage from an operated pancreas can involve pancreatic or peripancreatic vessels (Stanley et al. 1976; Manfredi et al. 2001). These conditions result in arterial complications, such as pseudoaneurysm, arterial disruption or venous complications, most frequently in the form of venous thrombosis (Bradley 1993b).

16.2.1 Arterial Complications

Major arterial hemorrhagic complications in pancreatitis are infrequent but can be life-threatening (Bresler et al. 1991; Frey et al. 1992; Procacci et al. 2002).

In severe acute pancreatitis, as defined by the 1992 Atlanta International Symposium on Acute Pancreatitis (Bradley 1993a), massive bleeding is a consequence of the erosion of peripancreatic arteries by active proteolytic enzymes (arterial disruption) (Bresler et al. 1991; Mansueto et al. 2006).

G. Mansueto, MD
R. Sante Murano, MD
A. Tognolini, MD
Department of Radiology, University of Verona, Policlinico "GB Rossi", Piazzale LA Scuro 10, 37134, Verona, Italy
G. Armatura, MD
Department of Surgery Sciences, University of Verona, Policlinico "GB Rossi", Piazzale LA Scuro 10, 37134, Verona, Italy
D. Cenzi, MD
Department of Radiology, Ospedale Borgo Trento, Piazzale Stefani 1, 37126 Verona, Italy

When acute or chronic pancreatitis is associated with a pseudocyst, the progressive enlargement of the pseudocyst induces necrotizing arteritis due to the added pressure on the vessel walls and the action of the proteolytic enzymes (Burke et al. 1986). Spontaneous bleeding frequently at the pancreatic tail, next to the spleen hilum or at the head of the pancreas. The splenic artery, the gastro-duodenal artery, the pancreatico-duodenal arcades and lastly, the left gastric artery are most frequently involved (Aranha et al. 1984; Brodsky and Turnbull 1991; Balladur et al. 1996; Rumstadt et al. 1998; Sato et al. 1998).

The precise site of bleeding can be further specified from knowledge of the splanchnic arterial anatomy (Mansueto et al. 2006, 2007). On the left side, arterial lesions usually involve the last portion of the splenic artery, immediately upstream from the origin of the left gastroepiploic artery and the collateral omental branches. Here, the retroperitoneal splenic branches become intraperitoneal, and are therefore more mobile in comparision with the retroperitoneal vessels; the site is susceptible to aneurysm formation (Fig. 16.1). On the right side, bleeding is most frequent from an analogous anatomic level where the gastroduodenal artery divides into the right gastroepiploic artery and the pancreatico-duodenal branches. Here, the gastroduodenal artery passes from the retroperitoneum into the omental root and becomes intraperitoneal (Fig. 16.2).

16.2.1.1 Arterial Disruption

Arterial bleeding in acute pancreatitis, not associated with a pseudocyst, is defined as "arterial disruption" and is caused by the auto digestion of the arterial wall by fluid collections. It usually occurs in the advanced phase of disease and in post-operative patients (Beattie et al. 2003; Mortele et al. 2004a,b). This critical condition corresponds to the so-called "necrotic hemorrhagic pancreatitis" and is considered the most severe vascular complication. The mortality rate is over 50% (Lendrum 1994). Survival depends greatly on prompt and accurate diagnostic and therapeutic intervention.

The most commonly involved is the splenic artery, but any of the peripancreatic vessels can be involved, depending on the location of the fluid collection. Bleeding from the right and middle colic arteries is common when the collection occupies the mesenteric root (Fig. 16.3). The superior mesenteric artery and the celiac trunk can also be involved, but to a lesser degree. Patients present in shock at the time of diagnosis. Bleeding can occur in the gastro-intestinal lumen, peritoneal cavity, retroperitoneum, or simultaneously in several anatomic cavities (Stroud et al. 1981; Balthazar and Fisher 2001; Testart et al. 2001).

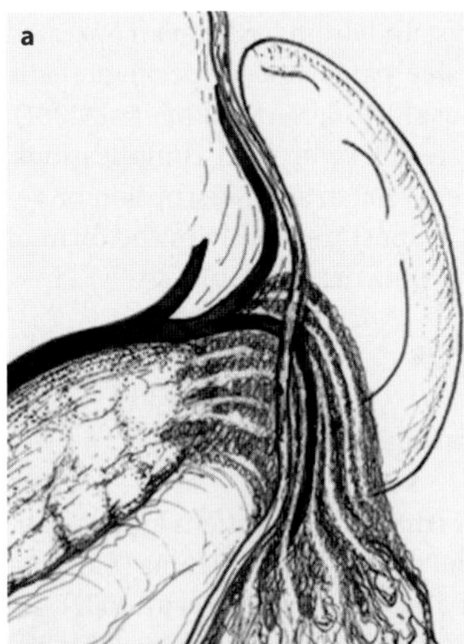

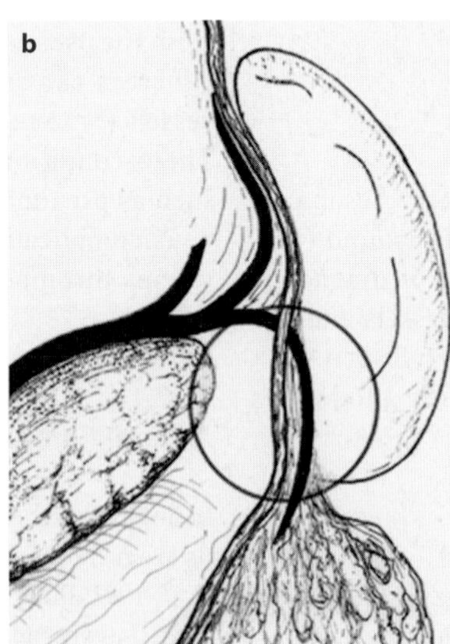

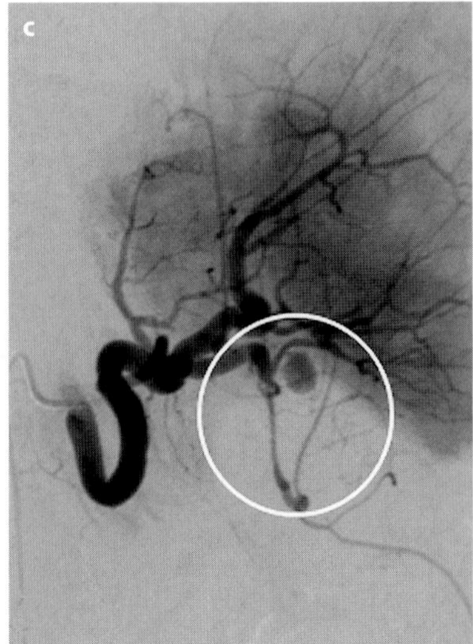

Fig. 16.1a–c. Pancreatic left-side arterial involvement in pancreatitis. The scheme highlights pancreatic left side arterial involvement (**a**). Arterial lesions usually occur in the last branch of the splenic artery, immediately upstream from the origin of the left gastroepiploic artery and the collateral branches (*circle*) (**b**). Selective angiography of the splenic artery in the anterior right oblique projection (**c**) displays a bleeding pseudocyst which develops just when these retroperitoneal branches become intraperitoneal (*circle*). (**a**,**b**: from Mansueto et al. 2006)

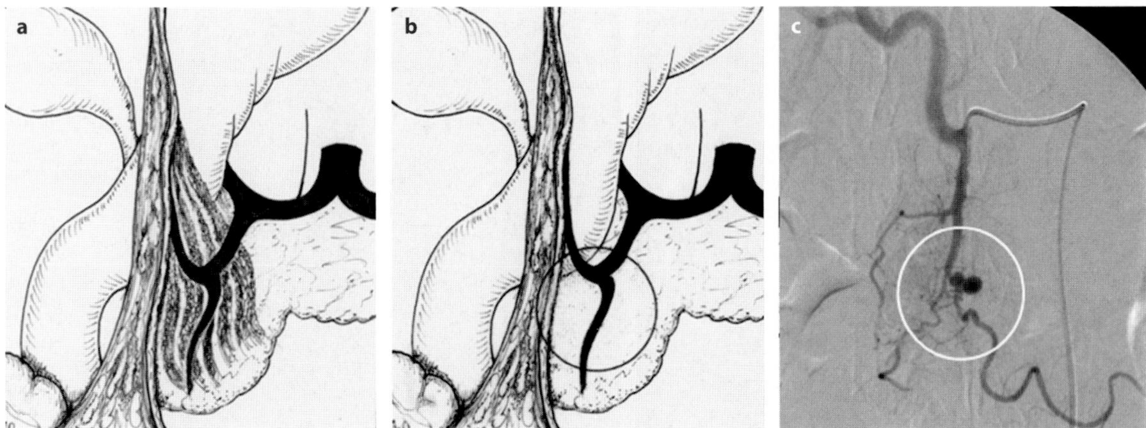

Fig. 16.2a–c. Pancreatic right side arterial involvement in pancreatitis. The scheme highlights pancreatic right side arterial involvement (**a**). At this site the gastroduodenal artery divides into the right gastroepiploic artery and the pancreatico-duodenal branches (*circle*) (**b**). Selective angiography of the common hepatic artery in the antero-posterior projection (**c**) demonstrates a small pseudoaneurysm which develops just at the origin of the right gastroepiploic artery (*circle*). (**a**,**b**: from Mansueto et al. 2006)

When pancreatitis related hemorrhage is suspected, MDCT is able to detect arterial vessels that might become completely involved by collections (Balthazar 2002a; Mansueto et al. 2006). In hemodynamically unstable patients, MDCT is often able to identify the hemorrhagic component inside the collection and possibly the source of bleeding (Fig. 16.4a). Nonetheless, diagnosis is still a considerable challenge. When immediate treatment is required, the gold standard imaging technique is catheter angiography, which has the advantage of being both a diagnostic and therapeutic tool (Fig. 16.4b–d).

Arterial bleeding in acute pancreatitis is a dramatic occurrence with a high mortality rate. Treatment of this condition may be very difficult for the surgeon or radiologist (Bergert et al. 2004, 2005; Mansueto et al. 2007). Emergency surgery is associated with a high degree of failure and mortality. A bleeding recurrence rate of more than 80% has been reported in the literature (Stanley et al. 1976; Stabile et al. 1983; El Hamel et al. 1991; de Perrot et al. 1999; Testart et al. 2001). The radiological treatment of arterial disruption in "necrotic hemorrhagic" pancreatitis can fail due to the excessive extent of maceration of the vessel or involvement of multiple arterial branches and vessel embolization has a 40% mortality rate.

Surgical resection has a mortality rate of more than 50% (Lendrum 1994).

16.2.1.2 Pseudoaneurysm and Bleeding Pseudocyst

When pancreatitis results in a pseudocyst, both the progressive enlargement and mass effect can cause necrotizing arteritis, leading to hemorrhage. Hemorrhage is initially contained by a fibrous tissue capsule that progressively enlarges due to the continous arterial pressure. This condition is known as a pseudoaneurysm or a bleeding pseudocyst in the literature (Burke et al. 1986; El Hamel et al. 1991). If the arterial bleeding fills the entire lumen of the pseudocyst, then the pseudocyst itself becomes the equivalent of a pseudoaneurysm, the wall of which is that of the cyst, not the vascular adventitia. If there is evidence of bleeding inside the pseudocyst, but a large amount of proteolytic enzymes still fills its lumen, this condition is better defined as a bleeding pseudocyst (Stabile et al. 1983; Carr et al. 2000).

The type of lesion that develops depends on the size of the pseudocyst: bleeding in a small pseudocyst remains contained resulting in the familiar pseudoaneurysm. In the case of a bleeding pseudocyst there is a significant risk of rupturing in the gastro-intestinal tract or into the peritoneal and/or retroperitoneal spaces. Angiography can identify an isolated non-bleeding pseudoaneurysm in 10%–21% of patients affected with chronic pancreatitis (Burke et al. 1986). The frequency of pseudoaneurysm is higher (10%–31%) in patients with pseudo-

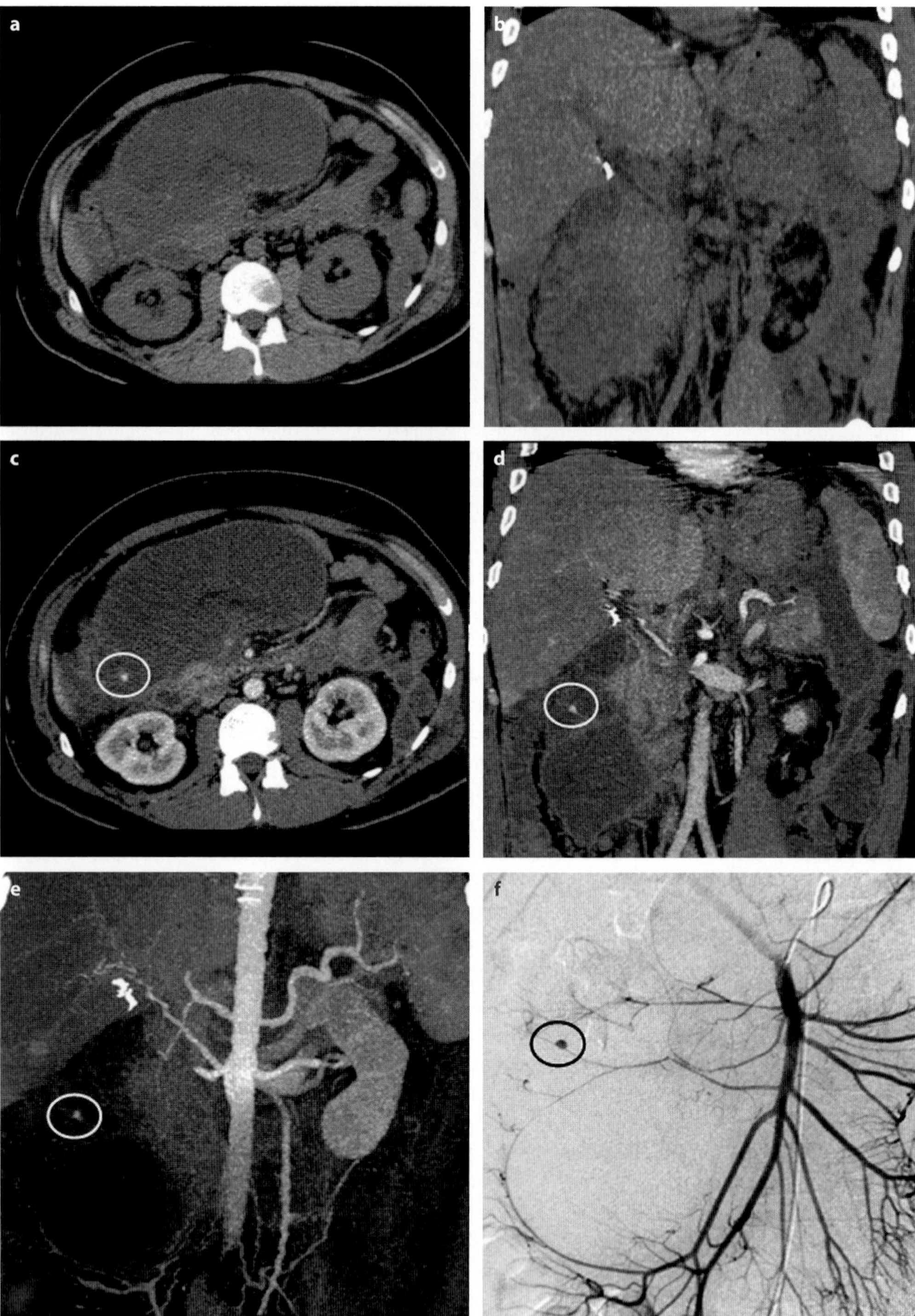

Fig. 16.3a–f. Arterial disruption in severe acute post-ERCP pancreatitis. Axial CT scans (**a**,**c**) and coronal MPR reconstructions (**b**,**d**) show a necrotic pancreatic collection which occupies mesenteric root. The pancreatic collection shows mild inhomogeneity with subtle hyperdensity at the non-enhanced CT scan in the most dependent portion (**a**,**b**). CT in the arterial phase displays a tiny hyperdensity (*circle*), suggestive of arterial disruption, even though the precise site of bleeding is not identified (**c**,**d**). MIP arterial reconstruction (**e**) demonstrates bleeding from the middle colic branch of the superior mesenteric artery which is displaced on the left by the pancreatic collection. Selective mesenteric artery angiography (**f**) confirms arterial disruption of middle colic artery (*circle*)

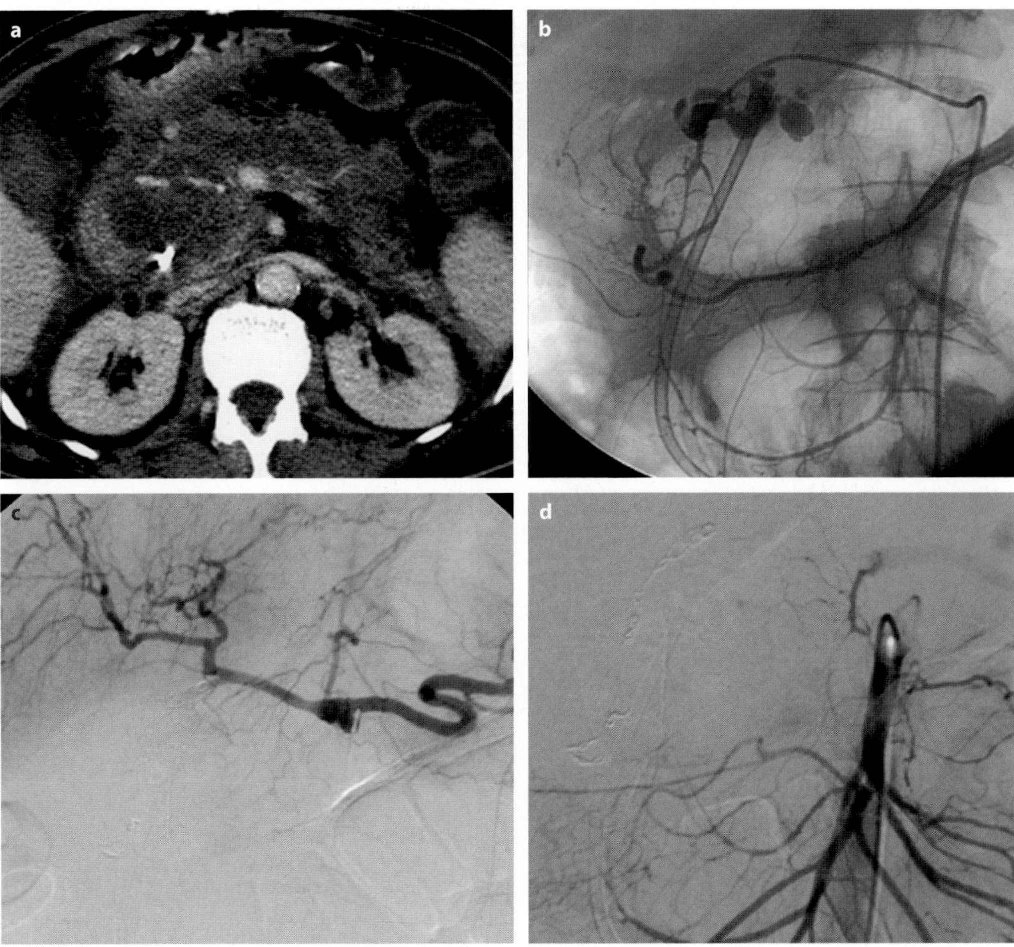

Fig. 16.4a–d. Emergency radiological treatment of arterial disruption in bleeding pancreatitis. **a** Contrast-enhanced CT scan highlights a fluid collection in the necrotic pancreatic head. A tiny hyperdensity inside the collection is suggestive of arterial disruption. **b** Selective angiography demonstrates active bleeding fronm the gastroduodenal artery, immediately proximal to the origin of the right gastroepiploic artery. The angiographic image is characteristic of arterial disruption in acute pancreatitis with leakage of contrast medium directly into the peripancreatic fluid collection. **c,d** Complete embolization achieved by placing coils along the inferior pancreatico-duodenal arcades. (From Mansueto et al. 2006)

cysts (Kiviluoto et al. 1989; Frey et al. 1992). Hemorrhagic complications are expected in 6%–31% of patients with pancreatic pseudocyst (Sankaran and Walt 1975) and in 7%–14% of those suffering from chronic pancreatitis (Bresler et al. 1991). Currently, non-invasive vascular imaging [Doppler US, MDCT, magnetic resonance angiography (MRA)] is almost as sensitive as angiography and should be the first choice in asymptomatic patients (Fig. 16.5) (Ammori et al. 1998; Dorffel et al. 2000). Because of the high frequency of these complications, all imaging protocols must include arterial phase aquisitions.

Doppler US immediately recognizes blood flow inside the pseudoaneurysm and, in some cases, may identify the vessel of origin. A bleeding pseudocyst may be suspected during a US examination if a cystic pancreatic mass rapidly enlarges or suddenly changes its echogenicity (Dorffel et al. 2000).

Its identification more often occurs during CT examination (Fig. 16.5a–d), where there is acute, usually gastro-intestinal pain and possible bleeding (Sankaran and Walt 1975). Multiple recurrences of gastro-intestinal hemorrhage, especially in association with transient pancreatic pain, must arouse the suspicion of a pseudoaneurysm or a bleeding pseudocyst.

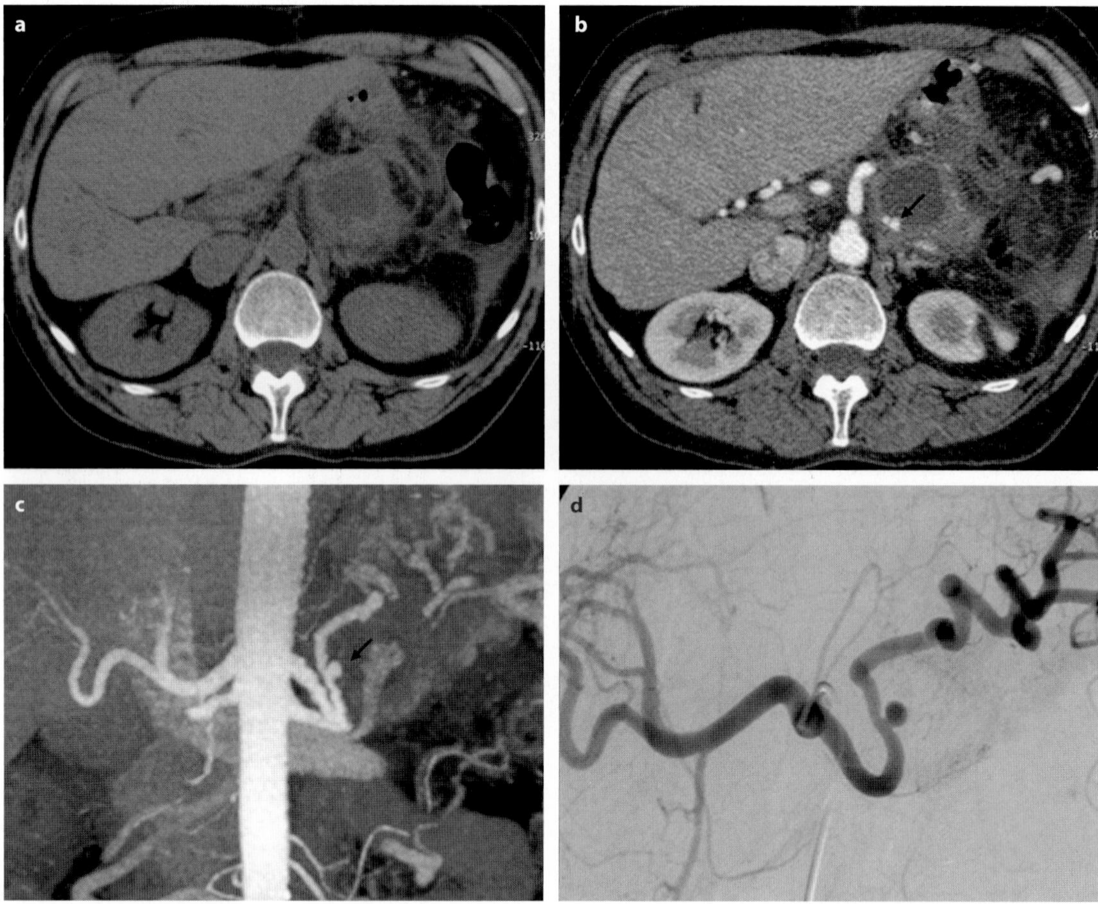

Fig. 16.5a–d. Bleeding pseudocyst in acute pancreatitis. **a** Unenhanced CT axial scan displays a pseudocyst at the pancreatic body; a small fluid collection occupies the retroperitoneal spaces. **b** At CT in the arterial phase, a small pseudoaneurysm of the splenic artery (*arrow*) inside the pseudocyst is shown. **c** MIP arterial reconstruction shows the site of the pseudoaneurysm (*arrow*), between the first and the second third of splenic artery. **d** Selective angiography of the celiac trunk confirms the CT findings

16.2.1.3 Haemosuccus Pancreaticus

"Haemosuccus pancreaticus" was first described by Lower and Farrell (1931). Patients present with intermittent bleeding, which on endoscopy is localized to the major papilla (Nabi Yattoo et al. 1999; Feng and Mauro 2003). In the case of chronic gastro-intestinal bleeding in pancreatic inflammatory disease associated with the diagnosis of pseudoaneurysm at CT scan (Fig. 16.6a), endoscopic retrograde cholangiopancreatography (ERCP) may be helpful in detecting an abnormal communication between the main pancreatic duct and the pseudoaneurysm. Diagnosis may be performed through a direct endoscopic visualization of wirsungorrhage or indirect confirmation due to the opacification of the pseudoaneurysm (Fig. 16.6b).

16.2.1.4 Acute Bleeding in Acute Pancreatitis

Acute bleeding in a patient with known pseudoaneurysm may occur as a consequence of a rupturing pseudoaneurysm or a bleeding pseudocyst. Clinical presentation is characterized by sudden hemorrhagic shock, with a mortality rate of 50% (Lendrum 1994). CT can easily identify the pseudoaneurysm and its contiguity with the gastro-intestinal tract or the presence of hemoperitoneum. To date, MDCT with image reconstruction (MPR, MIP, SSD, VR), or MR, with 3D acquisitions utilizimg contrast phases, are extremely effective in defining the bleeding point and outlining arterial anatomy (Fig. 16.7a–c).

Catheter angiography plays a fundamental role in the treatment of arterial complications identified

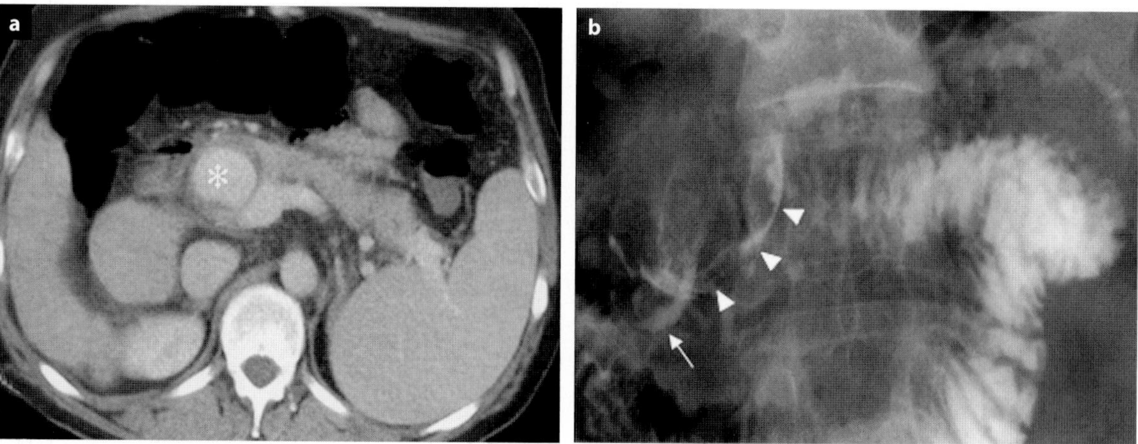

Fig. 16.6a,b. Pseudoaneurysm in chronic pancreatitis. Axial CT scan in the arterial phase (**a**) demonstrates a pseudoaneurysm (*asterisk*) embedded in the pancreatic head; ERCP (**b**) reveals the leakage of contrast medium from the main pancreatic duct (*arrow*) to the lumen of the pseudoaneurysm (*arrowheads*). (From Procacci et al. 2002)

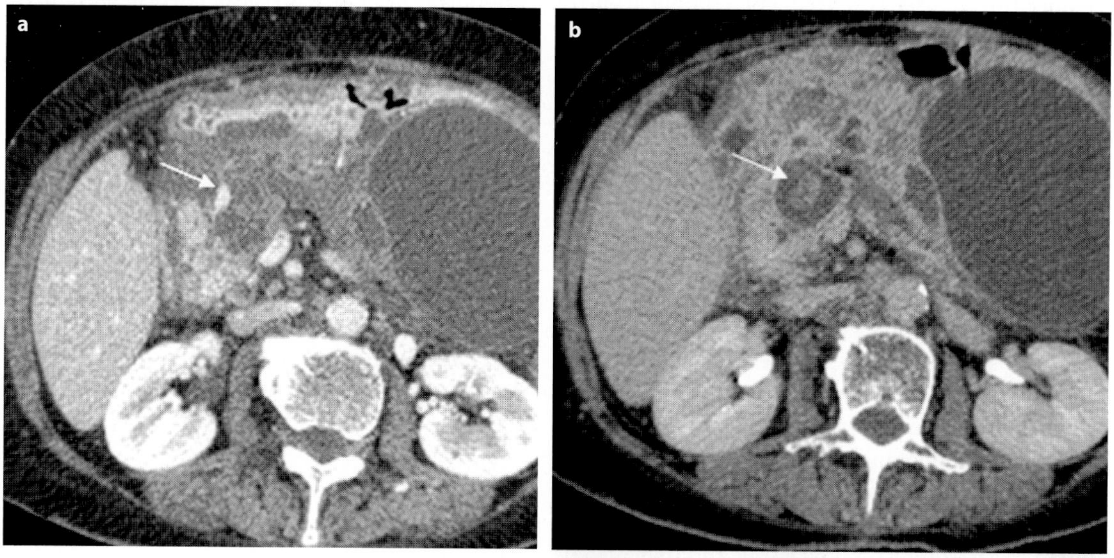

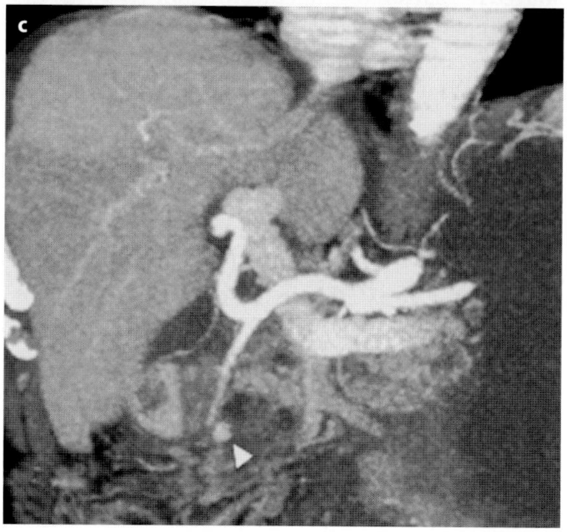

Fig. 16.7a–c. Pseudoaneurysm in acute pancreatitis. **a** The pancreas is enlarged and almost completely replaced by multiple pseudocysts. The largest is located in the pancreatic tail. A small hyperdense lesion at the pancreatic head is seen at CT in the arterial phase (*arrow*). **b** At delayed CT scans the lesion at the pancreatic head becomes enlarged and is still hyperdense: this is suggestive of a pancreatic pseudoaneurysm. **c** MIP arterial reconstruction demonstrates the source of bleeding from the gastroduodenal artery, just before the origin of the right gastroepiploic artery (*arrowhead*)

at non-invasive imaging. In particular, embolization reports high success rates in the treatment of these lesions (Beattie et al. 2003; Bergert et al. 2004, 2005; Mansueto et al. 2007). All the afferent and efferent arteries involved must be defined (Fig. 16.8a,b). Only by occluding all of these can the complete and definite exclusion of the pseudoaneurysm or bleeding pseudocyst from the arterial flow be achieved, with its resultant progressive collapse (Fig. 16.8c–f).

16.2.2 Venous Complications

16.2.2.1 Venous Thrombosis

Venous thrombosis is a frequent complication of pancreatitis. Thrombosis of the splenic vein is the most frequent because of its location in the groove along the upper posterior boundary of the pancreas (Sakorafas et al. 2000). Occlusion of the splenic vein has been reported in up to 45% of patients with pancreatitis. Chronic calcific pancreatitis is the most common cause of splenic vein thrombosis reported to occur in 5%–37% of patients (Vujic 1989) (Fig. 16.9). Usually there are also associated signs of a pre-hepatic segmental portal hypertension (Moossa and Gadd 1985). Splenic vein occlusion from pancreatitis can lead to the formation of gastric varices that may possibly lead to acute bleeding. US and/or CT imaging can easily demonstrate the presence of varices but not active bleeding. Endoscopy is the gold standard for directly detecting the source of gastrointestinal bleeding and may also be used to perform sclerotherapy of varices if needed. Splenic vein thrombosis and left hypertension may be treated by splenectomy (Vujic 1989).

16.2.2.2 Pancreatic Duct/Portal Vein Fistula

This complication results from a spontaneous rupture of a pancreatic pseudocyst into the portal vein. This complication is unusual: only a few cases have been reported in the literature (Willis and Brewer 1989; Procacci et al. 1995; Balthazar and Gollapudi 2000; Cho et al. 2003; Ko et al. 2003). Diagnosis of the fistula cannot be obtained by angiography, since the portal tree is excluded from the systemic circulation transformation. ERCP can highlight the fistula if the latter directly involves the pancreatic duct (Willis and Brewer 1989). Whenever the fistula is induced by a pseudocyst, ERCP may prove non-diagnostic. On contrast-enhanced CT, the portal lumen is replaced with fluid attenuation material (Fig. 16.10a–c). Communication between the venous lumen and the pseudocyst can sometimes be demonstrated. Confirmation of the fistula is obtainable by trans-hepatic portography carried out under US or CT guidance. MR imaging can also diagnose the development of pancreatic duct/portal vein fistula (Riddel et al. 2005).

16.2.2.3 Thrombophlebitis of the Peripancreatic Tributaries of the Portal Vein

This condition is defined as an acute infection of the portal system with associated hepatic involvement. It can arise from the extension of pancreatic necrosis infection along the portal venous tree. Abscess(es) may develop in the liver when infected necrosis seeds the portal system. At CT, intra-hepatic abscesses appear as poorly defined hypodense collections that may or may not contain small gas bubbles (Fig. 16.11). Early detection of septic ascending thrombophlebitis (Fig. 16.12) may decrease the mortality rate and improve the prognosis reported in the surgical literature (Balthazar and Gollapudi 2000).

16.3 Biliary Complications

Biliary complications are quite common in patients with acute or chronic pancreatitis. Because the common bile duct (CBD) runs within the head of the pancreas, common bile duct stenosis or obstruction with cholestasis, cholangitis, and even secondary biliary cirrhosis may occur (Rohrman and Baron 1989; Vijungco and Prinz 2003).

In acute pancreatitis, the necrotic action of lytic enzymes in the pancreatic and peri-pancreatic collections may cause fistulas resulting in bile leakage and extravasation (Vijungco and Prinz 2003) (Fig. 16.13). The incidence of this complication is higher in cases of operated necrotic-hemorrhagic pancreatitis. Often the bile collection spreads into the retroperitoneal space (Sarles and Sahel 1978;

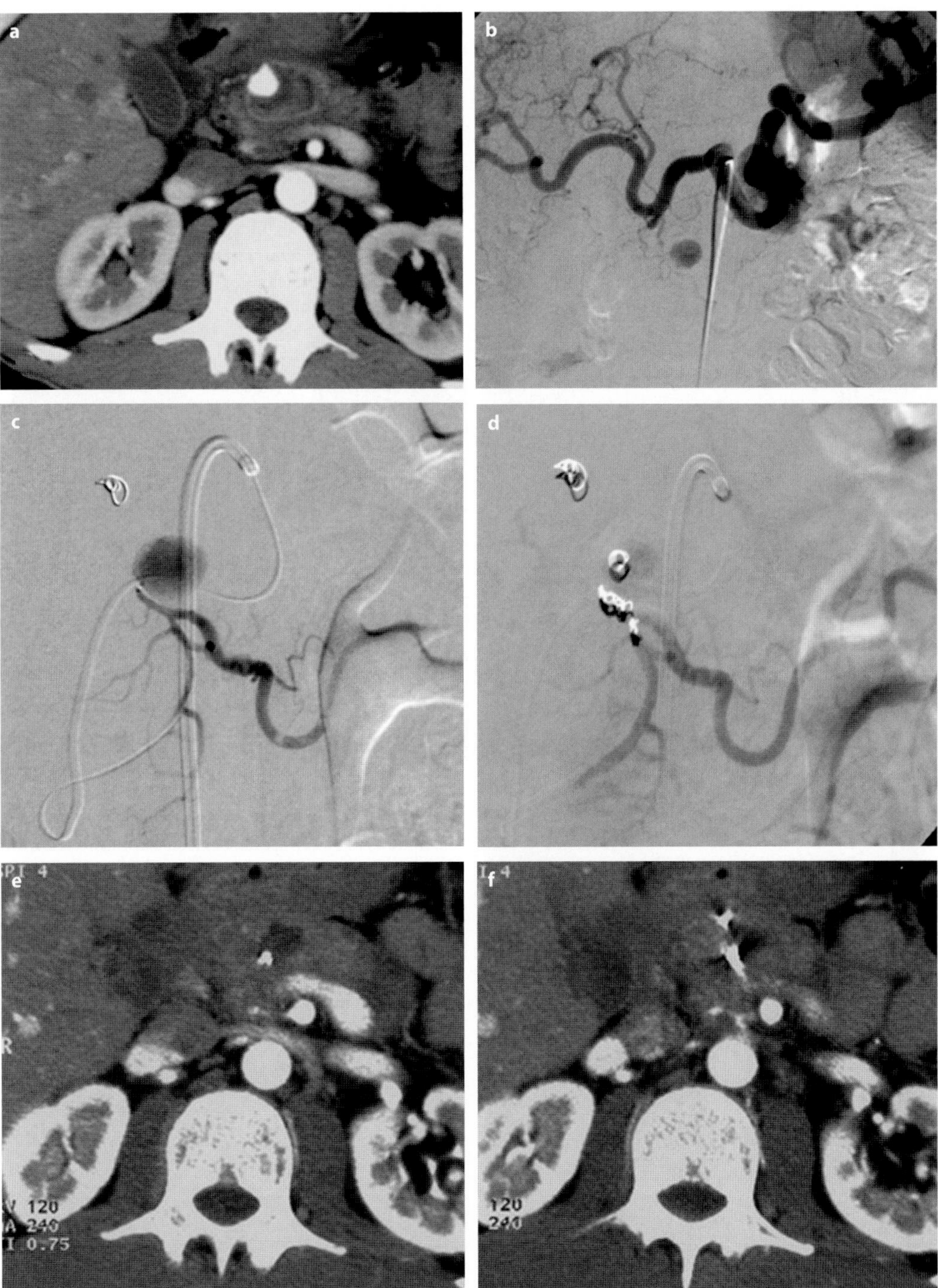

Fig. 16.8a–f. Pseudoaneurysm of the pancreatico-duodenal arcades in chronic pancreatitis: diagnosis and radiological treatment. **a** Axial CT scan in the arterial phase displays a pseudoaneurysm. **b** Angiography of the celiac trunk identifies the pseudoaneurysm, which communicates with the anterior and posterior pancreatico-duodenal arcades. **c** Selective angiography of the inferior pancreatico-duodenal artery defines a detailed vascular map of all the afferent and efferent vessels to the lesion (anterior and posterior pancreatico-duodenal arcades as well as some inferior afferent arteries). **d** Selective angiography after transcatheter embolization of the gastroduodenal artery demonstrates the complete exclusion of the arterial lesion. **e,f** Axial CT in the arterial phase 3 months after endovascular treatment, shows the coils occluding the afferent vessels. Pseudoaneurysm is completely excluded

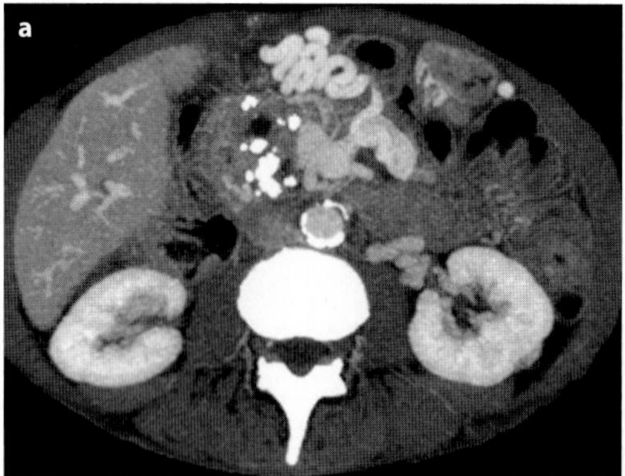

Fig. 16.9a–c. Splenic thrombosis in chronic pancreatitis. **a** CT axial scan in the portal venous phase demonstrates enlarged pancreatic head with multiple calcifications and dilatation of the main pancreatic duct. Multiple collateral venous branches around the pancreatic head are seen, while splenic vein is not clearly identified. This leads to the diagnosis of splenic vein thrombosis. **b,c** Volume rendering images in the anterior right (**b**) and anterior left projection (**c**) better demonstrate the extent of venous varices, the esophageal, gastric and splenorenal collateral venous branches

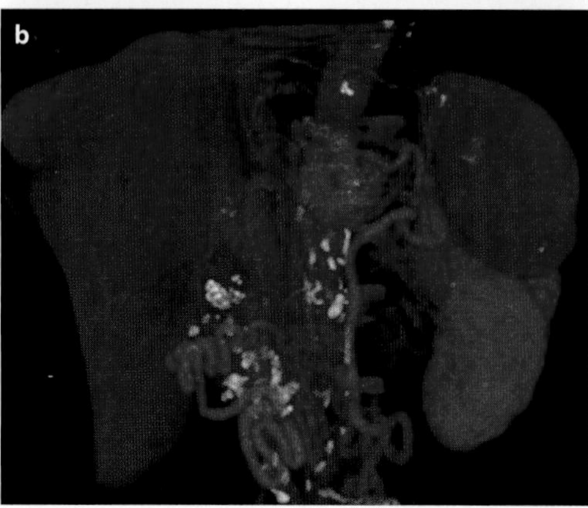

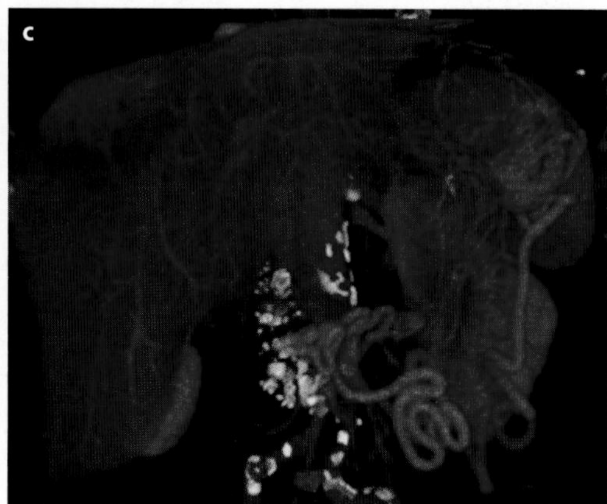

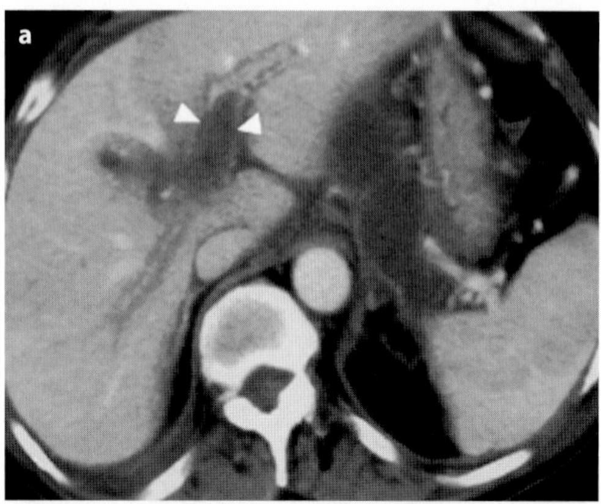

Fig. 16.10a–c. Thrombophlebitis of the spleno-portal venous axis. CT scans, carried out in the craniocaudal direction in the contrastographic phase, show hypodense hepatic areas, due to the reduced altered portal flow caused by the complete thrombosis of the portal tree (*arrowheads*), which is involved by a large pseudocyst of the pancreatic body (*asterisk*). The lumen of the portal vessels has the same density as the pseudocyst. (From Procacci et al. 2002)

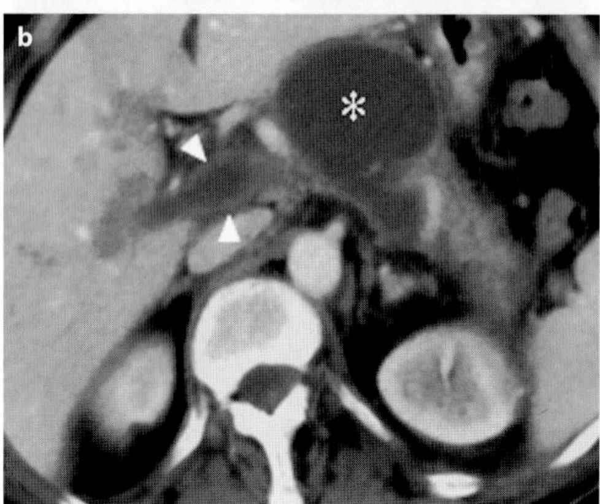

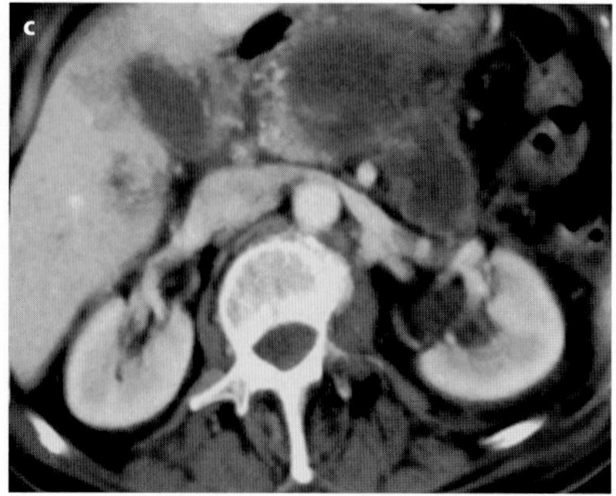

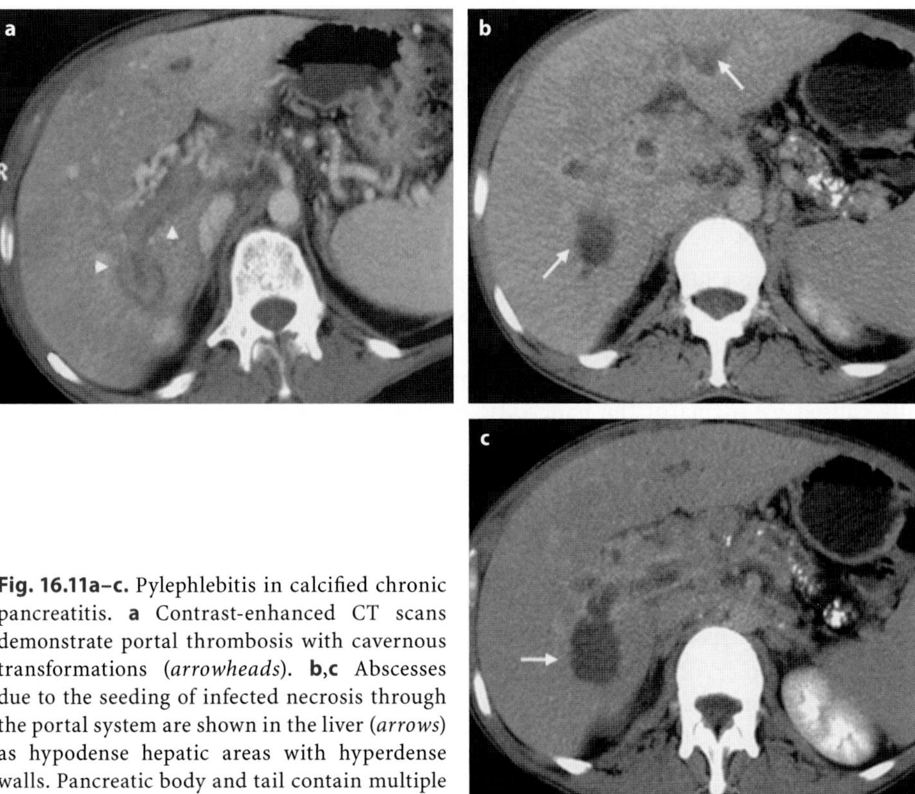

Fig. 16.11a–c. Pylephlebitis in calcified chronic pancreatitis. **a** Contrast-enhanced CT scans demonstrate portal thrombosis with cavernous transformations (*arrowheads*). **b,c** Abscesses due to the seeding of infected necrosis through the portal system are shown in the liver (*arrows*) as hypodense hepatic areas with hyperdense walls. Pancreatic body and tail contain multiple calcifications. (From Mansueto et al. 2006)

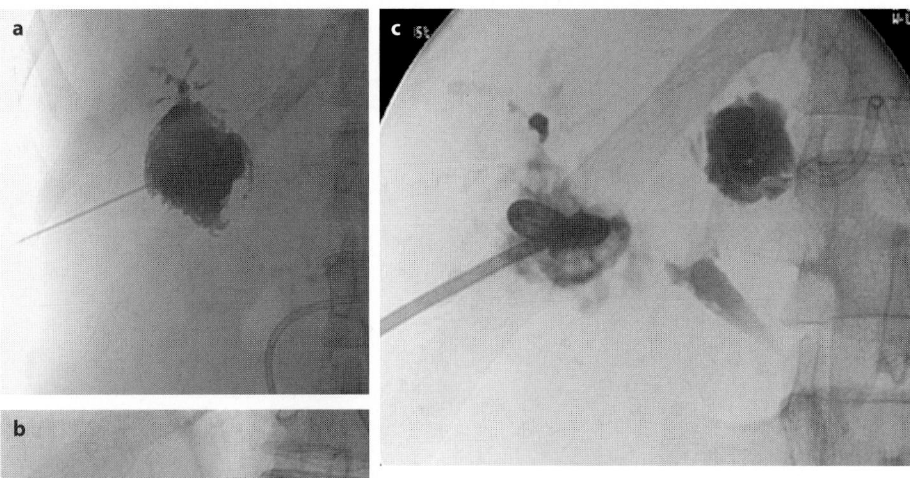

Fig. 16.12a–c. Percutaneous transhepatic drainage of liver abscesses in pylephlebitis in chronic pancreatitis (same patient as in Fig. 16.11). Definitive diagnosis and treatment of pylephlebitis is performed by percutaneous transhepatic drainage. The direct liver puncture is carried out with a fine needle (**a**) and then exchanged for a percutaneous catheter (**b**). The communication between fluid collections and thrombosed portal vein is demonstrated by the spreading of contrast medium directly into the portal tree (**b,c**). (From Mansueto et al. 2006)

Wilson et al. 1989). Pancreaticobiliary fistula in association with an underlying pseudocyst or abscess is much more unusual (Sakorafas et al. 2001).

16.3.1 Biliary Tract Obstruction

The incidence of CBD obstruction in patients with chronic pancreatitis has been described as ranging from 3% to 23% (Stabile et al. 1987).

In acute pancreatitis, biliary obstruction is usually caused by edema of the pancreatic head and is clinically characterized as transient jaundice (Fig. 16.14). Resolution of collections is associated with an improvement of jaundice.

In chronic pancreatitis, main biliary duct (MBD) obstruction is caused by irreversible fibrosis (Fig. 16.15). If there is a clinical suspicion of obstructed biliary tree, non-invasive imaging of the hepatobiliary tree, such as US or CT, may easily be able to diagnose biliary obstruction and the presence of a pseudocyst. At direct cholangiography, distal CBD structures from chronic pancreatitis may be indistinguishable from those caused by neoplasm. Thus, the advantage of CT is a better depiction of the pancreatic and retroperitoneal anatomy, as well as identification of calcifications as signs of chronic pancreatitis (Skellenger et al. 1983). In autoimmune pancreatitis, the differential diagnosis of biliary obstruction may mimic a lymphoma; a sign of the regression of pancreatic involvement and biliary stenosis after steroid therapy may be helpful in the differential diagnosis (Fig. 16.16). In autoimmune pancreatitis, differentiation from a pancreatic adenocarcinoma may be very difficult: in this case, if a non-invasive imaging technique such as CT or MRI is unable to differentiate pancreatitis and cancer, US- or CT- guided biopsy is mandatory (Stabile et al. 1987).

16.3.2 Pancreaticobiliary Fistula

Fistulization into the biliary tree secondary to pseudocyst or pancreatic necrosis is an unusual complication of pancreatic inflammatory disease. The

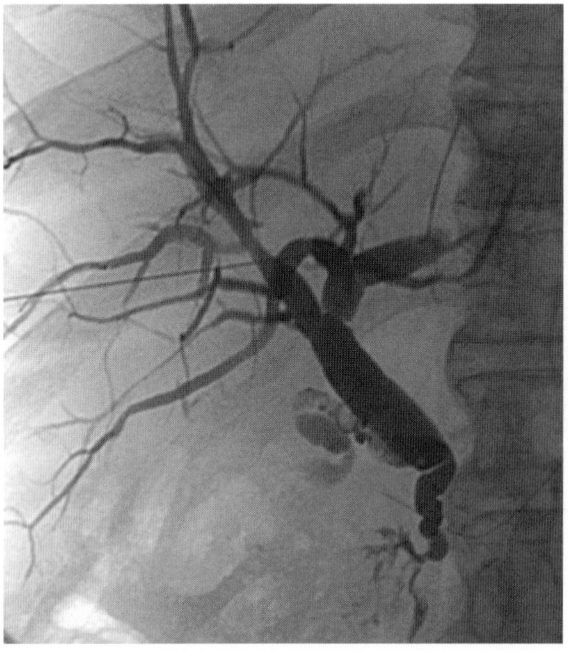

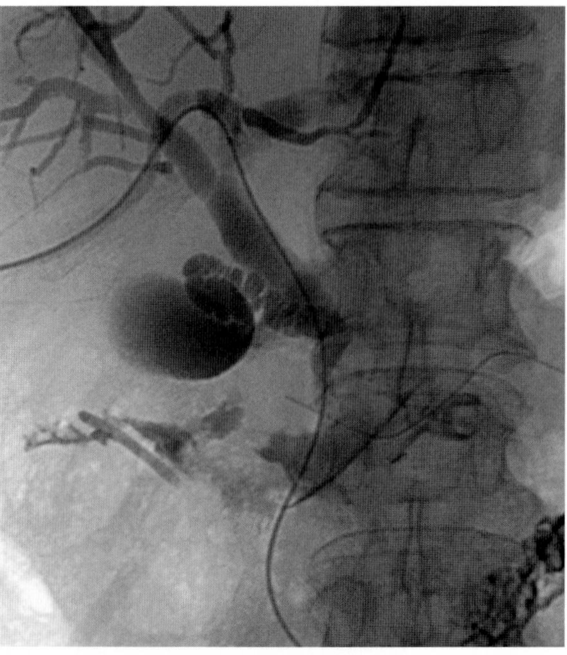

Fig. 16.13a,b. Main biliary duct rupture and leakage in severe acute pancreatitis: percutaneous diagnosis and treatment. **a** Direct puncture with a fine needle demonstrates dilatation of biliary intrahepatic ducts and biliary main duct, which reduces in diameter as it traverses the pancreatic head. Extravasation of contrast medium at the pancreatic head is suggestive of bile leakage. **b** The bile leakage spreads into the retroperitoneal spaces and it is treated by placing a percutaneous biliary drainage with the distal tip placed directly into the jejunum

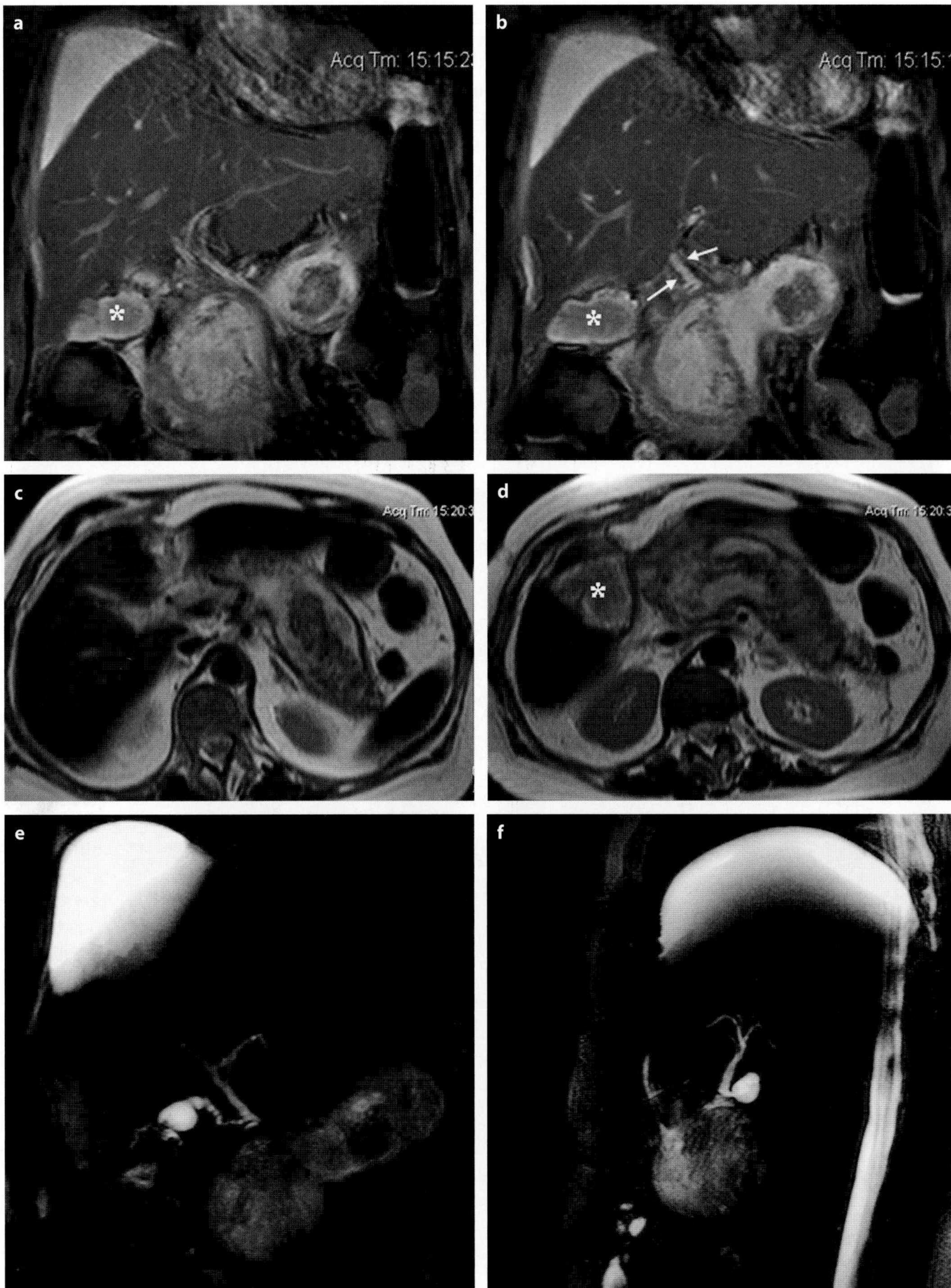

Fig. 16.14a–f. Main biliary duct obstruction in severe acute pancreatitis. **a,b** True FISP fat-suppressed coronal MR images display a huge non-homogenous collection surrounding the entire pancreas. The pancreas is enlarged with multiple necrotic collections. An heterogeneous fluid collection containing hemorrhagic debris is also seen next to the gallbladder (*asterisks*). Ascites is seen around the right hepatic lobe. Mild bile main duct dilatation is shown just immediately above the pancreatic collection (**b**) (*arrows*). **c,d** T2-weighted TSE MR axial images better defines the extent of the necrosis. **e,f** MRI images in coronal (**e**) and sagittal (**f**) projections demonstrate all the features previously demonstrated: the huge non-homogeneous collection around the pancreas, the abdominal perihepatic effusion and the main bile duct dilatation just above the intra-hepatic tract. Initial involvement of the intrahepatic ducts is also demonstrated

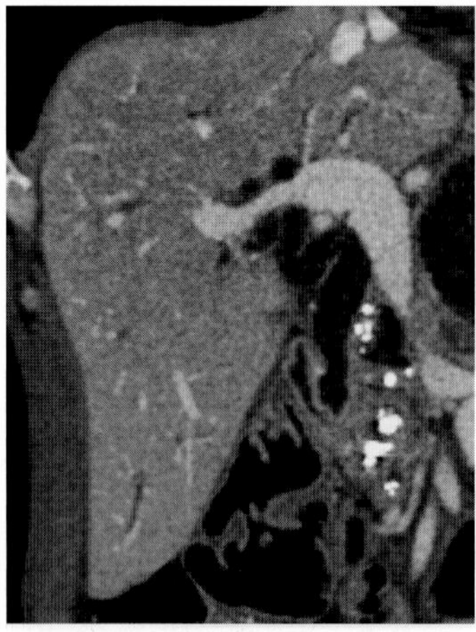

Fig. 16.15. Main biliary duct obstruction in chronic pancreatitis. MPR image from MDCT shows an enlarged and tortuous CBD with initial dilatation of the intrahepatic biliary ducts at the hepatic hylum. Fibrosis and multiple calcifications are visible at the pancreatic head causing bile duct obstruction and dilatation

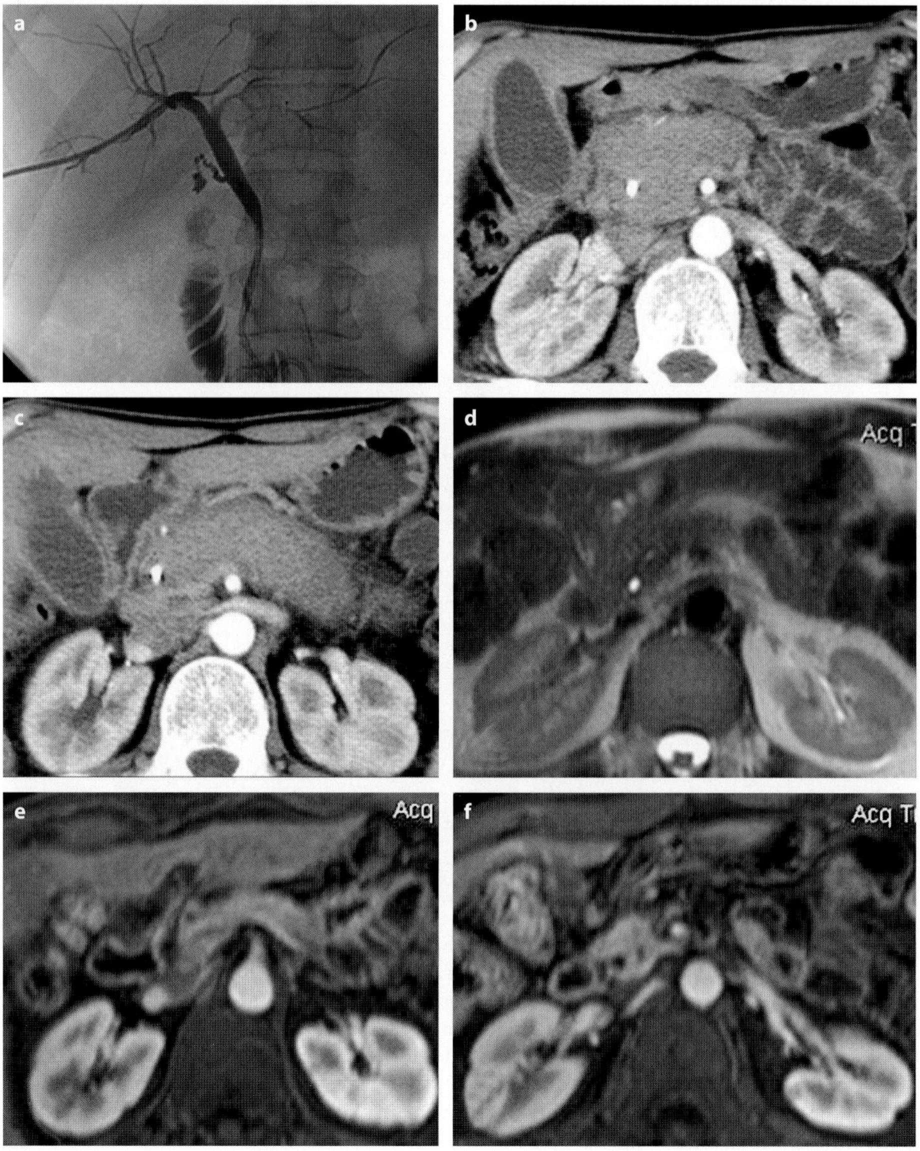

Fig. 16.16a–f. Main biliary duct obstruction in chronic autoimmune pancreatitis. **a** Percutaneous biliary drainage (PTBD) shows common bile duct stenosis with mild dilatation of the biliary tree. **b,c** CT axial scans in the arterial phase, performed after PTBD, display diffuse enlargement and slight hypodensity of the pancreas, suggestive of autoimmune pancreatitis. **d–f** T2-weighted TSE MR axial image (**d**) and T1 fat saturation post-gadolinium arterial images (**e**,**f**),performed following corticosteroid therapy show decrease in size of the pancreas which has a normal morphology, confirming the diagnosis of autoimmune pancreatitis

fistula may be caused by a necrotic process involving the pancreatic head or, in case of pancreatitis complicated by a pseudocyst, the narrowing of the CBD may be either secondary to stenosis from underlying pancreatitis, or due to pressure of the pseudocyst (Warshaw and Rattner 1980; Skellenger et al. 1983; Stabile et al. 1987). As a consequence of rupture of the pseudocyst in the biliary tree, suppurative cholangitis may occur (Rohrman and Baron 1989).

CT is useful in depicting the inflammatory involvement of the pancreatic gland and the extent of the peri-pancreatic collection. In the literature, biliary fistulization is reported to be discovered mostly at surgery (Warshaw and Rattner 1980; Skellenger et al. 1983; Nealon et al. 1989).

Both diagnostic and intra-operative ERCP are the gold standard in detecting a fistula: if there is a pancreatico-biliary fistula, contrast medium injected through the common bile duct is reported to leak into the main pancreatic duct. The presence of bile in a percutaneously or surgically drained pseudocyst or abscess is an indications of an underlying pancreatico-biliary fistula (Sakorafas et al. 2001). ERCP has been proposed in the follow up of patients with known pseudocysts to determine the status of the CBD and to demonstrate any possible pseudocyst communication with the main pancreatic duct or surrounding organs (Wong et al. 1980; Nealon et al. 1989).

References

Ammori BJ, Madan M, Alexander DJ (1998) Haemorrhagic complications of pancreatitis: presentation, diagnosis and management. Ann R Coll Surg Engl 80:316–325

Aranha GV, Prinz RA, Greenlee HB, Freeark RJ (1984) Gastric outlet and duodenal obstruction from inflammatory pancreatic disease. Arch Surg 119:833–835

Balladur P, Christophe M, Tiret E, Parc R (1996) Bleeding of pancreatic stump following pancreatoduodenectomy for cancer. Hepatogastroenterology 43:268–270

Balthazar EJ (2002a) Complications of acute pancreatitis: clinical and CT evaluation. Radiol Clin North Am 40:1211–1227

Balthazar EJ (2002b) Acute pancreatitis: assessment of severity with clinical and CT evaluation. Radiology 223:603–613

Balthazar EJ, Fisher LA (2001) Hemorrhagic complications of pancreatitis: radiologic evaluation with emphasis on CT imaging. Pancreatology 1:306–313

Balthazar EJ, Gollapudi P (2000) Septic thrombophlebitis of the mesenteric and portal veins: CT imaging. J Comput Assist Tomogr 24:755–760

Beattie GC, Hardman JG, Redhead D, Siriwardena AK (2003) Evidence for a central role for selective mesenteric angiography in the management of the major vascular complications of pancreatitis. Am J Surg; 185:96–102

Bergert H, Dobrowolski F, Caffier S, Bloomenthal A, Hinterseher I, Saeger HD (2004) Prevalence and treatment of bleeding complications in chronic pancreatitis. Langenbecks Arch Surg 389:504–510

Bergert H, Hinterseher I, Kersting S, Leonhardt J, Bloomenthal A, Saeger HD (2005) Management and outcome of hemorrhage due to arterial pseudoaneurysms in pancreatitis. Surgery 137:323–328

Bradley EL (1993a) A clinically based classification system for acute pancreatitis. Summary of the International Symposium on Acute Pancreatitis, Atlanta, Ga, September 11 through 13, 1992. Arch Surg 128:586–590

Bradley EL (1993b) A clinically based classification system for acute pancreatitis. Ann Chir 47:537–541

Bresler L, Boissel P, Grosdidier J (1991) Major hemorrhage from pseudocysts and pseudoaneurysms caused by chronic pancreatitis: surgical therapy. World J Surg 15:649–652; discussion 652–643

Brodsky JT, Turnbull AD (1991) Arterial hemorrhage after pancreatoduodenectomy. The "sentinel bleed". Arch Surg 126:1037–1040

Burke JW, Erickson SJ, Kellum CD, Tegtmeyer CJ, Williamson BR, Hansen MF (1986) Pseudoaneurysms complicating pancreatitis: detection by CT. Radiology 161:447–450

Carr JA, Cho JS, Shepard AD, Nypaver TJ, Reddy DJ (2000) Visceral pseudoaneurysms due to pancreatic pseudocysts: rare but lethal complications of pancreatitis. J Vasc Surg 32:722–730

Cho YD, Cheon YK, Cha SW et al (2003) Pancreatic duct-portal vein fistula. Gastrointest Endosc 58:415

de Perrot M, Berney T, Buhler L, Delgadillo X, Mentha G, Morel P (1999) Management of bleeding pseudoaneurysms in patients with pancreatitis. Br J Surg 86:29–32

Dorffel T, Wruck T, Ruckert RI, Romaniuk P, Dorffel Q, Wermke W (2000) Vascular complications in acute pancreatitis assessed by color duplex ultrasonography. Pancreas 21:126–133

El Hamel A, Parc R, Adda G, Bouteloup PY, Huguet C, Malafosse M (1991) Bleeding pseudocysts and pseudoaneurysms in chronic pancreatitis. Br J Surg 78:1059–1063

Feng DH, Mauro MA (2003) SIR 2003 film panel case 6: hemosuccus pancreaticus secondary to chronic pancreatitis. J Vasc Interv Radiol 14:803–805

Frey CF, Stanley JC, Eckhauser F (1992) Hemorrhage. In: Bradley EL (ed) Complications of pancreatitis. Saunders, Philadelphia, pp 96–123

Frey C (1993) Angiographic embolization therapy of pseudoaneurysm: comment on „arterial complications of pancreatitis“. Pancreas 8:742

Gadacz TR, Lillemoe K, Zinner M, Merrill W (1983) Common bile duct complications of pancreatitis evaluation and treatment. Surgery 93:235–242

Ito K, Koike S, Matsunaga N (2001) MR imaging of pancreatic diseases. Eur J Radiol 38:78–93

Kiviluoto T, Kivisaari L, Kivilaakso E, Lempinen M (1989) Pseudocysts in chronic pancreatitis. Surgical results in 102 consecutive patients. Arch Surg 124:240–243

Ko HS, Anders M, Diehl S, Dominguez E, Lohr M, Duber C (2003) Portal vein erosion and acute abdominal hem-

orrhage as a complication of acute pancreatitis. Abdom Imaging 28:700–702
Lendrum R (1994) Chronic pancreatitis. In: Misiewicz JJ, Pounder RE, Venables CW (eds) Diseases of the gut and pancreas. Blackwell, London, pp 441–454
Lower WE, Farrell TT (1931) Aneurysm of splenic artery: report of a case and review of literature. Ann Surg 23:182–190
Manfredi R, Brizi MG, Canade A, Vecchioli A, Marano P (2001) Imaging of acute pancreatitis. Rays 26:135–142
Mansueto G, Cenzi D, Gumbs AA, D'Onofrio M (2006) Imaging in acute pancreatic conditions. In: Emergency radiology. Marincek B, Dondelinger RF (eds) .Springer, Berlin, pp 493–522
Mansueto G, Cenzi D, D'Onofrio M et al (2007) Endovascular treatment of arterial bleeding in patients wih pancreatitis. Pancreatology 7:360–369
Moossa AR, Gadd MA (1985) Isolated splenic vein thrombosis. World J Surg 9:384–390
Mortele KJ, Mergo PJ, Taylor HM et al (2004a) Peripancreatic vascular abnormalities complicating acute pancreatitis: contrast-enhanced helical CT findings. Eur J Radiol 52:67–72
Mortele KJ, Wiesner W, Intriere L et al (2004b) A modified CT severity index for evaluating acute pancreatitis: improved correlation with patient outcome. AJR Am J Roentgenol 183:1261–1265
Nabi Yattoo G, Khuroo MS, Wani NA, Wani KA, Bhat FA (1999) Haemosuccus pancreaticus: a clinical challenge. J Gastroenterol Hepatol 14:172–175
Nealon WH, Townsend CM Jr, Thompson JC (1989) Preoperative endoscopic retrograde cholangiopancreatography (ERCP) in patients with pancreatic pseudocyst associated with resolving acute and chronic pancreatitis. Ann Surg 209:532–538; discussion 538–540
Procacci C, Mansueto GC, Graziani R et al (1995) Spontaneous rupture of a pancreatic pseudocyst into the portal vein. Cardiovasc Intervent Radiol 18:399–402
Procacci C, Mansueto G, D'Onofrio M, Gasparini A, Ferrara RM, Falconi M (2002) Non-traumatic abdominal emergencies: imaging and intervention in acute pancreatic conditions. Eur Radiol 12:2407–2434
Riddel A, Jhaveri K, Haider M (2005) Pseudocyst rupture into the portal vein diagnosed by MRI. Br J Radiol 78:265–268
Rohrmann CA Jr, Baron RL (1989) Biliary complications of pancreatitis. Radiol Clin North Am 27:93–104
Rumstadt B, Schwab M, Korth P, Samman M, Trede M (1998) Hemorrhage after pancreatoduodenectomy. Ann Surg 227:236–241
Sakorafas GH, Sarr MG, Farley DR, Farnell MB (2000) The significance of sinistral portal hypertension complicating chronic pancreatitis. Am J Surg 179:129–133
Sakorafas GH, Sarr MG, Farnell MB (2001) Pancreaticobiliary fistula: an unusual complication of necrotising pancreatitis. Eur J Surg 167:151–153
Sankaran S, Walt AJ (1975) The natural and unnatural history of pancreatic pseudocysts. Br J Surg 62:37–44
Sarles H, Sahel J (1978) Cholestasis and lesions of the biliary tract in chronic pancreatitis. Gut 19:851–857
Sato N, Yamaguchi K, Shimizu S, Morisaki T, Yokohata K, Chijiiwa K, Tanaka M (1998) Coil embolization of bleeding visceral pseudoaneurysms following pancreatectomy: the importance of early angiography. Arch Surg 133:1099–1102
Skellenger ME, Patterson D, Foley NT, Jordan PH Jr (1983) Cholestasis due to compression of the common bile duct by pancreatic pseudocysts. Am J Surg 145:343–348
Stabile BE, Wilson SE, Debas HT (1983) Reduced mortality from bleeding pseudocysts and pseudoaneurysms caused by pancreatitis. Arch Surg 118:45–51
Stabile BE, Calabria R, Wilson SE, Passaro E Jr (1987) Stricture of the common bile duct from chronic pancreatitis. Surg Gynecol Obstet 165:121–126
Stanley JC, Frey CF, Miller TA, Lindenauer SM, Child CG (1976) Major arterial hemorrhage: a complication of pancreatic pseudocysts and chronic pancreatitis. Arch Surg 111:435–440
Stroud WH, Cullom JW, Anderson MC (1981) Hemorrhagic complications of severe pancreatitis. Surgery 90:657–665
Testart J, Boyet L, Perrier G, Clavier E, Peillon C (2001) Arterial erosions in acute pancreatitis. Acta Chir Belg 101:232–237; discussion 237–239
Vijungco JD, Prinz RA (2003) Management of biliary and duodenal complications of chronic pancreatitis. World J Surg 27:1258–1270
Vujic I (1989) Vascular complications of pancreatitis. Radiol Clin North Am 27:81–91
Warshaw AL, Rattner DW (1980) Facts and fallacies of common bile duct obstruction by pancreatic pseudocysts. Ann Surg 192:33–37
Willis SM, Brewer TG (1989) Pancreatic duct-portal vein fistula. Gastroenterology 97:1025–1027
Wilson C, Auld CD, Schlinkert R et al (1989) Hepatobiliary complications in chronic pancreatitis. Gut 30:520–527
Wong DH, Schuman BM, Grodsinsky C (1980) The value of endoscopic retrograde cholangiopancreatography in the surgical management of chronic pancreatitis. Am J Gastroenterol 73:353–356

Imaging of Local Extension and Fistulas

17

Giovanni Carbognin, Chiara Calciolari, and Giovanni Foti

CONTENTS

17.1 **Introduction** *311*

17.2 **Pancreatic Complications** *311*
17.2.1 Pancreatic Necrosis *311*
17.2.2 Collections *312*
17.2.2.1 Sterile Collections *312*
17.2.2.2 Infected Necrosis *312*
17.2.2.3 Imaging Findings *312*
17.2.3 Pancreatic Abscess *316*
17.2.4 Hemorrhage *316*
17.2.5 Fistulas *317*
17.2.5.1 Internal Fistulas *318*
17.2.5.2 External Fistulas *321*

17.3 **Extrapancreatic Complications** *321*
17.3.1 Intestinal Stenosis *321*
17.3.2 Peptic Ulcer *324*
17.3.3 Ascites *324*
17.3.4 Splenic Involvement *325*

17.4 **Conclusions** *325*

References *326*

17.1 Introduction

Pancreatitis is a life-threatening disease with an overall mortality of 2%–10%, even considering the recent developments in diagnosis and treatment (Balthazar 2002).

Mortality is directly related to the development and extension of pancreatic necrosis. Mortality in patients affected by pancreatitis is due both to toxic-systemic manifestations associated with Multi Organ Failure (MOF) and to local complications, limited to the pancreas and/or peripancreatic tissues (Balthazar 2002).

Mild cases of acute pancreatitis usually improve in 48–72 h (Amano et al. 2001). There are no complications and patients can be observed and managed with diet and fluid support. Conversely, in severe acute pancreatitis local complications, such as fluid collections, pancreatic necrosis, pseudocysts, abscesses, and fistulas (Steinberg and Tenner 1994) can occur. These complications usually arise within 2–5 weeks from the resolution of the initial symptoms, and are important, accounting for 50% of the deaths caused by pancreatitis (Banks 2002; Balthazar 2002). Among local complications are also vascular complications and pancreatic ascites, which arise later, months or even years after the first episode of acute pancreatitis or in course of chronic pancreatitis (Balthazar 2002).

17.2 Pancreatic Complications

17.2.1 Pancreatic Necrosis

Pancreatic necrosis is an area of devascularized parenchyma that occurs in severe necrotizing pancreatitis (Balthazar et al. 1994). The necrotic areas are often multifocal, infrequently involve the entire gland. They may be confined to the periphery with sparing of the central portion of the pancreas. Necrosis develops early in the course of severe acute pancreatitis and is usually complete within 96 hours from the onset of symptoms (Balthazar et al. 1994).

The usefulness of transabdominal ultrasound (US) for identification of pancreatic necrosis is limited (Lecesne and Drouillard 1999).

G. Carbognin, MD; C. Calciolari, MD; G. Foti, MD
Department of Radiology, Policlinico "GB Rossi", University of Verona, Piazzale LA Scuro 10, 37134 Verona, Italy

However, with contrast enhanced ultrasound (CEUS) the role of US is being reassessed. Rickes has demonstrated that CEUS is comparable to contrast enhanced CT (CET) for the assessment of patients with acute pancreatitis, and can be recommended as a first choice imaging procedure, especially when iodinated contrast medium injection is contraindicated (Rickes et al. 2006). CEUS can accurately determine severity and predict clinical outcome during the course of acute pancreatitis. However, the impact of these findings on acute pancreatitis evaluation and management should be further investigated (Ozawa et al. 2002).

Contrast-enhanced CT can better define the extent of the necrosis and stage the disease. Contrast medium allows a differential diagnosis between interstitial and necrotizing pancreatitis. Edematous pancreatitis, with a normal microcirculation, displays homogeneous contrast-enhancement, while necrotizing pancreatitis, with destruction of normal microcirculation, shows diffuse areas of non-enhancement in the pancreatic parenchyma. While small non-enhancing areas may be a sign of the presence of intraparenchymal fluid, larger areas are a sign of marked microcirculation alterations and pancreatic necrosis (Banks 1997, 2002). Attenuation values of the pancreatic parenchyma during a contrast-enhanced study may be used as an indicator of necrosis and to predict the severity of the disease (Balthazar 2002).

Pancreatic necrosis can be better evaluated at MR than at CT due to the greater contrast sensitivity of gadolinium compared to iodinated CT contrast medium. The presence and extent of necrosis can be better evaluated in the images acquired 1–2 min after i.v. administration of Gadolinium-DTPA (Ward et al. 1997; Robinson and Sheridan 2000). T2-weighted (Fig. 17.1) and contrast-enhanced T1-weighted sequences allow a good evaluation of the extent of inflammation and necrosis (Lecesne and Drouillard 1999).

17.2.2 Collections

Pancreatic collections occur in 30%–50% of the patients affected by acute pancreatitis (Merkle and Gorich 2002). At 2–3 weeks after the onset of clinical symptoms, the inflammatory tissue around the necrotic area begins to organize, beginning the evolution to a pseudocyst (Merkle and Gorich 2002; Banks 2002).

Collections, which develop in the first 24 h from clinical onset, usually have irregular morphology and are located in the right anterior pararenal space, the transverse mesocolon or the mesentery root (Procacci et al. 2002), although they may involve the peritoneal cavity or the mediastinum (Balthazar et al. 1994).

Pancreatic necrosis is classified as either sterile or infected; this distinction is critical because of the significantly increased mortality associated with infected necrosis (Merkle and Gorich 2002).

17.2.2.1 Sterile Collections

Sterile collections form for liquefaction by pancreatic enzymes within 2–3 days from the onset of acute pancreatitis; the necrotic collection may persist and develop a pseudocyst or resolve spontaneously (Balthazar 2002).

17.2.2.2 Infected Necrosis

Necrotic tissue is an excellent medium for bacterial growth; infected necrosis occurs in 30%–70% of patients with necrotizing pancreatitis (Beger et al. 1997). The pathogens most commonly responsible of superinfection are *Escherichia coli* (35%), Enterococcus and Klebsiella (Beger et al. 1997). Anaerobes account for 10%–15% of the cases; fungal infections are constantly increasing (Beger et al. 1997). The most common source of contamination is usually the intestinal tract, especially the colon, with bacterial translocation through the bowel wall, microperforations, or with the direct passage of bacteria in the blood. Reflux of infected bile or of duodenal content in the pancreatic duct can be an unusual vehicle of infection (Balthazar 2002). Fine-needle aspiration of the collection content is necessary for a definite diagnosis and the identification of the infectious agent (Lecesne and Drouillard 1999). When the collection becomes infected –and the risk is proportional to necrosis extent and disease length – it gives onset to systemic symptoms, with a severe worsening of the prognosis (Balthazar 2002; Baril et al. 2000).

17.2.2.3 Imaging Findings

US in acute pancreatitis shows an enlarged, often hypoechoic, gland; less commonly the pancreatic

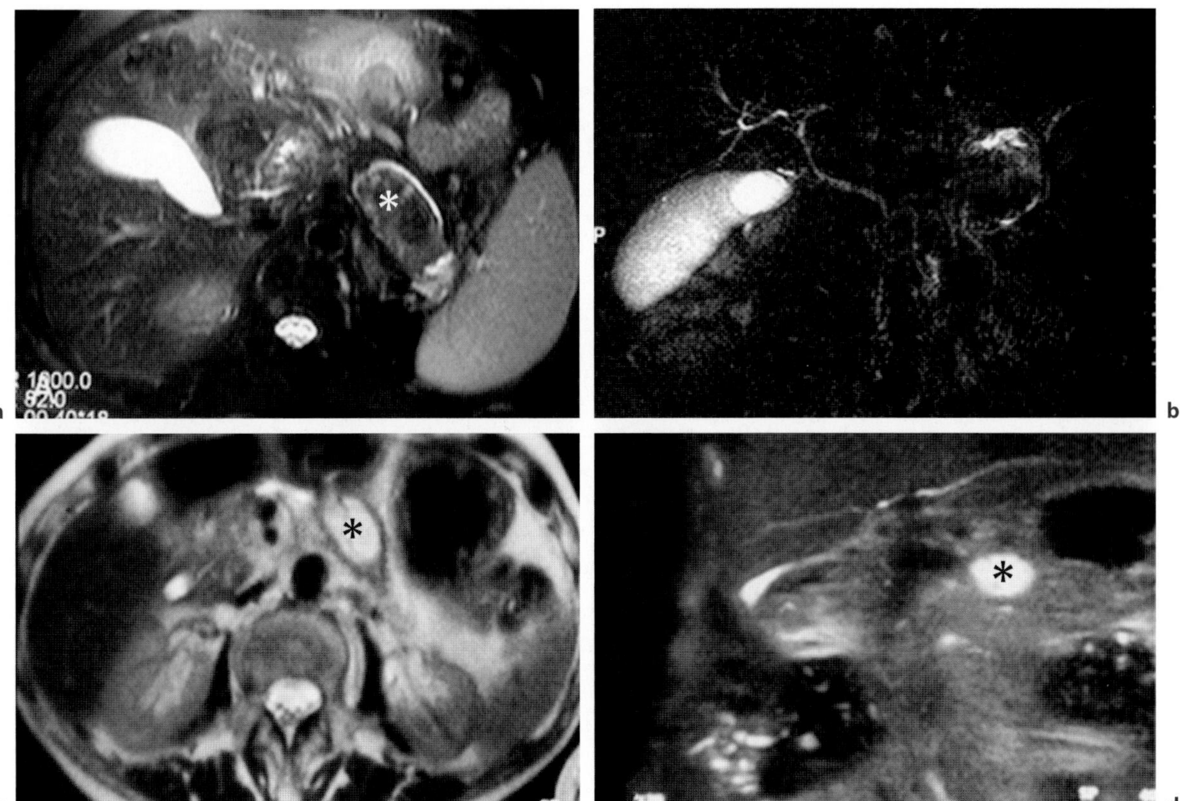

Fig. 17.1a–d. Patient 1: Axial T2 STIR image (**a**) shows an area of coagulative necrosis (*asterisk*) at the pancreatic tail. MRCP (**b**) reveals upstream dilation of the main pancreatic duct (*arrow* in **b**). The signal characteristics suggest that this collection is not amenable to percutaneous drainage. Patient 2: Axial (**c**) and coronal (**d**) T2 HASTE sequences show a homogeneous fluid collection (*asterisks*) . The "simple" collection should respond to drainage

parenchyma can be iso-echoic or hyper-echoic (Turner 2002). Collections appear as fluid areas, mostly hypoechoic, with irregular margins. Pancreatic necrosis and the eventual presence of gas in the collection are difficult to visualize at US (Turner 2002). Demonstration of gas bubbles, moreover, is not specific for a diagnosis of superinfection. US can be useful to guide the drainage of infectious collections when these do not include necrotic debris difficult to be removed (Procacci et al. 2002).

CT is the first choice examination in patients being evaluated with the clinical suspicion of acute pancreatitis (De Backer et al. 2002; Procacci et al. 2002) (Fig. 17.2).

Multidetector-row CT (MDCT) reduces acquisition times allowing breath-hold acquisitions with thinner slices of the pancreas and liver, optimizing intravenous contrast bolus utilization. For the evaluation of patients affected by pancreatitis, multiphasic (pancreatic and portal phase) acquisitions are recommended, following intravenous administration of 100–120 ml of non-ionic contrast medium at 4 ml/s. When MDCT is employed, acquisitions using narrow detector configurations are preferable to optimize 3-D evaluations.

With MDCT the pancreatic phase can be acquired with a 40-s delay from the initiation of the injection; a portal phase can be acquired approximately 20–30 s later.

Post-processing techniques such as multiplanar reformations (MPR), maximum intensity projection (MIP) and volume rendering (VR), provide useful information on the possible vascular involvement and the degree of dilatation of pancreatic and bile ducts (Kalra et al. 2002). MPR coronal reformats are useful in demonstrating local extension to stomach and duodenum (Kalra et al. 2002). Contrast-enhancement is fundamental, especially in severe acute pancreatitis, to differentiate viable parenchyma from heterogeneous fluid collections

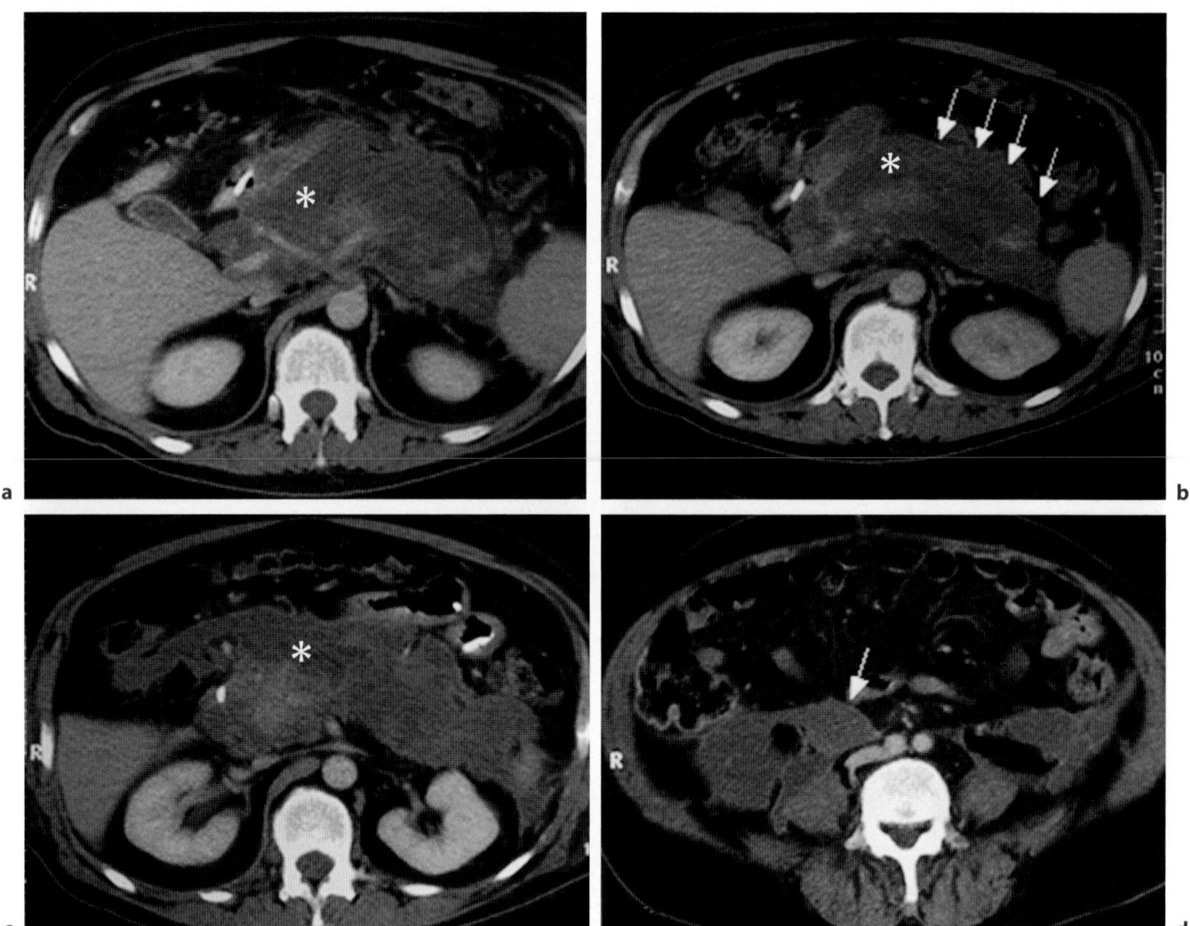

Fig. 17.2a–d. Peripancreatic collection in acute pancreatitis. Axial portal phase CT shows a large peripancreatic collection, with low and homogeneous attenuation (*asterisk* in **a–c**). Cranially the collection reaches the lateral recess of the lesser sac, while caudally reaches the left psoas muscle (**d**). The peripheral wall is thin, in the initial phase of organization (*arrows*)

Table 17.1. MDCT parameters utilized according to the scanner available

MDCT	Acquisition phase	Delay	Detector configuration	Reconstruction thickness
4-row	Pancreatic phase	150 HU threshold + 20 s delay	4 × 1 mm	3 mm
4-row	Portal-venous phase	150 HU threshold + 60 s delay	4 × 2.5 mm	5 mm
16-row	Pancreatic phase	150 HU threshold + 20 s delay	16 × 0.75 mm	3 mm
16-row	Portal-venous phase	150 HU threshold + 60 s delay	16 × 1.5 mm	5 mm
64-row	Pancreatic phase	150 HU threshold + 20 s delay	64 × 0.625 mm	3 mm
64-row	Portal-venous phase	150 HU threshold + 60 s delay	64 × 0.625 mm	5 mm

or peripancreatic inflammatory tissue. Arterial phase CT shows a non-enhancing area (Merkle and Gorich 2002) (Fig. 17.2). Visualization at CT of gas bubbles inside the lesion, product of anaerobes, is suggestive of superinfection (Procacci et al. 2002) (Fig. 17.3).

MR is especially useful in the evaluation of pancreatitis related fluid collections thanks to improved characterization of fluid content revealed by multiple sequences (Morgan et al. 1997). MR is especially useful in patients to whom iodated contrast medium administration is impossible due to allergy or renal failure.

At MR, visualization of a low signal region on unenhanced fat-suppressed T1 sequences (T1WFS) suggests collection. This sequence is also useful to identify hemorrhage, visible as a hyperintense region due to the presence of haemoglobin degradation products (Kalra et al. 2002).

Pancreatic edema and fluid collections are best demonstrated on T2 fat-suppressed Half-Fourier Single Shot Turbo Spin Echo (HASTE) and Single Shot Fast Spin Echo (SS-FSE) sequences (Ly and Miller 2002).

T2 sequences allow characterization of the collection content: necrotic tissue is hypointense (coagulative necrosis), while homogeneous fluid content is hyperintense compared to the normal pancreatic parenchyma (Morgan et al. 1997). Breath-hold and fat-suppression sequences are an excellent alternative imaging technique for patients in the acute phase.

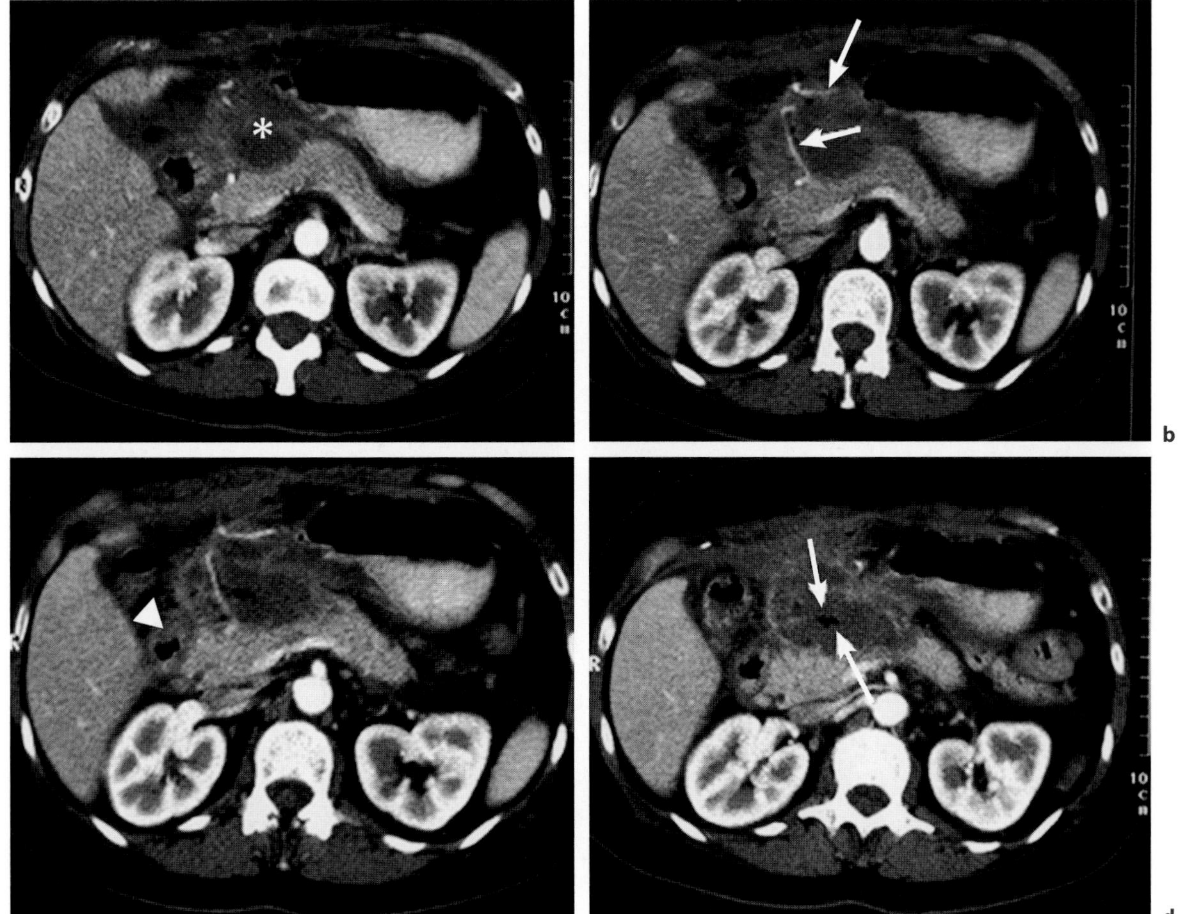

Fig. 17.3a–d. Infected collection in acute pancreatitis. Axial arterial phase CT shows an 8-cm fluid collection (*asterisk* in **a**) that separates and displaces branches of the pancreatico-duodenal arcades (*arrows* in **b**). The duodenum has a narrowed lumen and thickened wall (*arrowhead* in **c**). The collection has inhomogeneous fluid and gas bubbles (*arrows* in **d**)

17.2.3 Pancreatic Abscess

Pancreatic abscess is one of the most severe complications of acute pancreatitis with an estimated frequency of approximately 3% (Beger et al. 1997). The finding of a pancreatic abscess in chronic pancreatitis is extremely infrequent (Suzuki et al. 2002). A pancreatic abscess is distinguished from infected necrosis as a circumscribed intra-abdominal collection of pus in close proximity to the pancreas, with little or no pancreatic necrosis (Merkle and Gorich 2002). Abscesses require at least 4 weeks after the acute episode of severe acute pancreatitis to form. The prognosis in case of abscess is two times better than in case of infected necrosis (Baril et al. 2000; Park et al. 2002). Diagnosis is suggested when abdominal pain, fever, and leukocytosis or organ failure develop in a patient with a recent episode (3–4 weeks) of acute pancreatitis. The diagnosis of abscess is based both on clinical and imaging findings (Ferrucci and Mueller 2003).

US reveals a liquid hypo-anechoic lesion with thick walls, debris and possibly gas bubbles. CT shows a fluid collection with heterogeneous content and well defined margins, hypodense compared to the surrounding parenchyma, lined by a hyperdense wall (Procacci et al. 2002). Even though CT is the imaging technique most sensitive to the presence of gas (Ly and Miller 2002), the finding of gas inside the abscess is infrequent (Ferrucci and Mueller 2003) (Fig. 17.4). T2-weighted HASTE and SS-FSE sequences allow optimal visualization of abscesses on MRI. Gas bubbles and air-fluid levels appear on T2 sequences as areas of signal void, usually in non-dependent position (Morgan et al. 1997).

17.2.4 Hemorrhage

The incidence of all hemorrhagic complications in the course of acute and chronic pancreatitis is 1.3% (Balthazar 2002). Pancreatic and peripancreatic vessels involvement is due to the erosive action of activated proteolytic pancreatic enzymes, with disruption of the vessel wall and consequent hemorrhage (Procacci et al. 2002). An intraparenchymal hemorrhage involving arterial vessels causes shock and is associated with a mortality rate of 50% (Vujic 1989). Intermittent gastrointestinal bleeding is a characteristic finding in case of "hemosuccus pancreaticus", which presents as an intermittent bleeding from the major papilla. In this case ERCP allows direct endoscopic visualization (Procacci et al. 2002). This results from fistulization of a pancreatic vessel into the main pancreatic duct.

Doppler US examination can show a pulsatile arterial flow inside the cystic mass (Dorffel et al. 2000; Bennet and Hann 2001; Procacci et al. 2002).

CT can show the hemorrhagic collection as a high-attenuation fluid collection (Balthazar 2002) (Fig. 17.5). Sometimes CT can visualize the bleeding

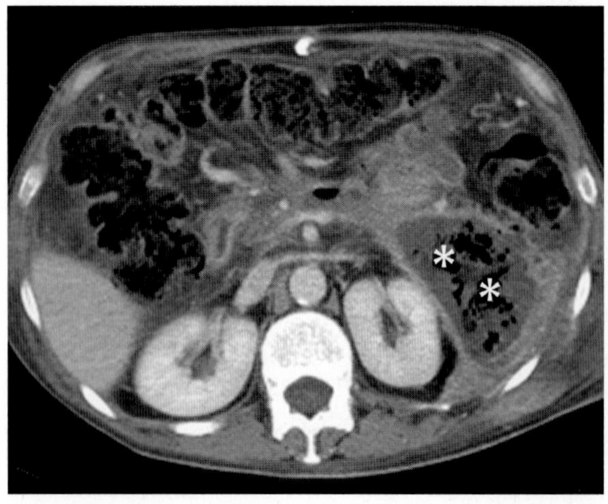

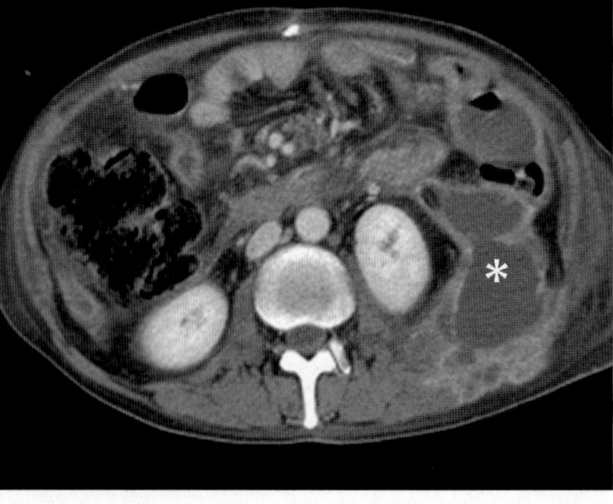

Fig. 17.4a,b. Abscess collection in necrotic-haemorrhagic AP. Delayed contrast-enhanced axial CT scans depict an abscess (*asterisk* in **b**) with a transverse diameter of 12 cm in the left anterior pararenal space. The abscess is hypoattenuating, with peripheral wall thickened due to organization processes. Inside, gas bubbles are clearly seen (*asterisks* in **a**)

inside the collection and the vessel from which the hemorrhage arises from (Procacci et al. 2002).

MR GRE T1 FS sequences on MR demonstrate high signal hemorrhagic foci within the pancreatic parenchyma (Piironen et al. 1997; Pedrosa and Rofsky 2003) (Fig. 17.6).

The ability of CT to detect hemorrhage in the course of acute pancreatitis is somewhat limited as a result of the rapid density variations in haematoma. MR signal alterations due to the presence of hemorrhage are maintained longer; therefore the sensitivity of MR in hemorrhage detection is greater (Ward et al. 1997). Moreover, contrast-enhanced 3D MR angiography allows an accurate depiction of the vascular map of the peripancreatic district and, sometimes, a direct visualization of the bleeding (Pedrosa and Rofsky 2003).

Angiography, which nowadays does not have a diagnostic role, is fundamental especially in the treatment, with selective embolization of bleeding vessels previously identified at non-invasive imaging (Procacci et al. 2002).

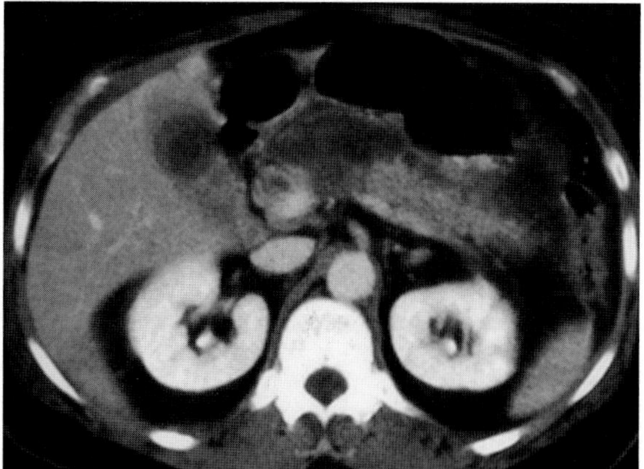

a

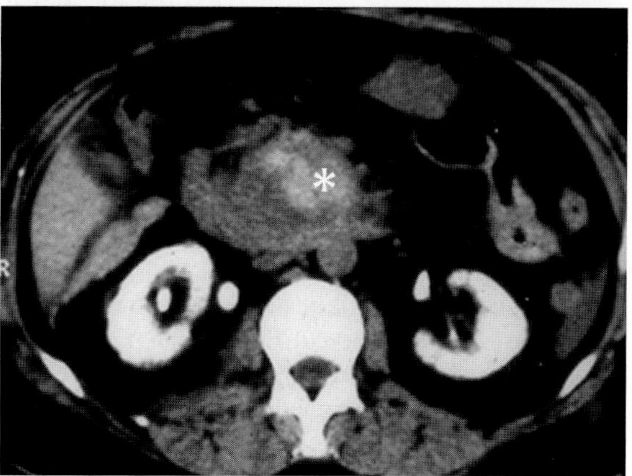

b

Fig. 17.5a,b. Hemorrhage in necrotic-hemorrhagic acute pancreatitis. Axial contrast-enhanced CT images show the pancreatitis and the hemorrhagic collection in the right anterior pararenal space

17.2.5 Fistulas

A pancreatic fistula is a non-anatomic communication between the pancreatic ductal system and a nearby structure. This can lead to complications such as infection, hemorrhage and erosion of adjacent viscera (Ridgeway and Stabile 1996). Pancreatic fistulas are classified according to their output: high output, when pancreatic fluid secretion is greater than 200 ml/day; low output, when the secretion is less than 200 ml/day. High output fistulas will ultimately require surgical intervention (Bassi et al. 2000; Ridgeway and Stabile 1996) for definitive control.

Fistulas are also classified as internal when the pancreatic fluid is released in the abdomen or thorax, or external, when the pancreatic fluid is released directly on the skin (Ridgeway and Stabile 1996). External fistulas are by far more common. Many patients will harbour *both* internal and external pancreatic fistulas.

Fistulography performed by injection of iodinated contrast medium into the tract(s) under fluoroscopic control provides direct visualization of the fistula and its ramifications (Pistolesi et al. 1992).

CECT allows direct visualization of the fistula and its track. Contrast can be instilled into ex-

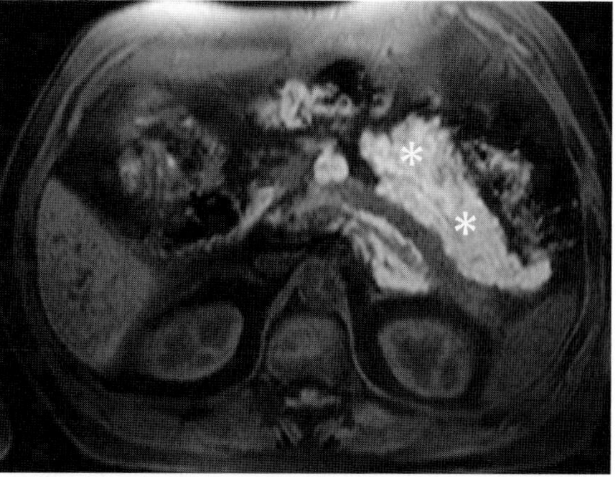

Fig. 17.6. Hemorrhage in acute pancreatitis. Axial T1 weighted MRI image reveals increased signal in the collection (*asterisks*) secondary to the presence of haemoglobin breakdown products within the collection

ternal tracts providing a cross-sectional display of the complex anatomic relationships. Of course CECT will also provide critical information about the status of the integrity of the pancreatic parenchyma.

Secretin enhanced MRCP is useful also to evaluate the main pancreatic duct, showing the site of duct disruption and aiding in determining the utility of stenting.

17.2.5.1
Internal Fistulas

Internal pancreatic fistulas can be classified into four types (Ridgeway and Stabile 1996).

17.2.5.1.1
Pancreatico-enteric Fistulas

Pancreatico-enteric fistulas are anomalous communications of the main pancreatic duct with the intestinal tract. These fistulas are uncommon complications of pancreatitis, external traumas, pseudocysts, abscesses, biopsies or pancreatic surgery (Wolfsen et al. 1992). Fistulization usually develops late (10–90 days after clinical onset) in the course of necrotizing acute pancreatitis (Herbert et al. 1992). The distal transverse colon near the splenic flexure is the most frequent site of involvement; less often other portions of the colon, stomach, duodenum or small bowel are involved (De Backer et al. 2001). The proximity of the transverse colon to the pancreas explains the relatively frequent formation of fistulas between these two sites. Fistulas secondary to rupture of a pseudocyst in the stomach, duodenum or small bowel may be large enough to allow a complete drainage and, unless bleeding occurs, may heal spontaneously (De Backer et al. 2001). If the rupture occurs in the colon, the risk of hemorrhage and sepsis is high (De Backer et al. 2001). Pancreatico-colonic fistulas may be associated with exocrine pancreatic failure and significant fluid and electrolyte imbalances (Ridgeway and Stabile 1996). Fistulas are also a preferential access route for intestinal bacteria that may infect a previously sterile pancreas (De Backer et al. 2001).

Fistulography, with the injection of water-soluble contrast medium through drainages usually already positioned in the pancreatic space, allows a direct visualization of the communication between the duct and the adjacent viscera, thus confirming the existence of a pancreatico-intestinal fistula (Ridgeway and Stabile 1996) (Fig. 17.7).

CT confirms the presence of inhomogeneous peripancreatic collections that may contain gas bubbles. Visualization of the tracts may be achieved passively using orally administered contrast material (Procacci et al. 2002; Ridgeway and Stabile 1996; Torres et al. 1981 (Fig. 17.8).

Secretin enhanced MRCP has proven useful in the evaluation of the duct rupture site, identifying the source of fluid collections and anomalous communications with bowel (Pederzoli et al. 1992) (Fig. 17.9).

3-D MRCP sequences allow a precise three-dimensional evaluation of the fistulous tract. Dilute gadolinium can be administered through drains, allowing demonstration of contrast medium passage from the collection to the bowel loops.

17.2.5.1.2
Pancreatico-biliary Fistulas

Pancreatico-biliary fistulas are unusual. They occur secondary to pancreatic duct disruption followed by an extension of the pancreatic necrosis to the bile duct or they may be associated to the rupture of a pseudocyst and its drainage in the adjacent bile ducts (Carrere et al. 2001).

Clinical symptoms include: pain, fever, jaundice and cholestasis from bile duct compression. Hemobilia, caused by vascular erosion, is the most severe complication (Carrere et al. 2001).

ERCP has been proposed as the first choice imaging technique for the study and evaluation of patients with pseudocysts and suspected pancreatico-biliary fistulas, to evaluate the common bile duct and demonstrate any possible communication with the main pancreatic duct or the adjacent organs (Hauptmann et al. 1992). This technique allows both diagnosis and therapeutic stent positioning (Carrere et al. 2001).

CT may accurately image pseudocysts and the site of pancreatico-biliary fistulas (Hauptmann et al. 1992). MR with MRCP can be useful for the diagnosis allowing an optimal visualization of the bile ducts. The use of 3D sequences can demonstrate fistulous tracts between bile ducts and pancreatic region (Cova et al. 2003); recent studies with MRCP at 3.0 T field strength have demonstrated the usefulness of 3D TSE sequences in depicting the biliary and pancreatic tree (Merkle et al. 2006).

17.2.5.1.3 Pancreatico-venous Fistulas

Pancreatico-vascular fistulas are extremely infrequent in pancreatitis. A necrotic collection or a pseudocyst may erode a vessel, allowing its direct communication with the main pancreatic duct (WILLIS et al. 1989; YOKOYAMA et al. 1984). Clinically, these fistulas are very severe, often lethal.

Pancreatico-vascular fistulas can be divided into venous and arterial, according to the type of vessel they communicate with; the arterial ones, however, are consequence of the rupture of an arterial pseudoaneurysm with bleeding in communication with the main pancreatic duct.

Pancreatico-venous fistulas are connections with a vein of the portal system. An unusual clinical syndrome of recurrent arthritis, subcutaneous fat necrosis, intramedullary aseptic bone necrosis and omental fat necrosis has been described in these patients (LEE et al. 1985; HAMMAR et al. 2002).

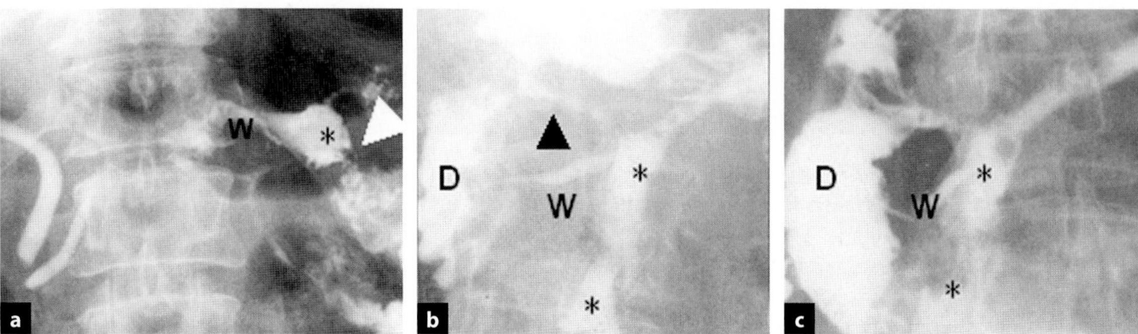

Fig. 17.7a–c. Pancreo-intestinal fistula. **a** ERCP: the main pancreatic duct (*W*) is interrupted and the contrast medium leaks into a pseudocyst (*asterisk*) from which, through a short tract (*white arrowhead*), the jejunal loops are opacified. **b,c** Small bowel follow-through (**b**) and ERCP (**c**) show the fistulous tract (*black arrowhead*) connecting the cephalic portion of the main pancreatic duct with the duodenum (*D*). The fistula communicates with the pseudocyst (*asterisks*)

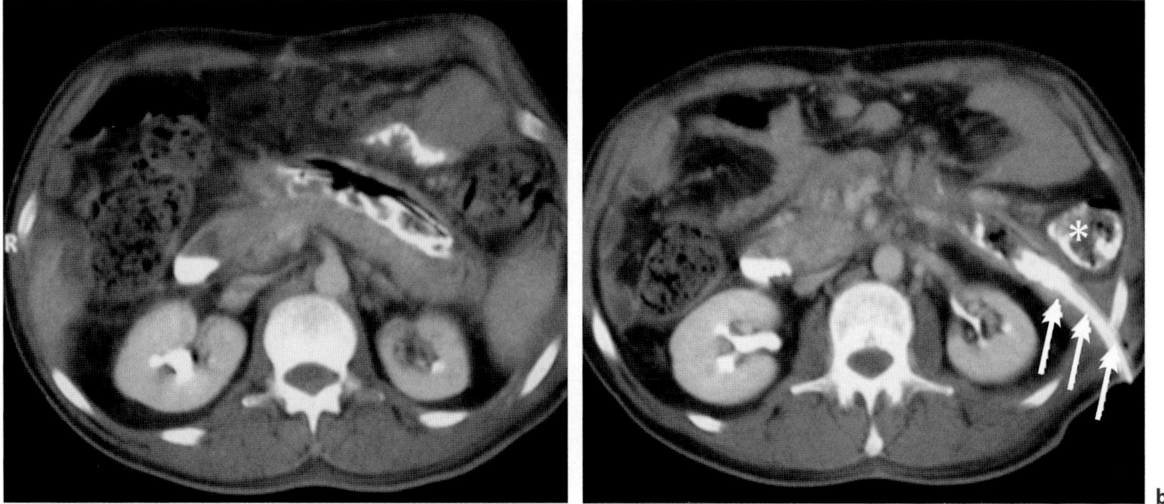

Fig. 17.8a,b. Colonic fistula in AP. Cranial (**a**) and caudal (**b**) CECT scans. A collection is seen ventral to the pancreas (**a**). Through a drainage tube in the left flank (*arrows* in **b**), contrast medium is injected which flows into the collection. Passage of contrast medium in the colonic lumen is visible (*asterisk* in **b**)

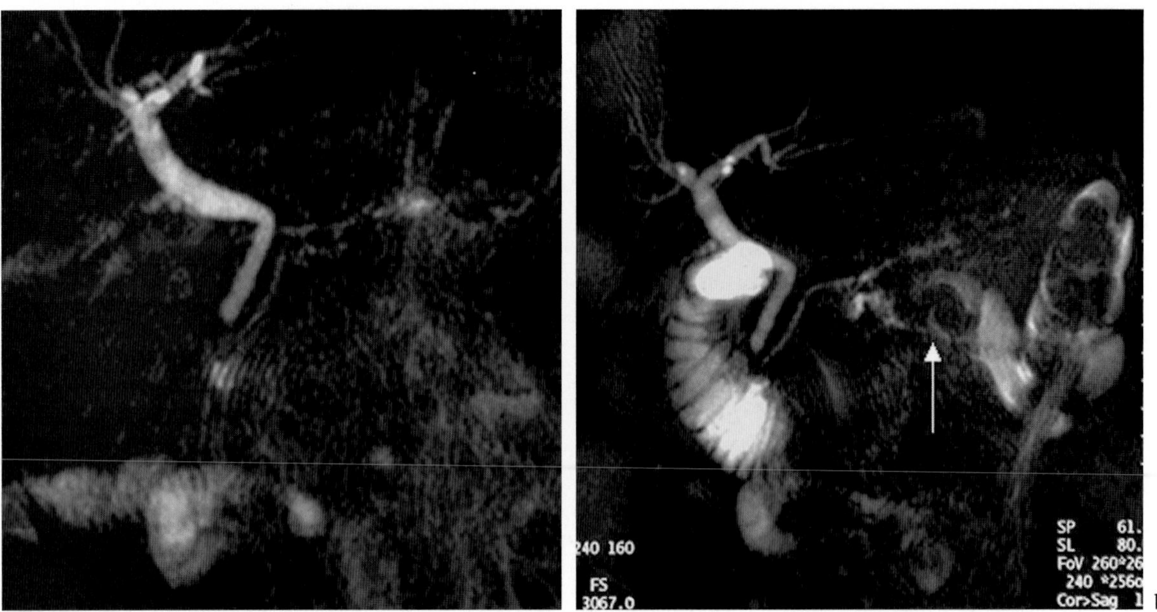

Fig. 17.9a,b. Colonic fistula in AP. Baseline MRCP (**a**) does not depict any fistula, while MRCP after secretin-stimulation (**b**) clearly depicts a fistula (*arrow* in **b**) connecting main pancreatic duct and left colon

CECT can visualize the pseudocyst and its communication with the portal vein: the vein lumen has fluid density and is usually easy to identify, while the communication between the vascular lumen and the pseudocyst is not always readily visualized (Skarsgard et al. 1995).

ERCP shows the continuity between the venous lumen and the pseudocyst and provides a dynamic view of the communication, but might not be diagnostic if the fistula does not involve the main pancreatic duct. Also trans-hepatic portography under CT or US guidance can confirm the fistula. MR can be an alternative. Angiography is not helpful for the diagnosis because the portal tree can be excluded from the systemic circulation because of its cystic transformation (Riddell et al. 2005; Takayama et al. 1986; McCormick et al. 1990; Procacci et al. 2002).

17.2.5.1.4 Pancreatico-pleural Fistulas

Pleuro-pulmonary involvement in acute pancreatitis is fairly common, occurring in 4%–17% of the patients. On the other hand, thoracic involvement in chronic pancreatitis is infrequent (pleural effusion occurs in 0.4% of chronic pancreatitis (Lanternier et al. 2002). Pancreatico-pleural fistulas are the result of a posterior disruption of the pancreatic duct into the retroperitoneal space and the subsequent creation of a fistulous tract between the pancreas and the pleural space through the aortic or the esophageal diaphragmatic hiatus (Materne et al. 2000). Pleural effusion has a high content in pancreatic amylase (Materne et al. 2000). Patients present with respiratory symptoms (e.g., dyspnea, cough or chest pain), while abdominal pain is often absent (Yanagie et al. 1997).

Effusion is readily diagnosed with plain film radiography, but accurate imaging study is necessary for a precise diagnosis, both with ERCP and CT (Lee et al. 1992; Verhaege et al. 1996).

US can demonstrate a clinically suspected pancreatico-pleural fistula non-invasively and without ionizing radiation (Kumar et al. 2002).

CT can show the signs of chronic pancreatitis, but can fail to show the track of the pancreatico-pleural fistula (Materne et al. 2000), unless a communication is demonstrated by injecting contrast medium into the drainages (Pottmeyer et al. 1987).

MR may accurately show the fistula, its relationship with the pancreatic duct and the precise site of entrance into the pleural space (Akahane et al. 2003). The use of coronal acquisitions is helpful for a better definition of the fistulous tract, which appears typically hyperintense in the dedicated sequences (T2 HASTE and MRCP) (Materne et al. 2000).

ERCP is the first choice examination for the diagnosis of fistulas, even though its sensitivity is not 100%. ERCP shows a dilation of the main pancreatic duct in its whole length, the possible presence of a pseudocyst and the fistulous tract between the pancreatic duct and the pleural space (Safadi and Marks 2000).

17.2.5.2 External Fistulas

External pancreatic fistulas are a complication after trauma, gastrointestinal surgery or pancreatitis (Cabay et al. 1998). Most external fistulas occur as a complication of surgery, with a 2–7 days delay. After elective pancreatico-duodenectomy, the estimated incidence is 6%–25% (Ridgeway and Stabile 1996; Lin et al. 2004) (Fig. 17.10).

External fistulas can be either simple, when communication between pancreatic duct and skin is direct, or complex, when there is interposition of other viscera, especially the intestinal ones (Fig. 17.11). Most external fistulas are high output, and therefore more difficult to treat (Cabay et al 1998).

17.2.5.2.1 Post-Traumatic Fistulas

External fistulas as a consequence of a trauma are quite common, accounting for approximately 9% of cases. Pancreatic duct disruption or resection are the two post-traumatic conditions most often associated with fistulization (Ridgeway and Stabile 1996).

In some cases the lesion is a complication of surgical treatment of other organs: in these cases the pancreatic fluid is secreted on the skin through the abdominal drains or directly through the surgical wound.

CT is a helpful technique for the evaluation of these fistulas, being used to monitor the patient and being also helpful in evaluating pancreatic lesions and the site and extent of the fistula (Procacci et al. 2002).

Fistulography is the first choice technique and usually sufficient for the demonstration of a post-traumatic external fistula, allowing also identification of the involved viscera (Procacci et al. 2002). Fistulo-CT (opacification of the fistulous tract and subsequent CT imaging) gives a more accurate evaluation of the abdominal recesses which the fistulous tract passes through and therefore of its relationship with the adjacent organs (Fig. 17.12).

When there is suspicion of main pancreatic duct disruption (an event that requires immediate surgery or preferably stenting), ERCP is able to evaluate whether there is total or partial disruption of the duct (Pederzoli et al. 1992). Currently, when a post-traumatic rupture of the main pancreatic duct is suspected in young patients, MR with MRCP can provide necessary information to the surgeon about pancreatic duct integrity (Fulcher et al. 2003) (Fig. 17.13).

17.2.5.2.2 Post-Surgical Fistulas

Pancreatico-cutaneous fistulas may be a complication of pancreatic surgery. The frequency of external fistulas is 4%–6% after pancreatic surgery, rising to 33% when the surgery is performed for abdominal trauma (Costamagna et al. 2001). Percutaneous drainage of peripancreatic collections after severe acute pancreatitis may result in a chronic fistula if the collection communicates with the ductal system.

The radiological approach to postsurgical external fistulas is based on fistulography, which allows definition of the lesion extent, visualizing also the communication with the pancreatic duct. CT, with contrast medium injection through abdominal drains, can correctly diagnose fistulas; in the suspicion of pancreatic duct disruption ERCP is the most useful examination.

17.3 Extrapancreatic Complications

Extrapancreatic local complications can involve hollow viscera, pleural space, spleen and peritoneal cavity in the form of pancreatic ascites.

17.3.1 Intestinal Stenosis

Intestinal stenosis is a late complication in pancreatitis. It is a consequence of the reabsorption of fluid collections in the transverse mesocolon or in the right anterior pararenal which causes fibrous retraction of the organ with subsequent partial or total luminal occlusion (Procacci et al. 2002). Intestinal complications of acute pancreatitis are uncommon (1% incidence for colonic complications), however,

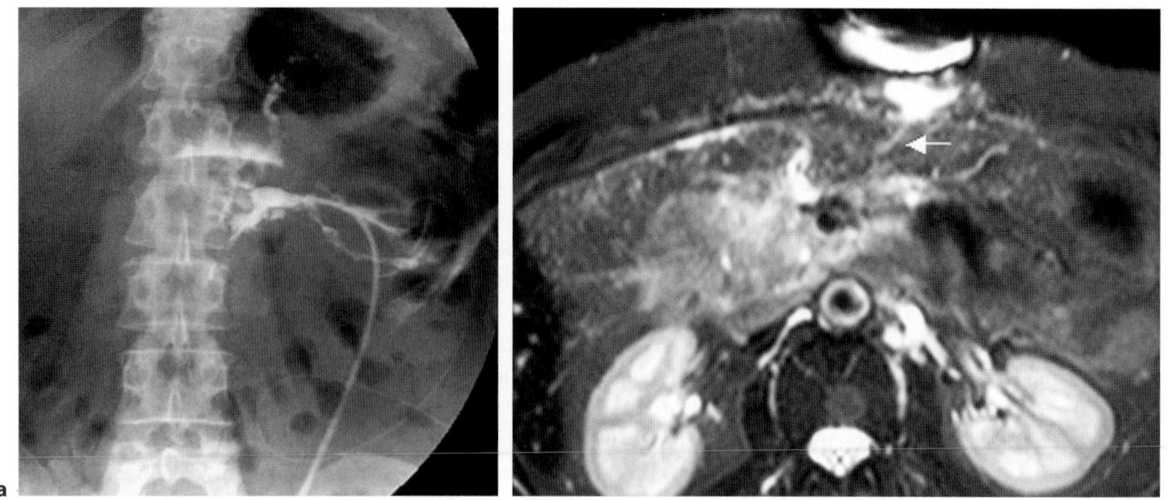

Fig. 17.10a,b. Cutaneous fistula in AP. Fistulography (**a**) shows the fistulous tract and the communication with the collection in the left hypochondrium. Four months later, at MR (**b**), the fistoulous tract (*arrow*) between the pancreatic region and the small subcutaneous collection is still seen

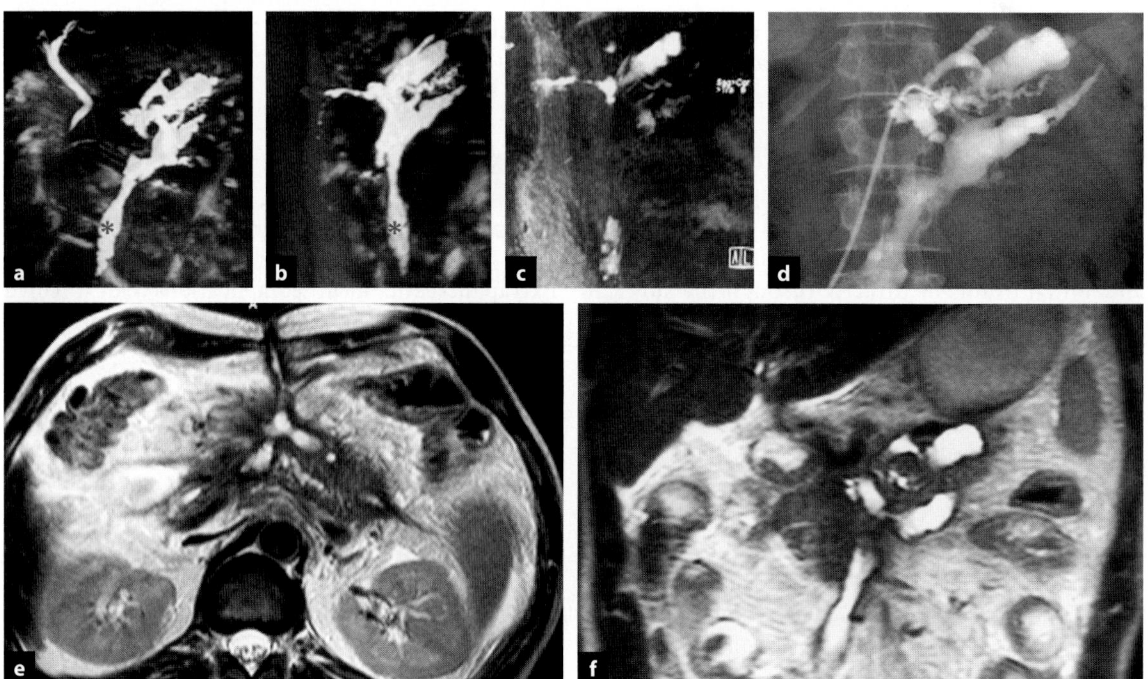

Fig. 17.11a–f. Complex cutaneous and intestinal fistula in AP, studied with MR (**a–c; e,f**) and fistulography (**d**). MR shows a fistulous tract (*asterisk*) connecting the collection, ventral to the pancreas and connected to the skin, and the main pancreatic duct at the tail. Contrast medium leaks into small bowel *(asterisks)*

they are associated to high morbidity and mortality (DE BACKER et al. 2001). Stenosis may involve the duodenum, colon or common bile duct.

Duodenal stenosis is an extremely infrequent complication of pancreatitis, both acute and chronic, and may be a consequence of severe pancreatic inflammation involving the duodenal wall, of extensive fibrosis of the pancreatic head or of a pseudocyst that compresses the duodenal lumen. It may produce symptoms of upper gastrointestinal obstruction including epigastric abdominal pain, nausea and vomiting. Diagnosis is obtained with barium studies or CT (LANKISCH and BANKS 1998).

Colonic stenosis occurs frequently near the splenic flexure (ARAKI et al. 1998). 3-D CT imaging will show the relationship of the colon to the pancreatitis and is the most effective way of confirming the diagnosis. Colonoscopy sometimes can visualize a colonic stenosis with normal mucosa, even though the stenosis may not allow passage of the endoscope (ARAKI et al. 1998).

The distal portion of the common bile duct may be involved in course of pancreatitis because it is positioned within the pancreatic head as it courses toward the duodenum. In chronic pancreatitis this portion of the common bile duct may be obstructed by an acute inflammatory episode, by pancreatic head fibrosis or by a close pancreatic pseudocyst. Severe complications are cholangitis in the short term and secondary biliary cirrhosis in the long term (LANKISCH and BANKS 1998). ERCP is the first choice examination, because it can often demonstrate main bile duct stenosis and allow placement of a stent (GREGG et al. 1981, ECKHAUSER et al. 1983)

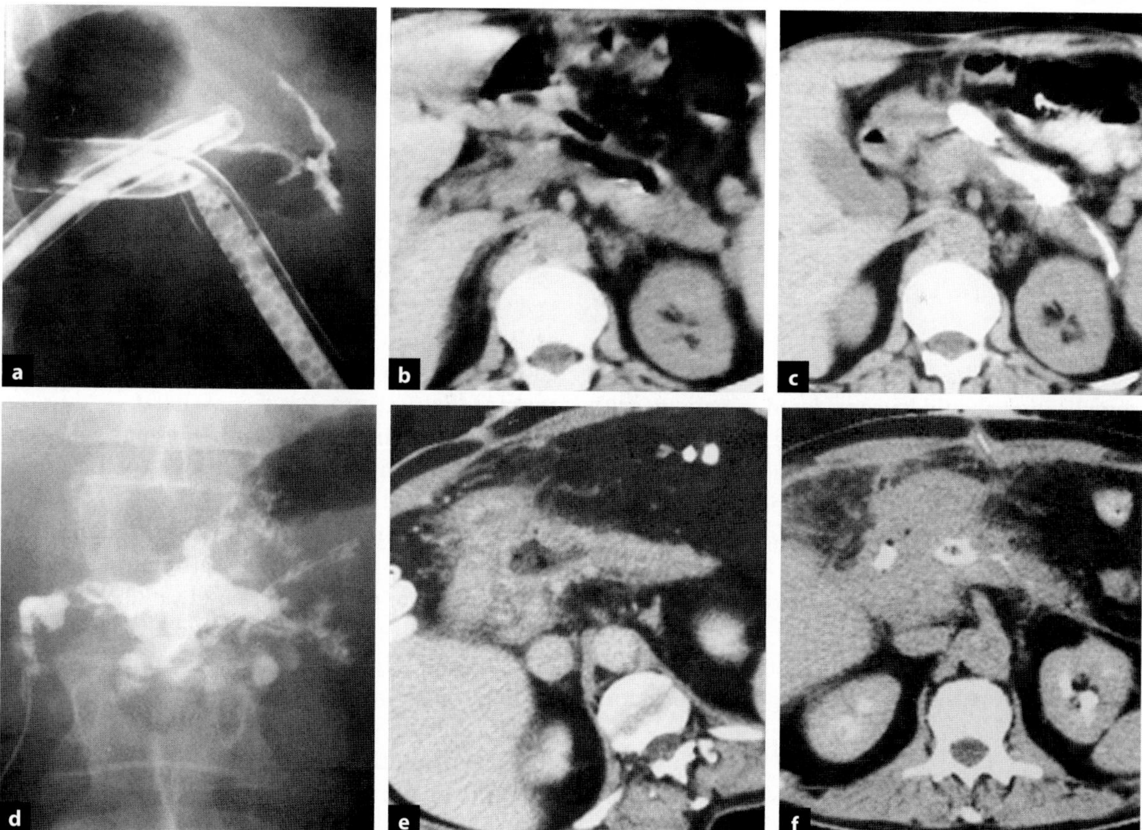

Fig. 17.12a–f. External fistula after drainage of necrotic-hemorrhagic acute pancreatitis: usefulness of fistulo-CT. **a–c** Case 1: at fistulography (**a**) the main pancreatic duct is not definitively opacified in the tail; axial unenhanced CT (**b**,**c**): the main pancreatic duct is not opacified. The fistulous tract develops along the anterior aspect of the pancreatic tail. **d–f** Case 2: fistulography shows an irregular collection in the pancreatic bed. The main pancreatic duct is not definitively opacified; at CT (**e**,**f**) the collection is located in the pancreatic neck; fistulo-CT shows communication with the main pancreatic duct

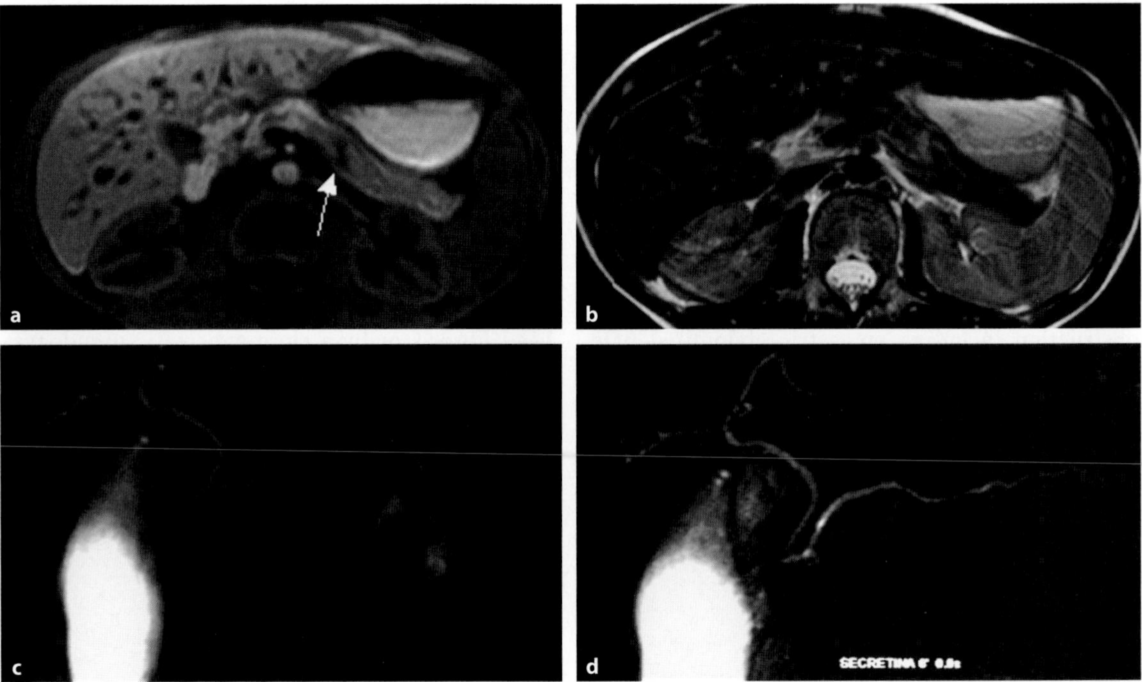

Fig. 17.13a–d. Traumatic rupture of the pancreatic body. Axial T1 FS sequence (**a**) clearly depicts the hypointense fracture rim (*arrow*). T2 FSE sequence (**b**) confirms the fracture (hyperintense), which appears to involve the main pancreatic duct. Baseline MRCP (**c**): main pancreatic duct is not well visualized. MRCP 6 min after secretin stimulation (**d**) confirms ductal integrity

17.3.2 Peptic Ulcer

Chronic pancreatitis and peptic ulcer coexist in 6.3%–37.5% of the cases (Vantini et al. 1982). This complication should be considered in patients with chronic pancreatitis and episodes of epigastric abdominal pain that differ in character and severity from the more chronic pain associated with pancreatitis. Diagnosis is confirmed with upper gastrointestinal endoscopy.

The pathological basis of this correlation is still obscure; it has been proposed that the reduced pancreatic ductal bicarbonate secretion may reduce the duodenal pH, thus promoting ulcer formation (Lankisch and Banks 1998).

17.3.3 Ascites

A transitory small amount of ascites in course of acute pancreatitis is a relatively common finding at CT (7%–12%). True pancreatic ascites, however, defined as a permanent disruption of the main pancreatic duct with communication between the pancreas and the peritoneal cavity, inducing massive chronic ascites, is rare (Balthazar 2002). It can also occur, with a high frequency (80%), after pseudocyst rupture (Fernandez-Cruz et al. 1993).

Clinically pancreatic ascites presents with abdominal swelling, pain, weight loss and occasionally nausea and vomiting (Johst et al. 1997). It is a severe and chronically debilitating complication, associated to a mortality rate around 20% and a recurrence rate of 15% (Balthazar 2002). Ascites is often massive, as the pancreatic exocrine secretion exceeds 1l/day. Diagnosis is confirmed with peritoneal aspiration, which must demonstrate a protein content greater than 3 g/dl and an amylase content greater than 1000 unities (Balthazar 2002; Kravetz et al. 1988).

Abdominal US is the first examination in a patient with ascites, allowing to evaluate easily the fluid amount in the abdomen (Balthazar 2002).

CT is the examination of choice, showing intraperitoneal fluid and specific signs of chronic pancreatitis (Balthazar 2002).

MR is not usually used in the study of pancreatic ascites, because the fluid degrades MR images, especially MRCP quality. ERCP is performed to define accurately ductal anatomy and disruption site (Balthazar 2002).

17.3.4 Splenic Involvement

Splenic involvement in the course of pancreatitis is expected because of the close anatomic proximity of the pancreatic tail to the splenic hilum. Patients with acute pancreatitis may present subcapsular or parenchymal fluid collections, intrasplenic pseudocysts, infarcts and hemorrhage (Balthazar 2002). Splenic hemorrhage and hematoma are consequence of the erosion of small intrasplenic vessels by activated pancreatic enzymes (Procacci et al 2002). Spontaneous spleen rupture may occur in course of chronic pancreatitis (Calvo et al. 1992). The most common splenic complication in chronic pancreatitis is thrombosis of the splenic vein (Lankisch and Banks 1998; Remer and Baker 2002).

Among the possible complication is splenic abscess. The consequence of splenic abscess is particularly severe because of increased risk of spontaneous splenic rupture with peritonitis and consequent high mortality. CT depicts abscesses as focal hypoattenuating splenic lesions with well-defined margins; the presence of gas is helpful for the diagnosis (Robertson et al. 2001).

US is especially useful in identifying parenchymal lesions and intraperitoneal collections and is used in the follow-up of non-surgical patients. The advantages of US are its repeatability and the absence of ionizing radiation (Robertson et al. 2001).

Contrast-enhanced CT is useful in the evaluation of abscesses and collections. They are visualized as areas of absent enhancement. CT is the first choice examination in case of trauma, infarct, cyst, tumor or abscess (Robertson et al. 2001; De Backer et al. 2002).

MR allows to the study of the splenic parenchyma and the vascular tree, and can be performed in younger patients for radiation safety reasons (Elsayes et al. 2005). Diagnostic splenic angiography has been replaced by CT, US and MR: its use is now exclusive to interventional radiology.

17.4 Conclusions

The radiological approach to the complications of pancreatitis, and especially to fistulas, is complex, and examinations should be chosen with particular attention to the clinical setting.

CT is the most common first choice in internal fistulas, allowing evaluation of the pancreatitis (acute or chronic), the presence of collections, pseudocysts, gas bubbles or air-fluid levels with direct visualization of the fistula.

a 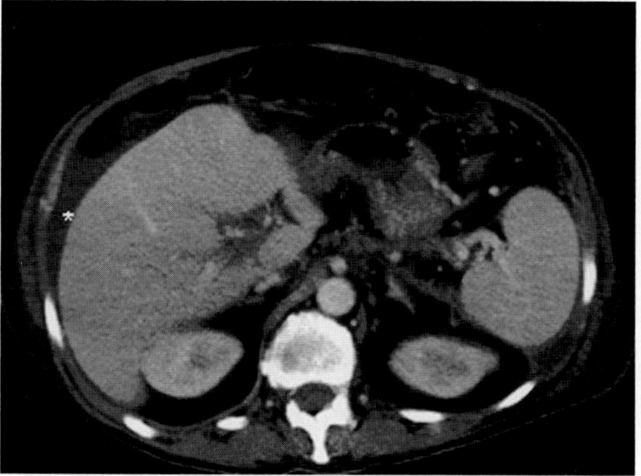

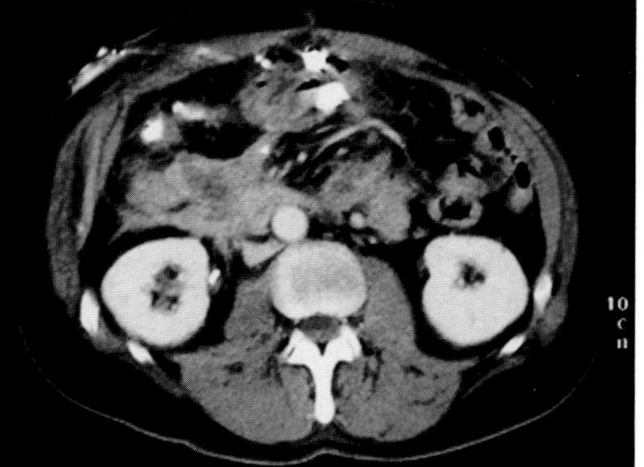 b

Fig. 17.14a,b. Small amount of fluid in acute pancreatitis. Axial contrast-enhanced CT images show a perihepatic and perisplenic fluid (ascites)

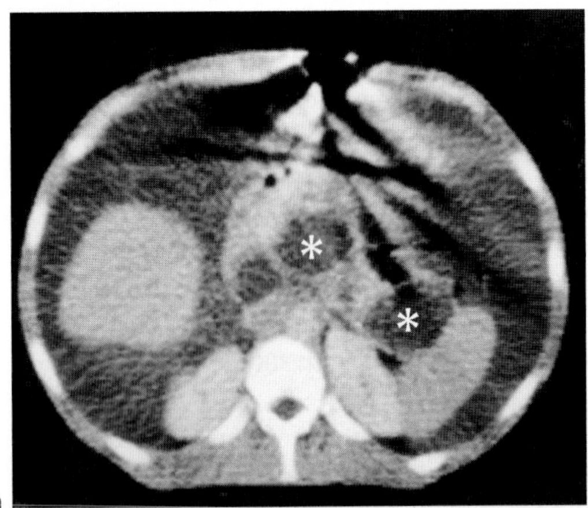
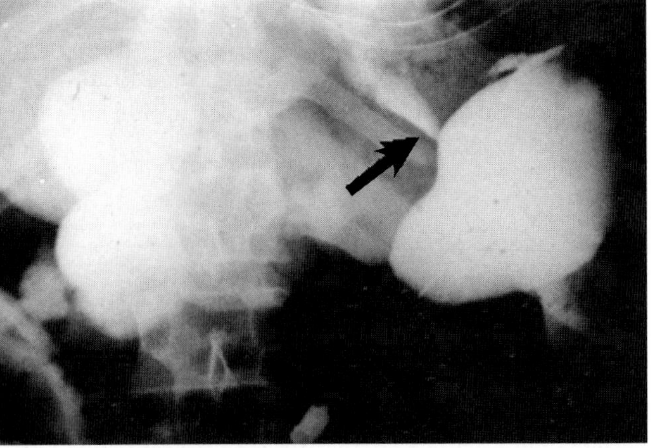

Fig. 17.15a,b. Pancreatic ascites. **a** Axial unenhanced CT shows a large amount of ascites. In the pancreatic bed two large pseudocysts are seen (*asterisks*). **b** Intra-operative cystography from the same patient shows contrast medium leaking into the peritoneal cavity from the cyst (*arrow*) at the pancreatic tail

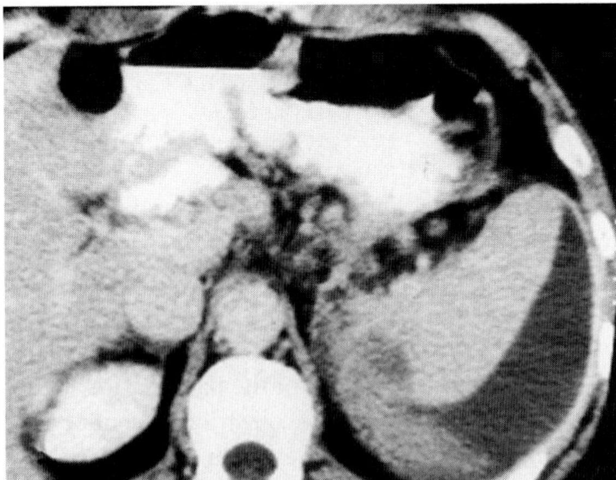
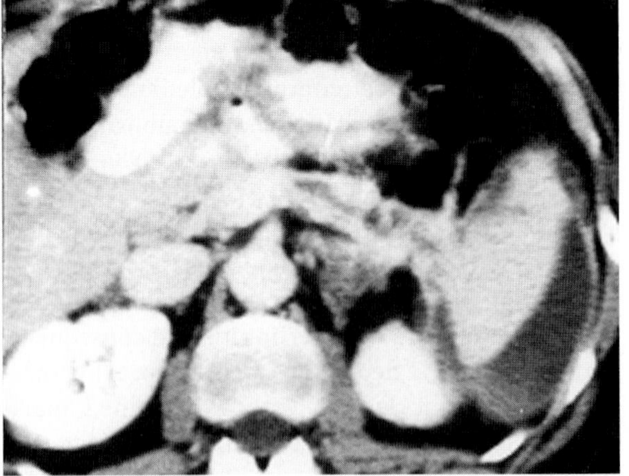

Fig. 17.16a,b. Retroperitoneal leakage of pancreatic juice with secondary involvement of the spleen. Axial contrast-enhanced CT images show a pseudocyst in the pancreatic tail which, through the splenic hilum, opens into the spleen with parenchymal laceration and subcapsular collection (**a**). The spleen is displaced anteriorly and medially by a large subcapsular collection, inhomogeneous for the presence of a hemorrhagic component (**b**)

For external fistulas, on the other hand, all techniques are considered complementary to fistulography, the first choice examination, to which fistulo-CT can be added for a more complete patient evaluation; CT is also useful for collection drainage.

MR can be a valid alternative to CT and fistulo-CT in the evaluation of the complications of pancreatitis. Moreover, the possibility of administration of diluted gadolinium through external orifices or drainages, similarly to what routinely performed in CT, makes this technique optimal in the evaluation of these complications, also thanks to the greater tissue resolution.

References

Akahane T, Kuriyama S, Matsumoto M, Kikuchi E, Kikukawa M, Yoshiji H, Masui K, Fukui H (2003) Pancreatic pleural effusion with a pancreatico-pleural fistula diagnosed by magnetic resonance cholangiopancreatography and cured by somatostatin analogue treatment. Abdom Imaging 28:92–95

Amano Y, Oishi T, Takahashi M, Kumazaki T (2001) Nonenhanced magnetic resonance imaging of mild acute pancreatitis. Abdom Imaging 26:59–63

Araki Y, Akahoshi K, Chijiiwa Y (1998) Case report: endosonographic evaluation of colonic stenosis associated with chronic pancreatitis. Clin Radiol 53:532–534

Balthazar EJ (2002a) Complications of acute pancreatitis: clinical and CT evaluation. Radiol Clin North Am 40:1211–1227

Balthazar EJ (2002b) Staging of acute pancreatitis. Radiol Clin North Am 40:1199–1209

Balthazar EJ (2002c) Acute pancreatitis: assessment of severity with clinical and CT evaluation. Radiology 223:603–613

Balthazar EJ, Freeny PC, van Sonnenberg E (1994) Imaging and intervention in acute pancreatitis. Radiology 193:297–306

Banks PA (1997) Practice guidelines in acute pancreatitis. Am J Gastroenterol 92:377–386

Banks PA (2002) Epidemiology, natural history, and predictors of disease outcome in acute and chronic pancreatitis. Gastrointest Endosc 56:226–230

Baril NB, Ralls PW, Wren SM, Selby RR, Radin R, Parekh D, Jabbour N, Stain SC (2000) Does an infected peripancreatic fluid collection or abscess mandate operation? Ann Surg 231:361–367

Bassi C, Butturini G, Salvia R, Contro C, Valerio A, Falconi M, Pederzoli P (2000) A single-institution experience with fistulojejunostomy for external pancreatic fistulas. Am J Surg 179:203–206

Beger HG, Rau B, Mayer J, Pralle U (1997) Natural course of acute pancreatitis. World J Surg 21:130–135

Bennett GL, Hann LE (2001) Pancreatic ultrasonography. Surg Clin North Am 81:259–281

Cabay JE, Boverie JH, Dondelinger RF (1998) Percutaneous catheter drainage of external fistulas of the pancreatic ducts. Eur Radiol 8:445–448

Calvo E, Ciguenza R, Alvarez-Sala JL, Massa B, Espinos D (1992) Spontaneous rupture of the spleen in chronic pancreatitis: an often forgotten complication. Gastroenterol Clin Biol 16:194

Carrere C, Heyries L, Barthet M, Bernard JP, Grimaud JC, Sahel J (2001) Biliopancreatic fistulas complicating pancreatic pseudocysts: a report of three cases demonstrated by endoscopic retrograde cholangiopancreatography. Endoscopy 33:91–94

Costamagna G, Mutignani M, Ingrosso M, Vamvakousis V, Alevras P, Manta R, Perri V (2001) Endoscopic treatment of postsurgical external pancreatic fistulas. Endoscopy 33:317–322

Cova M, Stacul F, Cester G, Ukmar M, Pozzi Mucelli R (2003) MR cholangiopancreatography: comparison of 2D single-shot fast spin-echo and 3D fast spin-echo sequences. Radiol Med 106:178–190

De Backer AI, Mortele KJ, Vaneerdeweg W, Ros PR (2001) Pancreatocolonic fistula due to severe acute pancreatitis: imaging findings. JBR-BTR 84:45–47

De Backer AI, Mortele KJ, Ros RR, Vanbeckevoort D, Vanschoubroeck I, De Keulenaer B (2002) Chronic pancreatitis: diagnostic role of computed tomography and magnetic resonance imaging. JBR-BTR 85:304–310

Dorffel T, Wruck T, Ruckert RI, Romaniuk P, Dorffel Q, Wermke W (2000) Vascular complications in acute pancreatitis assessed by color duplexultrasonography. Pancreas 21:126–133

Eckhauser FE, Knol JA, Strodel WE, Achem S, Nostrant T (1983) Common bile duct strictures associated with chronic pancreatitis. Am Surg 49:350–358

Elsayes KM, Narra VR, Mukundan G, Lewis JS Jr, Menias CO, Heiken JP (2005) MR imaging of the spleen: spectrum of abnormalities. Radiographics 25:967–982

Fernandez-Cruz L, Margarona E, Llovera J, Lopez-Boado MA, Saenz H (1993) Pancreatic ascites. Hepatogastroenterology 40:150–154

Ferrucci JT, Mueller PR (2003) Interventional approach to pancreatic fluid collections. Radiol Clin N Am 41:1217–1226

Fulcher AS, Turner MA, Yelon JA et al. (2003) Magnetic resonance cholangiopancreatography (MRCP) in the assessment of pancreatic duct trauma and its sequelae: preliminary findings. Am J Surg 185:251–255

Gregg JA, Carr-Locke DL, Gallagher MM (1981) Importance of common bile duct stricture associated with chronic pancreatitis. Diagnosis by endoscopic retrograde cholangiopancreatography. Am J Surg 141:199–203

Hammar AM, Sand J, Lumio J, Hirn M, Honkonen S, Tuominen L, Nordback I (2002) Pancreatic pseudocystportal vein fistula manifests as residivating oligoarthritis, subcutaneous, bursal and osseal necrosis: a case report and review of literature. Hepatogastroenterology 49:273–278

Hauptmann EM, Wojtowycz M, Reichelderfer M, McDermott JC, Crummy AB (1992) Pancreatic pseudocyst with fistula to the common bile duct: radiological diagnosis and management. Gastrointest Radiol 17:151–153

Kalra MK, Maher MM, Sahani DV, Digmurthy S, Saini S (2002) Current status of imaging in pancreatic diseases. J Comput Assist Tomogr 26:661–675

Kravetz GW, Cho KC, Baker SR (1988) Radiologic evaluation of pancreatic ascites. Gastrointest Radiol 13:163–166

Kumar A, Upreti L, Bhargava SK, Gupta S (2002) Sonographic demonstration of a pancreatopleural fistula. J Clin Ultrasound 30:503–505

Lankisch PG, Banks PA (1998) Acute pancreatitis: complications. In: Lankisch PG, Banks PA (eds) Pancreatitis. Springer, Berlin Heidelberg New York

Lanternier F, Valcke J, Hernigou A, Wermert D, Almeida F, Israel-Biet D (2002) Bilateral pleurisy and cardiac tamponade. A rare etiology: pancreatico-pleural fistula. Rev Mal Respir 19:795–797

Lecesne R, Drouillard J (1999) Acute pancreatitis. In: Baert AL, Delorme G, Van Hoe L (eds) Radiology of the pancreas. Springer, Berlin Heidelberg New York

Lee DH, Shin DH, Kim TH, Park SS, Park KN, Lee JH (1992) Mediastinal pancreatic pseudocyst with recurrent pleural effusion. Demonstration by endoscopic retrograde cholangiopancreatogram and subsequent computed tomography scan. J Clin Gastroenterol 14:68–71

Lin JW, Cameron JL, Yeo CJ, Riall TS, Lillemoe KD (2004) Risk factors and outcomes in postpancreatico-duodenectomy pancreatico-cutaneous fistula. J Gastrointest Surg 8:951–959

Ly JN, Miller FH (2002) MR imaging of the pancreas: a practical approach. Radiol Clin North Am 40:1289–1306

Materne R, Vranckx P, Pauls C, Coche EE, Deprez P, Van Beers BE (2000) Pancreaticopleural fistula: diagnosis with magnetic resonance pancreatography. Chest 117:912–914

McCormick PA, Chronos N, Burroughs AK, McIntyre N, McLaughlin JE (1990) Pancreatic pseudocyst causing portal vein thrombosis and pancreatico-pleural fistula. Gut 31:561–563

Merkle EM, Gorich J (2002) Imaging of acute pancreatitis. Eur Radiol 12:1979–1992

Merkle EM, Haugan PA, Thomas J, Jaffe TA, Gullotto C (2006) 3.0- Versus 1.5-T MR cholangiography: a pilot study. AJR Am J Roentgenol 186:516–521

Morgan DE, Baron TH, Smith JK, Robbin ML, Kenney PJ (1997) Pancreatic fluid collections prior to intervention: evaluation with MR imaging compared with CT and US. Radiology 203:773–778

Ozawa Y, Numata K, Tanaka K, Ueno N, Kiba T, Hara K, Morimoto M, Sakaguchi T, Sekihara H, Kubota T, Shimada H, Nakatani Y (2002) Contrast-enhanced sonography of small pancreatic mass lesions. J Ultrasound Med 21:983–991

Park JJ, Kim SS, Koo YS, Choi DJ, Park HC, Kim JH, Kim JS, Hyun JH (2002) Definitive treatment of pancreatic abscess by endoscopic transmural drainage. Gastrointest Endosc 55:256–262

Pedrosa I, Rofsky NM (2003) MR imaging in abdominal emergencies. Radiol Clin North Am 41:1243–1273

Piironen A, Kivisaari R, Pitkaranta P, Poutanen VP, Laippala P, Laurila P, Kivisaari L (1997) Contrast-enhanced magnetic resonance imaging for the detection of acute hemorrhagic necrotizing pancreatitis. Eur Radiol 7:17–20

Pistolesi GF, Procacci C, Residori E, Bicego E, Bertocco M, Moore F, Bergamo Andreis IA (1992) Radiologic imaging of pancreatic fistulas In: Pederzoli P, Bassi C, Vesentini S (eds) Pancreatic fistulas. Springer, Berlin Heidelberg New York

Pottmeyer EW, Frey CF, Matsuno S (1987) Pancreaticopleural fistulas. Arch Surg 122:648–654

Procacci C, Mansueto G, D'Onofrio M, Gasparini A, Ferrara RM, Falconi M (2002) Non-traumatic abdominal emergencies: imaging and intervention in acute pancreatic conditions. Eur Radiol 12:2407–2434

Remer EM, Baker ME (2002) Imaging of chronic pancreatitis. Radiol Clin North Am 40:1229–1242

Riddell A, Jhaveri K, Haider M (2005) Pseudocyst rupture into the portal vein diagnosed with MRI. Br J Radiol 78:265–268

Ridgeway MG, Stabile BE (1996) Surgical management and treatment of pancreatic fistulas. Surg Clin North Am 76:1159–1173

Robertson F, Leander P, Ekberg O (2001) Radiology of the spleen. Eur Radiol 11:80–95

Robinson PJ, Sheridan MB (2000) Pancreatitis: computed tomography and magnetic resonance imaging. Eur Radiol 10:401–408

Safadi BY, Marks JM (2000) Pancreatic-pleural fistula: the role of ERCP in diagnosis and treatment. Gastrointest Endosc 51:213–215

Skarsgard ED, Ellison E, Quenville N (1995) Spontaneous rupture of a pancreatic pseudocyst into the portal vein. Can J Surg 38:459–463

Soto JA, Barish MA, Yucel EK, Clarke P, Siegenberg D, Chuttani R, Ferrucci JT (1995) Pancreatic duct: MR cholangiopancreatography with a three-dimensional fast spin-echo technique. Radiology 196:459–464

Steinberg W, Tenner S (1994) Acute pancreatitis. N Engl J Med 330:1198–1210

Suzuki A, Matsunaga T, Aoki S, Hirayama T, Nakagawa N, Shibata K, Yabana T, Kawasaki H, Takasaka H, Sasaki K, Katsuramaki T, Mukaiya M, Hirata K, Imai K (2002) A pancreatic abscess 7 years after a pancreatojejunostomy for calcifying chronic pancreatitis. J Gastroenterol 37:1062–1067

Takayama T, Kato K, Sano H, Katada N, Takeichi M (1986) Spontaneous rupture of a pancreatic pseudocyst into the portal venous system. AJR Am J Roentgenol 147:935–936

Torres WE, Clements JL Jr, Sones PJ, Knopf DR (1981) Gas in the pancreatic bed without abscess. AJR Am J Roentgenol 137:1131–1133

Turner MA (2002) The role of US and CT in pancreatitis. Gastrointest Endosc 56:241–245

Van Sonnemberg E, Casola G, Varney RR, Wittich GR (1989) Imaging and interventional radiology for pancreatitis and its complications. Radiol Clin North Am 27:65–72

Vantini I, Piubello W, Scuro LA, Benini P, Talamini G, Benini L, Micciolo R, Cavallini G (1982) Duodenal ulcer in chronic relapsing pancreatitis. Digestion 24:23–28

Verhaeghe W, Meysman M, Opdebeeck B, Demey J, Naegels S, Osteaux M, Vincken W (1996) Pancreaticopleural fistula: a case report. Eur J Radiol 23:118–120

Vujic I (1989) Vascular complications of pancreatitis. Eur Radiol 1:81–91

Ward J, Chalmers AG, Guthrie AJ, Larvin M, Robinson PJ (1997) T2-weighted and dynamic enhanced in acute pancreatitis: comparison with contrast enhanced CT. Clin Radiol 52:109–114

Wolfsen HC, Kozarek RA, Ball TJ, Patterson DJ, Traverso LW, Freeny PC (1992) Pancreaticoenteric fistula: no longer a surgical disease? J Clin Gastroenterol. 14:117–121

Yanagie H, Tani T, Sairennji T, Ogata M, Eriguchi M (1997) A pancreatic pseudocyst with pancreatic pleural effusion: report of a case. Surg Today 27:1064–1068

Yokoyama I, Hashmi MA, Srinivas D, Shaikh KA, Levine SM, Sorokin JJ, Camishion RC (1984) Wirsungorrhagia or hemoductal pancreatitis: report of a case and review of the literature. Am J Gastroenterol 79:764–776

Chronic Pancreatitis vs Pancreatic Tumors

Alessandro Guarise, Niccolo' Faccioli, Giovanni Morana, and Alec J. Megibow

CONTENTS

18.1 **Introduction** *329*

18.2 **Focal Chronic Pancreatitis** *329*
18.2.1 Introduction *329*
18.2.2 Mass Forming Pancreatitis *330*
18.2.2.1 Introduction *330*
18.2.2.2 Differential Diagnosis at Imaging *330*
18.2.2.3 Role of US/EUS *331*
18.2.2.4 Role of CT *337*
18.2.2.5 Role of MR *338*
18.2.3 Autoimmune Chronic Pancreatitis *338*
18.2.3.1 Introduction *338*
18.2.3.2 Differential Diagnosis at Imaging *344*
18.2.3.3 Role of US *346*
18.2.3.4 Role of CT *346*
18.2.3.5 Role of MR *346*
18.2.3.6 Role of ERCP *346*
18.2.4 Cystic Duodenal Dystrophy (Solid Variant) *346*
18.2.4.1 Introduction *346*
18.2.4.2 Differential Diagnosis at Imaging *347*
18.2.4.3 Role of US and EUS *353*
18.2.4.4 Role of CT *353*
18.2.4.5 Role of MR *353*
18.2.5 Role of Nuclear Medicine *354*

18.3 **Diffuse Dilation of the Main Pancreatic Duct** *357*
18.3.1 Introduction *357*
18.3.2 OCP vs Ductal or Ampullary Adenocarcinoma *357*
18.3.3 CP vs IPMT of the Main Duct *357*
18.3.3.1 Role of US/EUS *361*
18.3.3.2 Role of CT and MR *363*
18.3.3.3 Role of Pancreatoscopy *365*

References *365*

A. Guarise, MD
Department of Radiology, San Bassiano Hospital, Via dei Lotti 41, 36024 Bassano del Grappa (VI), Italy
N. Faccioli, MD
Department of Radiology, University of Verona, Policlinico G.B. Rossi, Piazzale Scuro 10, 37134 Verona, Italy
G.Morana, MD
Department of Radiology, General Hospital Cà Foncello, Piazza Ospedale 1, 31100 Treviso, Italy
A. J. Megibow, MD, MPH, FACR
Professor, Department of Radiology, NYU-Langone Medical Center, 550 First Avenue, New York, NY 10016, USA

18.1 Introduction

The differential diagnosis between chronic pancreatitis (CP) and ductal adenocarcinoma adenocarcinomahas always been a c challenge for imaging. The greatest difficulties regard the following manifestations of CP:

- Focal forms ("mass forming pancreatitis", autoimmune pancreatitis, cystic dystrophy of the duodenal wall in the solid variant)
- Uniform dilatation of the main pancreatic duct (MPD)
- Cystic masses in CP

This chapter will consider the possible semeiotic radiological signs, that, if present allow a correct preoperative diagnosis. For the differential diagnosis of cystic lesions in chronic pancreatitis, please refer to Chapter 16 (Imaging of Pseudocyst).

18.2 Focal Chronic Pancreatitis

18.2.1 Introduction

CP in its classic form, involves the whole gland and characterized by the presence of widespread calcifications and/or "lake chain" dilatation of the MPD.

Imaging findings are often accompanied by the typical clinical picture (alcohol abuse, long history of recurrent abdominal pain, alterations in the laboratory indexes of pancreatic function). On the other hand, whenever the inflammatory diseases present focally within the pancreas, the proper recognition of the true abnormality by imaging is difficult.

The literature reports many large surgical series (Neff et al. 1984; Smith et al. 1994; Van Gulik et al. 1997) with percentages varying from 3% to 6% of Whipple interventions that were carried out due to non-neoplastic pancreatic pathology. In these cases imaging does not often bring clarity to this clinical inquiry. Resecting the lesion is the only definite way to establish the diagnosis (Neff et al. 1984; Smith et al. 1994; Van Gulik et al. 1997; Wharton et al. 1997). A correct preoperative and early diagnosis, on the one hand prevents patients with a benign pathology from being submitted to a pointless resection that, even if there is a low post-surgical mortality rate (< 5%) (Allema et al. 1995; Cameron et al. 1993; Baumel et al. 1994), has a significant morbidity rate (40%–50%) (Allema et al. 1995; Cameron et al. 1993; Baumel et al. 1994; Pitt 1995). On the other hand, there is a prognostic improvement in the case of adenocarcinomas that are identified while they are still confined to the gland (less than 2 cm in diameter) (Trede et al. 1990).

Chronic inflammatory focal glandular enlargement is found in three different non-neoplastic entities:

- Mass Forming Pancreatitis
- Autoimmune Chronic Pancreatitis
- Solid Variant Cystic Duodenal Dystrophy

18.2.2 Mass Forming Pancreatitis

18.2.2.1 Introduction

It has been reported that within a range of 27%–50% of cases of CP (Bennet and Hann 2001; Kroft et al. 1995; Luetmer et al. 1989) the disease presentes as a localized mass. This is also known as a "pseudotumor" (Lammer et al. 1985) or "mass forming pancreatitis" (MFP) (Shinozaki et al. 1987) to underline its similarity to ductal adenocarcinoma at imaging.

MFP is more frequently found at the head of the pancreas. According to Kim et al. (2001), the percentage is 71% of cases. From a clinical point of view the majority of patients with MFP have a typical past history with previous episodes of pancreatitis, alcohol abuse and recurrent abdominal pain for at least 2 years. Although the clinical history may be of help in directing the diagnosis, the MFP and adenocarcinomaductal adenocarcinoma imaging findings may be indistinguishable.

This is because both lesions are composed of extensive fibrosis. Moreover, adenocacinoma can also present with an indistinguishable array of symptoms (Van Gulik et al. 1999; Carter 1992). Finally, both entities may co-exist (Gabata et al. 2003). CP is a risk factor adenocarcinomafor the development of adenocarcinoma. (Van Gulik et al. 1997; Lowenfels et al. 1993). Conversely, an adenocarcinoma can cause upstream pancreatic inflammation. Therefore it is often impossible to establish which is the cause or the effect.

Although cyto-histological analysis may also be employed it has its limitations. Sampling errors may result in a false negative rate for tumor in as high as 60% of cases (Parsons and Palmer 1989; Rodriguez et al. 1992).. Even if sampling errors can be reduced to a certain extent by, for example, using EUS especially in cases of small focal lesions (Mallery et al. 2002), it can remain to bedifficult to differentiate MAP rom a well differentiated adenocarcinoma by cyto-histological alone (Van Gulik et al. 1997) (see Chap. 14).

From a laboratory point of view, the serum level of CA 19.9, using 40 U/mL as cut off, gives a sensitivity and specificity for adenocarcinoma of 70% and 98%–99% respectively (Nazli et al. 2000). Unfortunately, a adenocarcinoma is not often associated with an increase in CA 19.9 until it is advanced. Furthermore, when inflammation is in process, the normal value of this marker can change (Wiersema 2001; Carter 1992; DelMaschio et al. 1991; Gentiloni et al. 1995).

18.2.2.2 Differential Diagnosis at Imaging

As stated above, an MFP and a adenocarcinoma, can have a similar gross and microscopic appearance (Fig. 18.1), it should not be surprising that preoperative imaging diagnosis may be impossible (Fig. 18.2).

However, there are some elements of MFP that, if found, perhaps with different diagnostic techniques, can sometimes direct the diagnosis towards the inflammatory form rather than the neoplasm.

The presence of calcifications within the MFP, recognizable in about 50% of cases (Luetmer et al. 1989; Carter 1992; Kim et al. 2001) certainly favors CP (Karasawa et al. 1983; Luetmer et al. 1989; Carter 1992; Kim et al. 2001) (Figs. 18.3 and 18.4). This finding helps too when the twoentities co-exist in that, displacement of calcification may signal a co-existent tumor. (Elmas 2001) (Figs. 18.5 and 18.6).

The presence of collateral duct dilatation *within* the focal lesion strongly favors CP due to the traction effect that the fibrous tissue has on the ductal walls. MR, with MRCP s, is probably the best technique for displaying this finding (Figs. 18.7c–f and 18.8).

The concomitant presence of pseudocysts, in 25% of cases, according to Luetmer et al. (1989), is definitely a criterion that directs diagnosis towards the inflammatory form. However, it should not be forgotten that adenocarcinomas can have a cystic appearance (Fig. 18.9).

18.2.2.3
Role of US/EUS

Abdominal ultrasound (US) examination is the first diagnostic step to identifying and characterizing an MFP. The examination itself is sometimes limited by air in the bowel lumen and/or by the patient's body habitus.

At US examination an MFP appears irregularly hypoechoic (Figs. 18.2b and 18.3a), and is absolutely indistinguishable from a tumor (Fig. 18.2a) if not for the presence of calcifications, recognizable as clearly hyperechoic focuses with posterior shadowing (Fig. 18.3a,b) (Bennett and Hann

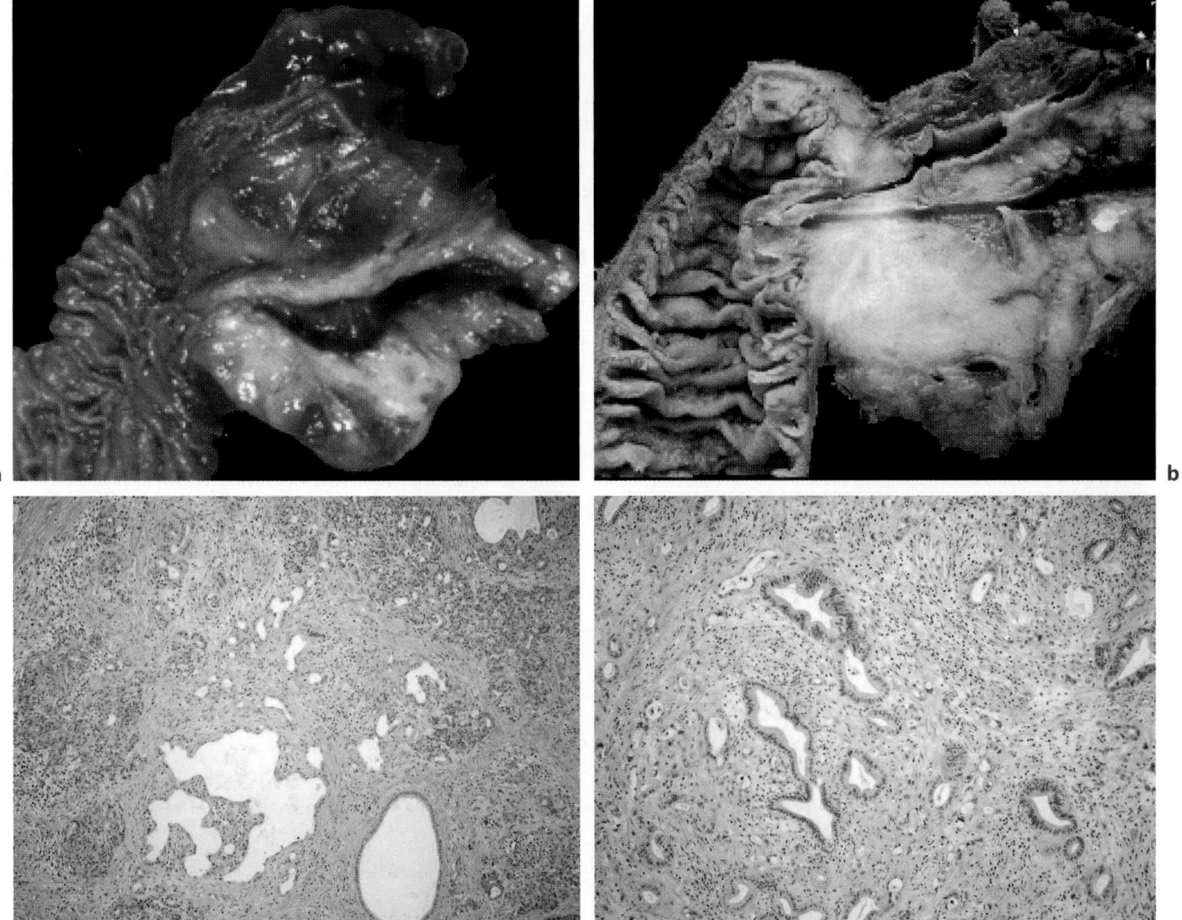

Fig. 18.1a–d. Cut sections of mass-forming pancreatitis (**a**) and ductal adenocarcinoma (**b**). Both forms show a similar appeareance as a focal lesion with scirrhous characteristics. Histologically (**c,d**) in both cases there is a rich fibrous component and poor vascularization

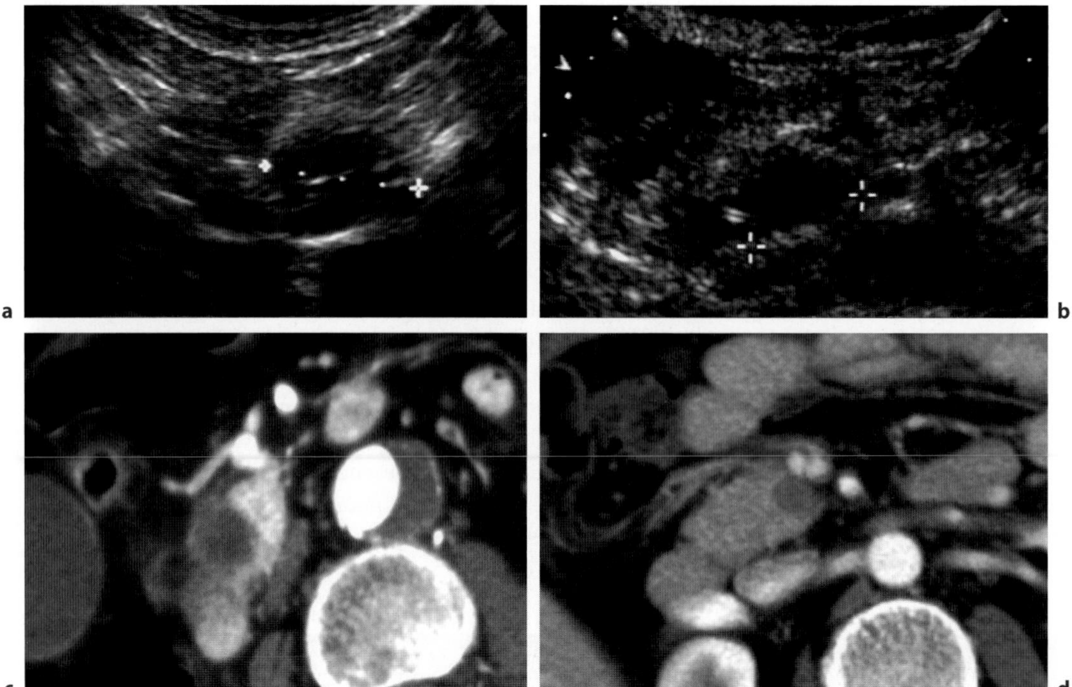

Fig. 18.2a–d. Ductal adenocarcinoma vs MFP (US and CT evaluation). **a,c** The ductal adenocarcinoma appears as a solid, clearly outlined, hypoechoic mass at US and hypodense at CT in the pancreatic phase. **b,d** The MFP is identical at both US and CT

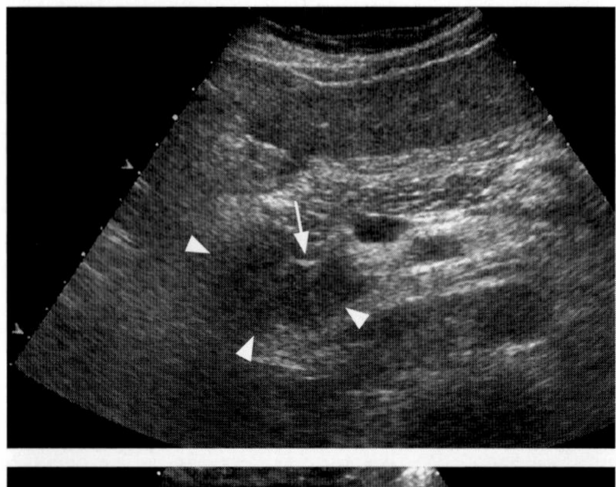

Fig. 18.3a–c. MFP (US and CT evaluation). First case (**a**): hypoechoic mass at US (*arrowheads*) located in the head of the pancreas where a slightly hyperechoic focus is recognizable (*arrow*) compatible with calcification. Second case (**b,c**): hypoechoic mass at US (**b**) located in the head of the pancreas with large calcifications (*arrows*). At CT (**c**), the mass located in the head of the pancreas appears hypodense in the pancreatic phase. The presence of large calcifications within is confirmed

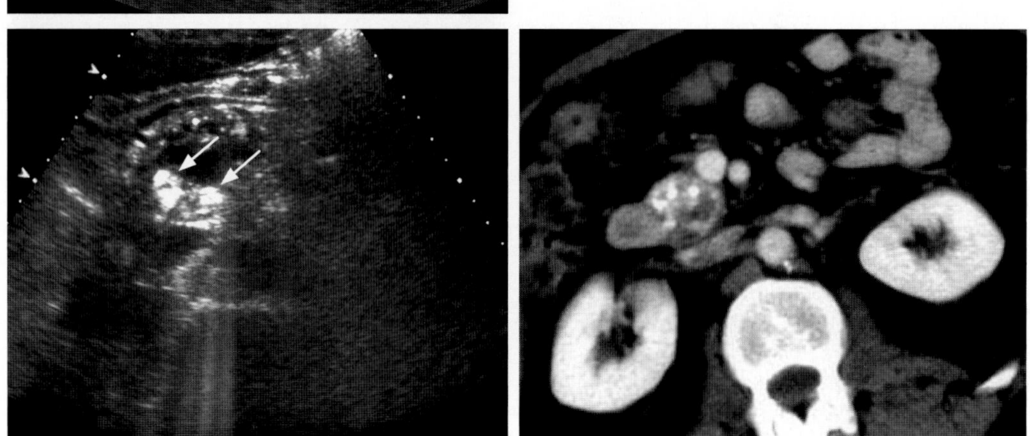

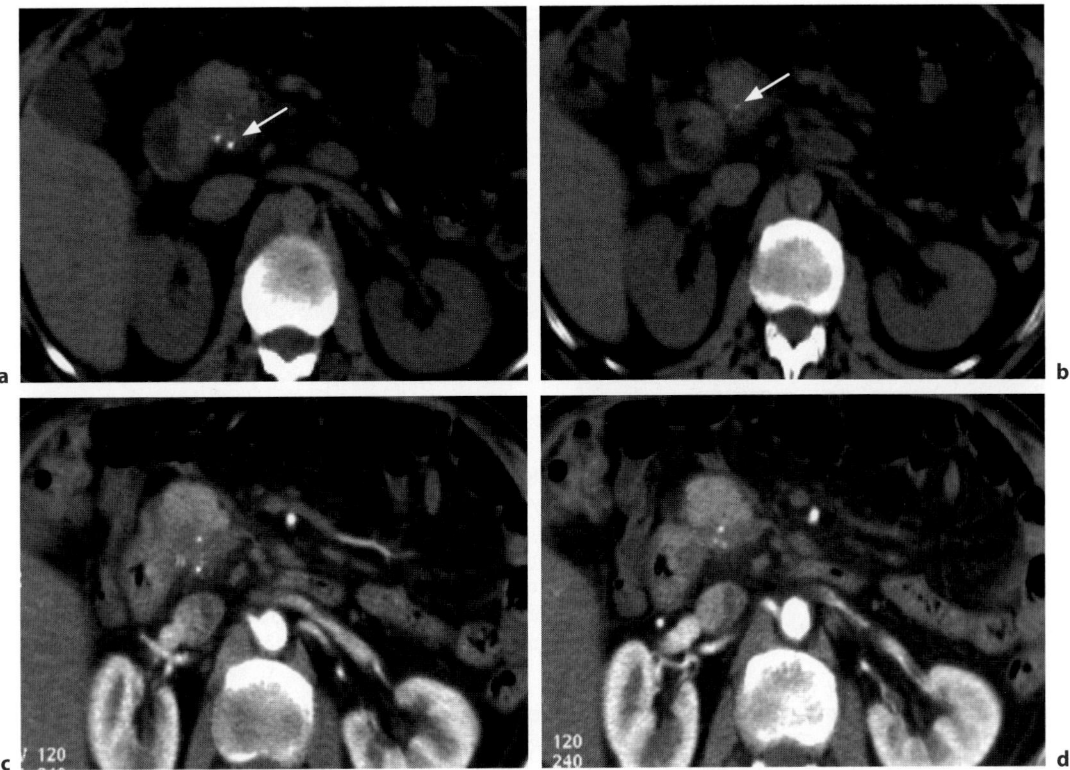

Fig. 18.4a–d. MFP (CT evaluation). The lesion, located in the pancreatic head, appears hypodense both before (**a**,**b**) and after c.m. administration (**c**,**d**). Small calcifications can be seen within it, especially before c.m. administration (*arrows* in **a**,**b**)

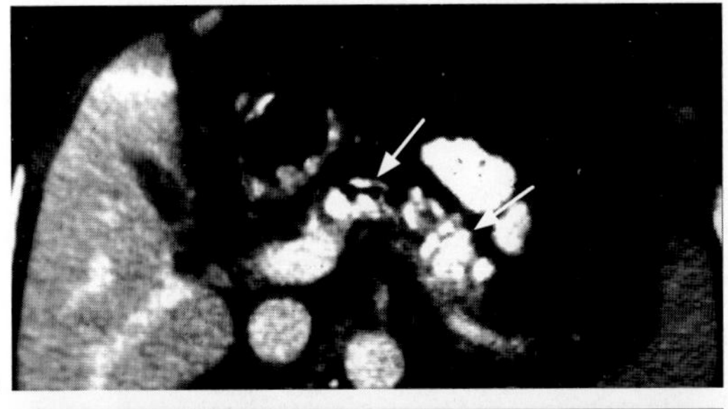

Fig. 18.5a–c. Ductal adenocarcinoma in CP (CT evaluation). Presence of large pancreatic calcifications (*arrows* in **a**); those located in the head appear displaced medially by the hypodense mass (*arrow* in **b**,**c**)

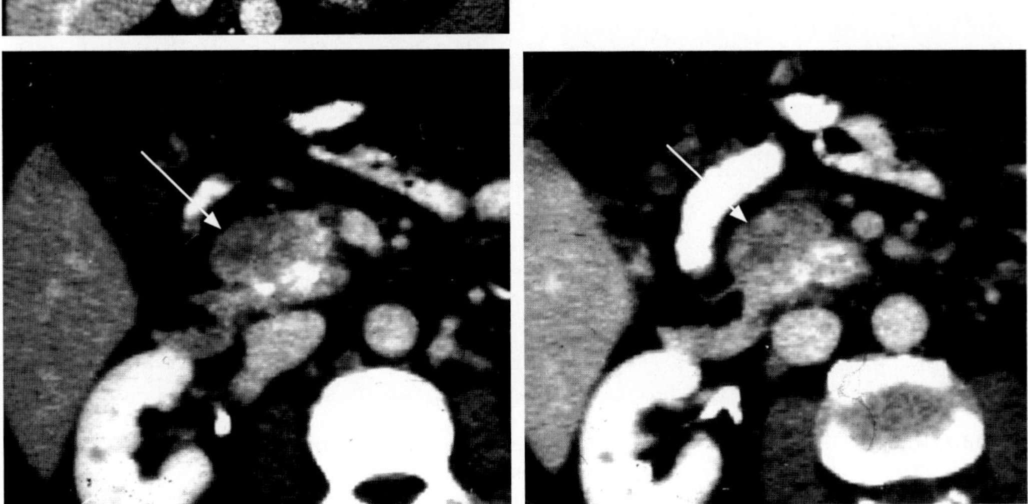

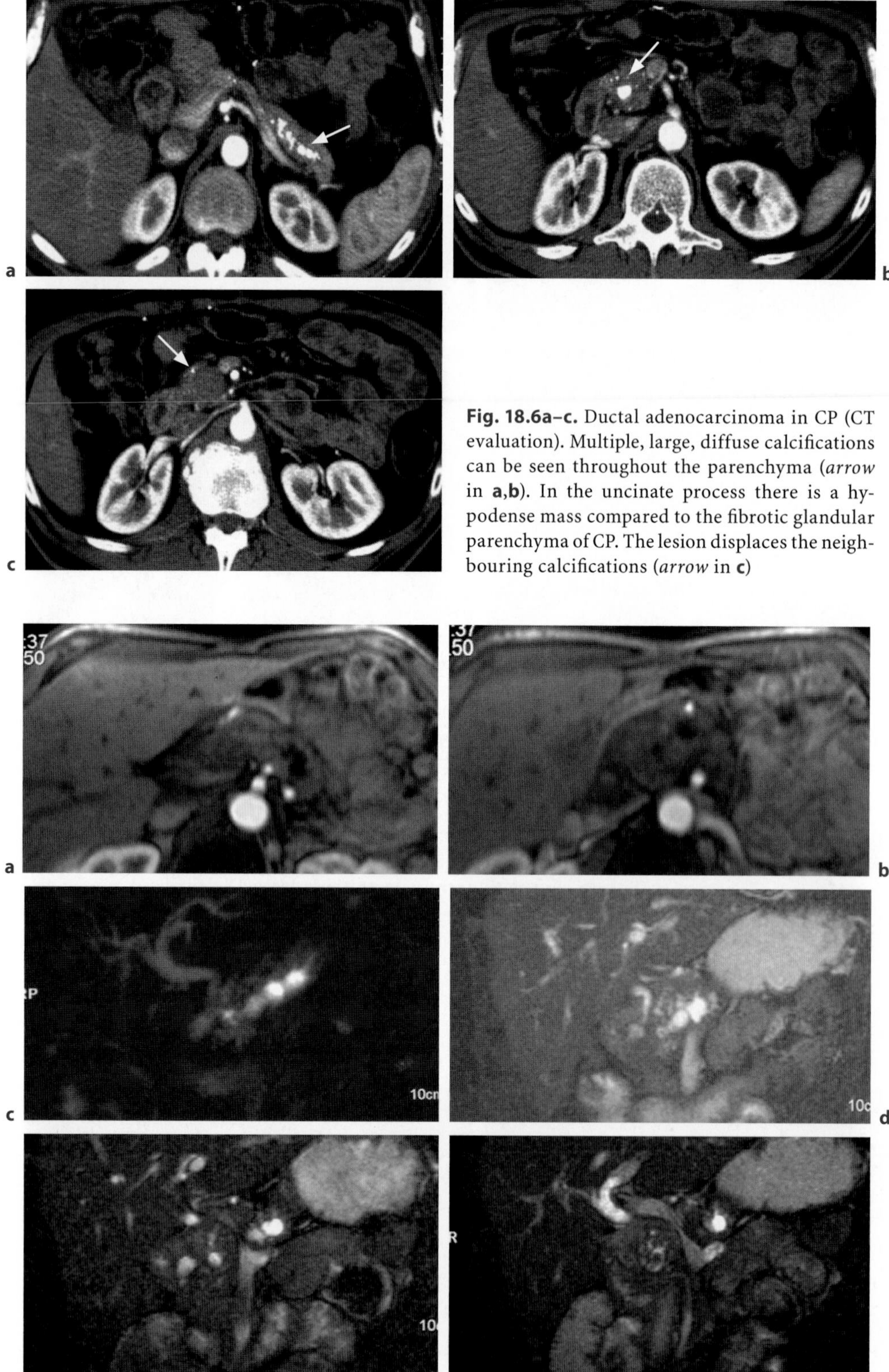

Fig. 18.6a–c. Ductal adenocarcinoma in CP (CT evaluation). Multiple, large, diffuse calcifications can be seen throughout the parenchyma (*arrow* in **a,b**). In the uncinate process there is a hypodense mass compared to the fibrotic glandular parenchyma of CP. The lesion displaces the neighbouring calcifications (*arrow* in **c**)

Fig. 18.7a–f. MFP (MR evaluation). The lesion, located in the head, appears hypovascularized (**a,b**) and produces dilation of both the cbd and the main pancreatic duct (double duct sign in **c,d**). TRUE-FISP sequences (**e,f**), the branch ducts can be recognized within the lesion (*arrow* in **e**)

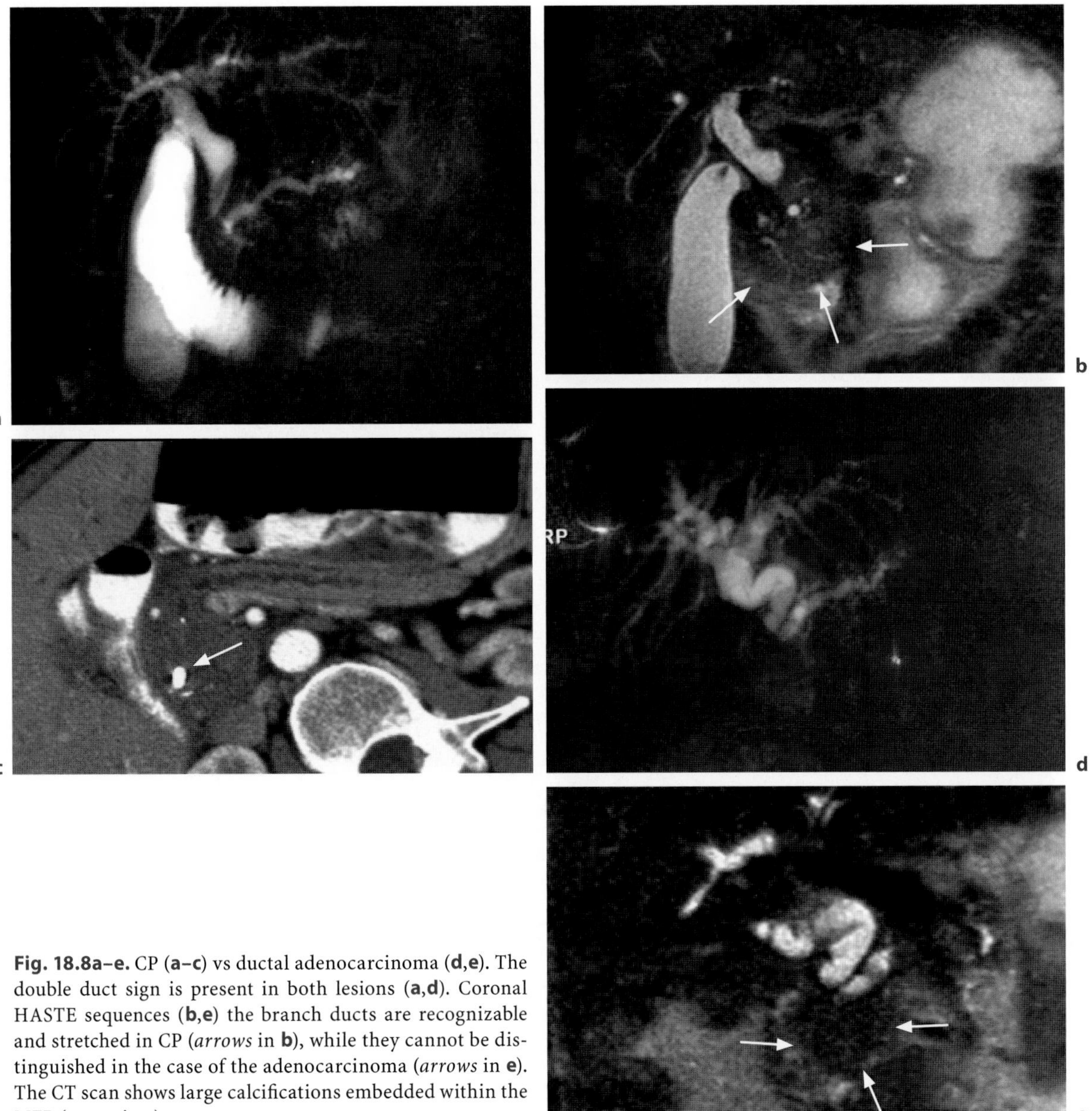

Fig. 18.8a–e. CP (**a–c**) vs ductal adenocarcinoma (**d,e**). The double duct sign is present in both lesions (**a,d**). Coronal HASTE sequences (**b,e**) the branch ducts are recognizable and stretched in CP (*arrows* in **b**), while they cannot be distinguished in the case of the adenocarcinoma (*arrows* in **e**). The CT scan shows large calcifications embedded within the MFP (*arrow* in **c**)

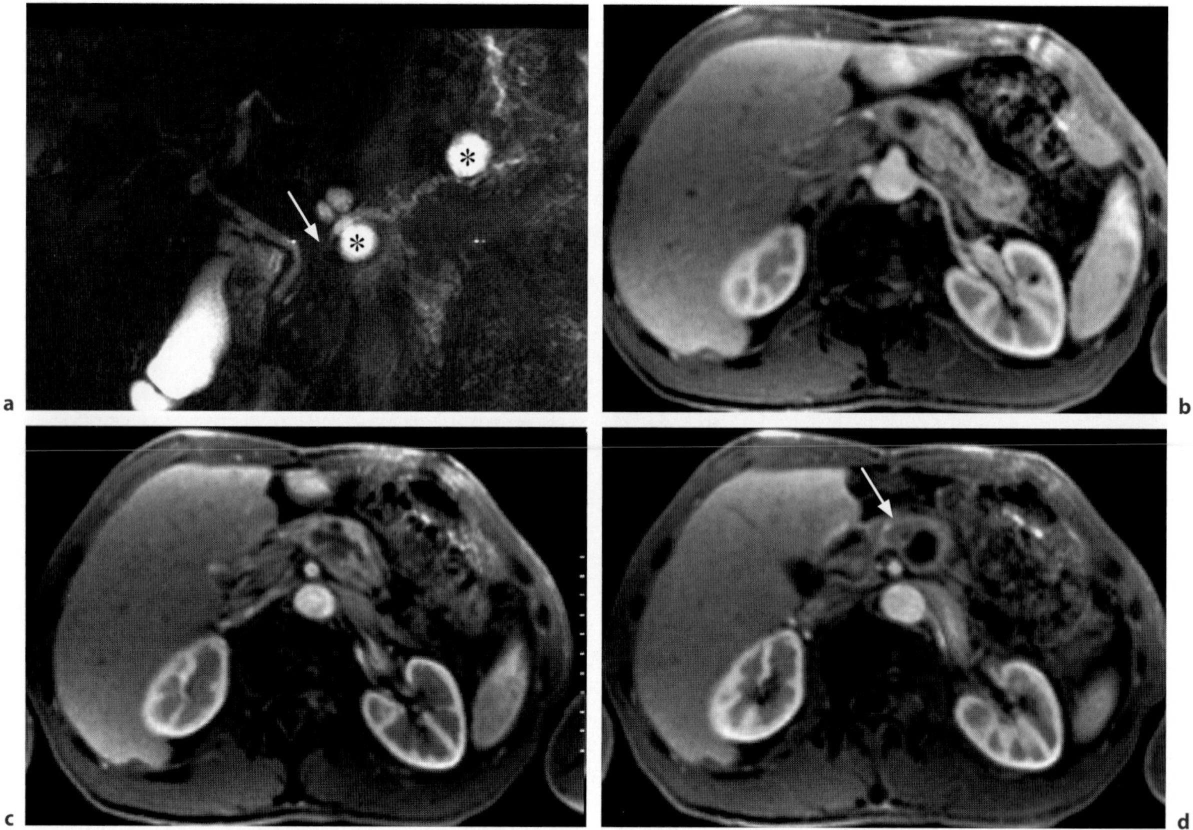

Fig. 18.9a–d. Ductal cystic adenocarcinoma (MR evaluation). MRCP (**a**) shows a slightly dilated main duct in the body-head with irregular morphology; associated cystic formations in the body and tail (*asterisks*). In the GRE T1 FS sequences carried out after c.m. administration (**b–d**), a solid component can be seen within the cystic formation located in the body which has an irregular enhancement (*arrow* in **d**) and is responsible for obstructing the main duct (*arrow* in **a**)

2001). According to some authors (Oshikawa et al. 2002), the MFP margins are quite clear compared to the more blurred outlines of an adenocarcinoma (Fig. 18.2a,b).

S US is limited and its diagnostic accuracy in differentiating between the two forms, according to the authors, varies from 72% to 79% (DelMaschio et al. 1991; DelHaze et al. 1989). Power Doppler US does not seem to have any advantages compared to the standard US examination (Rickes et al. 2002). This could be due to its low sensitivity in recognizing low velocity flow in small vessels in the pancreas. Recently, as already widely discussed in Chapter 10, contrast enhanced US (CE-US) and enhanced power Doppler have proved themselves to be competitive with CT and MR with sensitivity and specificity values in the diagnosis of adenocarcinoma of 87% and 94% respectively, and 85% and 99% respectively in CP diagnosis (Rickes et al. 2002). According to some authors (Ozawa et al. 2002), CE-US is actually better than CT and MR because the US contrast material remains in the intra-vascular compartment longer than CT and MR agents. CP has, no matter how hypovascularized, an average "contrast index" (CI = elevation of intensity in the lesion/elevation of intensity in the pancreatic parenchyma), higher than adenocarcinoma (Ozawa et al. 2002; Oshikawa et al. 2002; Takeda et al. 2003; Becker et al. 2001; Koito et al. 1997). This finding should lead to differentiation between the two pathologies. Recently, endoscopic ultrasound (EUS) is becoming widely used in pancreatic evaluation (Becker et al. 2001; Glasbrenner et al. 2000). The correct evaluation of the pancreatic head-uncinate process is carried out with the US probe positioned in the second duodenal portion while the body-tail sectors can be analyzed better with the probe alongside the greater curvature of the stomach. During the examination, cytological sampling can be carried out of suspicious areas (Fig. 18.10a) with minimal risk of complications (Becker et al. 2001; Mallery et al. 2002). At EUS, an MFP appears as a hypoechoic mass (Fig. 18.10a). Calcifications, pseudocysts and irregular dilatation of the branch ducts of the pancreas are easily recognized, all typical findings in CP. From early studies (Brand et al. 2000; Norton et al. 2001; Glasbrenner et al. 2000; Bennet and Hann 2001; Wiersema 2001; Yamao et al. 2003) sensitivity appears high (95%) especially in identifying solid intrapancreatic lesions, even when small, but the specificity range is still too broad (16%–93%) (Wiersema 2001; Yamao et al. 2003), and does not allow for a definite characterization of MFP (Fig. 18.10a).

Another recently introduced EUS procedure is the intra-ductal ultrasound (IDUS) which uses US micro probes, 2 mm in diameter, which can be introduced into the MPD. At IDUS, the pseudo-tumor appears as a clear, irregular hypoechoic area in which the normal glandular network is no longer recognizable (Yamao et al. 2003; Inui et al. 2002; Furukawa et al. 1994). This new technique, besides not being widely available because of its difficult and invasive nature, does not at the moment seem to significantly increase the accuracy of the other techniques in the differential diagnosis between MFP and adenocarcinoma, especially if less than 2 cm and still confined to the glandular parenchyma. It seems that in the near future, EUS and IDUS, thanks to their increasing confidence, will become the techniques of reference in evaluating CP and MFP in particular.

18.2.2.4 Role of CT

Although the use of single or multi-slice spiral CT (MDCT) has increased spatial and temporal resolution the accuracy (77%) reported by DelMaschio et al. (1991) and Delhaze et al. (1989) in differentiating between MFP from adenocarcinoma has remained substantially unchanged (Liao et al. 2003).

MDCT is better than US for demonstrating pancreatic calcifications (Figs. 18.3c and 18.4–18.6) their eventual dislocation due to a mass arising in the inflammatory process (Figs. 18.5b,c and 18.6c), the degree of atrophy and the morphology of the MPD. Karawasa et al. (1983) found a statistically significant difference in the ratio of duct diameter to pancreatic gland width, which is higher in patients with cancer. On unenhanced imagess both fibrous tissue and adenocarcinoma confined within the gland appear isodense compared to the surrounding tissue. The subsequent use of c.m. does not generally increase diagnostic accuracy, as both pathologies are hypodense compared with enhanced surrounding normal parenchyma(Figs. 18.2c,d, 18.3c, 18.4c,d, 18.5b,c and 18.6c) in the arterial and pancreatic phases (Kim et al. 2001; Johnson and Outwater 1999). Nevertheless, Robinson and Sheridan (2000) suggest that a neoplasm is less vascularized than fibrous tissue which would thus appear less hypodense in the pancreatic phase (Fig. 18.6) and

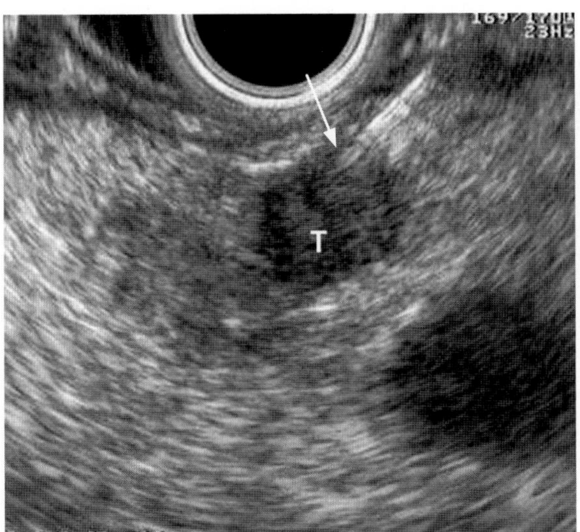

a

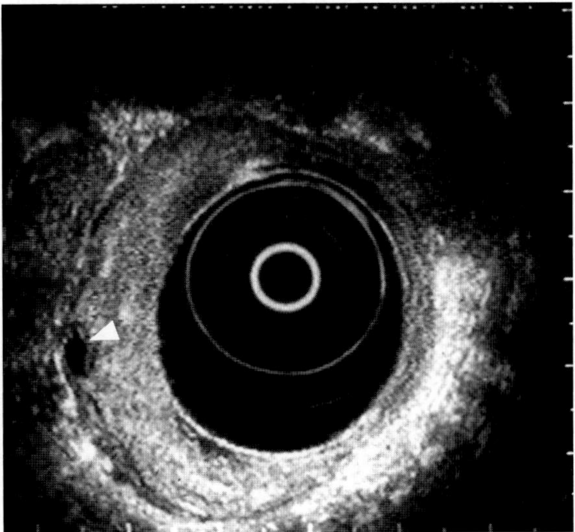

b

Fig. 18.10a,b. MFP and solid duodenal dystrophy (SDD) (EUS evaluation). At EUS, the MFP (**a**) located at the head appears hypoechoic (*T* in **a**) mimicking an adenocarcinoma. During the examination a needle aspiration of the lesion is carried out (*arrow* in **a**). At EUS it is possible to show the duodenal site of the SDD (**b**) and recognize its microcystic component (*arrowhead* in **b**), allowing for correct diagnosis.

substantially isodense in the late phase. The lack of absolute criteria of density limit the utility of the finding.

MDCT certainly makes it easier to recognize some typical signs of tumor such as extra-glandular spread (Figs. 18.11c and 18.12d) and vascular involvement (Figs. 18.11d and 18.12c,d). The demonstration of gastroduodenal artery encasement can be a helpful differentiating finding (Fig. 18.13). A relative increase in the size of the arterial vessels compared to the venous structure (artery-to-vein ratio greater than 1.0) (Elmas et al. 1996) favors tumor. Megibow et al. (1981) has described a thickening of the celiac tripod and/or superior mesenteric artery (Fig. 18.12c,d) when a tumor is present. More recently, on the other hand, Baker et al. (1990) and Schulte et al. (1991) reported infiltration of the peri-vascular fat in acute and chronic inflammatory forms.

Hough et al. (1999) highlights a deformation in the size of the superior mesenteric vein (teardrop sign: Fig. 18.12c) as an indirect sign of a locally infiltrating adenocarcinoma. Lastly, some authors (Mori et al. 1991; Hommeyer et al. 1995) maintain that a greater representation of the peri-pancreatic venous structure is an indirect sign of vascular involvement by a neoplastic process.

18.2.2.5 Role of MR

Because MR has a better tissue contrast resolution than CT, it is able to differentiate fibrosis from a healthy parenchyma. Both MFP and adenocarcinoma are partly made up of fibrous tissue and therefore appear equally hypointense in FS T1-weighted sequences (Fig. 18.14) compared to the adjacent parenchyma (Jenkins et al. 1987). Both entities behave in a similar fashion following c.m administration (Johnson and Outwater 1999; Sittek et al. 1995) (Figs. 18.14d,e and 18.15cMRCP however is extremely useful in evaluating the lesion's relationships with the ductal structures (Pavone et al. 1997) (Figs. 18.7c–f, 18.8 and 18.15a,b) and at dynamically demonstrating the distensibility of the ducts prior to intravenous secretin administration (Ichikawa et al. 2001; Matos et al. 2001). It is extremely easy with MRCP to demonstrate obliteration (Fig. 18.8d,e) and dislocation of the dilated collateral ducts caused by a tumor (Fig. 18.15a,b), and also to recognize duct distortion within the mass in CP (Figs. 18.7e,f and 18.8a,b). By administering secretin, as Ichikawa reports (Ichikawa et al. 2001), the main pancreatic duct remains irreversibly stenotic and obstructed due to the neoplastic process (Fig. 18.16e,f) while it appears patent, although narrowed, in an inflammatory condition (Fig. 18.17). This has been referred to as the "duct penetrating sign This sign has 86% sensitivity and 95% specificitiy in distinguishing between the two forms (Ichikawa et al. 2001).

Furthermore, the classic double duct sign (favouring adenocarcinoma) is certainly easily recognizable with MRCP (Figs. 18.7c, 18.9a and 18.15a). However this finding cannot be maintained as specific of a neoplastic pathology (Menges et al. 2000).

As previously said, thanks to the extreme sensitivity of MR in recognizing areas of parenchyma replaced by fibrosis, this method, more than the others, is able to identify and attribute congenital anomalies (pancreas divisum; pancreas divisum inversum), areas of irregular glandular parenchyma, hyperintense in T1 (Fig. 18.18a,b) compared to a parenchyma affected by CP, which is hypointense. These areas of the parenchyma are self-sufficient in terms of vascularization and drainage. Like a healthy pancreas, they are therefore notably hyperintense even after c.m. administration, mimicking, for example, neuroendocrine tumors. While in pancreas divisum it is quite easy to demonstrate with MRCP the typical ductal anomaly causing dorsal pancreatitis (Fig. 18.17), in the inverse form, only the site of the pseudo-lesion is cause for suspicion of this latter anatomical variant (Fig. 18.18).

18.2.3 Autoimmune Chronic Pancreatitis

18.2.3.1 Introduction

Autoimmune chronic pancreatitis (aCP), first described by Yoshida et al. (1995b). is a rare form of CP accounting for 1%–2% of all cases (Ito et al. 1997). In 30%–50% of cases (Yoshida et al. 1995b; Furukawa et al. 1998; Irie et al. 1998; Okazaki and Chiba 2002; Procacci et al. 2001b) it is associated with other autoimmune disorders (Hashimoto's thyroiditis, Sjogren's syndrome, rheumatoid arthritis, Crohn's disease, LES, primitive biliary cirrhosis, sclerosing cholangitis).

At pathology the gland almost always appears increased in size either focally or diffusely, and the ductal system is narrowed, compressed "*ab estrin-*

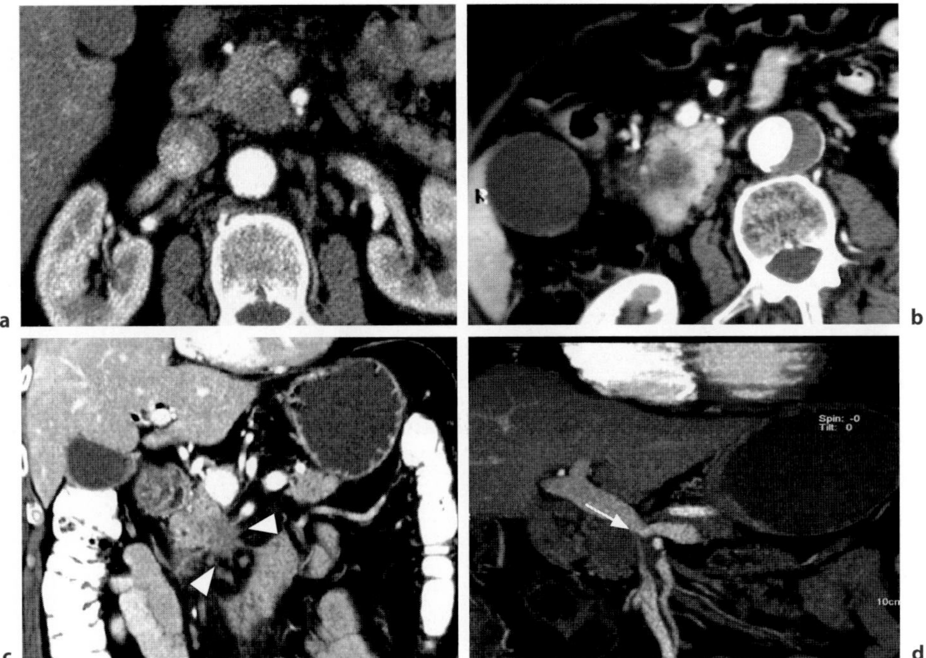

Fig. 18.11a–d. Ductal adenocarcinoma (MDCT evaluation). In the axial planes (**a**,**b**) a hypodense lesion is visible apparently embedded in the pancreatic gland. In the coronal reconstruction (**c**,**d**) the lesion infiltrates the peri-pancreatic adipose tissue (*arrowheads* in **c**) and causes "encasement" of the superior mesenteric vein (*arrow* in **d**).

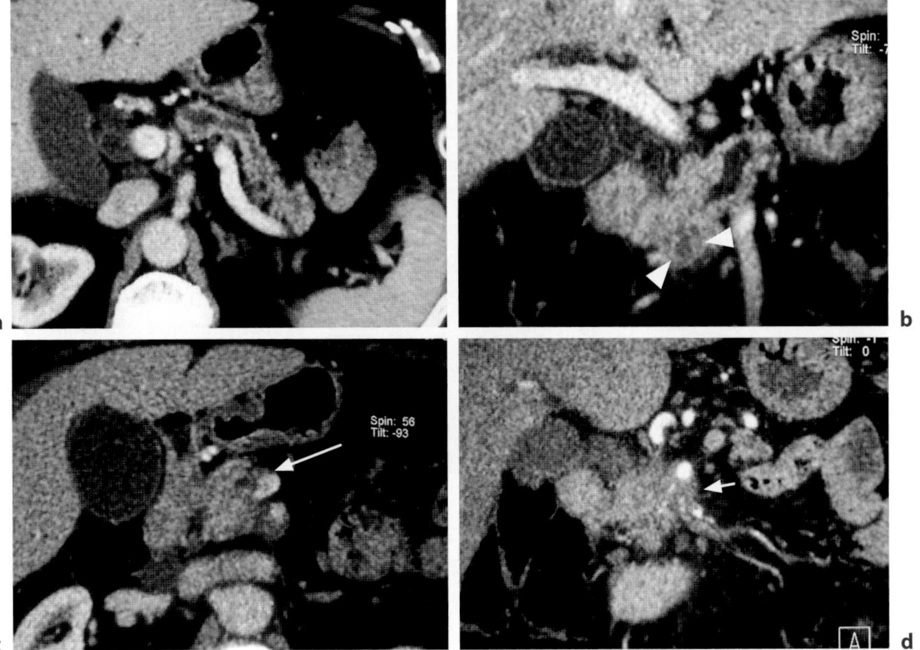

Fig. 18.12a–d. Ductal adenocarcinoma (MDCT evaluation). In the axial scan (**a**) the main duct abruptly stops in the neck of the pancreas. The lesion can be seen in the paracoronal plane reconstruction (**b**) where it appears irregularly hypodense (*arrowheads* in **b**). The soft extraglandular component is distinguishable around the superior mesenteric artery (*short arrow* in **d**) and the deformed superior mesenteric vein (teardrop sign: *long arrow* in **c**)

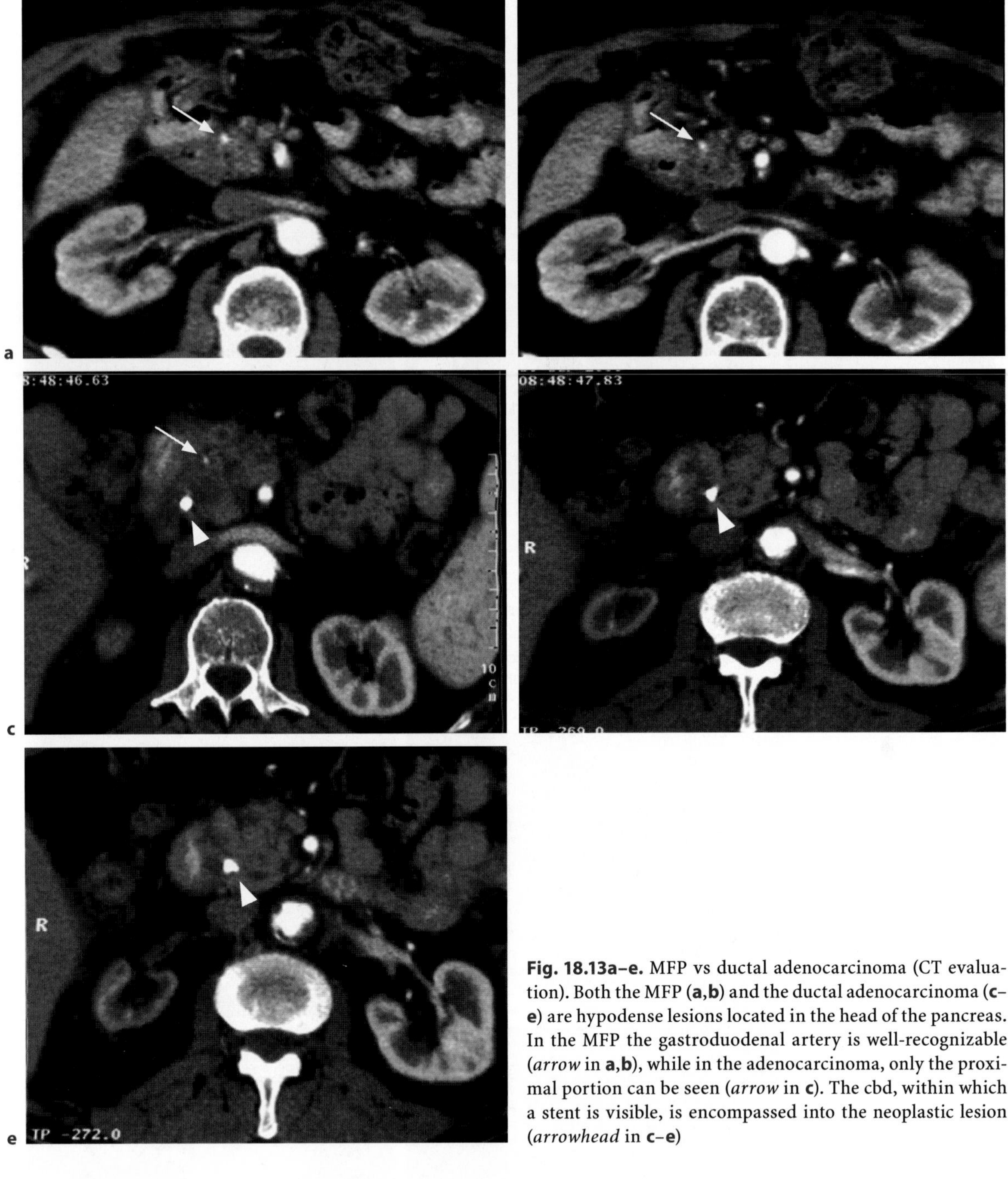

Fig. 18.13a–e. MFP vs ductal adenocarcinoma (CT evaluation). Both the MFP (**a**,**b**) and the ductal adenocarcinoma (**c**–**e**) are hypodense lesions located in the head of the pancreas. In the MFP the gastroduodenal artery is well-recognizable (*arrow* in **a**,**b**), while in the adenocarcinoma, only the proximal portion can be seen (*arrow* in **c**). The cbd, within which a stent is visible, is encompassed into the neoplastic lesion (*arrowhead* in **c**–**e**)

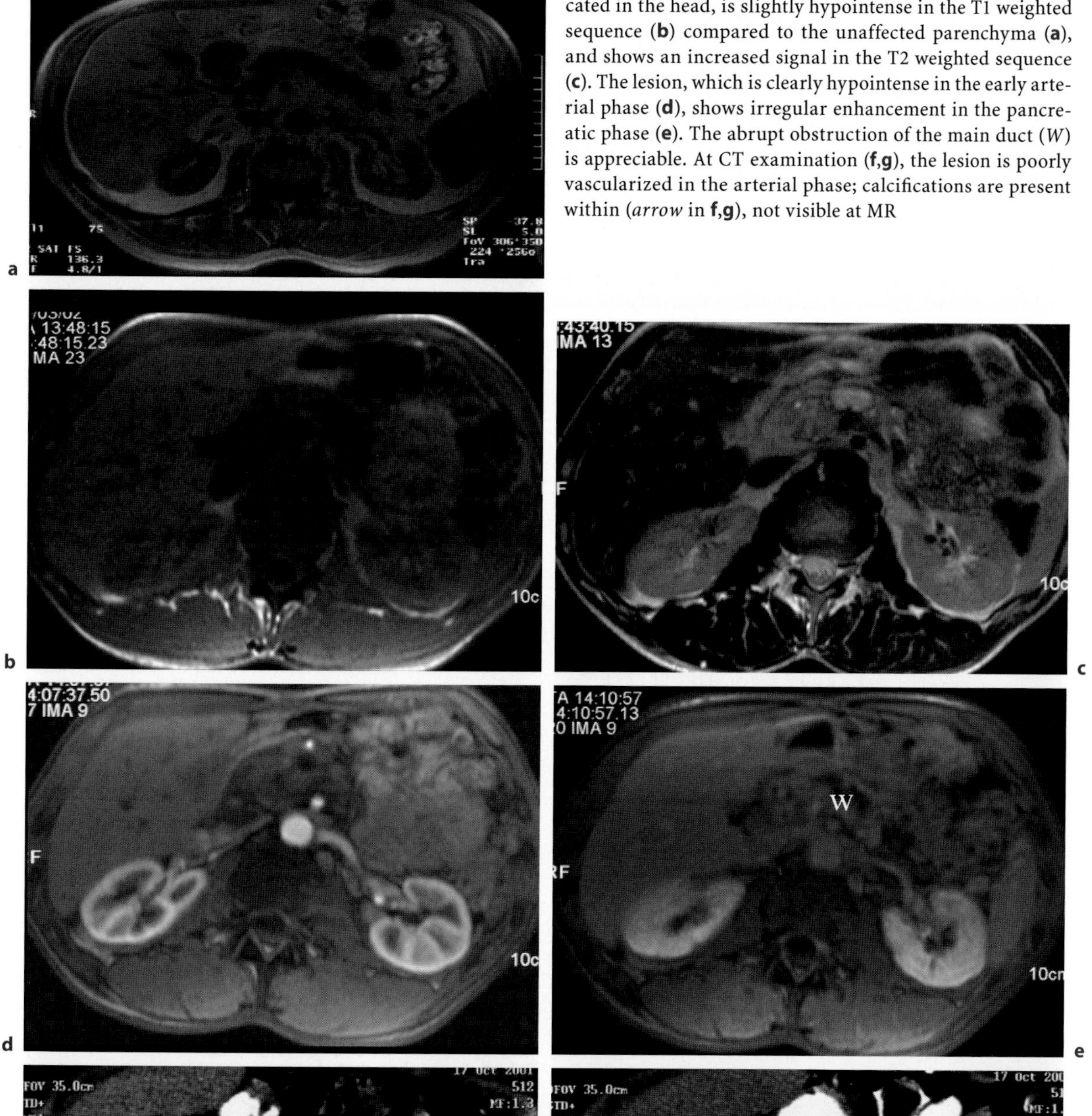

Fig. 18.14a–g. MFP (MR and CT evaluation). The MFP, located in the head, is slightly hypointense in the T1 weighted sequence (**b**) compared to the unaffected parenchyma (**a**), and shows an increased signal in the T2 weighted sequence (**c**). The lesion, which is clearly hypointense in the early arterial phase (**d**), shows irregular enhancement in the pancreatic phase (**e**). The abrupt obstruction of the main duct (*W*) is appreciable. At CT examination (**f,g**), the lesion is poorly vascularized in the arterial phase; calcifications are present within (*arrow* in **f,g**), not visible at MR

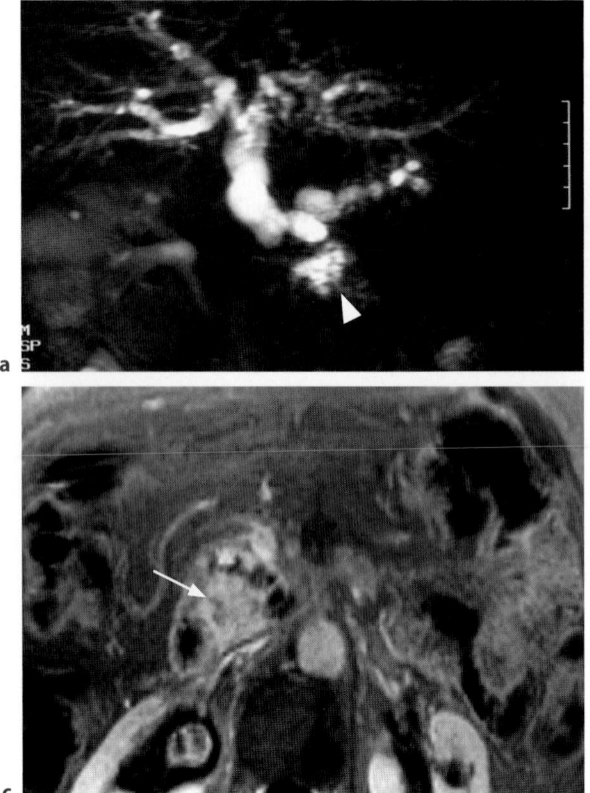

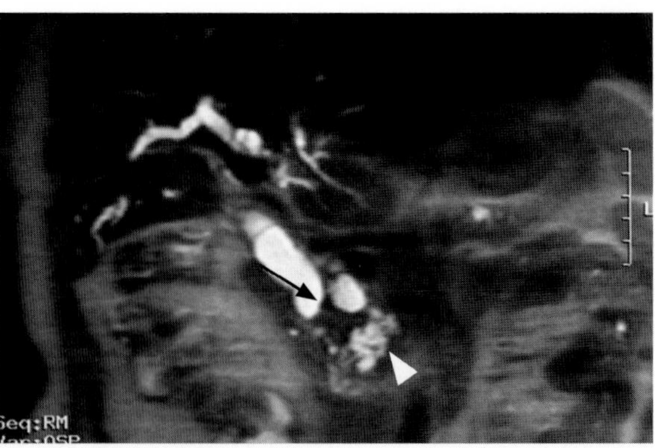

Fig. 18.15a–c. Ductal adenocarcinoma (MR/MRCP evaluation). MRCP (**a**) shows the double duct sign and dilation of the branch ducts (*arrowhead* in **a**,**b**) which are displaced by the solid mass (*arrow* in **b**,**c**) showing irregular enhancement in the pancreatic phase (**c**)

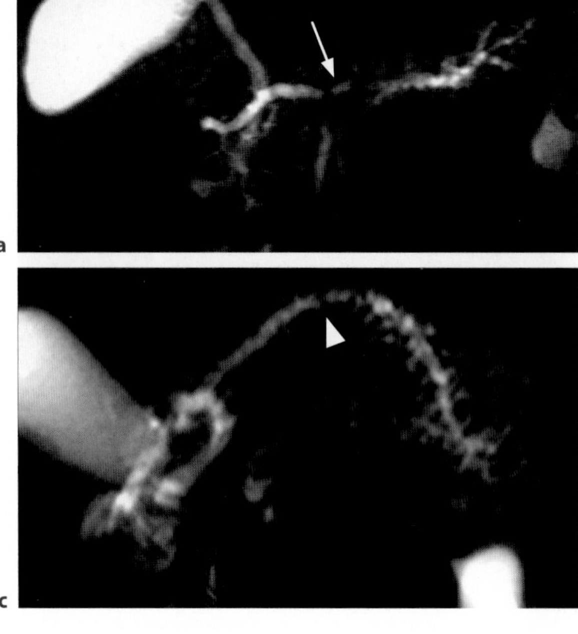

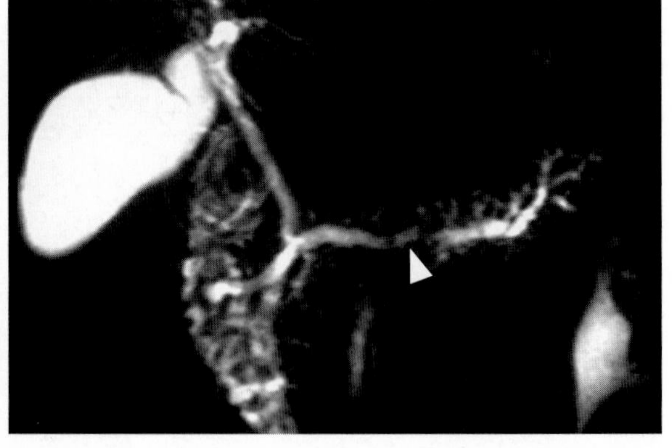

Fig. 18.17a–c. CP in pancreas divisum (MRCP evaluation). MRCP shows the presence of pancreas divisum with associated signs of obstructive chronic pancreatitis. Stenosis of the main duct can be seen at the body (*arrow* in **a**). After secretin stimulus (**b**,**c**), the stenosis becomes less evident (*arrowhead* in **b**,**c**) confirming its benign nature (duct penetrating sign).

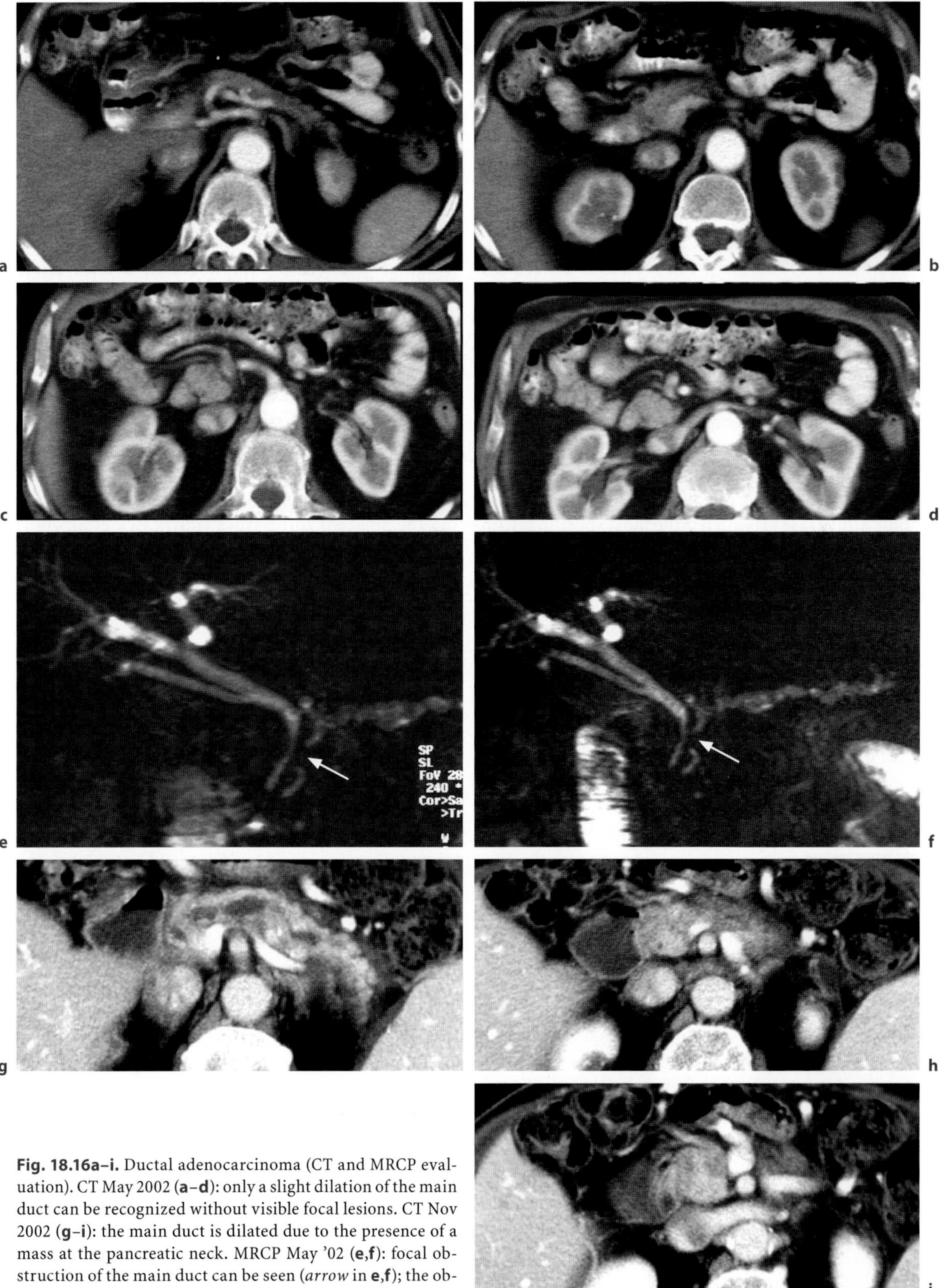

Fig. 18.16a–i. Ductal adenocarcinoma (CT and MRCP evaluation). CT May 2002 (**a–d**): only a slight dilation of the main duct can be recognized without visible focal lesions. CT Nov 2002 (**g–i**): the main duct is dilated due to the presence of a mass at the pancreatic neck. MRCP May '02 (**e**,**f**): focal obstruction of the main duct can be seen (*arrow* in **e**,**f**); the obstruction does not change after administration of secretin.

seco" by the lymphocytic infiltrate that plugs the glandular interstices. The gland appears to be surrounded by a wall made up of lympho-monocytic cells that, when found at imaging, are responsible for a imaging sign known as "capsule-like rim" practically pathognomical of aCP (Procacci et al. 2001b). In the more advanced phases of the disease, the gland is completely replaced by fibrous tissue within which one may find calcifications or pseudocysts (Okazaki and Chiba 2002).

Clinically (Table 18.1), aCP is never associated with specific symptoms (Okazaki and Chiba 2002). It is often serendipitously during imaging examinations performed for other reasons.

From the laboratory point of view (Table 18.1), there are no pathognomic markers of aCP. However, laboratory signs of an ongoing autoimmune disease are frequent, such as an increase in the titer of antinucleus antibodies (ANA and ENA), of the rheumatoid factor (RF) and, above all, of CA II (human carbonic anhydrase II) which is the most specific serum parameter for aCP (Okazaki and Chiba 2002).

The focal form of aCP is indistinguishable from adenocarcinoma (Koga et al. 2002; Tabata et al. 2003). Whenever imaging suggests aCP one can consider steroid treatment for at least 4 weeks with a daily dosage of 5–10 mg of prednisone. In the case of aCP the volume of the "pseudotumor" will be drastically reduced or disappear completely (Procacci et al. 2001b; Taniguchi et al. 2003).

18.2.3.2 Differential Diagnosis at Imaging

When aCP involves the whole gland, diagnosis at imaging is straightforward. Difficulties arise whenever faced with a "pseudotumor" (Fig. 18.19). In this case the radiological findings (Table 18.1), that aid in diagnosing CP, are not always present. US, In focal aCP, intra-lesional calcifications (Koga et al. 2002) (both intra-ductal and intra-parenchymal), irregular dilation of the pancreatic branch ducts or pseudocysts, are infrequent. The portion of the gland affected by the autoimmune inflammation is replaced by inflammatory tissue and therefore loses its normal lobulationand displays irregular and unclear borders due to the presence of the peri-glandular wall inflammation (Furukawa et al. 1998). The thickening due to inflammation of the adjacent fatty tissue in this case can be misleading giving the mistaken impression of a large process infiltrating the adjacent soft tissues (Ichikawa et al. 2001; Irie et al. 1998; Servais et al. 2001; Taniguchi et al. 2001). Only when there are clear signs of extra-pancreatic invasion or vessel involvement can aCP be definitively excluded (Fig. 18.20).

On the other hand, when facing the picture of a solid focal lesion of the pancreas without calcification and perhaps accompanied by homogeneous dilation upstream of the MPD, the diagnostic suspicion must be of adenocarcinoma until proved otherwise.

Table 18.1. Clinical-Laboratory-Radiological characteristics of aCP

Laboratory	Serum increase of pancreatic enzymes in Pts. with no or mild symptoms
	Eosinophilia
	Serum increase of γ-globulin (IgG4)
	Presence of auto-antibodies
	Increase in the cholestasis indexes
Clinical	Absence of, or only mild, pancreatic symptoms
	Possible association with other autoimmune disorders (Hashimoto's thyroiditis, Sjogren's syndrome, insulin dependent diabetes mellitus, Crohn's disease)
	No past history of alcoholism
	Steroid therapy efficiency
Imaging	Diffuse enlargement of the pancreatic gland
	Diffuse and irregular narrowing of the main duct
	Diffuse glandular and peri-glandular lymphocytic infiltration
	Dilation of the bile duct in the pre-pancreatic tract
	No pancreatic calcifications
	Peri-pancreatic pseudo-capsule made up of inflammatory tissue (capsule-like rim)
	No pancreatic pseudocysts

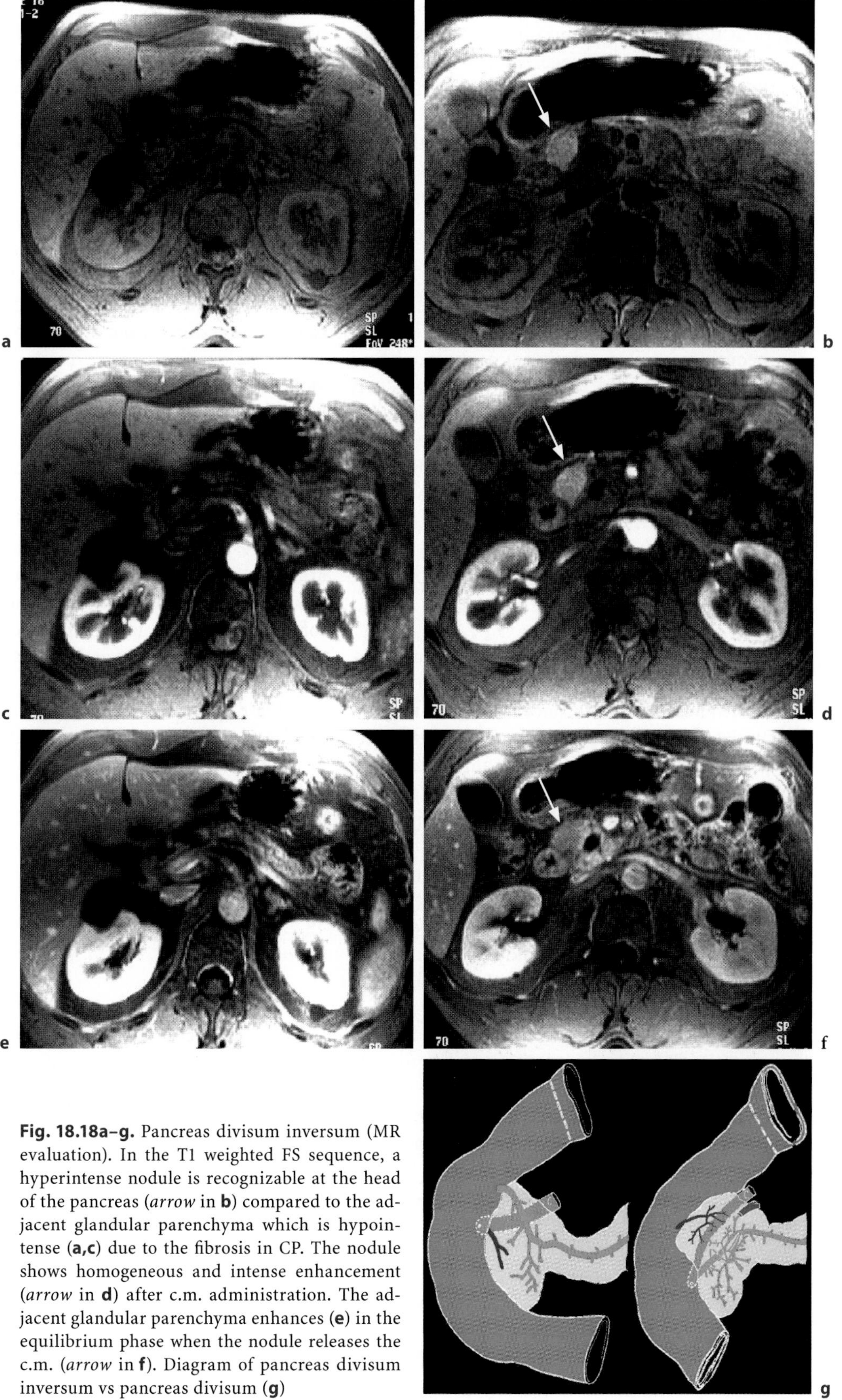

Fig. 18.18a–g. Pancreas divisum inversum (MR evaluation). In the T1 weighted FS sequence, a hyperintense nodule is recognizable at the head of the pancreas (*arrow* in **b**) compared to the adjacent glandular parenchyma which is hypointense (**a,c**) due to the fibrosis in CP. The nodule shows homogeneous and intense enhancement (*arrow* in **d**) after c.m. administration. The adjacent glandular parenchyma enhances (**e**) in the equilibrium phase when the nodule releases the c.m. (*arrow* in **f**). Diagram of pancreas divisum inversum vs pancreas divisum (**g**)

Therefore, in the case of diagnostic-clinical suspicion of aCP, in order to avoid unnecessary surgical resection, FNA is always suggested as it easily leads to a definite diagnosis (Fig. 18.21e). FNA can justify a simple follow-up of the disease, which, if treated accurately will no longer be recognizable at the next check-up (Fig. 18.21a–d). As stated above, a therapeutic trial of steroids may lead to the correct diagnosis.

18.2.3.3 Role of US

At US, the affected pancreas appears swollen and homogeneously hypoechoic mimicking adenocarcinoma (Ito et al. 1997; Koga et al. 2002; Taniguchi et al. 2001; Van Hoe et al. 1998). The MPD is not recognizable due to stenosis. In the cephalic areas is it not unusual to find co-existing dilation of the suprapancreatic CBD. It is likely that CE-US and EUS can provide a more refined characterization of the lesion.

18.2.3.4 Role of CT

The affected portion of the pancreas has no calcifications and is irregularly hypodense in the enhanced pancreatic phase, therefore, once again, it cannot be differentiated from a adenocarcinoma (Figs. 18.19d,e, 18.21a,b, 18.22b–d and 18.23a,d). The aforementioned "capsule-like rim", when present, is the only pathognomonic sign of aCP (Fig. 18.24). Its correct identification needs a multi-phase investigation of the pancreas. In the first phase, the inflamed wall looks like a hypodense frame while, in the late phase, it clearly and homogeneously enhances and is hyperdense (Fig. 18.24) compared to the glandular parenchyma which has lost contrast (wash out) (Irie et al. 1998; Koga et al. 2002; Procacci et al. 2001b).

The part of the main duct involved by the "pseudotumor" is almost always unrecognizable (Fig. 18.23c) due to the stenosis caused by the inflammatory process (Wakabayashi et al. 2003). Homogeneous dilation of the main duct upstream is rarely recognizable. Sometimes reactive lymphadenopathy is present in the peri-pancreatic, para-aortic and para-caval region (Fig. 18.22).

18.2.3.5 Role of MR

Focal aCP appears hypointense in T1-weighted sequences (Fig. 18.23b), and slightly hyperintense in T2-weighted ones (Robinson and Sheridan 2000). After paramagnetic c.m. administration, the lesion remains hypointense in the early phase with a slow progressive uptake of c.m. in the later phases (Ichikawa et al. 2001; Irie et al. 1998; Kim et al. 2001; Koga et al. 2002). The previously described "capsule-like rim" is also well visible in MR being hypointense in T2-weighted sequences with a weak enhancement in the late post-contrast phase (Irie et al. 1998). The use of MRCP sequences shows the irregularly stenotic segment of the MPD (Fig. 18.23c), and can precisely evaluate the extent and any eventual compression on the dilated cbd.

18.2.3.6 Role of ERCP

At ERCP in patients with aCP, one visualizes segmental or diffuse stenosis of the MPD (Horiuchi et al. 2002). Some authors maintain that the co-existing presence of segmental dilation of the pancreatic branch ducts favors the diagnosis of neoplasm (Karasawa et al. 1983). As previously mentioned for MRCP, if there is a "double duct" sign and a solid mass in the head area, the first diagnostic consideration must be of a neoplasm even though the "double-duct" has been described in aCP (Bennett and Hann 2001; Van Hoe et al. 1998; Menges et al. 2000).

18.2.4 Cystic Duodenal Dystrophy (Solid Variant)

18.2.4.1 Introduction

Cystic duodenal dystrophy (CDD), also known as "groove pancreatitis", is an inflammatory process that arises within islands of ectopic pancreatic parenchyma located within the wall of the second duodenal portion (Claudon et al. 1988; Mohl et al. 2001; Procacci et al. 1997). The secretion of pancreatic juice without an adequate ductal system allowing drainiage, produces acute pancreatitis within the pancreatic rest(s). With variable latency, CDD causes obstructive chronic pancreatitis (Procacci et al. 1997).

At pathology, the wall of the second duodenal segment appears to be made up of various sized, multiple cystic formations (macrocysts or microcysts), surrounded by fibrous tissue. The more common

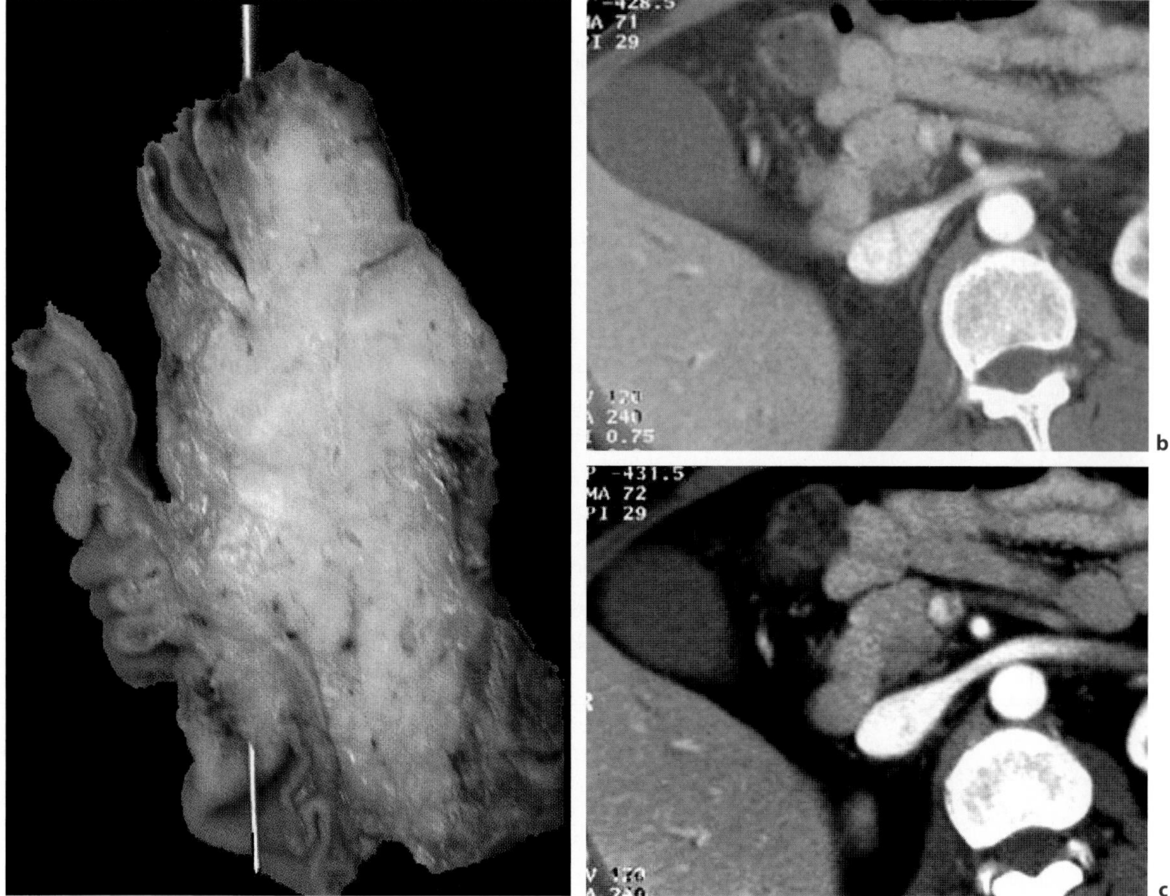

Fig. 18.19a–c. Focal aCP (CT evaluation).At the posterior edge of the head of the pancreas, a hypodense lesion (**b,c**) is recognizable which turned out to be an aCP after surgical resection (**a**) and which was absolutely indistinguishable in aspect from a ductal adenocarcinoma at imaging

cystic variant (about 65%–70% of cases) is made up of macrocysts (>1 cm in size).

The solid variant is composed of cysts with diameters at the lower limits of imaging resolution and for this reason it takes on a solid appearance. The two pathological entities can co-exist.

Fibrosis that results from the inflammatory process results in stenosis of the common bile-pancreatic duct outlet producing jaundice and relapsing obstructive acute pancreatitis (Vullierme et al. 2000). The inflammatory tissue itself can also cause narrowing of the duodenal lumen and obstructive symptoms.

Serum tests are (Table 18.2) the same as for CP, including the increase in pancreatic amylase and lipase to which can be associated any serum increases of the direct bilirubin, the transaminase and the γGT.

18.2.4.2 Differential Diagnosis at Imaging

The cystic form (Table 18.2) does not usually cause problems of differential diagnosis due to the typical location of the macrocysts and associated thickening of the duodenal wall. When the cysts are large, the complex can be mistaken for an intraductal tumor (IPMT) of the branch ducts (Fig. 18.25). Even if rather rare, adenocarcinomas, located in the groove region, can have a mixed solid and cystic component mimicking CDD (Fig.18.26).

The solid form (Table 18.2) appears at imaging as solid tissue located in the groove with characteristic fibrous “sheet-like” thickening (Figs. 18.27 and 18.28b,d). Both the location and appearance can be identical to adenocarcinoma (Fig. 18.28e,f).

Table 18.2. Clinical-Laboratory-Radiological characteristics of CDD

Laboratory	No correlation with the CA 19.9 plasma tumoral marker	
Clinical	Variable past history of prior pancreatitis	
Imaging	Located in the groove region	
	Fibrous, hypovascularized tissue	
	Frequent co-existence of radiological signs of CP	
	Anterior and leftward displacement of the gastroduodenal artery	
	Possible narrowing of the duodenal lumen	
	Possible displacement of the CBD and dilation of the intra- and extra-hepatic biliary tracts	
	Cystic variant	Presence of cysts with an average diameter larger than 1 cm in the duodenal wall
		The shape is more often elongated and bilobular
		The peri-cystic tissue is fibrous and hypovascularized
	Solid variant	Presence of microcysts (diameter <5 mm)
		Localized thickening of the duodenal wall, hypovascularized compared to the adjacent regions

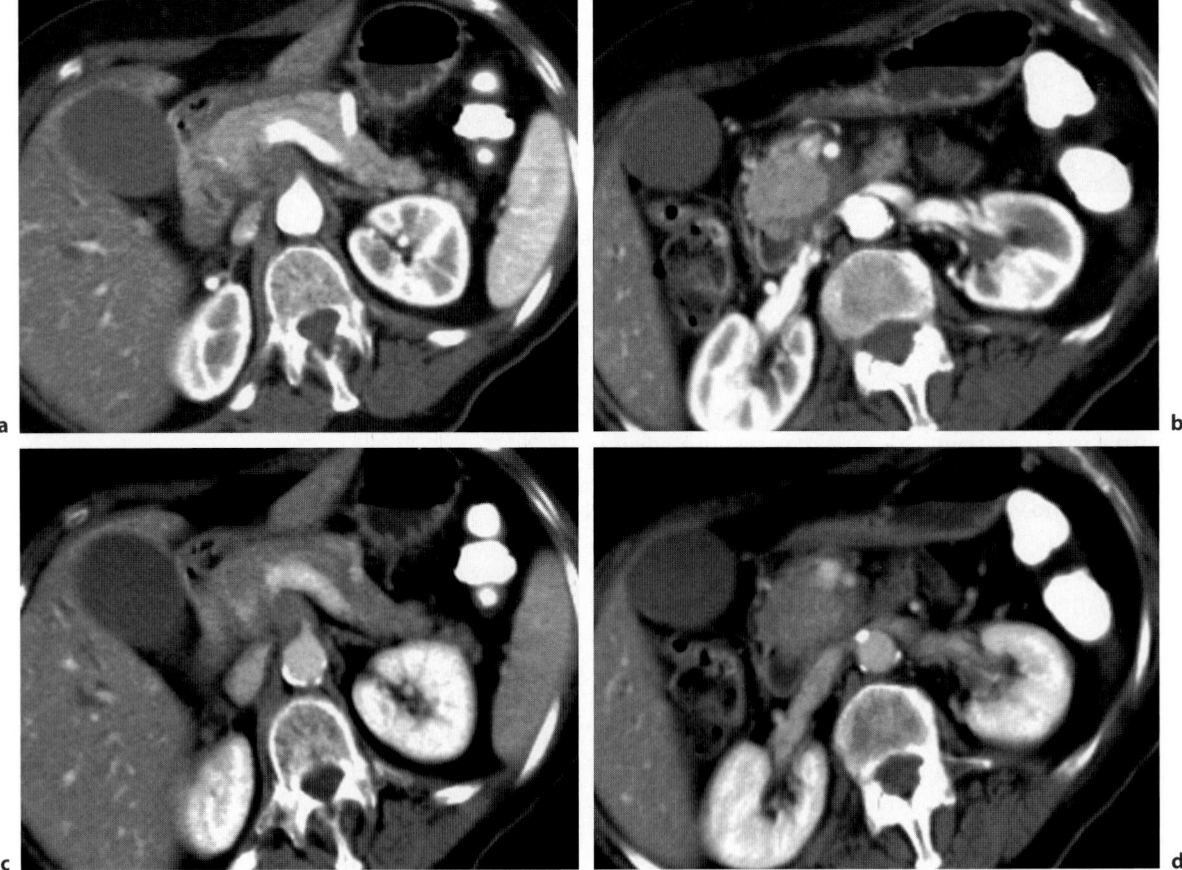

Fig. 18.20a–d. Ductal adenocarcinoma mistakenly interpreted as aCP (CT evaluation). Arterial phase (**a,b**); pancreatic phase (**b,c**). The head of the pancreas appears enlarged (**b,d**) with no evident change in its density. Along its posterior edge, a hypodense structure is recognizable (**a,c**), which turned out to be neoplastic tissue infiltrating the peri-pancreatic fat

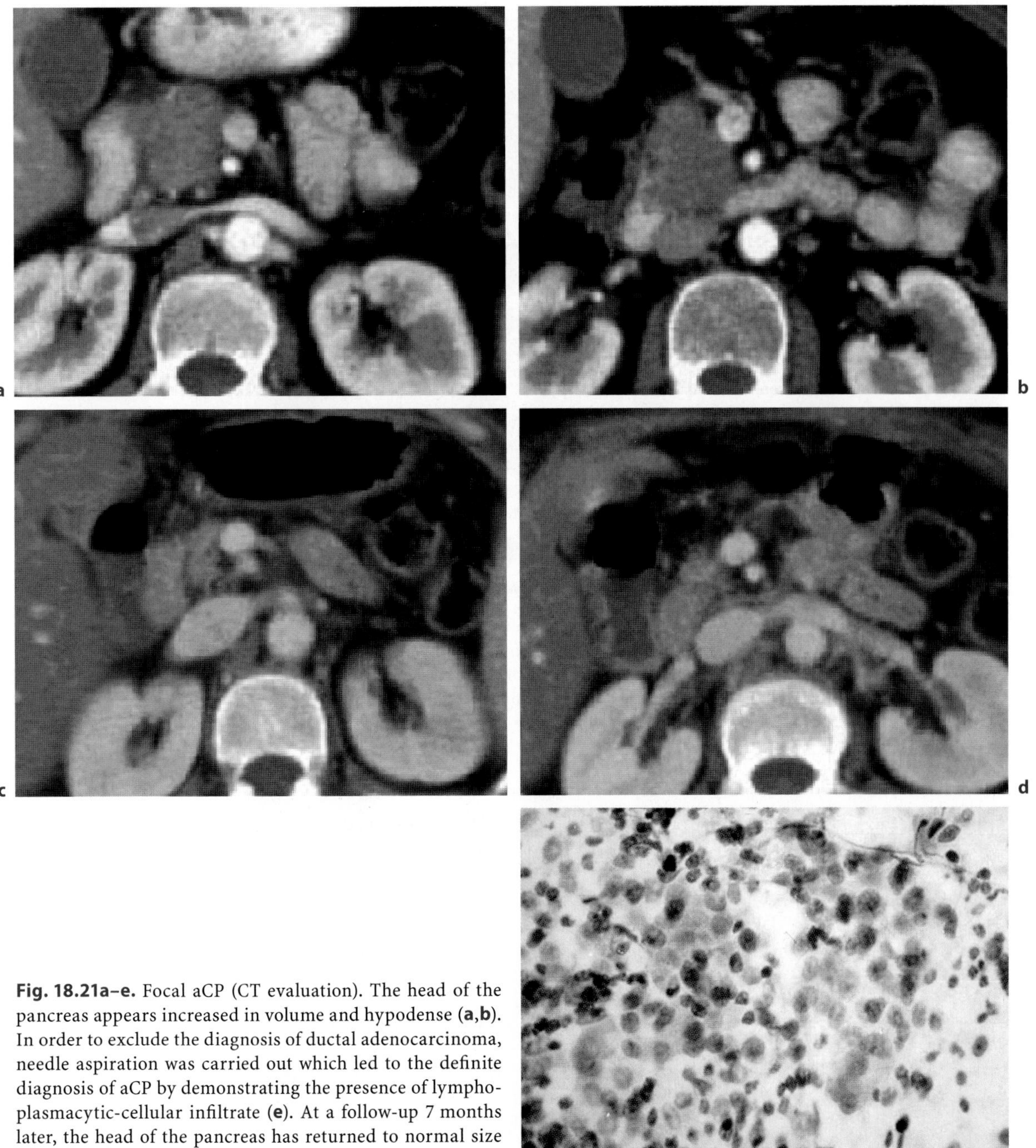

Fig. 18.21a–e. Focal aCP (CT evaluation). The head of the pancreas appears increased in volume and hypodense (**a**,**b**). In order to exclude the diagnosis of ductal adenocarcinoma, needle aspiration was carried out which led to the definite diagnosis of aCP by demonstrating the presence of lympho-plasmacytic-cellular infiltrate (**e**). At a follow-up 7 months later, the head of the pancreas has returned to normal size and density (**c**,**d**)

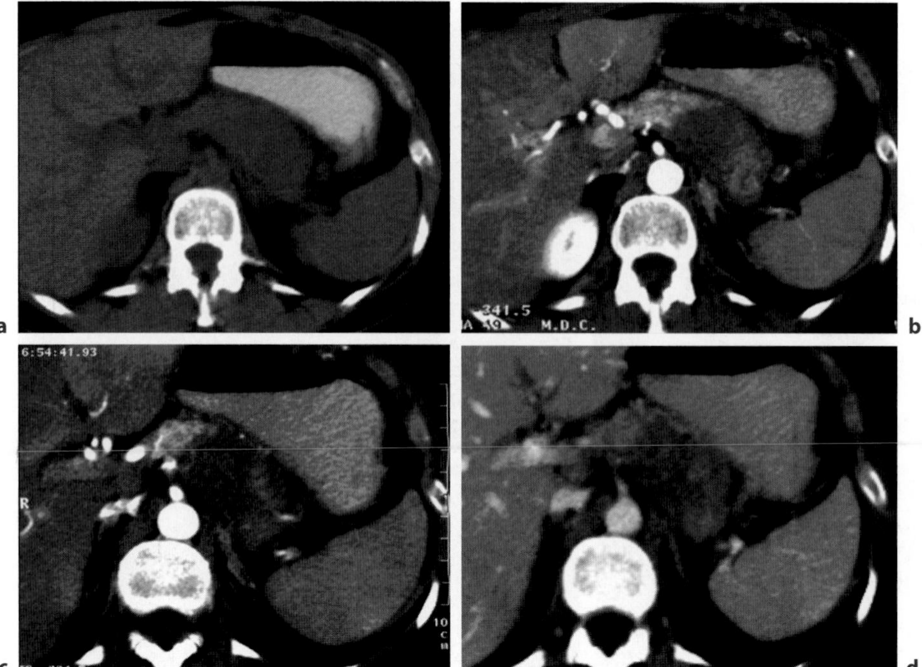

Fig. 18.22a–d. Focal aCP (CT evaluation). The disease can be suspected when focal enlargement of the gland is found. In this case the tail is involved showing really poor enhancement after c.m. Small nodes are present in the peri-pancreatic area (*arrow*). CLINICAL DATA: a 33-year-old male, affected by ulcerative colitis, recurrent abdominal pain, weight loss, Ca 19.9: normal, presence of anti Human Carbonic Anhydrase II Antibodies

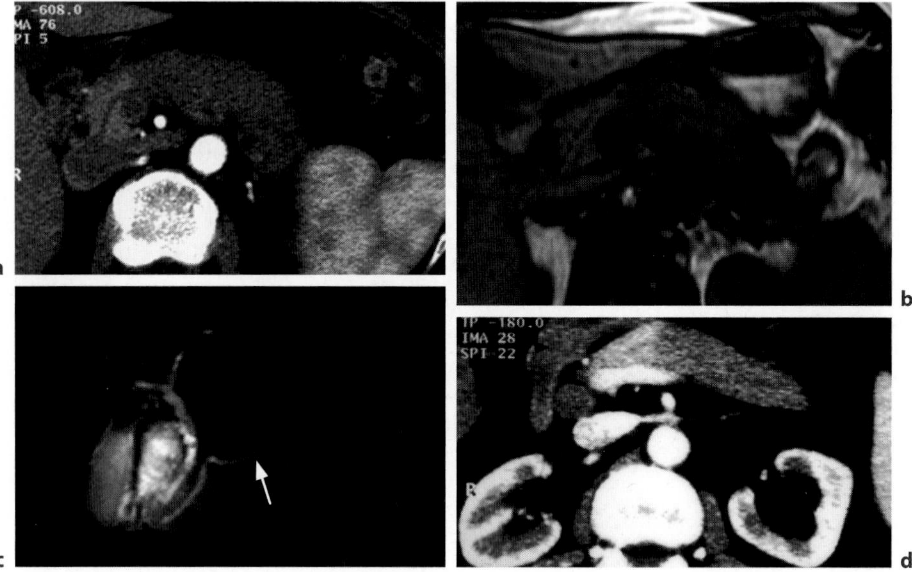

Fig. 18.23a–d. Focal aCP vs ductal adenocarcinoma. First case (**a–c**): Large lesion in the body-tail, hypodense at CT (**a**) and hypointense in the T1 weighted sequence (**b**). The mass compresses the main duct which cannot be seen in the body-tail at MRCP (*arrow* in **c**). Clinical data: a 37-year-old male, with ulcerative colitis and recurrent episodes of abdominal pain, Ca 19.9: normal. Conclusion: Autoimmune pancreatitis. Second case (**d**): The CT identical to the previous case. Clinical data: a 65-year-old male, persistent and deep abdominal pain, weight loss, Ca 19.9: 30,000 U/ml. Conclusion: Ductal adenocarcinoma

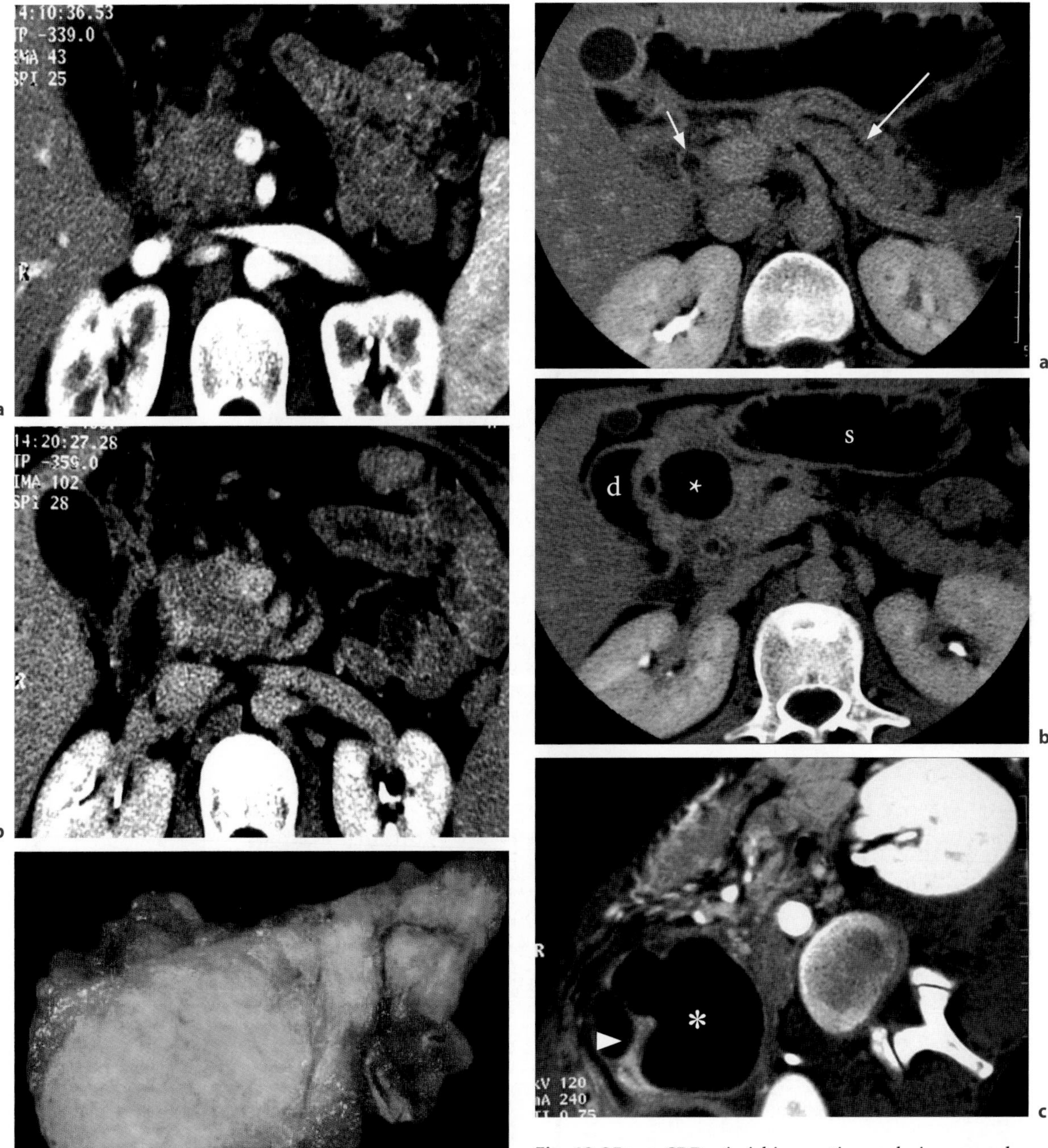

Fig. 18.24a–c. Focal aCP (CT evaluation). Focal enlargement of the head of the pancreas: the hypovascularized lesion in the pancreatic phase (**a**) has a hyperdense rim in the equilibrium phase (*arrow* in **b**). The patient underwent surgical resection of the lesion; cut section in **c**

Fig. 18.25a–c. CDD mimicking cystic neoplasia or pseudocyst (CT evaluation). Dilation of the main duct (*long arrow* in **a**) and the cbd is displaced to the left (*short arrow*); there is a cystic formation (*asterisks* in **b,c**) adjacent to the pancreatic head responsible for narrowing of the duodenal lumen (*d*), and gastric distention (*s*)

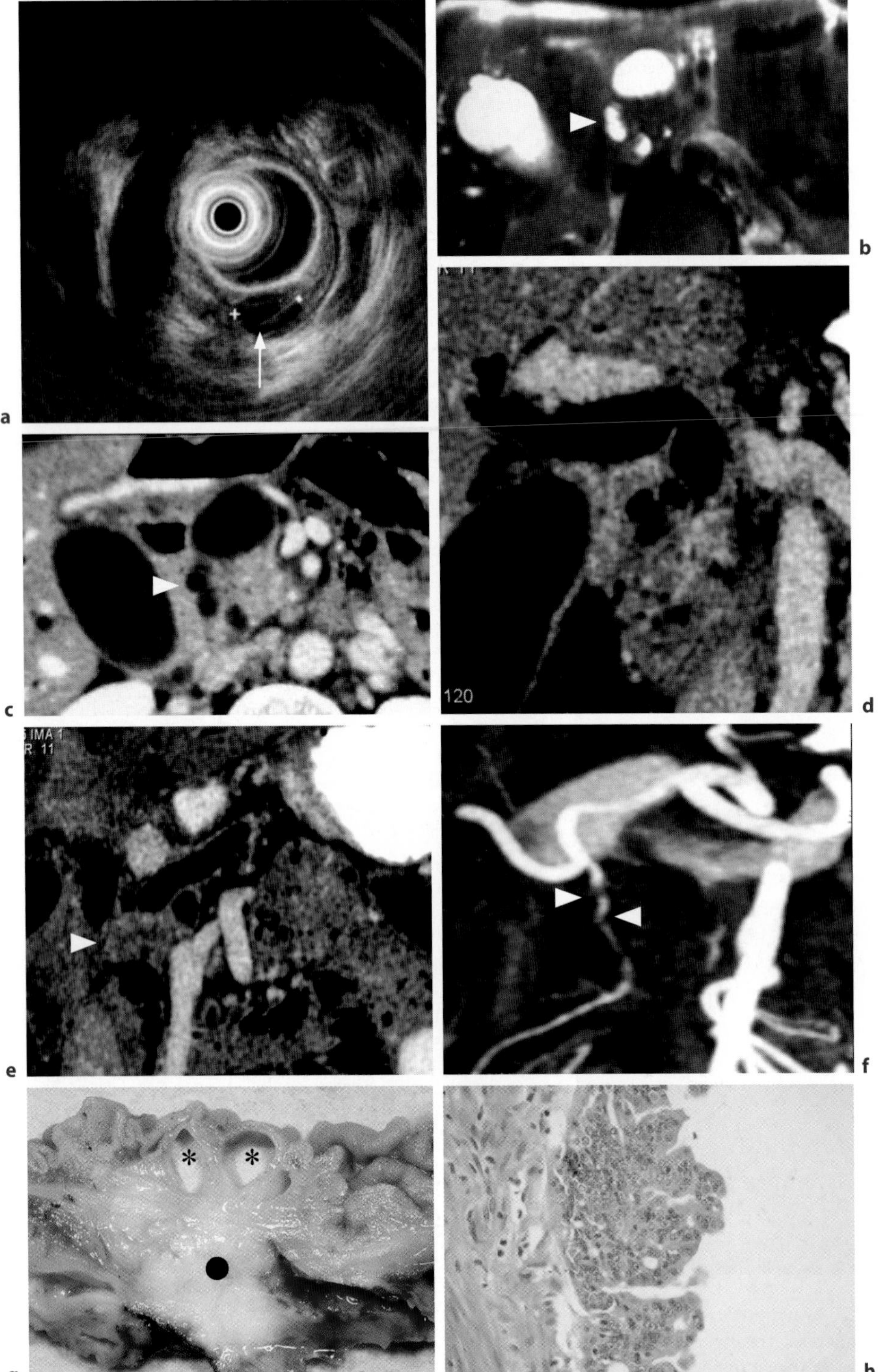

Fig. 18.26a–h. Ductal adenocarcinoma mimicking CDD (EUS, MDCT and MR evaluation). In the groove region, multiple cystic formations are recognizable (*arrowhead* in **b**,**c**), some of which are embedded in the duodenal wall (*arrow* in **a**). In the curved reconstruction (**d**), the cysts imprint the CBD. After c.m. administration, a nodule can be seen in the head of the pancreas which is slightly hypodense compared to the gland (*arrowhead* in **e**) and which causes the double duct sign (**e**) and infiltrates the gastroduodenal artery, the walls of which show multiple irregularities (*arrowheads* in **f**). The cut section (**g**) shows the cystic formations in the duodenal wall (*asterisks*) and the adenocarcinoma in the head of the pancreas (*dot*); histological analysis (**h**) confirms the presence of a mixed solid and cystic ductal adenocarcinoma

The position of the gastroduodenal artery can significantly aid differential diagnosis. Anterior and leftward displacement favors (Fig. 18.27a). The cbd can also be displaced to the left (Fig. 18.27b) if the duodenal wall has become considerably thick. Another finding to look for is the presence of a fatty cleavage plane between the solid mass and the pancreatic head (Fig. 18.27a).

"Groove" pancreatitis is almost always associated to obstructive chronic pancreatitis of the body-tail with the presence of typical parenchymal and ductal calcifications (Fig. 18.29).

18.2.4.3 Role of US and EUS

CDD (solid variant) appears as a hypoechoic expansive mass located between the head of the pancreas and the duodenal wall. Therefore, there are no distinct echo-structural elements visualized by transabdominal US compared to a adenocarcinoma. EUS, thanks to his high resolution, can identify tiny cysts inside the mass representing a useful sign for the correct diagnosis (Fig. 18.10b).

18.2.4.4 Role of CT

Under standard conditions and after c.m. administration, CDD (solid variant) behaves in the same way as pancreatic "groove" carcinoma (Gabata et al. 1994) being clearly hypodense, after c.m. administration, in the arterial phase, and becoming isodense in the late phase (Fig. 18.28a–d). In the early phase the fatty cleavage plane can sometimes be clearly seen, thus excluding the pancreatic origin of the large mass (Fig. 18.27a). In this phase the site of the gastroduodenal artery can be evaluated which, in CDD (solid variant) is displaced to the left (Fig. 18.27a), while in the case of an adenocarcinoma, is usually encased, irregular (Fig. 18.26f) or even obliterated by the mass (Fig. 18.13c–e).

When CP involves the head of the pancreas it also appears hypodense in both the arterial and pancreatic phases, the fatty cleavage plane no longer recognizabletherefore indistinguishable from a adenocarcinoma of the pancreatic head infiltrating the duodenal wall. In this case the definitive diagnosis is impossible and, in the majority of cases, can only be made on examination of the following resection.

18.2.4.5 Role of MR

Fibrosis in the duodenal wall, typical of CDD (solid variant), like adenocarcinoma, appears hypointense in T1-weighted sequences (Fig. 18.30d) but is iso to hyperintense in the T2-weighted sequences (Fig. 18.30a), depending on the amount of microcysts within. After intravenous paramagnetic c.m. administration the pseudotumoral mass appears hypointense in the early phase (Fig. 18.30e), and shows progressive enhancement in the later phases (Fig. 18.30b,f) showing the fibrous nature (Irie et al. 1998). This behavior, as for CT, is absolutely in-

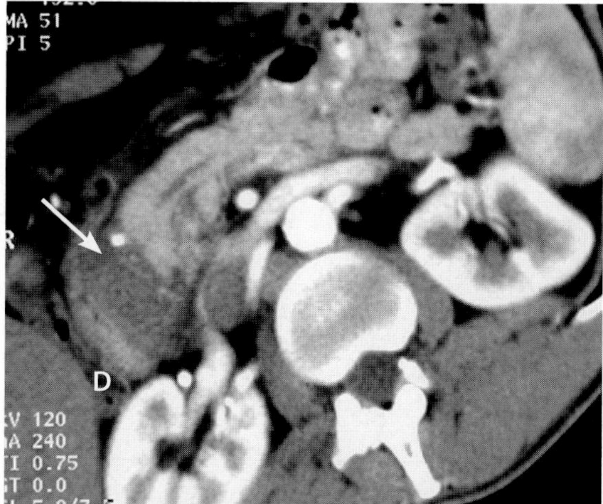

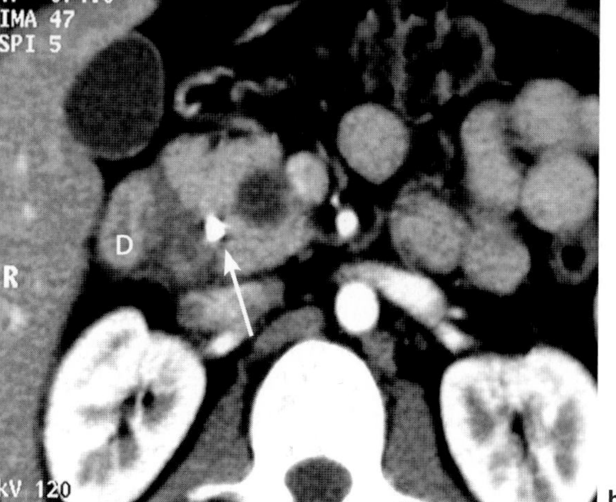

Fig. 18.27a,b. CDD (solid variant) (CT evaluation: typical findings). Recognizable sheet-like mass in the groove region separated from the head of the pancreas by a hypodense fatty cleavage plane. the gastroduodenal artery is displaced to the left (*arrow* in **a**), as is the cbd towards the left (*arrow* in **b**), away from the duodenum (*D*).

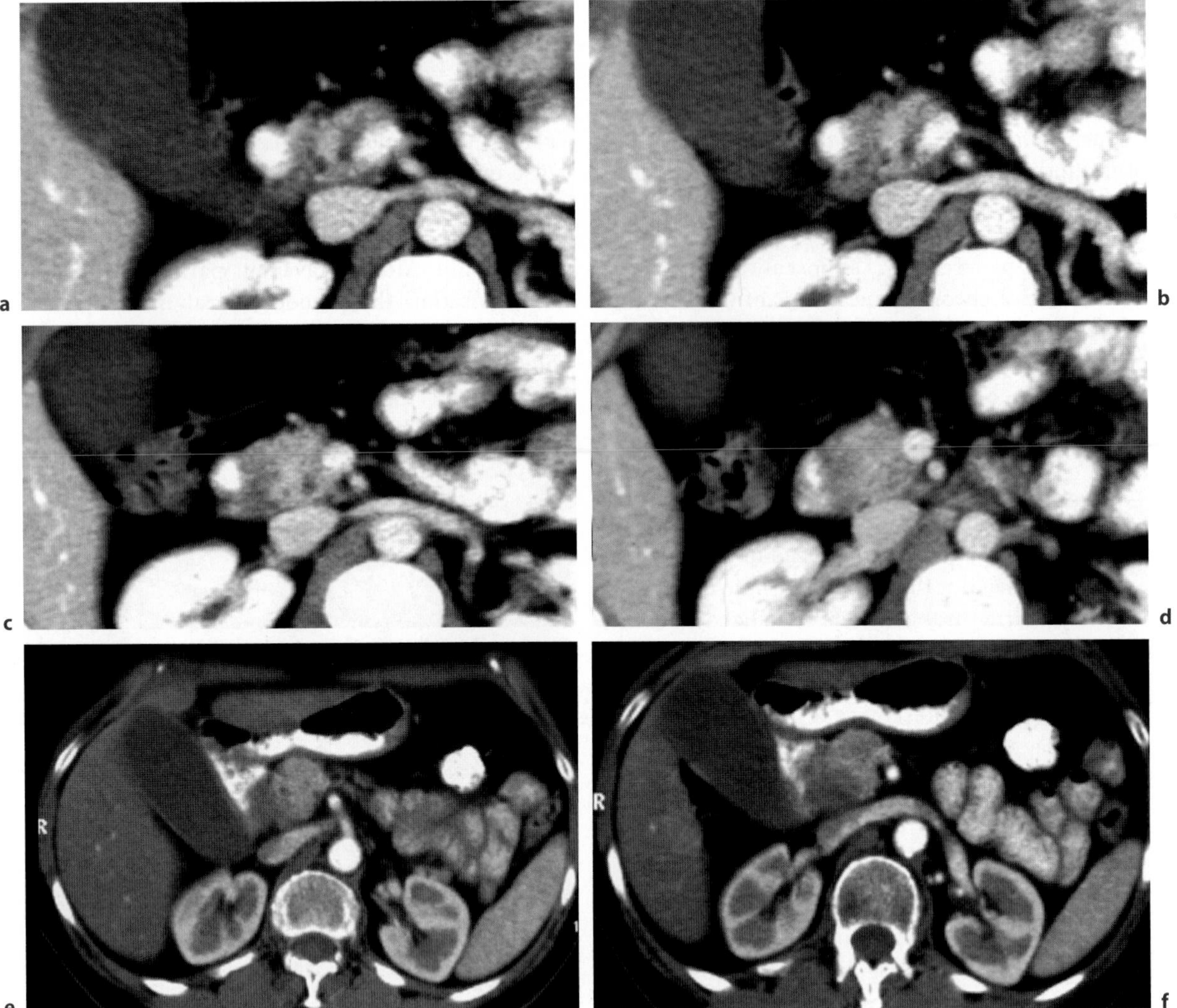

Fig. 18.28a–f. CDD (solid variant) (**a–d**) vs groove adenocarcinoma (**e,f**). Both lesions show the same hypodense sheet-like mass aspect in the pancreatic phase. In adenocarcinoma (**e,f**) the cbd is not recognizable due to its infiltration.

distinguishable from a adenocarcinoma. MR, more effectively than CT, on T1 fat suppressed sequences, can differentiate the normal pancreatic parenchyma of the head of the pancreas, which is hyperintense from fibrosis with its typical hypointense "sheet-like" appearance (Fig. 18.30d,e). In the same way as CT, it is possible to recognize the changes in position of the gastroduodenal artery.

At MRCP the dislocation of the cbd to the left is easily recognizable (Fig. 18.30a,c). In contrast, with adenocarcinoma, the cbd is in "normal" position, infiltrated and has an abrupt obstruction (Fig. 18.13c–e). Both "groove" pancreatitis and adenocarcinoma can produce the double duct sign that therefore is not specific (Fig. 18.28e,f).

18.2.5 Role of Nuclear Medicine

Positron emitting tomography (PET) is an advanced imaging technique for the diagnosis, staging and monitoring of a wide variety of processe – both inflammatory and neoplastic.

PET bases its specificity on the ability to identify an increase in the glycolysis in malignant cells (McGowan et al. 1995; Wahl 1996). The glucose analog, the 2-[fluorine-18] fluorine-2-deoxi-D-glucose (FDG), is the most widely used tracer in clinical PET and therefore in the study of pancreatic disease. The 2-[fluorine-18] fluorine-2-deoxi-D-glucose (FDG), metabolic analogue of glucose, collects inside the

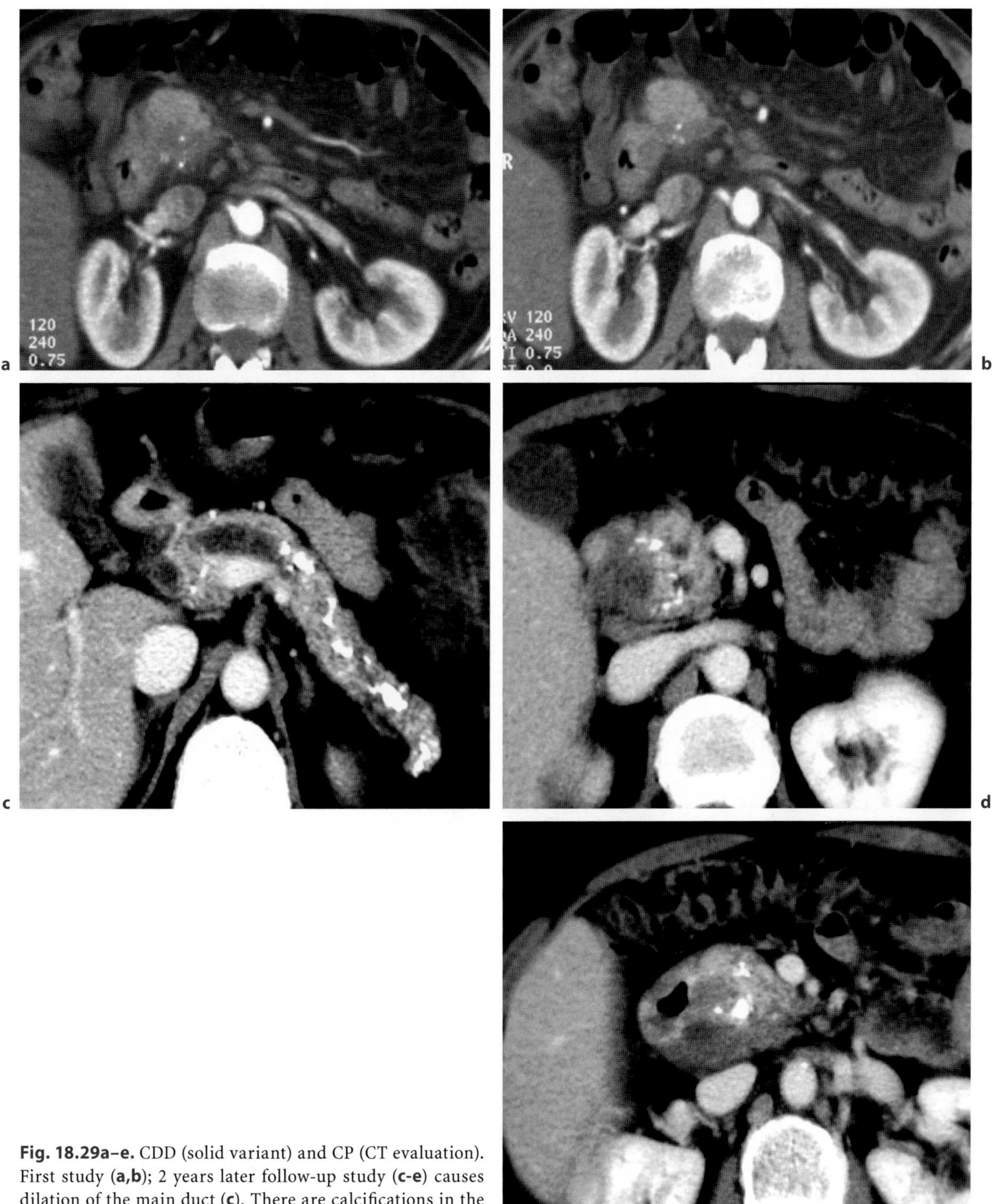

Fig. 18.29a–e. CDD (solid variant) and CP (CT evaluation). First study (**a,b**); 2 years later follow-up study (**c-e**) causes dilation of the main duct (**c**). There are calcifications in the duct (**c**) and in the gland (**a,b,d,e**)

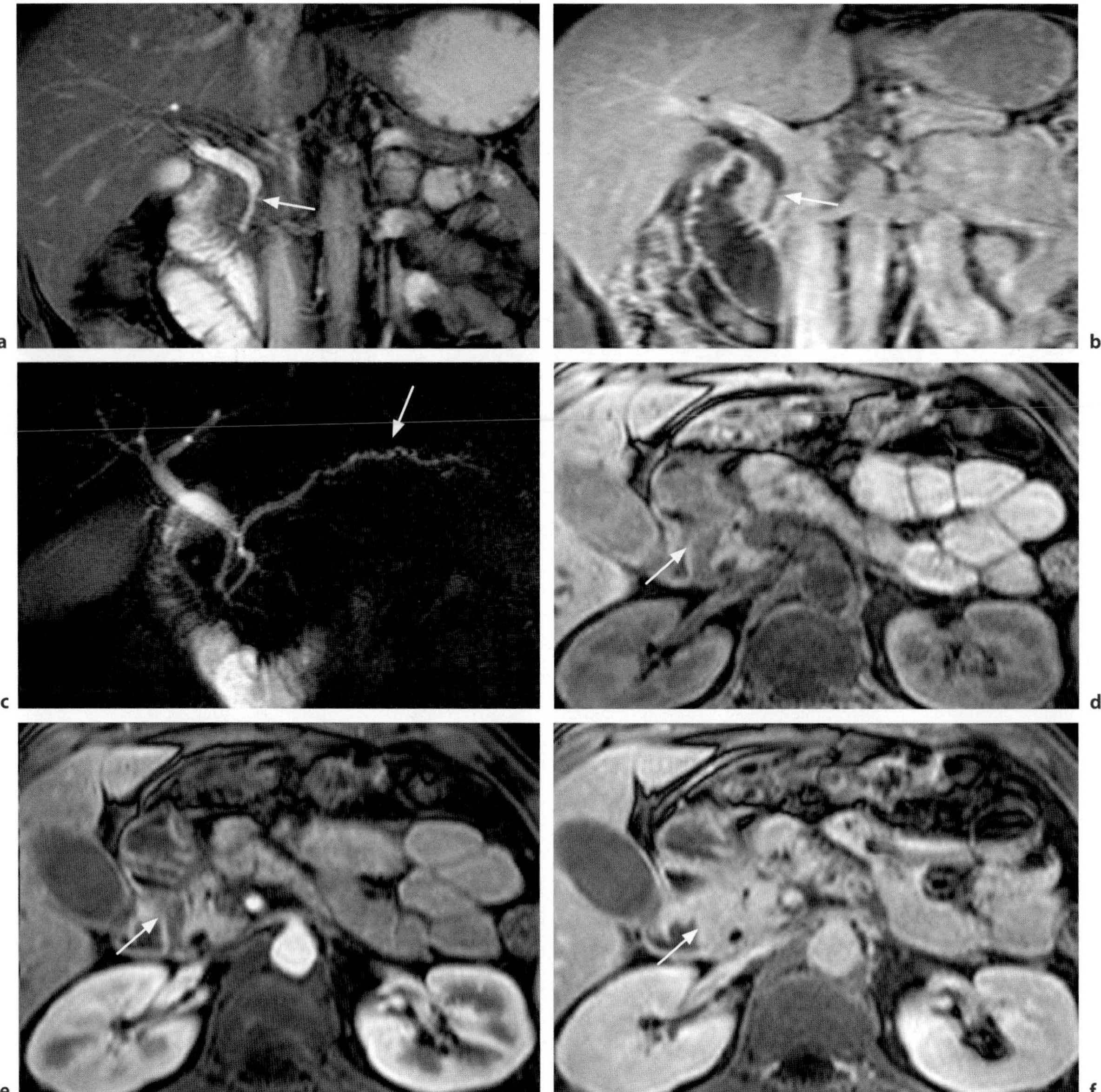

Fig. 18.30a–f. CDD (solid variant) (MR/MRCP evaluation). In the T1 weighted sequences performed in the axial plane before (**d**) and after c.m. administration (**e**,**f**), tissue thickening is recognizable in the groove with a sheet-like appearance which demonstrates progressive enhancement (*arrow* in **d–f**). The cbd is displaced to the left (*arrow* in **a**,**b**). At MRCP (**c**) the main duct is dilated with alterations of the wall due to CP (*arrow* in **c**)

tumor cells and is phosphorylated by the glycolysis in FDG 6-phosphate that, not being effectively metabolized, tends to concentrate in the target cells. This "metabolic entrapment" process of FDG 6-phosphate, is the basis for identifying pathological collections of the tracer. This technique is highly sensitive for identifying the tracer collection in the primary pathology site but is also just as sensitive for identifying metastatic foci, as it is possible to acquire images of the whole body in one single study session.

Recently, some authors (Reske et al. 1997; Higashi et al. 1998) have demonstrated how some glucose transporters (glucose transporter 1 GLUT-

1) are particularly over-expressed in pancreatic originating malignant cells, thus giving good reason for the potential use of this technique not only for identification, but above all for characterizing the pancreatic mass.

In the literature (Hanley and McNeil 1982; Inokuma et al. 1995b, Rose et al. 1999; Kubota et al. 1992; Jadvar and Fischman 2001), PET is thought to be a useful technique for pre-operative staging, post-operative monitoring and evaluating the effectiveness of chemo-radiotherapy (Nakata et al. 1997; Higashi et al. 1999) in tumors of the pancreas as it is able to demonstrate both pathological lymph node collections and distant metastases (Valinas et al. 2002). Its efficiency in making a differential diagnosis between an inflammatory process and a tumor is, however, not yet proven (Shreve 1998).

The tracer collection throughout the gland and in the fat surrounding the pancreas is a typical finding observed in acute pancreatitis. Clinical correaltion facilitates the correct appropriate diagnosis. Nitzsche et al. (2002) maintains that it is possible to distinguish inflammatory processes that show a homogeneous and diffuse tracer distribution throughout the gland from an adenocarcinoma where the tracer would tend to collect more focally, in greater quantities and persist in time. Clearly, in cases where CP and adenocarcinoma are simultaneously present, the problem of differential diagnosis goes unsolved. The same is true for focal CP (Shreve 1998).

18.3 Diffuse Dilation of the Main Pancreatic Duct

18.3.1 Introduction

In cases of CP, where the MPD has a "lake-chain" morphology, radiological diagnosis is reliable. If the MPD has a uniform and diffuse appearance, the diagnosis it is necessary to differentiate between the obstructive CP form (OCP) and ductal obstructions caused by juxta-papillary neoplasms of either the pancreatic head or duodenum. Even if a mass has been excluded, the possible presence of an intraductal papillary mucinous tumor (IPMT) of the MPD must also be considered.

18.3.2 OCP vs Ductal or Ampullary Adenocarcinoma

Identifying small juxtapapillary neoplasms (Fig. 18.31) that result in uniform dilation of the MPD, can prove difficult at imaging. With CT, in particular, the tumor may appear isodense (Prokesch et al. 2002) compared to the pancreatic parenchyma and is therefore difficult to identify, even after c.m. administration (Fig. 18.31). Furthermore, small hypervascularized tumors (endocrine tumors, metastases: Fig. 18.32a,b) responsible for ductal dilation upstream, can go unrecognized at CT (Fig. 18.32a) and at MR whenever the arterial phase is excluded. According to some authors (Minniti et al. 2003; Yasuda et al. 1995; Rösch et al. 1991), US and EUS are more sensitive than CT in identifying small, solid, ductal lesions (Figs. 18.31d, 18.32b and 18.33e).

MR seems to have the advantage over CT thanks to a better contrast resolution (Figs. 18.33c and 18.34a,c) and the possibility of using organ-specific c.m. (Schima and Fugger 2002; Rieber et al. 2000).

Therefore, when there is a ductal obstruction it is sometimes necessary to perform several Imaging techniques in order to exclude with certainty the presence of small-sized or isodense tumors at CT with the adjacent parenchyma.

The co-existence of dilation of both the cbd (Fig. 18.35) and the MPD strongly favors a diagnosis of neoplasm, although inflammatory disease can produce this finding in highly unusual circumstances. In these cases the use of ERCP together with biopsy is undoubtedly justified (Axon 1989).

Sometimes ductal obstruction can be sustained by stones located in the main duct outlet into the papilla. In this case, MRCP is the most sensitive and specific technique (Hintze et al. 1997) for diagnosis (Fig. 18.36) and ERCP plays a therapeutic role by allowing for extraction.

18.3.3 CP vs IPMT of the Main Duct

Once the presence of a solid mass obstructing the main duct has been excluded, the differential diagnosis takes into consideration obstructive CP on the one hand, and main duct IPMT. As well as ductal dilation, both pathologies produce atrophy of the glandular parenchyma (Ito et al. 2001; Warshaw et al. 1990) and stones, usually found in CP, but

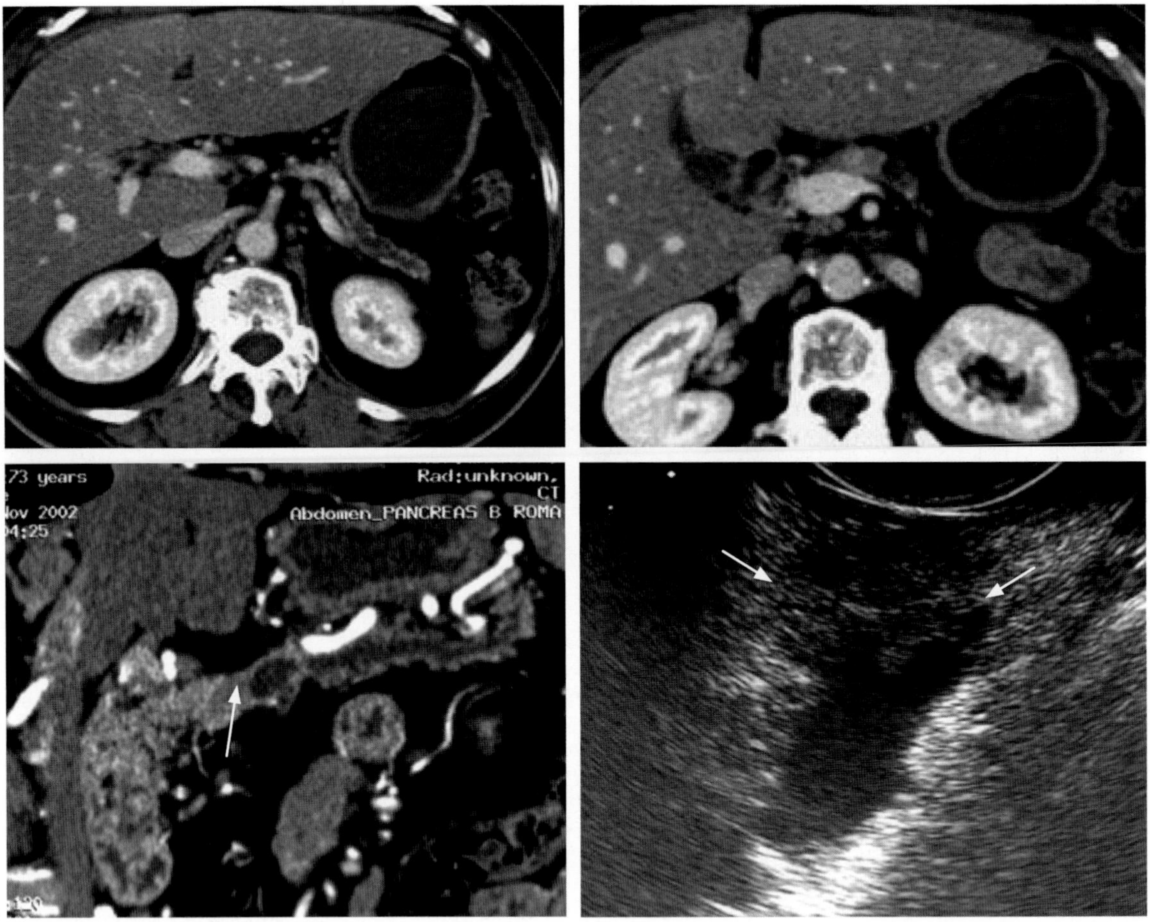

Fig. 18.31a–d. Ductal adenocarcinoma vs CP (MSCT and US evaluation). In the axial scans the dilated main duct is obstructed by the neck and no lesions are visible (**a,b**). The slightly hypodense lesion, obstructing the main duct, is only appreciable in the curved para-coronal reconstruction (*arrow* in **c**). The lesion can be seen better at US jutting into the dilated duct (*arrows* in **d**)

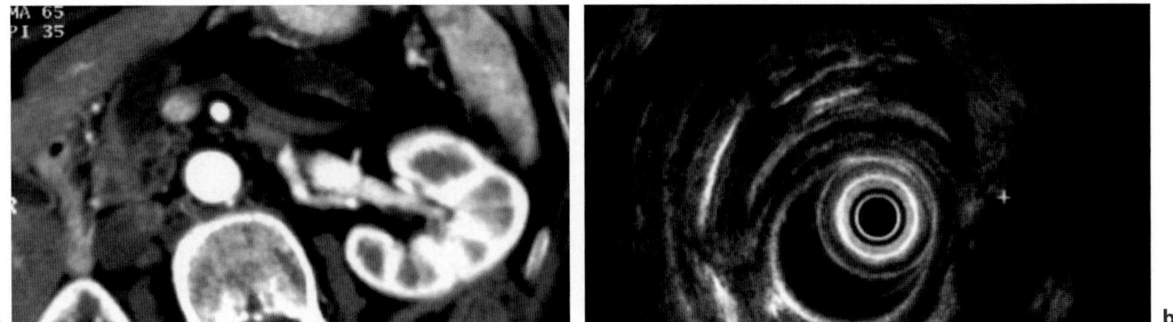

Fig. 18.32a,b. OCP vs solid neoplasm (CT and EUS evaluation). CT carried out in the pancreatic phase (**a**), shows dilation of the main duct without evidence of any mass. The presence of a solid lesion (metastasis from renal carcinoma) is demonstrated only with EUS (**a**)

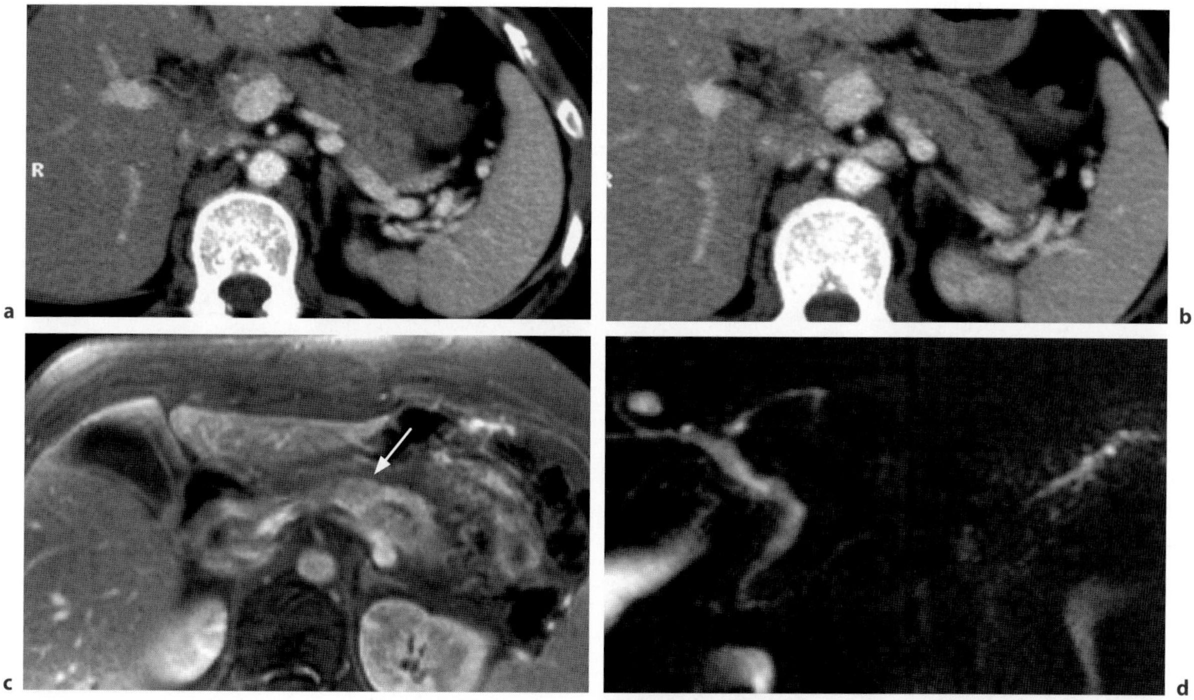

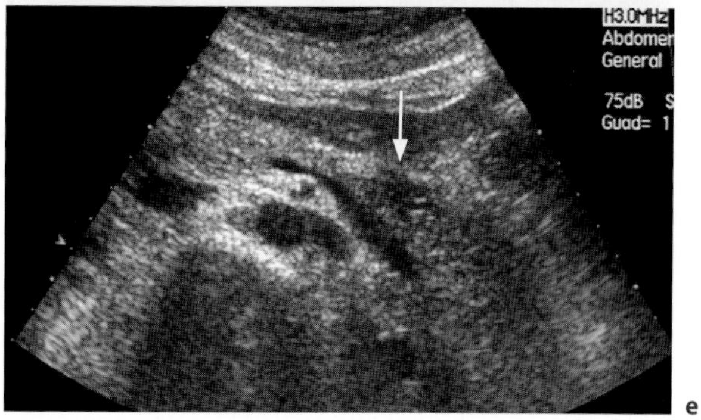

Fig. 18.33a–e. OCP vs solid neoplasm (CT, MR and US evaluation). At CT (**a,b**) only the irregular dilation of the main duct in the body-tail is recognizable with no change in gland density. MRCP (**d**) confirms ductal obstruction and, in the T1 weighted sequence taken in the equilibrium phase (**c**), an unclear, slightly hypointense lesion can be recognized (*arrow* in **c**). US clearly shows a hypoechoic lesion in the body of the pancreas (*arrow* in **e**)

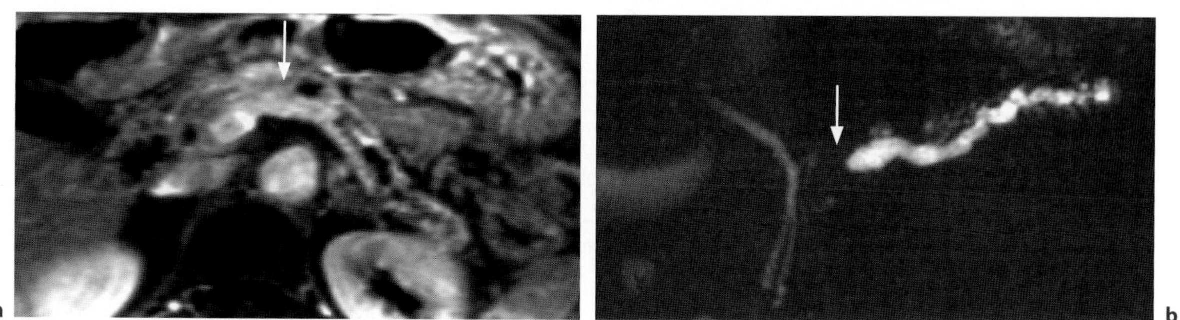

Fig. 18.34a,b. OCP vs adenocarcinoma (MR evaluation). FS GRE T1 weighted image in the equilibrium phase (**a**) shows a slightly hypointense mass (*arrow* in **a**) responsable for dilation of MPD and chronic obstructive pancreatitis upstream. MRCP (**b**) documents the abrupt obstruction of the main duct (*arrow* in **b**).

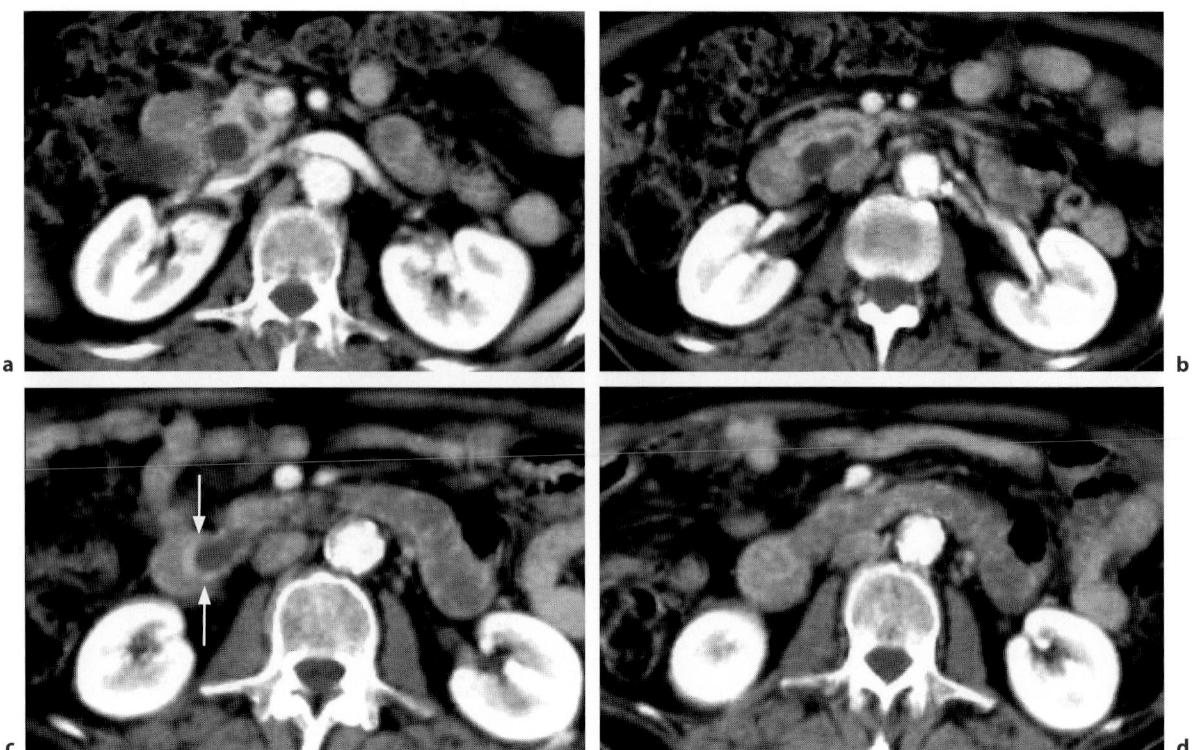

Fig. 18.35a–d. OCP vs adenocarcinoma of the papilla (CT evaluation). Axial CT sections show marked and uniform dilation of the main duct without mass (**c,d**) and with dilation of the major papilla seen protruding into the duodenum (*arrows* in **c**). The presence of the double duct sign (**a,b**) and the parietal enhancement suggested the correct diagnosis of periampullary neoplasm

which can also be present in IPMT and especially in the areas of chronic pancreatitis, secondary to ductal obstruction, or as precipitates of mucin collections (Procacci et al. 1999, 2001a). Protrusion of the major papilla into the duodenum is a critical sign for distinguishing between the two forms, as it is a pathognomonic finding of IPMT. Ampullary adenocarcinoma can also cause papillary protrusion into the duodenum but in this case enhancement can be recognized in the mass (Fig. 18.35).

IPMT must be diagnosed as quickly as possible as these tumors are potentially malignant and pancreatitectomy is the appropriate surgical treatment (Tenner et al. 1996; Kobari et al. 1999; Lim et al. 2001). If misinterpreted as CP, patients can be mistakenly submitted to a pancreatic-jejunal diversion. Over time, it is possible that the disease progresses to invasive carcinoma and by the time the correct diagnosis of an IPMT made, there is no therapeutic option (Fig. 18.37).

The patient's clinical history does not always help in diagnosis. 60% of cases of IPMTs have the same clinical symptoms as CP (McDonald et al. 2000). Differential diagnosis is easier if dilation of the MPD is found without a history of previous episodes of pancreatitis. However, definite diagnosis requires ERCP confirmation. Making a differential diagnosis between a segmental type IPMT (Fig. 18.38) and CP is often a challenge at imaging as the two forms are indistinguishable (Figs. 18.39). ERCP is the best technique in these cases and is able to demonstrate the eventual presence of mucin as well as to opacify the whole duct showing patency and/or parietal proliferations (Farrell and Brugge 2002). Sometimes ERCP cannot be diagnostic due to the abundant presence of mucin obstructing the duct or the excessive enlargement of the papillary orifice. In these cases, if the patient is sent for surgery, it is essential to carry out serial frozen sections on the resected specimen.

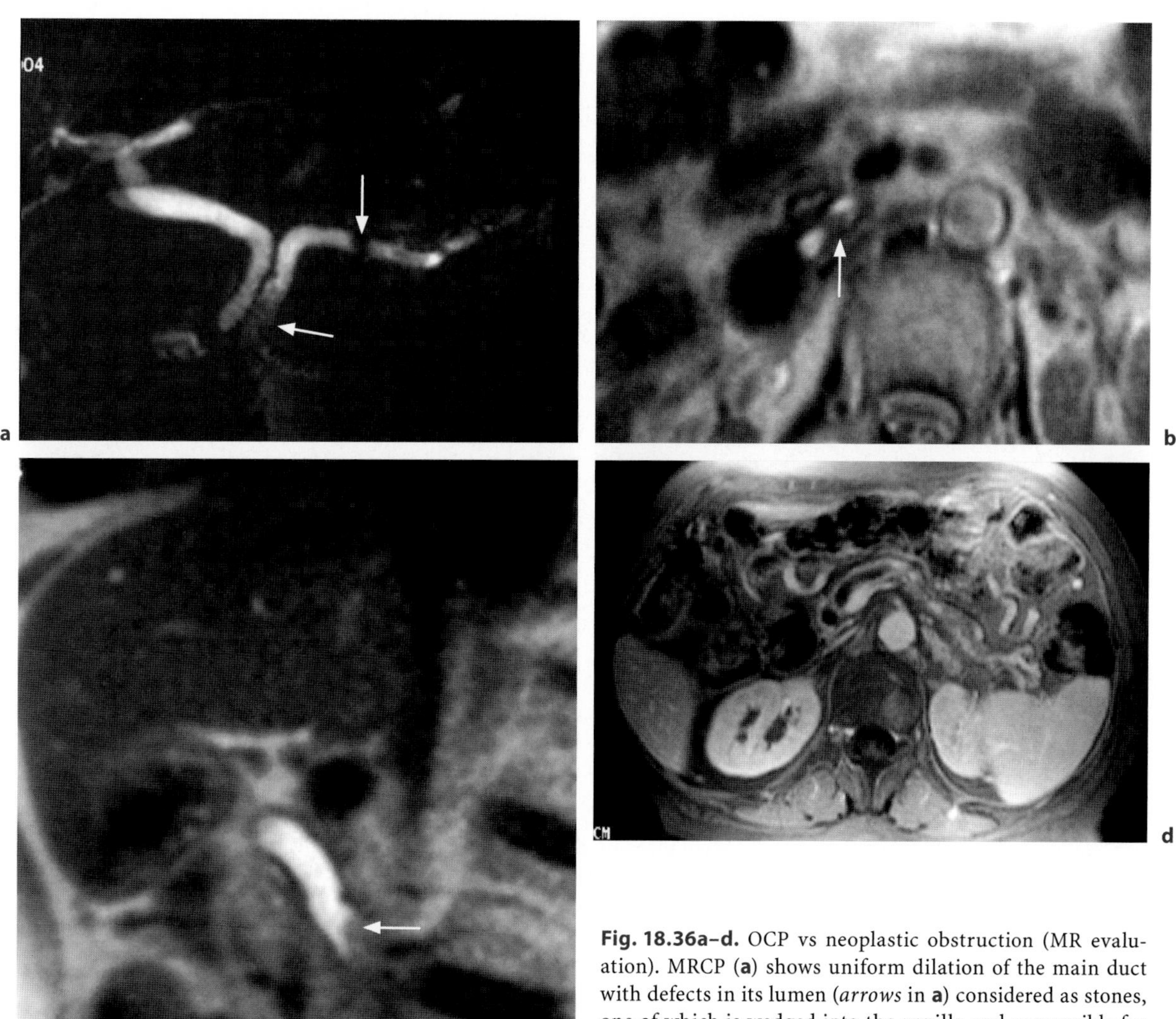

Fig. 18.36a–d. OCP vs neoplastic obstruction (MR evaluation). MRCP (**a**) shows uniform dilation of the main duct with defects in its lumen (*arrows* in **a**) considered as stones, one of which is wedged into the papilla and responsible for the obstruction (*arrow* in **b**,**c**). After c.m. administration (**d**), the absence of an mass lesion is confirmed

18.3.3.1 Role of US/EUS

Trans-abdominal US easily shows uniform focal or diffuse dilation of the MPD (Figs. 18.40) (Itai et al. 1987; Kaneko et al. 2001). Nevertheless, it is not always easy with this technique to establish the cause. While cystic ectasia of the branch ducts, a quite typical sign of the combined form of an IPMT, can be generally recognized, the same cannot be said of papillary proliferations (Kaneko et al. 2001) (Fig. 18.40a,b) or for the demonstration of the dilated papilla protruding into the duodenum (Fig. 18.40e,f) (Procacci et al. 1999). Mucin deposits may also not be easily recognizable with the exception of cases where they are particularly echoic due to the presence of calcium (Itai et al. 1987; Procacci et al. 1999).

EUS has led to promising results in the differential diagnosis between CP and IPMT, proving to be an accurate diagnostic technique in terms of type and extent of IPMT (Kubo et al. 2001) and is also able to demonstrate intra-ductal nodules. With this technique FNA of mural nodules and cytological sampling of the pancreatic secretion can also be performed.

The use of high frequency probes (15–30 MHz) allows for intra-ductal ultrasound examination that, even if it is an invasive and little used technique, is accurate in diagnosing IPMT due to its higher resolution.

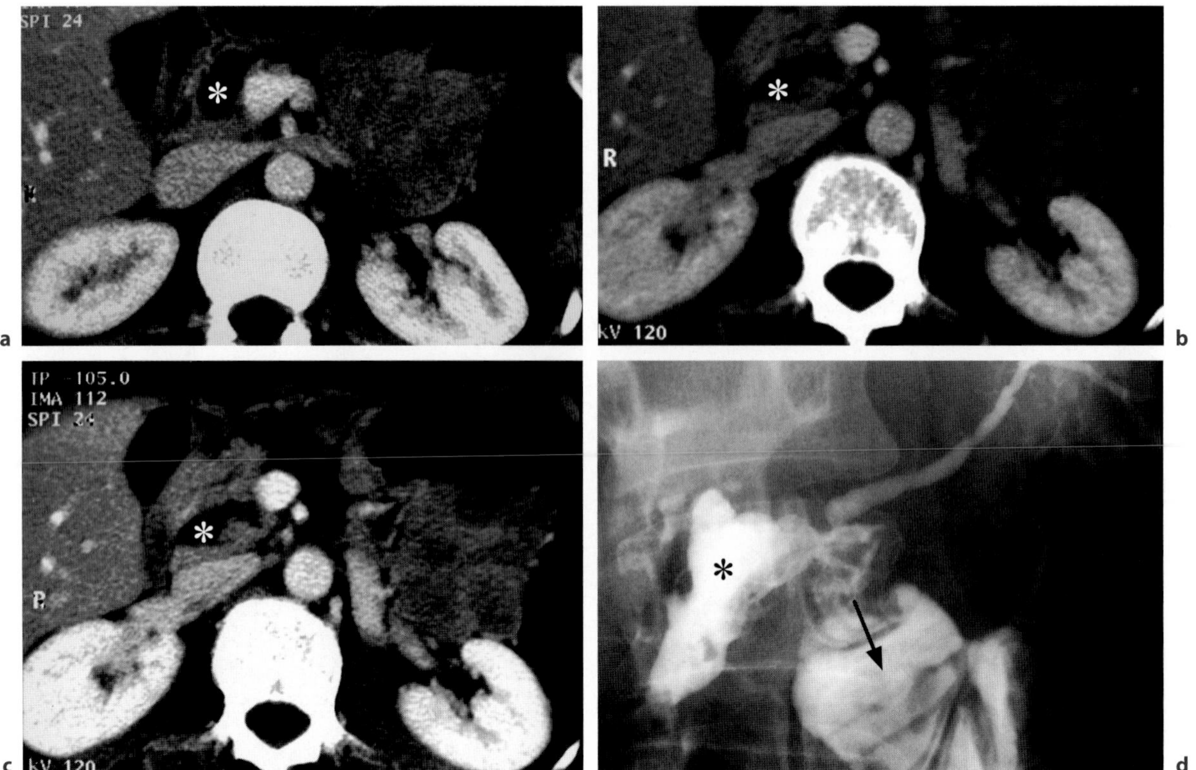

Fig. 18.37a–d. Mixed type IPMT (CT and ERCP evaluations). The CT scans (**a**,**b**) carried out in the iv contrast-enhanced pancreatic phase reveal cystic dilation (*asterisk*) of the main duct in the head and neck of the pancreas. ERCP (**c**) confirms the cystic dilation of the duct within the head (*asterisk*). This patient had undergone previous pancreatojejunostomy, and contrast material opacifies the jejunal loop

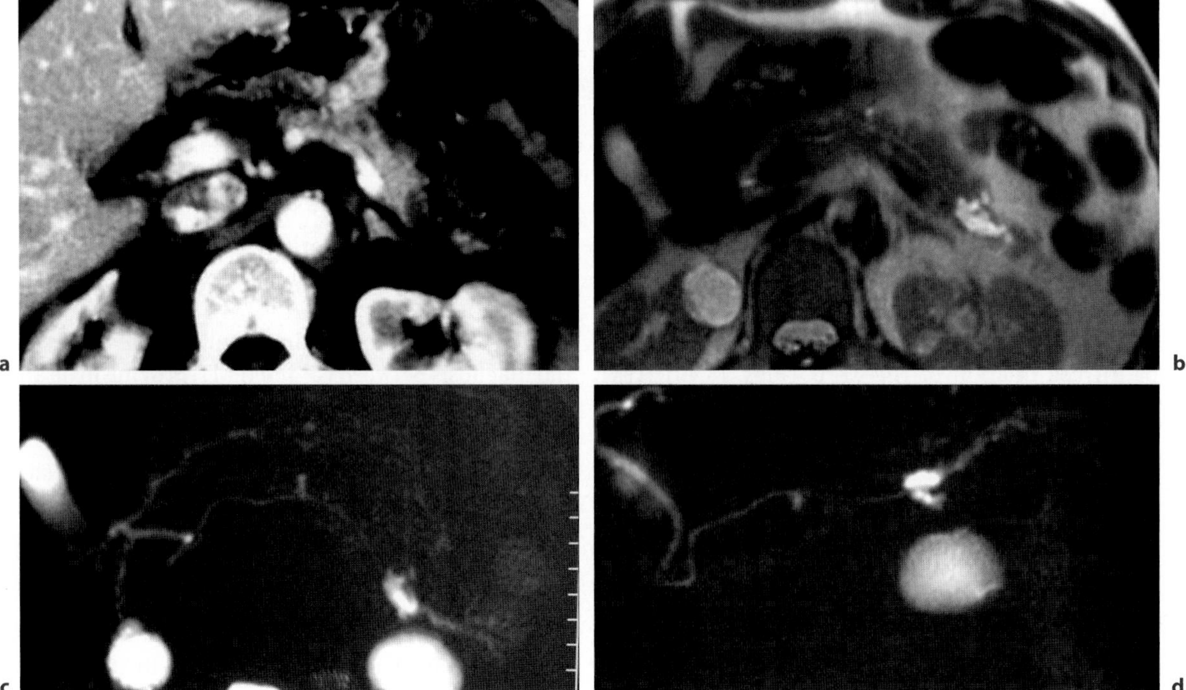

Fig. 18.38a–d. CP vs segmental IPMT (CT and MR evaluation). At CT (**a**) and MR (**b**) in the axial planes, dilation of the main duct is found in the body-tail. This finding is more evident at MRCP in the axial (**c**) and coronal (**d**) planes. The two pathologies are indistinguishable at imaging

18.3.3.2
Role of CT and MR

With current day CT and MR/MRCP, it is possible to recognize the following findings, the presence of which favors IPMT:

- Small nodulations and/or solid papillary proliferations of the ductal walls (Fig. 18.40b).
  These are seen more clearly with CT and MR after c.m. administation thanks to their enhancement. The presence of such nodulations suggests the malignancy of the tumor.
- Mucin deposits within the ductal lumen
  The content of an IPMT is usually homogeneous and is non-specific as displayed on different imaging techniques: hypoechoic at US, hypodense at CT, hyperintense in T2w and hypointense in T1w MR images (Koito et al. 1998; Sugiyama et al. 1998, Onaya et al. 1998). Thick mucin deposits are well visible especially with MR, as hypoin-

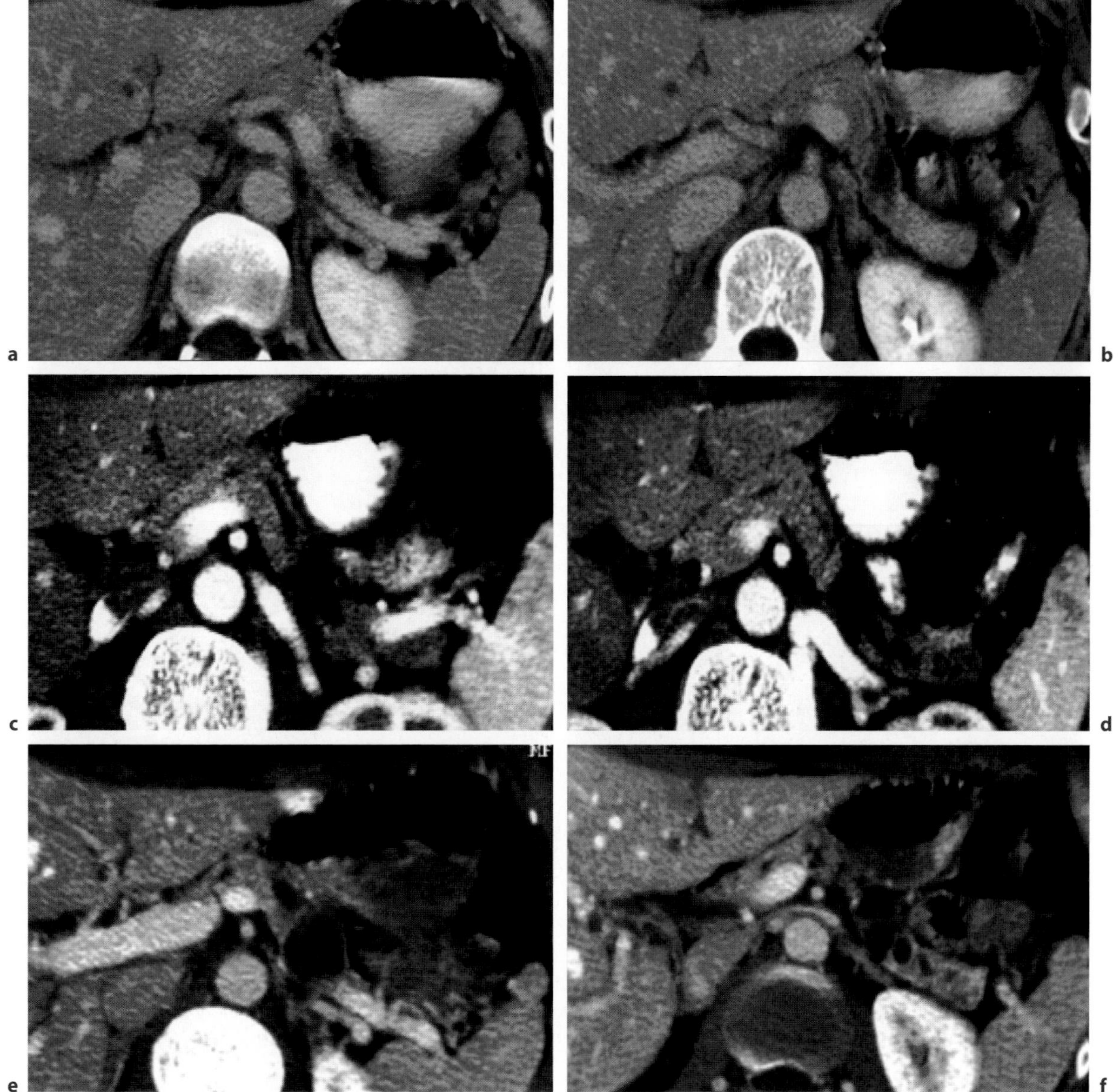

Fig. 18.39a–f. CP vs segmental IPMT (CT evaluation). Initially there is mild dilation of the main duct (**a**,**b**) compatible with segmental chronic pancreatitis. The diagnosis could have been suspected when the main duct became progressively larger in a relatively short period (**c**–**f**)

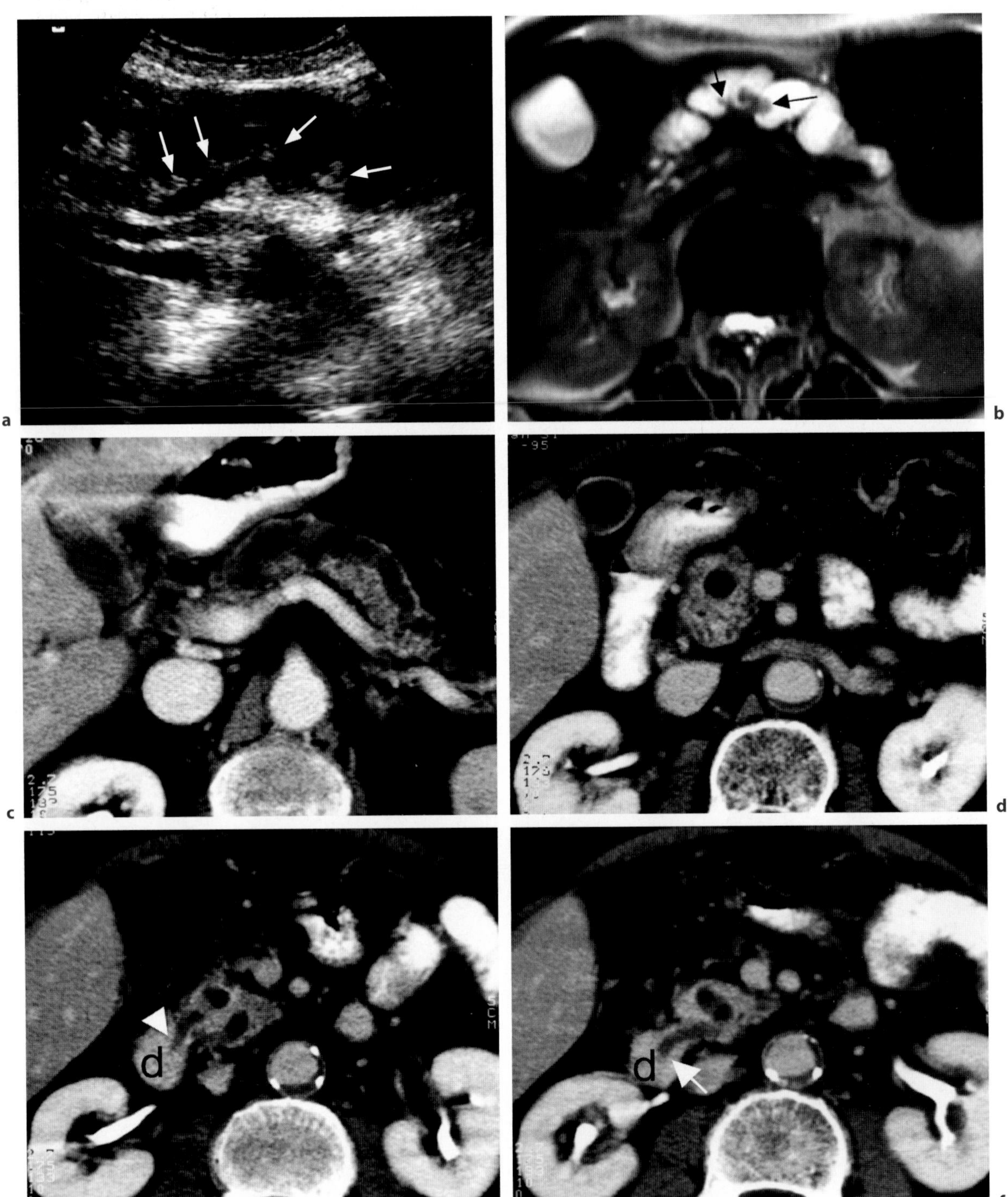

Fig. 18.40a–f. IPMT of the main duct (US, CT and MR evaluation). All the imaging techniques can demonstrate the typical signs of IPMT in the same way: uniform dilation of the main duct (**a–c**), parietal vegetation (*arrows* in **a**,**b**), ectasia of the branch ducts (**b**,**e**) and protrusion of the papilla (*arrowhead* in **e**,**f**) into the duodenal lumen (**d**)

tense defects in the T2w sequences. Sometimes at CT, it is possible to differentiate the mucin from papillary proliferations by changing the patient's position (Procacci et al. 2001a). Papillary proliferations inside the dilated duct are hypointense in the T2 weighted sequences (Fig. 18.40b) and, unlike mucin collections, enhance after c.m. administration (Irie et al. 2000).
Attention should, however, be paid in distinguishing such endoluminal defects from non-calcified stones that may be present in hereditary forms of CP, for example, in patients with cystic fibrosis.
Yamashita et al. (1998) has suggested the use of diffusion weighted MR sequences for differentiating an IPMT from CP. This is due to the lower diffusion coefficient of the mucin present in an IPMT compared to other fluids. However, there is no agreement to this in literature. In particular, in the more advanced stages of CP, the content of the ducts can be highly viscous due to the high protein content and therefore this also would be indistinguishable (Irie et al. 2002).

- Dilated major papilla protruding into the duodenal lumen (Fig. 18.40e,f).
  This finding is as well recognizable in CT, as in MR, during the pancreatic enhancement phase, before duodenal distension (Procacci et al. 1999).
- Cystic ectasia of the branch ducts.
  Although the branch ducts may also be dilated in CP, they do not usually take on a cystic morphology.

18.3.3.3 Role of Pancreatoscopy

Some authors (Nickl et al. 1991; Raijman et al. 1994) have recently maintained that the use of the pancreatoscopy is more effective than ERCP in differentiating CP and IPMT. Furthermore, with this technique the true extent of the IMPT can be evaluated better and it is also easy to distinguish between the small parietal proliferations and mucin collections (Nickl et al. 1991; Raijman et al. 1994; Kaneko et al. 1998).

Hara et al. (2002) propose the combined use of the pancreatoscopy and intra-ductal US in the preoperatory strategy of IPMT in order to differentiate benign and malignant forms.

References

Allema JH, Reinders ME, Van Gulik TM, Koelemay MJ, Van Leeuwen DJ, De Wit LT, Gouma DJ, Obertop H (1995) Prognostic factors for survival after pancreatico-duodenectomy for patients with carcinoma of the pancreatic head region. Cancer 75(8):2069–2076

Axon AT (1989) Endoscopic retrograde cholangiopancreatography in chronic pancreatitis. Cambridge classification. Radiol Clin North Am 27(1):39–50

Baker ME, Cohan RH, Nadel SN, Leder RA, Dunnick NR (1990) Obliteration of the fat surrounding the celiac axis and superior mesenteric artery is not a specific CT finding of carcinoma of the pancreas. AJR Am J Roentgenol 155(5):991–994

Baumel H, Huguier M, Manderscheid JC, Fabre JM, Houry S, Fagot H (1994) Results of resection for cancer of the exocrine pancreas: a study from the French Association of Surgery. Br J Surg 81(1):102–107

Becker D, Strobel D, Bernatik T, Hahn EG (2001) Echo-enhanced color- and power-Doppler EUS for the discrimination between focal pancreatitis and pancreatic carcinoma. Gastrointest Endosc 53(7):784–789

Bennet GL, Hann LE (2001) Pancreatic ultrasonography. Surg Clin North Am 81(2):259–280

Brand B, Pfaff T, Binmoeller KF, Sriram PV, Fritscher-Ravens A, Knofel WT, Jackle S, Soehendra N (2000) Endoscopic ultrasound for differential diagnosis of focal pancreatic lesions, confirmed by surgery. Scand J Gastroenterol 35(11):1221–1228

Cameron JL, Pitt HA, Yeo CJ, Lillemoe KD, Kaufman HS, Coleman J (1993) One hundred and forty-five consecutive pancreatico-duodenectomies without mortality. Ann Surg 217(5):430–435

Carter DC (1992) Cancer of the head of pancreas or chronic pancreatitis? A diagnostic dilemma. Surgery 111(6):602–603

Claudon M, Verain AL, Bigard MA, Boissel P, Poisson P, Floquet J, Regent D (1988) Cyst formation in gastric heterotopic pancreas: report of two cases. Radiology 169(3):659–660

Delhaze M, Jonard P, Gigot JF, Descamps C, Dive C (1989) Pancréatite chronique et cancer du pancréas. Un diagnostic différentiel parfois difficile. Acta Gastroenterol Belg 52:458–466

DelMaschio A, Vanzulli A, Sironi S, Castrucci M, Mellone R, Staudacher C, Carlucci M, Zerbi A, Parolini D, Faravelli A (1991) Pancreatic cancer versus chronic pancreatitis: diagnosis with CA 19-9 assessment, US, CT, and CT-guided fine-needle biopsy. Radiology 178(1):95–99

Elmas N (2001) The role of diagnostic radiology in pancreatitis. Eur J Radiol 38(2):120–132

Elmas N, Oran I, Oyar O, Ozer H (1996) A new criterion in differentiation of pancreatitis and pancreatic carcinoma: artery-to-vein ratio using the superior mesenteric vessels. Abdom Imaging 21(4):331–333

Farrell JJ, Brugge WR (2002) Intraductal papillary mucinous tumor of the pancreas. Gastrointest Endosc 55(6):701–714

Furukawa N, Muranaka T, Yasumori K, Matsubayashi R, Hayashida K, Arita Y (1998) Autoimmune pancreatitis: radiologic findings in three histologically proven cases. J Comput Assist Tomogr 22(6):880–883

Furukawa T, Tsukamoto Y, Naitoh Y, Hirooka Y, Hayakawa T (1994) Differential diagnosis between benign and malignant localized stenosis of the main pancreatic duct by intraductal ultrasound of the pancreas. Am J Gastroenterol 89(11):2038–2041

Gabata T, Matsui O, Kadoya M, Yoshikawa J, Miyayama S, Takashima T, Nagakawa T, Kayahara M, Nonomura A (1994) Small pancreatic adenocarcinomas: efficacy of MR imaging with fat suppression and gadolinium enhancement. Radiology 193(3):683–688

Gabata T, Kadoya M, Terayama N, Sanada J, Kobayashi S, Matsui O (2003) Groove pancreatic carcinomas: radiological and pathological findings. Eur Radiol 13(7):1679–1684

Gentiloni N, Caradonna P, Costamagna G, D'Ostilio N, Perri V, Mutignani M, Febbraro S, Tinari N, Iacobelli S, Natoli C (1995) Pancreatic juice 90K and serum CA 19-9 combined determination can discriminate between pancreatic cancer and chronic pancreatitis. Am J Gastroenterol 90(7):1069–1072

Glasbrenner B, Schwarz M, Pauls S, Preclik G, Beger HG, Adler G (2000) Prospective comparison of endoscopic ultrasound and endoscopic retrograde cholangiopancreatography in the preoperative assessment of masses in the pancreatic head. Dig Surg 17(5):468–474

Hanley JA, McNeil BJ (1982) The meaning and use of the area under a receiver operating characteristic (ROC) curve. Radiology 143(1):29–36

Hara T, Yamaguchi T, Ishihara T, Tsuyuguchi T, Kondo F, Kato K, Asano T, Saisho H (2002) Diagnosis and patient management of intraductal papillary-mucinous tumor of the pancreas by using peroral pancreatoscopy and intraductal ultrasonography. Gastroenterology 122(1):34–43

Higashi T, Tamaki N, Torizuka T, Nakamoto Y, Sakahara H, Kimura T, Honda T, Inokuma T, Katsushima S, Ohshio G, Imamura M, Konishi J (1998) FDG uptake, GLUT-1 glucose transporter and cellularity in human pancreatic tumors. J Nucl Med 39(10):1727–1735

Higashi T, Sakahara H, Torizuka T, Nakamoto Y, Kanamori S, Hiraoka M, Imamura M, Nishimura Y, Tamaki N, Konishi J (1999) Evaluation of intraoperative radiation therapy for unresectable pancreatic cancer with FDG PET. J Nucl Med 40(9):1424–1433

Hintze RE, Adler A, Veltzke W, Abou-Rebyeh H, Hammerstingl R, Vogl T, Felix R (1997) Clinical significance of magnetic resonance cholangiopancreatography (MRCP) compared to endoscopic retrograde cholangiopancreatography (ERCP). Endoscopy 29(3):182–187

Hommeyer SC, Freeny PC, Crabo LG (1995) Carcinoma of the head of the pancreas: evaluation of the pancreaticoduodenal veins with dynamic CT – potential for improved accuracy in staging. Radiology 196(1):233–238

Horiuchi A, Kawa S, Hamano H, Hayama M, Ota H, Kiyosawa K (2002) ERCP features in 27 patients with autoimmune pancreatitis. Gastrointest Endosc 55(4):494–499

Hough TJ, Raptopoulos V, Siewert B, Matthews JB (1999) Teardrop superior mesenteric vein: CT sign for unresectable carcinoma of the pancreas. AJR Am J Roentgenol 173(6):1509–1512

Ichikawa T, Sou H, Araki T, Arbab AS, Yoshikawa T, Ishigame K, Haradome H, Hachiya J (2001) Duct-penetrating sign at MRCP: usefulness for differentiating inflammatory pancreatic mass from pancreatic carcinomas. Radiology 221(1):107–116

Inokuma T, Tamaki N, Torizuka T, Fujita T, Magata Y, Yonekura Y, Ohshio G, Imamura M, Konishi J (1995a) Value of fluorine-18-fluorodeoxyglucose and thallium-201 in the detection of pancreatic cancer. J Nucl Med 36(2):229–235

Inui K, Yoshino J, Okushima K, Miyoshi H, Nakamura Y (2002) Intraductal EUS. Gastrointest Endosc 56(4 Suppl):S58–62

Irie H, Honda H, Baba S, Kuroiwa T, Yoshimitsu K, Tajima T, Jimi M, Sumii T, Masuda K (1998) Autoimmune pancreatitis: CT and MR characteristics. AJR Am J Roentgenol 170(5):1323–1327

Irie H, Honda H, Aibe H, Kuroiwa T, Yoshimitsu K, Shinozaki K, Yamaguchi K, Shimada M, Masuda K (2000) MR cholangiopancreatographic differentiation of benign and malignant intraductal mucin-producing tumors of the pancreas. AJR Am J Roentgenol 174(5):1403–1408

Irie H, Honda H, Kuroiwa T, Yoshimitsu K, Aibe H, Shinozaki K, Masuda K (2002) Measurement of the apparent diffusion coefficient in intraductal mucin-producing tumor of the pancreas by diffusion-weighted echo-planar MR imaging. Abdom Imaging 27(1):82–87

Itai Y, Kokubo T, Atomi Y, Kuroda A, Haraguchi Y, Terano A (1987) Mucin-hypersecreting carcinoma of the pancreas. Radiology 165(1):51–55

Ito K, Koike S, Matsunaga N (2001) MR imaging of pancreatic disease. Eur J Radiol 38:78–93

Ito T, Nakano I, Koyanagi S, Miyahara T, Migita Y, Ogoshi K, Sakai H, Matsunaga S, Yasuda O, Sumii T, Nawata H (1997) Autoimmune pancreatitis as a new clinical entity. Three cases of autoimmune pancreatitis with effective steroid therapy. Dig Dis Sci 42(7):1458–1468

Jadvar H, Fischman AJ (2001) Evaluation of pancreatic carcinoma with FDG PET. Abdom Imaging 26(3):254–259

Jenkins JP, Braganza JM, Hickey DS, Isherwood I, Machin M (1987) Quantitative tissue characterisation in pancreatic disease using magnetic resonance imaging. Br J Radiol 60(712):333–341

Johnson PT, Outwater EK (1999) Pancreatic carcinoma versus chronic pancreatitis: dynamic MR imaging. Radiology 212(1):213–218

Kaneko T, Nakao A, Nomoto S, Furukawa T, Hirooka Y, Nakashima N, Nagasaka T (1998) Intraoperative pancreatoscopy with the ultrathin pancreatoscope for mucin-producing tumors of the pancreas. Arch Surg 133(3):263–267

Kaneko T, Nakao A, Inoue S, Sugimoto H, Hatsuno T, Ito A, Hirooka Y, Nagasaka T, Nakashima N (2001) Intraoperative ultrasonography by high-resolution annular array transducer for intraductal papillary mucinous tumors of the pancreas. Surgery 129(1):55–65

Karasawa E, Goldberg HI, Moss AA, Federle MP, London SS (1983) CT pancreatogram in carcinoma of the pancreas and chronic pancreatitis. Radiology 148(2):489–493

Kim T, Murakami T, Takamura M, Hori M, Takahashi S, Nakamori S, Sakon M, Tanji Y, Wakasa K, Nakamura H (2001) Pancreatic mass due to chronic pancreatitis: correlation of CT and MR imaging features with pathologic findings. AJR Am J Roentgenol 177(2):367–371

Kobari M, Egawa S, Shibuya K, Shimamura H, Sunamura M, Takeda K, Matsuno S, Furukawa T (1999) Intraductal papillary mucinous tumors of the pancreas comprise 2 clinical subtypes: differences in clinical characteristics and surgical management. Arch Surg 134(10):1131–1136

Koga Y, Yamaguchi K, Sugitani A, Chijiiwa K, Tanaka M (2002) Autoimmune pancreatitis starting as a localized form. J Gastroenterol 37(2):133–137

Koito K, Namieno T, Nagakawa T, Morita K (1997) Inflammatory pancreatic masses: differentiation from ductal carcinomas with contrast-enhanced sonography using carbon dioxide microbubbles. AJR Am J Roentgenol 169(5):1263–1267

Koito K, Namieno T, Ichimura T, Yama N, Hareyama M, Morita K, Nishi M (1998) Mucin-producing pancreatic tumors: comparison of MR cholangiopancreatography with endoscopic retrograde cholangiopancreatography. Radiology 208(1):231–237

Kroft SH, Stryker SJ, Winter JN, Ergun G, Rao MS (1995) Inflammatory pseudotumor of the pancreas. Int J Pancreatol 18(3):277–283

Kubo H, Chijiiwa Y, Akahoshi K, Hamada S, Harada N, Sumii T, Takashima M, Nawata H (2001) Intraductal papillary-mucinous tumors of the pancreas: differential diagnosis between benign and malignant tumors by endoscopic ultrasonography. Am J Gastroenterol 96(5):1429–1434

Kubota K, Yamada K, Yoshioka S, Yamada S, Ito M, Ido T (1992) Differential diagnosis of idiopathic fibrosis from malignant lymphadenopathy with PET and F-18 fluorodeoxyglucose. Clin Nucl Med 17(5):361–363

Lammer J, Herlinger H, Zalaudek G, Hofler H (1985) Pseudotumorous pancreatitis. Gastrointest Radiol 10(1):59–67

Liao Q, Zhao YP, Wu WW, Li BL, Li JY (2003) Diagnosis and treatment of chronic pancreatitis. Hepatobiliary Pancreat Dis Int 2(3):445–448

Lim JH, Lee G, Oh YL (2001) Radiologic spectrum of intraductal papillary mucinous tumor of the pancreas. Radiographics 21(2):323–337

Lowenfels AB, Maisonneuve P, Cavallini G, Ammann RW, Lankisch PG, Andersen JR, Dimagno EP, Andren-Sandberg A, Domellof L (1993) Pancreatitis and the risk of pancreatic cancer. International Pancreatitis Study Group. N Engl J Med 328(20):1433–1437

Luetmer PH, Stephens DH, Ward EM (1989) Chronic pancreatitis: reassessment with current CT. Radiology 171(2):353–357

Mallery JS, Centeno BA, Hahn PF, Chang Y, Warshaw AL, Brugge WR (2002) Pancreatic tissue sampling guided by EUS, CT/US, and surgery: a comparison of sensitivity and specificity. Gastrointest Endosc 56(2):218–224

Matos C, Winant C, Delhaye M, Deviere J (2001) Functional MRCP in pancreatic and periampullary disease. Int J Gastrointest Cancer 30(1/2):5–18

Mcdonald JM, Williard W, Mais D, Beitler A (2000) The incidence of intraductal papillary mucinous tumors of the pancreas. Curr Surg 57(6):610–614

McGowan KM, Long SD, Pekala PH (1995) Glucose transporter gene expression: regulation of transcription and mRNA stability. Pharmacol Ther 66(3):465–505

Megibow AJ, Bosniak MA, Ambos MA, Beranbaum ER (1981) Thickening of the celiac axis and/or superior mesenteric artery: a sign of pancreatic carcinoma on computed tomography. Radiology 141(2):449–453

Menges M, Lerch MM, Zeitz M (2000) The double duct sign in patients with malignant and benign pancreatic lesions. Gastrointest Endosc 52(1):74–77

Minniti S, Bruno C, Biasiutti C, Tonel D, Falzone A, Falconi M, Procacci C (2003) Sonography versus helical CT in identification and staging of pancreatic ductal adenocarcinoma. J Clin Ultrasound 31(4):175–182

Mohl W, Hero-Gross R, Feifel G, Kramann B, Puschel W, Menges M, Zeitz M (2001) Groove pancreatitis: an important differential diagnosis to malignant stenosis of the duodenum. Dig Dis Sci 46(5):1034–1038

Mori H, Miyake H, Aikawa H, Monzen Y, Maeda T, Suzuki K, Matsumoto S, Wakisaka M (1991) Dilated posterior superior pancreatico-duodenal vein: recognition with CT and clinical significance in patients with pancreatico-biliary carcinomas. Radiology 181(3):793–800

Nakata B, Chung YS, Nishimura S, Nishihara T, Sakurai Y, Sawada T, Okamura T, Kawabe J, Ochi H, Sowa M (1997) 18F-fluorodeoxyglucose positron emission tomography and the prognosis of patients with pancreatic adenocarcinoma. Cancer 79(4):695–699

Nazli O, Bozdag AD, Tansug T, Kir R, Kaymak E (2000) The diagnostic importance of CEA and CA 19-9 for the early diagnosis of pancreatic carcinoma. Hepatogastroenterology 47(36):1750–1752

Neff CC, Simeone JF, Wittenberg J, Mueller PR, Ferrucci JT Jr (1984) Inflammatory pancreatic masses. Problems in differentiating focal pancreatitis from carcinoma. Radiology 150(1):35–38

Nickl NJ, Lawson JM, Cotton PB (1991) Mucinous pancreatic tumors: ERCP findings. Gastrointest Endosc 37(2):133–138

Nitzsche EU, Hoegerle S, Mix M, Brink I, Otte A, Moser E, Imdahl A (2002) Non-invasive differentiation of pancreatic lesions: is analysis of FDG kinetics superior to semi-quantitative uptake value analysis? Eur J Nucl Med Mol Imaging 29(2):237–242

Norton ID, Zheng Y, Wiersema MS, Greenleaf J, Clain JE, DiMagno EP (2001) Neural network analysis of eus images to differentiate between pancreatic malignancy and pancreatitis. Gastrointest Endosc 54(5):625–629

Okazaki K, Chiba T (2002) Autoimmune related pancreatitis. Gut 51(1):1–4

Onaya H, Itai Y, Niitsu M, Chiba T, Michishita N, Saida Y (1998) Ductectatic mucinous cystic neoplasms of the pancreas: evaluation with MR cholangiopancreatography. AJR Am J Roentgenol 171(1):171–177

Oshikawa O, Tanaka S, Ioka T, Nakaizumi A, Hamada Y, Mitani T (2002) Dynamic sonography of pancreatic tumors: comparison with dynamic CT. AJR Am J Roentgenol 178(5):1133–1137

Ozawa Y, Numata K, Tanaka K, Ueno N, Kiba T, Hara K, Morimoto M, Sakaguchi T, Sekihara H, Kubota T, Shimada H, Nakatani Y (2002) Contrast-enhanced sonography of small pancreatic mass lesions. J Ultrasound Med 21(9):983–991

Parsons L Jr, Palmer CH (1989) How accurate is fine-needle biopsy in malignant neoplasia of the pancreas? Arch Surg 124(6):681–683

Pavone P, Panebianco V, Laghi A, Catalano C, Messina A, Lobina L, Pirillo S, Passariello R (1997) Cholangiopancreatography with magnetic resonance in the assessment of pancreatic ducts Radiol Med (Torino) 94(1/2):61–67

Pitt HA (1995) Curative treatment for pancreatic neoplasms. Standard resection. Surg Clin North Am 75(5):891–904

Procacci C, Graziani R, Zamboni G, Cavallini G, Pederzoli P, Guarise A, Bogina G, Biasiutti C, Carbognin G, Bergamo-Andreis IA, Pistolesi GF (1997) Cystic dystrophy of the duodenal wall: radiologic findings. Radiology 205(3):741–747

Procacci C, Megibow AJ, Carbognin G, Guarise A, Spoto E, Biasiutti C, Pistolesi GF (1999) Intraductal papillary mucinous tumor of the pancreas: a pictorial essay. Radiographics 19(6):1447–1463

Procacci C, Carbognin G, Biasiutti C, Guarise A, Ghirardi C, Schenal G (2001a) Intraductal papillary mucinous tumors of the pancreas: spectrum of CT and MR findings with pathologic correlation. Eur Radiol 11(10):1939–1951

Procacci C, Carbognin G, Biasiutti C, Frulloni L, Bicego E, Spoto E, el-Khaldi M, Bassi C, Pagnotta N, Talamini G, Cavallini G (2001b) Autoimmune pancreatitis: possibilities of CT characterization. Pancreatology 1(3):246–253

Prokesch RW, Chow LC, Beaulieu CF, Bammer R, Jeffrey RB Jr (2002) Isoattenuating pancreatic adenocarcinoma at multi-detector row CT: secondary signs. Radiology 224(3):764–768

Raijman I, Kortan P, Walden D, Kandel G, Marcon NE, Haber GB (1994) Mucinous ductal ectasia: cholangiopancreatographic and endoscopic findings. Endoscopy 26(3):303–307

Reske SN, Grillenberger KG, Glatting G, Port M, Hildebrandt M, Gansauge F, Beger HG (1997) Overexpression of glucose transporter 1 and increased FDG uptake in pancreatic carcinoma. J Nucl Med Sep;38(9):1344–1348

Rickes S, Unkrodt K, Neye H, Ocran KW, Wermke W (2002) Differentiation of pancreatic tumours by conventional ultrasound, unenhanced and echo-enhanced power Doppler sonography. Scand J Gastroenterol 37(11):1313–1320

Rieber A, Tomczak R, Nussle K, Klaus H, Brambs HJ (2000) MRI with mangafodipir trisodium in the detection of pancreatic tumours: comparison with helical CT. Br J Radiol 73(875):1165–1169

Robinson PJ, Sheridan MB (2000) Pancreatitis: computed tomography and magnetic resonance imaging. Eur Radiol 10(3):401–408

Rodriguez J, Kasberg C, Nipper M, Schoolar J, Riggs MW, Dyck WP (1992) CT-guided needle biopsy of the pancreas: a retrospective analysis of diagnostic accuracy. Am J Gastroenterol 87(11):1610–1613

Rösch T, Lorenz R, Braig C, Feuerbach S, Siewert JR, Schusdziarra V, Classen M (1991) Endoscopic ultrasound in pancreatic tumor diagnosis. Gastrointest Endosc 37(3):347–352

Rose DM, Delbeke D, Beauchamp RD, Chapman WC, Sandler MP, Sharp KW, Richards WO, Wright JK, Frexes ME, Pinson CW, Leach SD (1999) 18Fluorodeoxyglucose-positron emission tomography in the management of patients with suspected pancreatic cancer. Ann Surg 229(5):729–737

Schima W, Fugger R (2002) Evaluation of focal pancreatic masses: comparison of mangafodipir-enhanced MR imaging and contrast-enhanced helical CT. Eur Radiol 12(12):2998–3008. Epub 2002 Jul 12

Schulte SJ, Baron RL, Freeny PC, Patten RM, Gorell HA, Maclin ML (1991) Root of the superior mesenteric artery in pancreatitis and pancreatic carcinoma: evaluation with CT. Radiology 180(3):659–662

Servais A, Pestieau SR, Detry O, Honore P, Belaiche J, Boniver J, Jacquet N (2001) Autoimmune pancreatitis mimicking cancer of the head of pancreas: report of two cases. Acta Gastroenterol Belg 64(2):227–230

Shinozaki M, Saisho H, Tokinaga K (1987) Tumor-forming pancreatitis on ultrasonography: follow-up study of the images and relation to clinical features. Jpn J Med Ultrasonics 14:189–198

Shreve PD (1998) Focal fluorine-18 fluorodeoxyglucose accumulation in inflammatory pancreatic disease. Eur J Nucl Med 25(3):259–264

Sittek H, Heuck AF, Folsing C, Gieseke J, Reiser M (1995) Static and dynamic MR tomography of the pancreas: contrast media kinetics of the normal pancreatic parenchyma in pancreatic carcinoma and chronic pancreatitis. Rofo Fortschr Geb Rontgenstr Neuen Bildgeb Verfahr 162(5):396–403

Smith CD, Behrns KE, Van Heerden JA, Sarr MG (1994) Radical pancreatoduodenectomy for misdiagnosed pancreatic mass. Br J Surg 81(4):585–589

Sugiyama M, Atomi Y, Hachiya J (1998) Intraductal papillary tumors of the pancreas: evaluation with magnetic resonance cholangiopancreatography. Am J Gastroenterol 93(2):156–159

Tabata M, Kitayama J, Kanemoto H, Fukasawa T, Goto H, Taniwaka K (2003) Autoimmune pancreatitis presenting as a mass in the head of the pancreas: a diagnosis to differentiate from cancer. Am Surg 69(5):363–366

Takeda K, Goto H, Hirooka Y, Itoh A, Hashimoto S, Niwa K, Hayakawa T (2003) Contrast-enhanced transabdominal ultrasonography in the diagnosis of pancreatic mass lesions. Acta Radiol 44(1):103–106

Taniguchi T, Seko S, Azuma K, Asagoe K, Tamegai M, Nishida O, Inoue F, Okamoto M, Mizumoto T, Kobayashi H (2001) Autoimmune pancreatitis detected as a mass in the head of the pancreas with contiguous fibrosis around the superior mesenteric artery. Dig Dis Sci 46(1):187–191

Taniguchi T, Tanio H, Seko S, Nishida O, Inoue F, Okamoto M, Ishigami S, Kobayashi H (2003) Autoimmune pancreatitis detected as a mass in the head of the pancreas without hypergammaglobulinemia, which relapsed after surgery: case report and review of the literature. Dig Dis Sci 48(8):1465–1471

Tenner S, Carr-Locke DL, Banks PA, Brooks DC, Van Dam J, Farraye FA, Turner JR, Lichtenstein DR (1996) Intraductal mucin-hypersecreting neoplasm „mucinous ductal ectasia": endoscopic recognition and management. Am J Gastroenterol 91(12):2548–2554

Trede M, Schwall G, Saeger HD (1990) Survival after pancreatoduodenectomy. 118 consecutive resections without an operative mortality. Ann Surg 211(4):447–458

Valinas R, Barrier A, Montravers F, Houry S, Talbot JN, Huguier M (2002) 18 F-fluorodeoxyglucose positron emission tomography for characterization and initial staging of pancreatic tumors. Gastroenterol Clin Biol 26(10):888–892

Van Gulik TM, Reeders JW, Bosma A, Moojen TM, Smits NJ, Allema JH, Rauws EA, Offerhaus GJ, Obertop H, Gouma DJ (1997) Incidence and clinical findings of benign, inflammatory disease in patients resected for presumed pancreatic head cancer. Gastrointest Endosc 46(5):417–423

Van Gulik TM, Gerhards M, De Vries J, Van Geenen R, De Wit LT, Obertop H, Gouma DJ (1999) Local resection of biliopancreatic cancer. Ann Oncol 10 Suppl 4:243–246

Van Hoe L, Gryspeerdt S, Ectors N, Van Steenbergen WV, Aerts R, Baert AL, Marchal G (1998) Nonalcoholic duct – destructive chronic pancreatitis: imaging findings. AJR Am J Roentgenol 170:643–647

Vullierme MP, Vilgrain V, Flejou JF, Zins M, O'Toole D, Ruszniewski P, Belghiti J, Menu Y (2000) Cystic dystrophy of the duodenal wall in the heterotopic pancreas: radiopathological correlations. J Comput Assist Tomogr 24(4):635–643

Wahl RL (1996) Targeting glucose transporters for tumor imaging: "sweet" idea, "sour" result. J Nucl Med 37(6):1038–1041

Wakabayashi T, Kawaura Y, Satomura Y, Watanabe H, Motoo Y, Okai T, Sawabu N (2003) Clinical and imaging features of autoimmune pancreatitis with focal pancreatic swelling or mass formation: comparison with so-called tumor-forming pancreatitis and pancreatic carcinoma. Am J Gastroenterol 98(12):2679–2687

Warshaw AL, Compton CC, Lewandrowski K, Cardenosa G, Mueller P (1990) Cystic tumors of the pancreas. Ann Surg 212 (4):432–443

Wharton SM, Rahman Z, Johnson CD (1997) Missed curable carcinoma of the pancreas presenting as chronic pancreatitis. Postgrad Med J 73(863):577–579

Wiersema MJ (2001) Accuracy of endoscopic ultrasound in diagnosing and staging pancreatic carcinoma. Pancreatology 1(6):625–632

Yamao K, Okubo K, Sawaka A, Hara K, Nakamura T, Suzuki T, Shimizu Y, Ozden I (2003) Endolumenal ultrasonography in the diagnosis of pancreatic diseases. Abdom Imaging 28(4):545–555

Yamashita Y, Namimoto T, Mitsuzaki K, Urata J, Tsuchigame T, Takahashi M, Ogawa M (1998) Mucin-producing tumor of the pancreas: diagnostic value of diffusion-weighted echo-planar MR imaging. Radiology 208(3):605–609

Yasuda K, Mukai H, Nakajima M (1995) Endoscopic ultrasonography diagnosis of pancreatic cancer. Gastrointest Endosc Clin N Am 5(4):699–712

Yoshida EM, Scudamore CH, Erb SR, Owen DA, Silver HK (1995a) Markedly elevated serum CA 19-9 levels in a case of chronic pancreatitis. Can J Surg 38(1):83–86

Yoshida K, Toki F, Takeuchi T, Watanabe S, Shiratori K, Hayashi N (1995b) Chronic pancreatitis caused by an autoimmune abnormality. Proposal of the concept of autoimmune pancreatitis. Dig Dis Sci J40(7):1561–1568

The Role of Endoscopy in Acute and Chronic Pancreatitis

19

David L. Diehl

CONTENTS

19.1 **General Issues** *371*

19.2 **Biliary Obstruction in Acute and Chronic Pancreatitis** *372*

19.3 **Pancreatic Pseudocysts** *373*

19.3.1 Endoscopic Transmural Drainage – Candidates *374*

19.3.2 Endoscopic Pseudocyst Drainage – Technique *374*

19.3.3 Transpapillary Drainage of Pseudocysts *377*

19.3.4 Outcomes of Endoscopic Drainage *377*

19.3.5 Complications of Endoscopic Pseudocyst Drainage *378*

19.3.6 Recurrence After Endoscopic Pseudocyst Drainage *379*

19.4 **Endoscopic Management of Other Pancreatic Fluid Collections** *379*

19.4.1 Endoscopic Management of Pancreatic Duct Leaks *380*

19.5 **Conclusions** *381*

References *381*

D. L. Diehl, MD, FACP
Adjunct Associate Clinical Professor of Medicine, NYU-Langone School of Medicine, Geisinger Medical Center, Department of Gastroenterology and Nutrition, 100 North Academy Ave, 21-11 Danville, PA 17822, USA

19.1 General Issues

Acute and chronic pancreatitis can develop complications within the first few days or weeks of the illness, or be delayed by weeks to months. Acute pancreatitis can lead to peripancreatic fluid collections, which then may resolve, or organize into cystic fluid collections. Most fluid collections that have organized into pseudocysts will spontaneously resolve over time, they are typically followed by serial CT scans to prove resolution. Some cysts may not resolve, or may even increase in size, and require intervention. A subset of these non-resolving pseudocysts may be amenable to endoscopic management.

Biliary obstruction also may occur with acute or chronic pancreatitis. Early in the course of acute pancreatitis, pancreatic head inflammation can lead to a temporary biliary stenosis. A subtype of acute pancreatitis called “groove pancreatitis” can occur in the groove between the duodenum and pancreatic head and can lead to biliary and even duodenal obstruction (Balakrishnan et al. 2007). Later in the course of an acute episode of pancreatitis, biliary obstruction may be related to a pseudocyst in the head of the pancreas. Vigilance must be maintained in cases of biliary obstruction that arise after acute pancreatitis, because some of these cases may turn out to be a pancreatic neoplasm that presents initially with acute pancreatitis and then later with biliary obstruction.

The role of endoscopic retrograde pancreatography (ERCP) in the management of chronic pancreatitis and pancreatic strictures is discussed elsewhere in this issue (Chap. 13). The role of ERCP in the initial management of acute pancreatitis is also covered elsewhere.

19.2 Biliary Obstruction in Acute and Chronic Pancreatitis

Biliary obstruction can occur in the setting of chronic pancreatitis. Cholangiography reveals a smooth distal bile duct stricture as it passes through the pancreatic head (Fig. 19.1). Most of these strictures only mildly elevate the serum alkaline phosphatase, but jaundice can occur in a minority of patients. Because of the risk of cholangitis or secondary biliary cirrhosis, patients with jaundice are typically referred for biliary drainage.

Successful biliary drainage is rather easily accomplished with endoscopic methods of plastic stent placement. However, permanent resolution of the biliary strictures of chronic pancreatitis is not easily accomplished with a standard approach to endoscopic stent placement. While benign biliary strictures due to other causes can be typically resolved with a regimen of stent changes over a period of months, this does not seem to be the case with biliary strictures due to chronic pancreatitis.

Smits et al. (1996) carried out a retrospective review of 58 patients with chronic pancreatitis and biliary stricture who received endoscopic insertion of a plastic 10-Fr biliary endoprosthesis. About 80% of the patients were jaundiced, with the remainder having persistent cholestasis without jaundice. The majority (71%) had calcific pancreatitis. The patients underwent repeat ERCPs every 3–9 months. Patients underwent a median of three ERCPs over the follow-up period (median 14 months).

All patients had relief of jaundice or cholestasis from the stent placement. There was a 9% complication rate associated with the procedure. The temporary stent placement resulted in regression of the stricture in 28%. However, 37 out of 58 patients (64%) had stent related complications, mainly due to stent clogging. A total of 28% of the patients eventually underwent surgical drainage procedures.

Kahl et al. (2003) analyzed reasons for failure of biliary stenting to resolve benign biliary strictures in chronic pancreatitis. The presence of calcifications in the head of the pancreas was predictive of a poor response. Only 8% of the patients with this finding showed resolution of the common bile duct (CBD) stricture even after 1 year of serial stenting, compared to 59% stricture resolution in the absence of head calcifications.

Similar results were demonstrated by Draganov et al. (2002) in a review of their experience with retention of two or three 10-Fr biliary stents over a period of about 1 year to try to achieve permanent dilation of benign biliary strictures. Their series of 29 patients included nine with biliary strictures due to chronic pancreatitis (three were noncalcific and

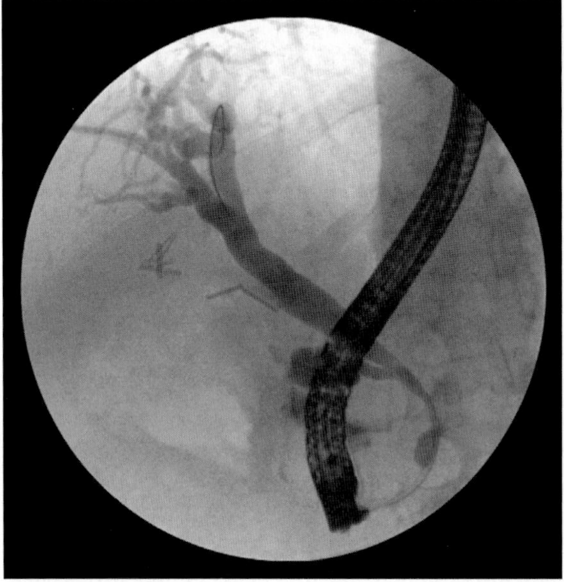

a

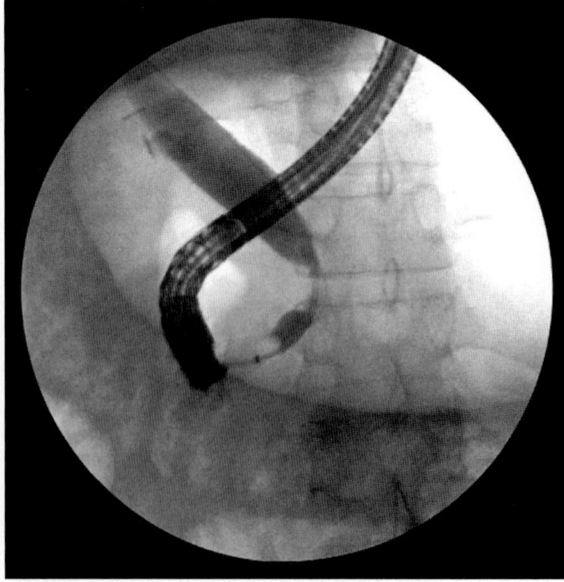

b

Fig. 19.1a,b. Distal common bile duct stricture from chronic pancreatitis. ERCP images from two different patients illustrate common bile duct strictures secondary to chronic pancreatitis. The appearance can be indistinguishable from a malignant biliary stricture due to a pancreatic or primary biliary neoplasm

six were calcific). The two stents were inserted during two ERCP procedures done 12 weeks apart. Of the patients with chronic pancreatitis, only one out of the six with calcific pancreatitis had resolution of the stricture after prolonged stenting, whereas all three with non-calcific pancreatitis responded to the prolonged stenting.

Catalano et al. (1995) looked at the benefit of placement of several simultaneous stents in patients with CBD strictures from chronic pancreatitis. They compared patients managed with a single 10-Fr stent, to patients treated with multiple 10-Fr stents in place. All patients had stent exchanges every 3–6 months. Of the patients, 12 had additional stents placed at 3-month intervals (eight patients had four stents, and four patients had five stents). Follow-up was carried out over approximately 4 years. After the treatment period (mean of 14 months), there was improvement of the biliary stenosis from 1.0 to 3.0 mm in diameter.

Because of the promising results of multiple stenting, several investigators looked at the feasibility of using self-expanding metal stents (SEMS) for the treatment of CBD stenosis in chronic pancreatitis. Eickhoff et al. (2003) found good initial response to the SEMS, but stent dysfunction occurred in two-thirds of patients, necessitating additional endoscopic procedures. Since SEMS are not removable, this may necessitate surgical therapy. Partially covered SEMS have also been investigated (Cantu et al. 2005). Similar results were found: initial improvement in cholestasis was good, and stent patency at 1 year was 100% in 14 patients. However, stent patency at 2 years and 3 years was only 40% and 37.5%, respectively, and necessitated retreatment. Slightly better results with SEMS were found by van Berkel et al. (2004). A total of 13 patients received SEMS, and were followed for a mean length of 50 months. Nine patients (69%) were adequately treated, although three patients needed a second SEMS placed within the first, and one patient needed the SEMS cleaned out endoscopically. SEMS occluded early in three patients, and there was a stent migration in one.

More recently, fully covered and "removable" SEMS have become available. The goals of using such a device would be large diameter dilation for a prolonged period, followed by successful endoprosthesis removal. Cahen et al. (2008) looked at the feasibility of using such a stent in this clinical scenario in six patients. In all cases, the stents were successfully placed. The fully covered SEMS could be removed in only four out of six of the cases. All of these patients achieved stricture resolution. A recurrent stenosis occurred in one patient. Proximal stent migration occurred in two patients. The authors correctly conclude that before fully covered SEMS can become an acceptable treatment option for benign CBD strictures, removability must be proven, and other design modifications instituted.

Taken together, these studies and others suggest that biliary stenting, while technically quite feasible and highly successful at resolving jaundice, necessitates repeated procedures and exposure of the patient to bacterial cholangitis from clogged stents. It is reasonable to initially manage the stricture with multiple plastic endoprostheses for perhaps 6 months to 1 year. Investigation continues for the use of fully covered metal stents that are removable. After the period of stenting, the stricture can be re-evaluated for resolution. If there is non-resolution (which is likely to be the case for most patients with calcific pancreatitis), or if the patient requires additional pancreatic surgery (for example, for pain management due to an obstructed pancreatic duct), surgical drainage should be performed if the patient is otherwise a good surgical candidate.

19.3 Pancreatic Pseudocysts

Pancreatic pseudocysts that are symptomatic or increasing in size should be treated. Biliary or bowel obstructions from a pseudocyst are complications that also dictate therapy. Some complications of pseudocysts, including infection or hemorrhage need intervention, but endoscopic management is usually not possible. The standard therapy for management of symptomatic or persistent pseudocysts has been surgical drainage of the cyst. In cases of pseudocyst associated with chronic pancreatitis (Fig. 19.2) and a dilated main pancreatic duct, many surgeons have added a lateral pancreaticojejunostomy (the so-called "Puestow" procedure) to the surgical management, in an attempt to reduce pseudocyst recurrence.

With advances in percutaneous radiologic access techniques, percutaneous drainage of pseudocysts became a more widely used technique in lieu of surgical drainage. It was established early that aspiration alone was often insufficient for complete resolu-

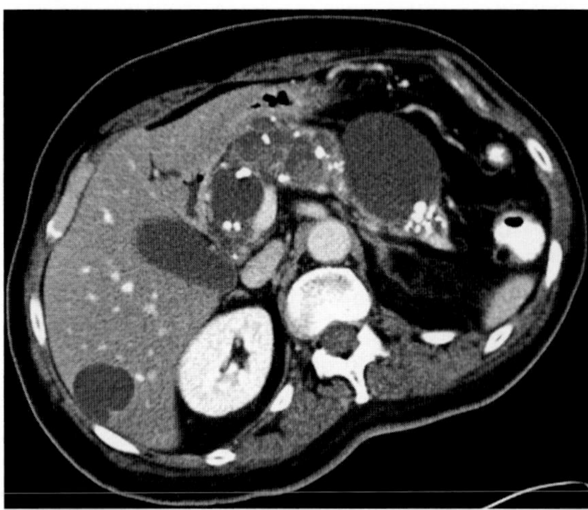

Fig. 19.2. Chronic pancreatitis with pseudocyst: multiple pseudocysts are seen, with the largest being at the pancreatic tail. Coarse calcifications are noted in the pancreatic parenchyma, indicative of chronic pancreatitis

tion; in addition, it had an unacceptable incidence of complications, including infection and cyst leakage. Placement of a percutaneous drain into a pseudocyst is still occasionally done, mainly as a temporizing intervention in selected cases (infected cyst, or immature cyst wall). Complications include introduction of infection, rupture of the cyst, and development of persistent pancreatic fistula.

Endoscopic transmural drainage of pseudocysts was first described by Rogers et al. in 1975. Following this initial experience, many groups have described case series of pseudocysts treated by endoscopic drainage. Endoscopic drainage does take special expertise, and should be carried out only by experienced pancreatico-biliary endoscopists. However, it appears that endoscopic drainage has a definite role in the management of selected pseudocysts.

19.3.1 Endoscopic Transmural Drainage – Candidates

To be amenable for endoscopic drainage, the pancreatic pseudocyst should have a "mature" wall and be in close apposition to the stomach or duodenum. A recent pre-procedure CT scan is mandatory. The cyst should in general not be loculated or septated, since this procedure may not completely accomplish drainage.

A visible bulge of the pseudocyst against the wall is generally favored if no endoscopic ultrasound (EUS) guidance is going to be used. However, EUS guidance is being used more frequently to help guide suitable puncture sites. The linear EUS system can find a suitably "thin" part of the pseudocyst wall. Most advanced endoscopists prefer that the wall has a thickness of less than 1 cm in the region of proposed cyst puncture. Using the Doppler capability of the linear EUS allows identification of intervening gastric wall vessels that should be avoided with the cyst puncture. This is a particularly important in some cases of chronic pancreatitis, in which splenic vein thrombosis can lead to collateral veins in a perigastric and periduodenal location.

EUS-guided cyst puncture can be accomplished through the EUS endoscope. A linear echoendoscope with a larger channel is available (GF-UCT160-OL5, Olympus Medical, Center Valley, PA, or FG38 UX, Pentax Medical, Montvale, NJ) to allow for passage of larger drainage stents (10 Fr) into the cyst. Most EUS units will not have this echoendoscope, however. A recently developed prototype front-viewing curvilinear echoendoscope has been used in seven patients (Voermans et al. 2007). It appears to have some advantages in regard to ease of stent passage into the cyst that is being drained. This is because the cyst can be approached en-face rather than tangentially, giving better "pushability" of the accessories that are being introduced into the cyst. This device has received 501(k) FDA clearance, but is still in the prototype stages, and is not available outside of centers with an ongoing research protocol.

Biliary or duodenal obstruction by the pseudocyst is not a contraindication for endoscopic cyst drainage. Significant coagulopathy should be corrected prior to the procedure. Prophylactic antibiotics are typically given. Notification of a surgical team prior to the procedure should be considered, since some complications of the procedure may require emergent surgical management.

19.3.2 Endoscopic Pseudocyst Drainage – Technique

Review of the CT scan will give a preliminary identification of a cyst that may be a candidate for transmural drainage. Pre-procedure antibiotics are strongly recommended, as their use seems to decrease the incidence of infective complications. The patient is brought into the fluoroscopy unit and sedated in the usual manner for an ERCP or EUS (moderate sedation with benzodiazepine and opiate or equivalent). In some cases, there is an advantage to positioning the patient in decubitus or supine position rather than the typical prone position of ERCP. This is because the anterior gastric wall is compressed when the patient is prone, and in some cases can interfere with identification of a gastric bulge. A front-viewing endoscope is often used initially to assess the location of the bulging pseudocyst (Fig. 19.3). The actual cyst drainage can be done with a front-viewing or side-viewing endoscope, depending on which gives the most en-face approach to the proposed point of puncture.

In cases where EUS guidance is used, puncture can be accomplished through the EUS endoscope (Fig. 19.4). It should be remembered that this will limit the diameter of the stent that can be placed to 7 Fr. EUS may lead to safer endoscopic cysto-enterostomy by allowing the endoscopist to select the best point of puncture by avoiding intervening vessels and decreasing the risk of bleeding, particularly in cases of portal hypertension. A visible "bulge" of the pseudocyst should be present if endoscopic drainage alone (that is, without EUS guidance) is going to be pursued. An alternative approach that has been described is the initial use of EUS to identify a suitable puncture site, followed by "marking" of the proposed site, for example, with a biopsy forceps. Then, a duodenoscope is used to initiate the endoscopically created fistula.

At the selected point of puncture, a "needle-knife" sphincterotome or a special instrument with a 0.038" cautery wire (Cystotome, Cook Medical, Winston-Salem, NC) is used with cautery to literally burn a hole through the gastric or duodenal wall and into the cyst cavity. The catheter portion of the needle-knife is then advanced into the cyst. Contrast can be instilled and observed fluoroscopically to confirm entry into the cyst. A hydrophilic guidewire can then be introduced which can be seen

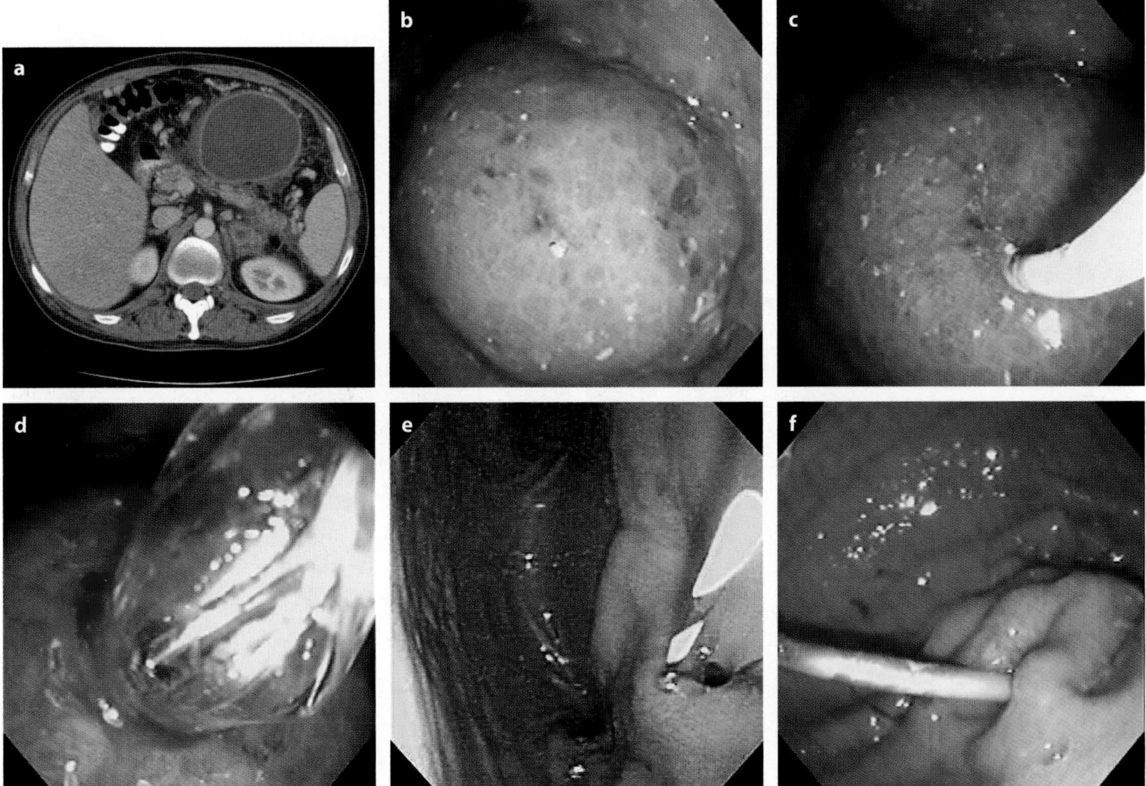

Fig. 19.3 a–f. Endoscopic trans-gastric drainage of pancreatic pseudocyst. **a** A mid-body pancreatic pseudocyst is seen on the CT. **b** Endoscopy shows a visible bulge into the gastric lumen. **c** This is punctured with a needle-knife sphincterotome, and a guidewire placed into the cyst. **d** The fistula that is made is then dilated with a hydrostatic dilation balloon. **e** After removal of the balloon, a brisk flow of cyst contents can be seen coming through the enlarged fistula. **f** The first stent is inserted, usually followed by one or more additional stents

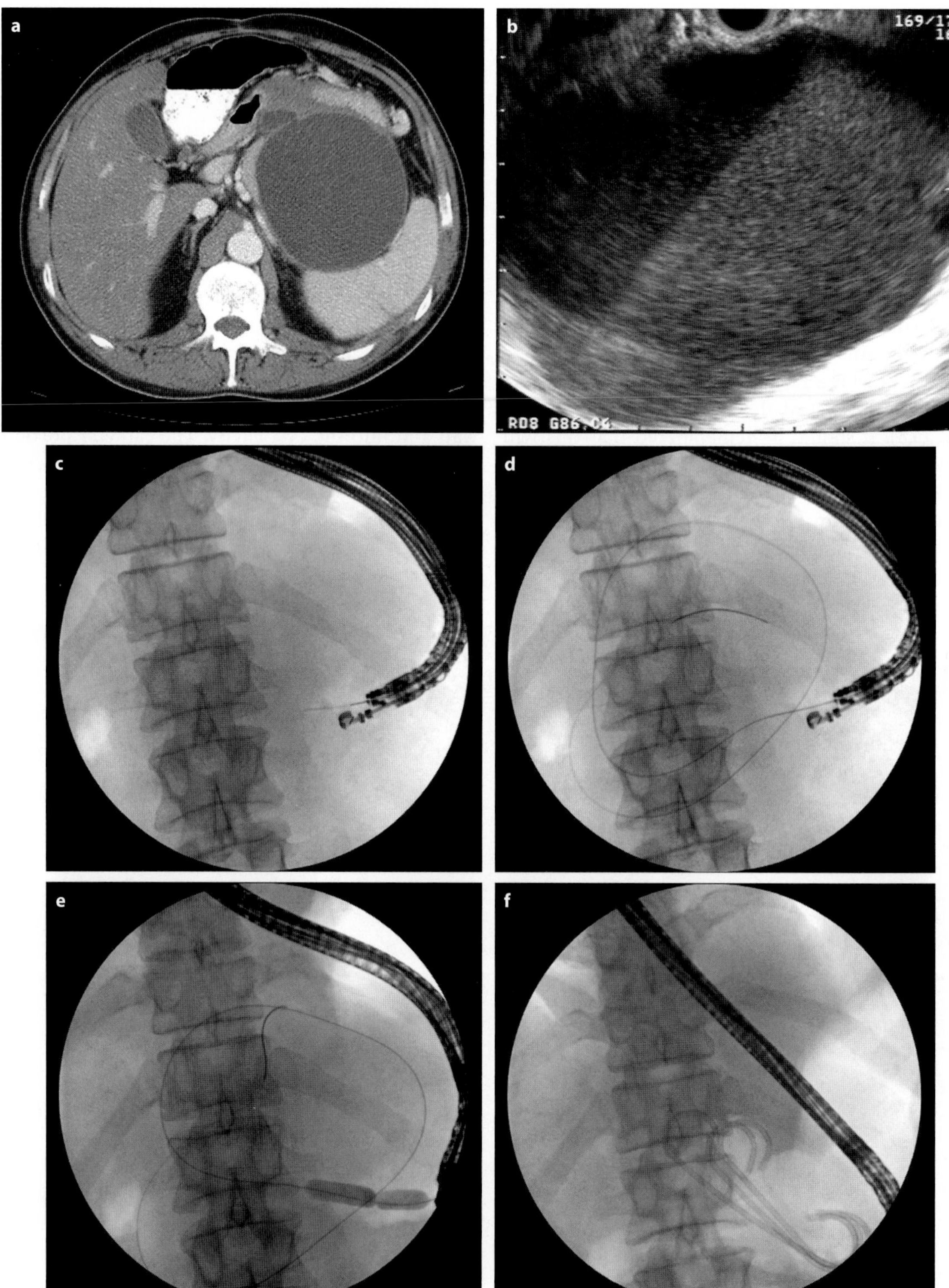

Fig. 19.4a–f. EUS-guided pseudocyst drainage. **a** On CT, a pseudocyst is apparent in the region of the pancreatic tail. **b** EUS imaging shows the cyst with some layering debris, but no large pieces of solid material. **c** The echoendoscope is positioned against the pseudocyst, and an EUS needle is used for initial cyst puncture. **d** A guidewire is coiled into the cyst. **e** The dilation balloon is used to enlarge the fistula; note the "waist" on the dilation balloon. **f** Three double pigtail stents are inserted into the cyst, across the gastric wall

to coil within the cyst. An 8- to 12-mm hydrostatic balloon is used to expand the fistula.

Creation of the cyst-enterostomy can also be done without use of a needle-knife access device. In this case, an EUS needle is used to puncture the cyst under EUS control. After puncture, the stylet of the EUS needle is removed, and a guidewire inserted into the cyst as described above. Use of a 19-gauge EUS needle allows insertion of a 0.035" guidewire; the 22-gauge needle requires a 0.025" guidewire. A biliary-type dilator is used to enlarge the opening,. Finally further dilation is achieved with the hydrostatic balloon.

After balloon expansion of the enterocystic fistula, one or more plastic biliary-type stents (usually double-pigtail) are placed to allow drainage from the cyst to the lumen. Double pigtail stents are less likely to migrate, and are probably better than straight stents (Cahen et al. 2005). If the cyst contents are thick or highly particulate, the inserted stents can rapidly clog and cyst infection can occur. In these situations, it is often recommended that a nasocystic drain be inserted along with the double-pigtail drains (Baron 2007). The nasocystic drain can be irrigated on a regular basis. Daily or twice-daily irrigation through the nasocystic tube will facilitate drainage and cyst resolution.

Initial studies described endoscopic removal of the stents 2 weeks after documented resolution of the pseudocyst. The rationale for this practice was subjected to a prospective randomized review by Arvanitakis et al. (2007). Their data suggest that early removal of the pseudocyst stents leads to a higher rate of pseudocyst recurrence; these authors suggested leaving the stents in place. There was no increased rate of complication, such as cyst infection. In some cases, the stents can stay in for a prolonged period of time (in this study, beyond 2 years of follow-up). In about a third of patients, pseudocyst stents will extrude on their own. In summary, it seems reasonable to leave pseudocyst stents in place indefinitely.

Non-bulging pseudocysts can also be treated endoscopically (Cortes et al. 2002). Of 34 non-bulging fluid collections, 18 cystostomies were performed with fluoroscopy alone, and 14 were drained by EUS together with fluoroscopy (there were two unsuccessful attempts). Fockens et al. (1997) reported on their experience of drainage of bulging and non-bulging pseudocysts. In their series, a prominent bulge was approached by endoscopy and fluoroscopy, while EUS was used in cases without endoscopic bulge.

19.3.3 Transpapillary Drainage of Pseudocysts

If a communication can be demonstrated between the cyst and the main pancreatic duct, then transpapillary drainage may be adequate to allow resolution of the pseudocyst. In this technique, a pancreatic stent is placed through the papilla, and bridges the defect in the pancreatic duct (Fig. 19.5). Some endoscopists favor placing the stent into the cyst itself. The stent allows pancreatic juice to be redirected into the duodenum instead of refilling the cyst. In some patients, additional pancreatic endotherapy may be required, such as pancreatic sphincterotomy, pancreatic stone extraction, or pancreatic ductal stricture dilation.

Multiple pancreatic cysts have also been treated with transpapillary drainage. Bhasin et al. (2006) used a nasopancreatic drain (5 Fr or 7 Fr) to bridge pancreatic ductal disruption in a series of 11 patients. Technical success was achieved in 10/11. Initial nasopancreatic drains were then changed to pancreatic stents. Complete resolution was seen in 4–8 weeks in cases of partial ductal disruption that could be bridged by the drain. In cases of complete ductal disruption, surgery was required for management of the pseudocyst.

19.3.4 Outcomes of Endoscopic Drainage

Several groups have performed endoscopic cyst drainage on large numbers of patients, and there is long-term follow up data available (Table 19.1). In general, the results are fairly uniform, with a high degree of initial technical success (usually 80%–90%), an acceptable complication rate (3%–24%), and a low but apparently irreducible recurrence rate (9%–24%). Much of the recent literature has examined outcomes of EUS-guided versus non-EUS-guided drainage. Kahaleh et al. (2006) retrospectively looked at the outcomes of 99 patients undergoing endoscopic pseudocyst drainage. Patients with visible endoscopic bulge and without portal hypertension (n=53) underwent direct endoscopic drainage without EUS. All of the other patients (n=46) had EUS-guided drainage. No difference between these groups was noted in complications (18% with endoscopic vs 19% with EUS-guided techniques), immediate success, or recurrence rate.

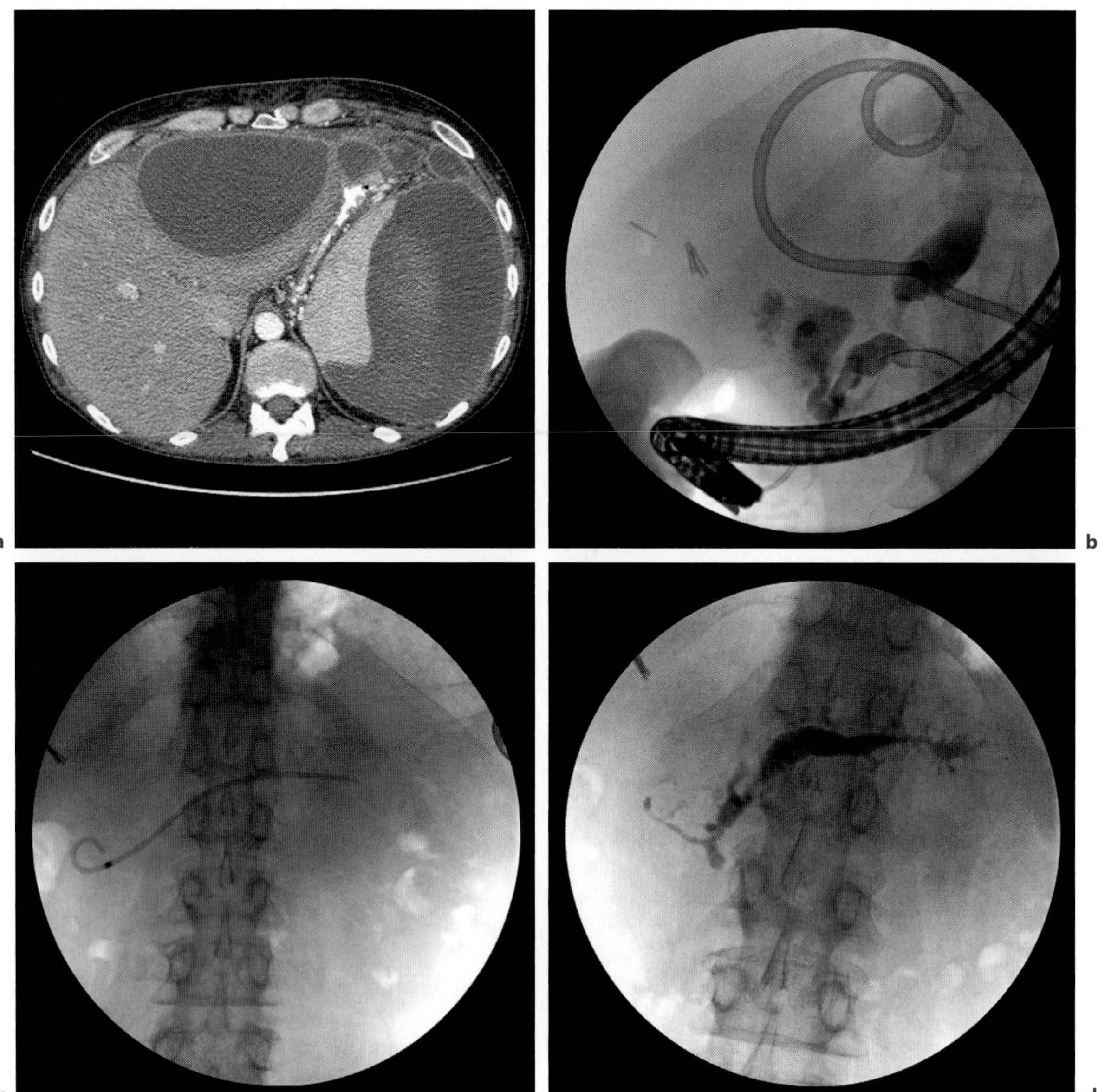

Fig. 19.5a–d. Transpapillary pseudocyst drainage. **a** CT shows two large fluid collections. The large fluid collection near the pancreatic tail was drained percutaneously. **b** Pancreatogram shows a dilated and irregular pancreatic duct with filling defects. Two areas of ductal disruption are evident in the head and neck of the pancreas. A guidewire has been advanced to the tail of the pancreas. An external drain which is draining the tail collection is visible. **c** A long pancreatic duct stent is placed. **d** After removal of the pancreatic stent 1 month later, the ductal disruptions are no longer present, and there is no pseudocyst filling. Typical ductal changes of chronic pancreatitis are evident

Varadarajulu et al. (2008) prospectively randomized 30 patients to EUS- versus esophagogastroduodenoscopy (EGD)-directed transmural drainage. This group found technical success in 100% of EUS-directed drainages, versus only 33% in the EGD group. In addition, bleeding complications (one fatal) occurred in two patients, both in the EGD group

19.3.5 Complications of Endoscopic Pseudocyst Drainage

Complications of endoscopic pseudocyst drainage include bleeding, perforation, and infection. Bleeding in earlier series occurred when a regular sphincterotome was used to expand the initial fistula; the

Table 19.1. Endoscopic management of pancreatic pseudocysts (includes transpapillary drainage and transmural drainage into stomach or duodenum)

Ref	Initial success	Complications	Resurrence
Cremer et al. 1989	32/33(97%)	6%	9%
Smits et al. 1995	24/37 (65%)	16%	12.5%
Barthet et al. 1995	26/30 (87%)	13%	27%
Binmoeller et al. 1995	50/53 (94%)	12%	22%
Catalano et al. 1995	17/21 (81%)	5%	6%
Beckingham et al. 1999	24/34 (71%)	-	38%
Venu et al. 2000	20/22 (90%)	5%	74%
Giovannini et al. 2001	31/35 (88.5%)	3%	8.5%
Norton et al. 2001	13/17 (76%)	14%	15%
Sanchez-Cortes et al. 2002	32/34 (94%)	8%	3%
DePalma et al. 2002	43/49 (88%)	24.5%	24.5%
Sharma et al. 2002	32/33 (97%)	15%	15%
Cahen et al. 2005	89/92 (97%)	34%	29%
Hookey et al. 2006	-	11%	12%
Kahaleh et al. 2006	92% (93%)	18%	18%
Lopes et al. 2007	48/51 (94%)	17%	18%
Barthet et al. 2008	49/50 (98%)	18%	4%

current practice of expanding the fistula with a dilating balloon without further cutting has served to greatly lower intraprocedural bleeding. EUS guidance can be helpful to avoid intervening blood vessels between the cyst and stomach or duodenal wall, but may not be strictly necessary in the absence of portal hypertension. Perforation is rare, but can happen when the cyst is not firmly adherent to the wall of the stomach or duodenum, and "falls away" after some of the cyst contents have drained out. This may result in cyst contents or gastric/intestinal contents spilling into the peritoneum with resulting chemical or infected peritonitis. Alternatively, pneumoperitoneum may occur, which also usually requires surgical repair.

Infectious complications typically occur as a result of stent clogging which is why multiple stents are typically used. Double pigtail stents are far less likely to migrate into or out of the cyst as compared to straight stents. Although 10-Fr stents will stay patent longer than 7 French stents, they cannot be placed through a standard linear echoendoscope. Self-expanding metallic stents which can maintain patency of the endoscopically created cystoenteric fistula are under development, but are not currently available. The other factor that can promote stent clogging is the presence of a large amount of debris within a pseudocyst. This may actually be a contraindication to endoscopic cystenterostomy.

19.3.6 Recurrence After Endoscopic Pseudocyst Drainage

A subgroup of patients undergoing endoscopic cystenterostomy will have recurrence of the cyst. This appears to be irrespective of drainage technique (EUS versus no EUS guidance), and is between 6% and 27%. These recurrences are due to "downstream" anatomic issues with the pancreatic duct. It has been borne out by clinical experience that downstream obstruction of the pancreatic duct, either by strictures or by intraductal pancreatic stones, will lead to recurrence. A large communication between the pancreatic duct and the pseudocyst may also be indicative of cases which may not respond to endoscopic therapy. Nealon and Walser (2002, 2005) described seven subtypes of pancreatic pseudocysts depending on whether there is or is not communication with the main duct, and on the presence of pancreatic ductal changes (strictures or chronic pancreatitis). Recurrence is highest in those cysts that are associated with communication and downstream pancreatic ductal stricture. In some cases of extensive necrosis of the body of the pancreas, a "disconnected pancreatic tail" can remain (Fig. 19.6.). In these cases, recurrence after endoscopic drainage is high (Deviere and Antaki 2008).

Rarely, a cystic lesion strongly resembles a pseudocyst, but is actually a cystic neoplasm. These lesions would of course not be expected to resolve. Sending a sample of cyst fluid for CEA has been recommended to rule out this possibility.

19.4 Endoscopic Management of Other Pancreatic Fluid Collections

Techniques that are used for drainage of pancreatic pseudocysts have also been used to drain other peripancreatic fluid collections. These include organized pancreatic necrosis and pancreatic abscesses. It has also been used for endoscopic pancreatic necrosectomy. Baron et al. (2002) carried out a retrospective

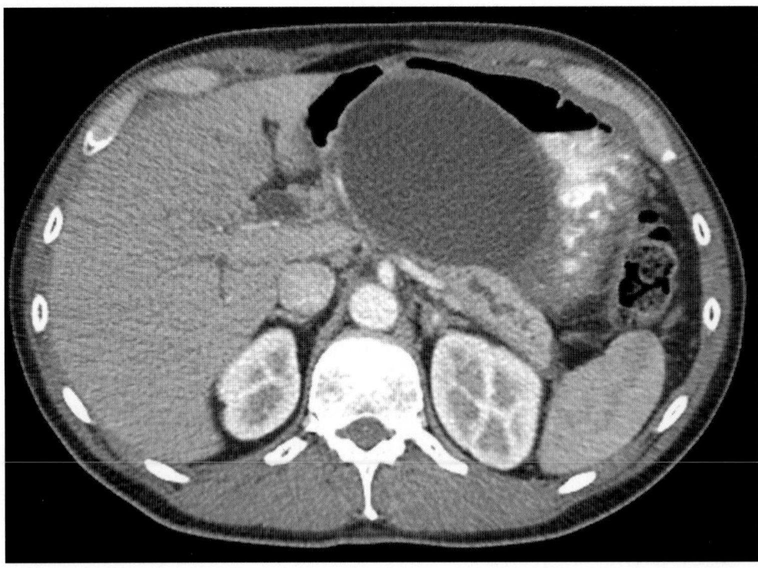

Fig. 19.6. Pseudocyst with disconnected pancreatic tail. A large mid-body pseudocyst is seen. A large section of pancreatic tail is still present, with a dilated pancreatic duct within it. This situation is associated with a high frequency of cyst recurrence after transmural drainage

review of their experience with 138 cases, including 31 acute pseudocysts, 64 chronic pseudocysts, and 43 cases of pancreatic necrosis. Drainage of pancreatic necrosis was associated with the highest complication rate (37%), the lowest percentage of successful resolution (72%), and the highest rate of recurrence (29%).

Pancreatic abscesses may be drained, if the anatomy is favorable (Venu et al. 2000). Successful outcome may require multiple procedures, placement of nasopancreatic drains, and intracavitary instillation of antibiotics. More recently, a technique has been described in which, after an EUS-guided fistula into the infected necrotic area has been made, an endoscope is used to access the interior of the cavity. Endoscopic accessories, including snares and baskets, are then used to debride the interior and walls of the cavity (Charnley et al. 2006; Seewald et al. 2006). The results of this technique are encouraging, and appear to be safe. The major drawback is the need for multiple procedures, sometimes repeated daily.

19.4.1 Endoscopic Management of Pancreatic Duct Leaks

In some cases, pancreatic duct disruption does not lead to pseudocyst formation, but to persistent pancreatic duct leaks. These may lead to spillage of pancreatic juice into the peritoneal cavity ("pancreatic ascites"), which is diagnosed by high amylase content in peritoneal fluid. Pancreatic fluid can also track into the pleural space, leading to high amylase pleural effusion. Post-operative pancreatic duct leaks are not rare. While most resolve with conservative therapy, some will result in persistent pancreatico-cutaneous fistulae or in continued high output of amylase-rich fluid from surgical drains. Similar leaks can be the result of post-traumatic pancreatic injury.

Pancreatic stenting for PD leaks and fistulae has been found to be highly useful. In some cases downstream pancreatic duct strictures can be found that are "driving" the fistula. These will need to be addressed if long-term success is to be achieved. The reader is referred to Chap. 13 for details on techniques and equipment for pancreatic duct stenting.

Kozarek et al. (1997) described a series of nine patients with pancreatic duct leaks from a variety of causes including two post-operative cases. All had failed other management. Eight of nine cases resolved with transpapillary stenting. Bridging of the leak point was not necessary to effect closure of the leak. Cicek et al. (2006) retrospectively looked at 28 cases of leak, including four cases of pancreatic ascites. Pancreatic stents were successful in closing 94% of leaks from partial or side branch ductal disruption. Complete ductal disruption responded in only one of five cases.

In a series of 16 consecutive patients with post-surgical pancreatic fistulas, Costamagna et al. (2001) attempted nasopancreatic drain placement (or pancreatic stent in one case) to aid in fistula closure. Placement of the drain was possible in 12 (technical success of 75%). In all of these patients, fistulas closed in a mean time of 8.8 days, and there were no recurrences after a mean follow-up of 25 months.

19.5 Conclusions

Endotherapy for chronic pancreatitis and its complications has made considerable progress over the past 20 years. Careful case selection appears to be able to lead to better outcomes in terms of clinical resolution. Several leading endoscopy centers have pushed the envelope on what can be accomplished through the endoscope. The addition of EUS is a major advance in the management of pseudocysts. As therapeutic endoscopists become more "adventurous," pancreatic problems that were once thought to be off-limits to endoscopic therapy have become "fair game." Clearly, there are clinical situations in which surgical management will remain the best choice. There are other situations in which endoscopic management is feasible, but probably not the most efficient treatment given the number of repeat ERCPs and possible extracorporeal shock wave lithotripsy sessions that may be necessary to achieve a good outcome. Application of the research methodology used in the field of outcome research will hopefully be able to better define cases which are best managed with endotherapy versus the more traditional surgical approach.

References

Arvanitakis M, Delhaye M, Bali MA, et al. (2007) Pancreatic-fluid collections: a randomized controlled trial regarding stent removal after endoscopic transmural drainage. Gastrointest Endosc 65:609–619

Balakrishnan V, Chatni S, Radhakrishnan L, et al. (2007) Groove pancreatitis: a case report and review of literature. JOP 7:592–597

Baron TH (2007) Treatment of pseudocysts, pancreatic necrosis, and pancreatic duct leaks. GI Endosc Clin North Am 17:559–579

Baron TH, Harewood GC, Morgan DE, Yates MR (2002) Outcome differences after endoscopic drainage of pancreatic necrosis, acute pancreatic pseudocysts, and chronic pancreatic pseudocysts. Gastrointest Endosc 56:7–17

Barthet M, Sahel J, Bodiou-Bertei C, Bernard JP (1995) Endoscopic transpapillary drainage of pancreatic pseudocysts. Gastrointest Endosc 42:208–213

Barthet M, Lamblin G, Gasmi M, et al. (2008) Clinical usefulness of a treatment algorithm for pancreatic pseudocysts. Gastrointest Endosc 67:245–252

Beckingham IJ, Krige JEJ, Bornman PC, et al. (1999) Long term outcome of endoscopic drainage of pancreatic pseudocysts. Am J Gastroenterol 94:71–74

Bhasin DK, Rana SS, Udawat HP, et al. (2006) Management of multiple and large pancreatic pseudocysts by endoscopic transpapillary nasopancreatic drainage alone. Am J Gastroenterol 101:1780–1786

Binmoeller KF, Seifert H, Walter A, Soehendra N (1995) Transpapillary and transmural drainage of pancreatic pseudocysts. Gastrointest Endosc 42:219–224

Cahen D, Rauws E, Fockens P, et al. (2005) Endoscopic drainage of pancreatic pseudocysts: long-term outcome and procedural factors associated with safe and successful treatment. Endoscopy 37:977–983

Cahen Dl, Rauws EA, Gouma Dj et al. (2008) Removable fully covered self-expandable metal stents in the treatment of common bile duct strictures due to chronic pancreatitis: a case series. Endoscopy 40:697–700

Cantu P, Hookey LC, Morales A, et al. (2005) The treatment of patient with symptomatic common bile duct stenosis secondary to chronic pancreatitis using partially covered metal stents: a pilot study. Endoscopy 37:735–739

Catalano MF, Geenen JE, Schmalz MJ, et al. (1995) Treatment of pancreatic pseudocysts with ductal communication by transpapillary pancreatic duct endoprosthesis. Gastrointest Endosc 42:214–218

Charnley RM, Lochan R, Gray H, et al. (2006) Endoscopic necrosectomy as primary therapy in the management of infected pancreatic necrosis. Endoscopy 38:925–928

Cicek B, Parlak E, Oguz D, et al. (2006) Endoscopic treatment of pancreatic fistulas. Surg Endosc. 20:1706–1712.

Cortes ES, Maalai A, Le Moine O, et al. (2002) Endoscopic cystenterostomy of nonbulging pancreatic fluid collections. Gastrointest Endosc 56:380–386

Costamagna G, Mutignani M, Ingrosso M, et al. (2001) Endoscopic treatment of postsurgical external pancreatic fistulas. Endoscopy 33:317–322.

Cremer M, Deviere J, Engelhom L (1989) Endoscopic management of cysts and pseudocysts in chronic pancreatitis: long-term follow-up after 7 years of experience. Gastrointest Endosc 35:1–9

DePalma GD, Galloro G, Puzziello A, et al. (2002) Endoscopic drainage of pancreatic pseudocysts: a long-term follow-up study of 49 patients. Hepatogastroenterology 49:1113–1115

Devière J, Antaki F (2008) Disconnected pancreatic tail syndrome: a plea for multidisciplinarity. Gastrointest Endosc 67:680–682.

Draganov P, Hoffman B, Marsh W, et al. (2002) Long-term outcome in patients with benign biliary strictures treated endoscopically with multiple stents. Gastrointest Endosc 55:680–686

Eickhoff A, Jakobs R, Leonhardt et al. (2003) Self-expandable metal mesh stents for common bile duct stenosis in chronic pancreatitis: retrospective evaluation of long-term follow-up and clinical outcome pilot study. Z Gastroenterol 41:649–654

Fockens P, Johnson TG, VanDullemen HM, et al. (1997) Endosonographic imaging of pancreatic pseudocysts before endoscopic transmural drainage. Gastrointest Endosc 46:412–416

Giovannini M, Pesenti C, Rolland AL, et al. (2001) Endoscopic ultrasound-guided drainage of pancreatic pseudocysts or pancreatic abscesses using a therapeutic echo endoscope. Endoscopy 33:473–477

Hookey LC, Debroux S, Delhaye M, et al. (2006) Endoscopic drainage of pancreatic fluid collections in 116 patients: a comparison of etiologies, drainage techniques, and outcomes. Gastrointest Endosc 63:635–643

Kahaleh M, Shami WM, Conaway M, et al. (2006) Endoscopic ultrasound drainage of pancreatic pseudocyst: a prospective comparison with conventional endoscopic drainage. Endoscopy 38:355–359

Kahl S, Zimmermann S, Genz I, et al. (2003) Risk factors for failure of endoscopic stenting of biliary strictures in chronic pancreatitis: a prospective follow-up study. Am J Gastroenterol 98:2448–2453

Kozarek RA, Ball TJ, Patterson DJ, et al. (1997) Transpapillary stenting for pancreatico-cutaneous fistulas. J Gastrointest Surg 1:357–361

Lopes CV, Pesenti C, Bories, et al. (2007) Endoscopic-ultrasound-guided endoscopic transmural drainage of pancreatic pseudocysts and abscesses. Scand J Gastroenterol 42:524–529

Nealon WH, Walser E (2002) Main pancreatic ductal anatomy can direct choice of modality for treating pancreatic pseudocysts (surgery versus percutaneous drainage). Ann Surg 235:751–758

Nealon WH, Walser E (2005) Surgical management of complications associated with percutaneous and/or endoscopic management of pseudocyst of the pancreas. Ann Surg 241:948–960

Norton ID, Clain JE, Wiersema MJ, et al. (2001) Utility of endoscopic ultrasonography drainage of pancreatic pseudocysts in selected patients. Mayo Clin Proc 76:794–798

Rogers BH, Cicurel NJ, Seed RW (1975) Transgastric needle aspiration of pancreatic pseudocyst through an endoscope. Gastrointest Endosc 21:133–134

Sanchez Cortes, E, Maalak A, LeMoine O, et al. (2002) Endoscopic cystenterostomy of non-bulging pancreatic fluid collections. Gastrointest Endosc 56:380–386

Seewald S, Groth S, mar S, et al. (2006) Aggressive endoscopic therapy for pancreatic necrosis and pancreatic abscess: a new safe and effective treatment algorithm. Gastrointest Endsoc 62:92–100

Sharma SS, Bhargawa N, Govil A (2002) Endoscopic management of pancreatic pseudocyst: a long-term follow-up. Endoscopy 34:203–207

Smits ME, Rauws EAJ, Tytgat GNJ, Huibregtse K (1995) The efficacy of endoscopic treatment of pancreatic pseudocysts. Gastrointest Endosc 42:202–207

Smits ME, Rauws EAJ, Van Gulik TM, et al. (1996) Long-term results of endoscopic stenting and surgical drainage for biliary strictures due to chronic pancreatitis. Br J Surg 83:764–768

van Berkel AM, Cahen DL, van Westerloo DJ, et al. (2004) Self-expanding metal stents in benign biliary strictures due to chronic pancreatitis. Endoscopy 36:381

Varadarajulu S, Christein JD, Tamhane A, et al. (2008) Prospective randomized trial comparing EUS and EGD for transmural drainage of pancreatic pseudocysts. Gastrointest Endosc 68:1102–1111

Venu RP, Brown RD, Marrero JA, et al. (2000) Endoscopic transpapillary drainage of pancreatic abscess: technique and results. Gastrointest Endosc 51:391–395

Voermans RP, Eisendrath P, Bruno MJ, et al. (2007) Initial evaluation of a novel prototype forward-viewing ultrasound endoscope in transmural drainage of pancreatic pseudocysts. Gastrointest Endosc 66:1013–1017

Surgical and Interventional Perspective in Chronic Pancreatitis

20

Massimo Falconi, Letizia Boninsegna, Nora Sartori, Claudio Bassi, and Paolo Pederzoli

CONTENTS

20.1 **Introduction and Therapeutic Indications** 383
20.1.1 Signs and Symptoms 383
20.1.2 Development of the Disease 384
20.1.3 Morphological Aspects Evaluated with Imaging 384
20.2 **Clinico-morphologic Correlation and Therapeutic Choices** 384
20.2.1 Pain 384
20.2.1.1 Pain Associated with Uniform Dilatation of the Wirsung Duct 385
20.2.1.2 Pain Associated with "Chain-of-Lake" Dilatation of the Wirsung Duct 385
20.2.1.3 Pain Asscociated with Segmental Dilatation of the Wirsung Duct 386
20.2.1.4 Pain and Groove Pancreatitis 386
20.2.1.5 Pain and Suspected Tumor 386
20.2.2 Pseudocysts 387
20.2.3 Biliary Obstruction 387
20.2.4 Duodenal Obstruction 388
20.3 **Conclusions** 388
References 389

M. Falconi, MD; L. Boninsegna, MD; N. Sartori, MD
C. Bassi, MD; P. Pederzoli, MD
Chirurgia B, Surgical and Gastroenterological Department, Hospital "GB Rossi", University of Verona, Piazzale LA Scuro 10, 37134 Verona, Italy

20.1 Introduction and Therapeutic Indications

Chronic pancreatitis (CP) is characterised by the progressive destruction of the pancreatic parenchyma with coincident replacement by fibrous tissue (Di Magno et al. 1993; Kloeppel and Maillet 1993). As the disease evolves, clinical manifestations and anatomic changes progress forcing an evolving therapeutic approach, be it surgical or interventional, to these comlex patients (Cavallini et al. 1998). In recent years, the level of sophistication of our knowledge of the epidemiology, etiological factors, and concurrent increasing availability of new therapeutic options has significantly altered our approach. The following chapter will attempt to reassess the role of surgery for patients with CP.

Clinical and therapeutic decisions are made based on: (1) the presence of determined signs and symptoms; (2) the natural history of the disease, its physical impact and effect on the quality of life (QOL) and (3) the presence or absence of morphologic alterations that are amenable to surgical intervention.

20.1.1 Signs and Symptoms

During the course of the disease, the most frequent treatment indication is the presence of pain defined as severe and disabling (Pederzoli et al. 1994). Less common indications of treatment are the presence of a pseudocyst, biliary tract and/or duodenum involvement and the suspicion of a tumor (Russel 1998). Infrequent (although compelling) indications for rapid treatment include haemorrhage and portal hypertension (Seiler et al. 1998), stenosis of the colon (Bradley 1982a) and the onset of pancreatic ascites, pleural effusion and internal fistulas (Neoptolemos and Winslet 1990). It is evident from the varied spectrum of complications that no single or "universal" approach to the disease exists and that treatment must be based on other factors.

20.1.2 Development of the Disease

The goal of surgical or interventional therapy is to improve the patient's quality of life (Knoefel et al. 1997). This has lead to the steady increase of minimally invasive (e.g. endoscopic) therapies replacing "traditional" surgical treatments (Bassi et al. 1998). The two approaches are complementary. Guidelines are continually being outlined to help the clinician towards an optimal therapeutic choice; however, endoscopic approaches will be favored over surgical when the outcome of treatment is equivalent (Binmoeller et al. 1995). Nevertheless, there are few controlled short or long term clinical trials that have compared the results and impacts of the different therapeutic options. Not surprisingly, therapeutic choices are still based on local experience and expertise rather than on medical evidence. Moreover, the absence of a more precise definition of a "painful and disabling" symptom actually makes comparison of inter-institutional experiences considerably less reliable. Many scores and/or questionnaires have been proposed to attempt to make evaluation of pain in CP more "objective" (Beger et al. 1989; Knoefel et al. 1997).

20.1.3 Morphological Aspects Evaluated with Imaging

Further important information to help determine which therapeutic choice to adopt can be obtained from imaging, especially computed tomography (CT) and magnetic resonance (MRI) (Freney 1998). Imaging studies have not only contributed substantially to the recognition of the disease and its complications, but have also "added" further disease classification and pathogenetic elements. The radiologist can diagnose the illness, and his description becomes a guide in choosing the therapy.

One complication of CP that cross-sectional imaging greatly aided in defining is the entity of Groove pancreatitis. It has been reported that in about 20% of CP cases a scarring in the "groove" region (between the medial duodenal wall and the pancreatic head) occurs (Becker and Mischke 1991; Ioth et al. 1994). We have observed a distinct entity of cystic dystrophy of the duodenal wall as a "subset" of complications occurring in patients with chronic groove pancreatitis (Colardelle et al. 1994; Procacci et al. 1997; Falconi et al. 2000).

As of today, however, there is poor correlation between the imaging findings of dilatation of the pancreatic duct and patient symptoms (Nealon et al. 1988; Nealon and Thompson 1993). In truth, there is not enough clinical information at the moment to warrant surgical therapy or endoscopic stenting of every dilated duct in CP patients.

20.2 Clinico-morphologic Correlation and Therapeutic Choices

It has been highlighted how the same symptom, for example pain, can occur in patients with a wide spectrum of morphological alterations to the pancreas and how a careful radiological description can help the clinician in deciding on the therapy that is best tailored to the particular pattern of the disease. The aim of this section is to outline the different approaches to the disease in relation to the symptoms and the morphology.

20.2.1 Pain

Pain, typically debilitating and overwhelming, is the most common clinical manifestation occurring during the course of the disease. There are two hypotheses offered to explain the source of this pain. The first relates the pain to an increase in intraductal and/or parenchymal pressure related to difficulty in discharging pancreatic juice in the duodenum (Bradley 1982b; Ebbehoj et al. 1984; Ebbehoj 1993). The second and more recent, however, maintains that pain is linked to the release of neurotransmitters into the inflamed mass (Bockmann et al. 1988). If the clinician believes the first hypothesis, he will opt for any therapy that can relieve ductal pressure whereas, if the clinician believes the second hypothesis, he maintain that this objective can only be reached by resection of the part of the gland principally involved. What is true is that both theories are probably complementary: in fact, the long-term results of both "removers" and "diverters", in terms of patient pain, are practically the same. BEGER et al. (1989) found that more than two thirds of the patients they observed had a "mass forming" CP, while, in our experience, this ratio is reversed (PEDERZOLI et al. 1994; FALCONI et al. 2000). The relation of morphologic change to the types and proportions of alcohol abuse has never been investigated.

To further complicate matters the intensity of the pain over the course of the patient's illness follows a "bimodal" pattern (CAVALLINI et al. 1998). In the initial years of the disease the pain gradually intensifies but then it tends to spontaneously disappear once the gland is totally atrophied (AMMAN et al. 1984). This aspect makes it particularly difficult to establish whether the pain relief is directly related to surgical intervention or the natural progression of the disease (LANKISH 1998); however, reports document that up to 50% of patients attain pain relief from surgical therapy (TALAMINI et al. 1996). Table 20.1 summarizes how our surgical therapies for CP patients with severe pain are based on specific morphologic alterations as defined by imaging.

20.2.1.1
Pain Associated with Uniform Dilatation of the Wirsung Duct

This condition occurs when the fibrosis directly involves the papilla of Vater. Papillary stenosis leads to uniform and progressive dilatation of the main duct (chronic obstructive pancreatitis). The stasis of the pancreatic juice promotes the formation of calculi. These patients can be effectively treated endoscopically by stenting the papilla with or without lithotripsy, as a first line therapeutic intervention (DELHAYE et al. 1992; SAUERBRUCH et al. 1992). The published endoscopic series reports good results, even in the long term (CREMER et al. 1991; BINMOELLER et al. 1995; SMITS et al. 1995). These patients should be referred to the surgeon only after an endoscopic attempt has failed (BASSI et al. 1998).

20.2.1.2
Pain Associated with "Chain-of-Lake" Dilatation of the Wirsung Duct

This is the classical duct morphology associated with CP often caused by alcohol abuse. It is characterised by the dilatation of the main pancreatic duct associated with numerous stenoses, intraductal and intraparenchymal calcification. If the pancreatic duct is dilatated, with or without enlargement of the pancreatic head, the intervention of choice should be one of the procedures that is directed at widening the pancreatic duct to improve drainage. As opposed to simple drainage (as achieved by stenting), these procedures offer the highest likelihood of relief of intraductal pressure and clearance of intraductal calculi.. Pain relief is achieved in more than 80% of cases with minimal sacrifice of the parenchyma (IZBICKI et al. 1995). We prefer lateral pancreatico-jejunostomy according to Frey (FREY and SMITH 1987). This operation provides drainage of the pancreatic duct at the head-tail and removal of a small portion of the pancreatic head in order to connect, and therefore drain, all the Wirsung and Santorini ducts and, at the same time, remove that part of the pancreatic area that is principally expected to produce neurotransmitters. The quantity of the gland removed is equal to about 5 g of tissue. An alternative method combines partial removal of the pancreatic head and

Table 20.1. Relationship between radiological findings and type of surgical procedures in the presence of disabling pain in CP

Dilatation of the Wirsung duct not limited to the body-tail	Pancreaticojejunostomy according to Frey
Stenosis[a] with dilatation of the Wirsung duct at the tail	Pancreaticojejunostomy according to Partington-Rochelle
Pseudocyst that does not involve the splenic hilum	Cysto-jejunostomy\pancreatico-cysto-jejunostomy
Pseudocyst that involves the splenic hilum	Left-pancreatectomy
Cystic dystrophy of the duodenal wall	PPPD[b]
Pancreatic head mass	PPPD[b]
Multiple cephalic calcifications	PPPD[b]

[a] Single calculus – cicatricial stenosis post acute severe pancreatitis or trauma
[b] A classic PD according to Whipple or Longmire-Traverso can be performed

widespread ductal drainage, the duodenum preserving pancreatic head resection (DPPHR) (Beger et al. 1985). Compared to the Frey method, more of the head of the pancreas is resected (including part of the uncinate process), extending as far as the neck of the gland. However, in a prospective randomized clinical trial the surgical outcomes are identical although the DPPHR had a higher morbidity (Izbicki et al. 1995). Successful DPPHR requires pancreatic transection in front of the portal vein, which is often difficult in CP patients. Preservation of the duodenum, part of both techniques, is of particular importance. It guarantees, in the long-term, better control of glucose metabolism (Izbicki et al. 1998).

20.2.1.3 Pain Asscociated with Segmental Dilatation of the Wirsung Duct

This condition is a late consequence of acute necrotizing pancreatitis (ANP). The repairing-scarring process results in a stenosis of the main (Wirsung) duct leading to upstream dilatation with or without ductal casts. A history of a past episode of ANP or of a trauma are particularly important to differentiate the upstream dilatation resulting from intraductal papillary mucinous tumor (IPMT), or even a small "strategically located' neoplasm. If the diagnosis of chronic pancreatitis is established, we perform a Partington-Rochelle pancreatico-jejunostomy (PJ) (Partington and Rochelle 1960) in this select group of patients. This involves bivalving the affected Wirsung duct over an approximately 6 cm length and creating an anastomosis with an excluded jejunal Y loop. Mortality and morbidity rates are extremely low. Most authors consider a Wirsung duct of at least 8 mm as sufficiently dilatated.

20.2.1.4 Pain and Groove Pancreatitis

A scarring in the region of the "groove" between the duodenum and the head of the pancreas has been described in 20% of CP cases (Becker and Mischke 1991; Ioth et al. 1994). The reported frequency reflects our experience as well. When the scarring results in the coalescence of a cystic collection in this region, we have introduced the term cystic dystrophy of the duodenal wall (Procacci et al. 1997; Falconi et al. 2000). The pathogenesis is believed to be related to development of acute, and then chronic pancreatitis in pancreatic rests embedded in the duodenal wall. Alcohol abuse, particularly beer, is found in most patients who develop this complication. The portion of the pancreatic head between the duodenum laterally, and the choledochus medially, is involved, while in about 20% of cases, the pancreas appears normal (Colardelle et al. 1994). Symptoms of the onset of pain are associated with symptoms of gastric outlet obstruction alternating with cystic formations in the duodenal part that obstruct the lumen. Morphologically, either a "cystic" variant, requiring differentiation from pseudocyst, or a "solid" variant, requiring differentiation from neoplasm, will occur. Generally, the head of the pancreas is enlarged by up to three to four times its normal size. Surgical treatment requires pancreatico-duodenectomy (PD) utilizing, if possible, pyloric sparing reconstruction (pylorus-preserving pancreatico-duodenectomy; PPPD) (Traverso and Longmire 1978). PPPD, compared to the traditional Whipple resection (Whipple et al. 1935), decreases recovery time and more rapidly improves nutrition (Di Carlo et al. 1999). However, local conditions, such as an extensive inflammatory process or adhesions between the pancreatic head and the splenoporto-mesenteric vessels, increase surgical morbidity and mortality.

20.2.1.5 Pain and Suspected Tumor

Imaging differentiation of CP and tumor (Rosch et al. 2000), whether ductal carcinoma (Taylor 2003) or cystic forms (IPMT), remains difficult in individual cases (Falconi et al. 2001). The clinical history of alcohol and additional tobacco abuse should heighten suspicion of tumor in an older CP patient with recent onset of pain (Talamini et al. 1999a,b). CP in and of itself carries a greater risk of pancreatic cancer development (Lowenfels et al. 1993; Talamini et al. 1999a,b). At operation, the surgeon must perform needle aspiration and/or biopsy, even opening the main duct (Witz et al. 1989) to exclude tumor. If doubt persists, the surgical choice should be to assume tumor is present and perform the appropriate resection based on the size and location (Smith et al. 1994; Thompson et al. 1994; Bottger et al. 1999); lesions in the head of the pancreas are treated with PPPD (Kozuscheck et al. 1994). This is true even if the final histological examination on the resected tissue should confirm CP (Martin et al. 1996). A Frey pancreatico-jejunostomy or DPPHR is not optimal in the case of a suspected tumor (Izbicki et al. 1995).

If there is clinical suspicion of tumor in the body or tail of the pancreas, the best intervention is a classic left-pancreatectomy (LP), removing the body-tail of the pancreas and the spleen. In these cases, the presence of simultaneous morphologic changes that also involve the head (calcifications, dilatation of the main duct) should prompt performing a pancreatico-jejunostomy as well (Puestow and Gillesby 1958).

20.2.2 Pseudocysts

This is a common complication during CP occurring in between 10%–20% of patients. The development of a pseudocyst is due to acute pancreatic inflammation that leads to rupture in the pancreatic duct system and spillage of pancreatic juices into the peritoneum. This results in the creation of a pseudowall and consequently the formation of a pseudocyst (Pederzoli et al. 1994). Unlike acute pancreatitis, in CP the pseudocysts are significantly less frequently reabsorbed because they are generally connected to the ductal system and cause further complications (Yeo et al. 1990). When pseudocysts develop in CP patients, there are three possible treatments: percutaneous drainage, endoscopic drainage or surgery. Percutaneous drainage, given the frequent communication between the pseudocyst and the ductal system, should be reserved for infected pseudocysts only (Contasdemir et al. 2003). Endoscopic drainage may be taken into consideration for those pseudocysts that impinge on the stomach or duodenum with no other surgical indications (Bassi et al. 1998; Beckingham et al. 1999). Surgery, however, is indicated in those cases where a pseudocyst is not accessible to endoscopic approach. If the pseudocyst has a readily demonstrable connection with the main duct, a cystojejunostomy (CJ) may suffice. If it is isolated or if communication is not evident but the Wirsung duct is dilatated, it will be necessary to perform a pancreo-cysto-jejunostomy (PCJ) (Pederzoli et al. 1994). If the pseudocyst involves the spleen or if there is clinical suspicion that the mass might in fact be a mucinous cystic tumor, optimal surgical treatment is to perform a left-pancreatectomy with a possible pancreatico-jejunal anastomosis on the stump (Prinz 1993; Sawyer and Frey 1994).

20.2.3 Biliary Obstruction

Biliary obstruction occurs in 10%–30% of CP patients. The distal common bile duct (CBD) passes inside the substance of the head of the pancreas. The bile duct becomes stenotic due to progressive fibrosis in the surrounding affected parenchyma. An obstruction in the main biliary duct rarely presents as an isolated symptom of the disease; it is often associated with pain or the presence of pseudocysts (Falconi et al. 1999). Clinical jaundice does not always occur despite the biliary obstruction; however, an elevation in the serum alkaline phosphatase may signal biliary obstruction (Stahl et al. 1998; Falconi et al. 1999). Stenosis in CP can be differentiated from neoplasm in that CP induced biliary stenosis generally involves the entire intra-pancreatic protion of the CBD.

The surgical procedure is determined by symptoms and co-morbidities (Table 20.2). There is no problem if the head of the pancreas is to be resected as a choledocho-enterostomy is routinely performed. When the cholestasis indexes are altered, any narrowing of the bile ducts should be addressed. The best intervention is a hepatic or choledoco-jejunostomy on the same excluded Y-Roux

Table 20.2. Relationship between radiological findings and type of surgical procedures in the presence of biliary tract involvement in CP patients

Dilatation of the choledochus and the Wirsung duct due to cephalic calcifications	Pancreaticojejunostomy according to Frey or alternatively PPPD[a]
Dilatation of the choledochus and the Wirsung duct due to pancreatic head mass	PPPD[a]
Cystic dystrophy of the duodenal wall	PPPD[a]
Pseudocyst conditioning dilation of the biliary tree	Pancreaticojejunostomy or cysto-jejunostomy

[a] Depending on the anatomical conditions, a PD according to Whipple or Longmire-Traverso can be performed

jejunal loop used for the pancreatico-jejunostomy (Prinz et al. 1985; Sugerman et al. 1986; Warshaw 1988; Pederzoli et al. 1994). This operation, unlike a choledo-duodeno-anastomosis, offers the advantage of fewer risks of cholangitis in the follow-up from reflux of foodstuffs in the biliary tract (Rothlin et al. 1998). A cholecysto-jejunostomy should always be avoided due to the high risk of malfunction (Sarfeh et al. 1988). Cholecystectomy should always be performed after choledocho-enterostomy. In specific cases, endoscopic stenting can be performed. Stenting is performed for patients with significant portal hypertension due to mesenteric thrombosis, when the biliary tract is surrounded by a cavernoma and surgical access is not possible (Kahl et al. 2002). Surgery is ultimately definitive and avoids multiple procedures necessary to replace the stents, improving the QOL of these patients.

20.2.4 Duodenal Obstruction

An isolated duodenal stenosis is also a rare occurrence. When it does occur, it is usually associated with a cystic dystrophy of the duodenal wall or groove pancreatitis (see Sect. 2.1.4). If surgical resection is not indicated or possible, a bypass procedure for the stomach should be considered (Table 20.3). Clinical history should be directed at assessing for symptoms of gastric outlet obstruction. If in doubt, an endoscopic or barium assessment of the stomach and duodenum is useful.

There are several surgical techniques for performing a digestive by-pass, the most common of which is latero-lateral, retrogastric, transmesocholic gastro-entero-anastomosis (GEA). Gastric transposition with pylorus preservation is a possible alternative (Falconi et al. 2004). In this intervention, a duodenal transection is performed as in PPPD, leaving the pancreatic head and carrying out an anastomosis between the remaining duodenal stump with the stomach and the first jejunal loop after the Treitz. Compared to a traditional GEA, this operation has the advantage of avoiding a possible recirculation of the food bolus between the duodenum and the stomach and of being able to make a possible biliary anastomosis on the excluded duodenum, thus reducing the risk of cholangitis (Falconi et al. 2004).

20.3 Conclusions

Considering the wide range of interventional therapeutic options and the different types of operations that can be proposed, the radiologist's role in the management of CP patients is crucial in defining the correct anatomic status of the patient allowing for the choice of the most optimal intervention. The results are improved in centers where there is a team approach to pancreatic disease. These teams are composed of surgeons, gastroenterologists, radiologists, endoscopists and nutritionists. In this way either interventional percutaneous or endoscopic or surgical management can be assigned based on individual patient parameters. If surgical intervention is indicated, the choice of procedure should be based both on the reasons that have led to the treatment indication and the morphological aspects that imaging has brought to light. Increasing reports in the literature comparing therapeutic alternatives will lead to the rapid abandonment of those techniques that can no longer be justified in terms of morbidity and therapeutic failure.

Table 20.3. Relationship between morphological radiological findings and type of surgical procedures in the presence of gastrointestinal symptoms

Annular pancreas with stenosis of the duodenum	Gastro-entero-anastomosis or gastric transposition [a]
Cystic dystrophy of the duodenal wall	Pancreaticoduodenectomy [b]
Pseudocyst conditioning delayed gastric and/or duodenal discharge	Pancreatico-cysto-jejunostomy, pancreatico-gastro-jejunostomy or cysto-jejunostomy

[a] Depending on the anatomical conditions (see text)

[b] Depending on the anatomical conditions, a PD according to Whipple or Longmire-Traverso can be performed

References

Amman RW, Akovbiantz A, Largiader F, Schueler G (1984) Course and outcome of chronic pancreatitis. Longitudinal study of a mixed medical-surgical series of 254 patients. Gastroenterology 86:820–828

Bassi C, Falconi M, Caldiron E et al. (1998) To what extent is surgery superior to endoscopic therapy in the management of chronic pancreatitis. Ital J Gastroenterol Hepatol 30:571–578

Becker V, Mischke U (1991) Groove pancreatitis. Int J Pancreatol 10:173–182

Beckingham IJ, Krige JE, Bormman PC, Terblanche J (1999) Long term outcome of endoscopic drainage of pancreatic pseudocysts. Am J Gastroenterol 94:71–74

Beger HG, Krautzberger W, Bittner R et al. (1985) Duodenum-preserving resection of the head of the pancreas in patients with severe chronic pancreatitis. Surgery 98:467–472

Beger HG, Buechler MW, Bittner RR et al. (1989) Duodenum-preserving resection of the head of the pancreas in severe chronic pancreatitis. Ann Surg 209:273–278

Binmoeller KF, Jue P, Seifert H et al. (1995) Endoscopic pancreatic stent drainage in chronic pancreatitis and dominant stricture: long term results. Endoscopy 27 638–644

Bockmann DE, Buechler MW, Malfertheiner P, Beger HG (1988) Analysis of nerves in chronic pancreatitis. Gastroenterology 94:1459–1469

Bottger TC, Junginger T (1999) Treatment of tumors of the pancreatic head with suspected but unproved malignancy: is a nihilistic approach justified? World J Surg 23:158–162

Bradley EL III (ed) (1982a) Complications of chronic pancreatitis: medical and surgical management. WB Saunders, Philadelphia, pp 265–292

Bradley EL III (1982b) Pancreatic duct pressure in chronic pancreatitis. Am J Surg 144:313–316

Cavallini G, Frulloni L, Pederzoli P et al. (1998) Long term follow-up of patients with chronic pancreatitis in Italy. Scand J Gastroenterol 33:880–889

Colardelle P, Chochon M, Larvon L et al. (1994) Dystrophie kystique sur pancreas aberrant antro-bulbaire. Gastroenterol Clin Biol 42:277–280

Contasdemir M, Kara B, Kantarci F, Mihmanli I, Numan F, Egurney S (2003) Percutaneous drainage of infected pancreatic pseudocysts. South Med J 96:136–140

Cremer M, Deviere J, Delhaye M et al. (1991) Stenting in severe chronic pancreatitis: results of medium-term follow-up in seventy-six patients. Endoscopy 23:171–176

Delhaye M, Vandermeeren A, Baize M, Cremer M (1992) Extracorporeal shockwave lithotripsy of pancreatic calculi. Gastroenterology 102:610–620

Di Carlo V, Zerbi A, Balzano, Corso V (1999) Pylorus-preserving pancreatico-duodenectomy versus conventional Whipple operation. World J Surg 23:920–925

Di Magno EP, Layer P, Clain JE (1993) Chronic pancreatitis. In: Go VLW, Di Magno EP, Gardner JD et al (eds) The pancreas: biology, pathobiology and disease. Raven Press, New York, pp 1433–1437

Ebbehoj N (1993) Pancreatic tissue fluid pressure and pain in chronic obstructive pancreatitis. Danish Med Bull 39:128–133

Ebbehoj N, Svendsen LB, Madsen P (1984) Pancreatic tissue pressure in chronic obstructive pancreatitis. Scand J Gastroenterol 19:1066–1068

Falconi M, Sartori N, Caldiron E et al. (1999) La pancreatite cronica: linee guida per un razionale approccio terapeutico endoscopico e chirurgico. Giornale Aggiornamenti Patologia Digestiva 2:17–35

Falconi M, Valerio A, Caldiron E et al. (2000) Changes in pancreatic resection for chronic pancreatitis over 28 years in a single institution. Br J Surg 87:428–433

Falconi M, Salvia R, Bassi C, Zamboni G, Talamini G, Pederzoli P (2001) Clinicopathological features and treatment of intraductal papillary mucinous tumour of the pancreas. Br J Surg 88:376–381

Falconi M, Hilal MA, Salvia R, Sartori N, Bassi C, Pederzoli P (2004) Prophylactic pylorus-preserving gastric transposition in unresectable carcinoma of the pancreatic head. Am J Surg 187:564–566

Freney PC (1998) Radiology. In: Beger HG, Warshaw AL, Buechler MW, et al (eds) The pancreas. Blackwell Science, London, pp 728–739

Frey CF, Smith GJ (1987) Description and rationale for a new operation for chronic pancreatitis. Pancreas 2:701–707

Ioth S, Yamakawa K, Shimamoto K et al. (1994) Groove pancreatitis. J Computed Assit Tomogr 18:911–915

Izbicki JR, Bloechle C, Knoeffel WT et al. (1995) Duodenum preserving resections of the head of the pancreas in chronic pancreatitis. A prospective randomized trial. Ann Surg 221:350–358

Izbicki JR, Bloechle C, Broering DC et al. (1998) Extended drainage versus resection in surgery for chronic pancreatitis. Prospective randomized trial comparing the longitudinal pancreatico-jejunostomy combined with local pancreatic head excision with the pylorus-preserving pancreatico-duodenectomy. Ann Surg 228:771–779

Kahl S, Zimmermann S, Glasbrenner B et al. (2002) Treatment of benign biliary strictures in chronic pancreatitis by self-expandable metal stents. Dig Dis 20:199–203

Kloeppel G, Maillet B (1993) Pathology of acute and chronic pancreatitis. Pancreas 8:659–670

Knoefel WT, Bloechle C, Limmer JC et al. (1997) Pathogenesis of pain and quality of life in chronic pancreatitis. In: Izbicki JR, Binmoeller KF, Soehendra N (eds)Chronic pancreatitis an interdisciplinary approach. De Gruyter, Berlin, pp 15–30

Kozuscheck W, Reith HB, Waleczech H et al. (1994) A comparison of long term results of the standard Whipple procedure and the pylorus preserving pancreatico-duodenectomy. J Am Coll Surg 178:443–453

Lankish PG, Lohr-Happe A, Otto J, Creutzfeldt W (1993) Natural course in chronic pancreatitis. Pain, exocrine and endocrine pancreatic insufficiency and prognosis of the disease. Digestion 54:148–155

Lankish PG (1998) Prognosis. In: Beger HG, Warshaw AL, Buechler MW, et al (eds) The pancreas. Blackwell Science, London, pp 740–747

Lowenfels AB, Maisonneuve P, Cavallini G et al. (1993) Pancreatitis and the risk of pancreatic cancer. International Pancreatitis Study Group. N Engl J Med 328:1433–1437

Martin RF, Rossi RL, Leslie KA (1996) Long term results of pylorus-preserving pancreatico-duodenectomy for chronic pancreatitis. Arch Surg 131:247–252

Nealon WH, Townsend CM, Thompson JC (1988) Operative drainage of the pancreatic duct delays functional impairment in patients with chronic pancreatitis. Ann Surg 208:321–329

Nealon WH, Thompson JC (1993) Progressive loss of pancreatic function in chronic pancreatitis is delayed by main pancreatic duct decompression. Ann Surg 217:458–468

Neoptolemos JP, Winslet MC (1990) Pancreatic ascites. In: Beger HG, Buechler MW, Ditschuneit H, Malferthainer P (eds) Chronic pancreatitis. Springer-Verlag, Berlin Heidelberg New York, pp 269–279

Partington PF, Rochelle RE (1960) Modified Puestow procedure for retrograde drainage of the pancreatic duct. Ann Surg 152:1037–1042

Pederzoli P, Falconi M, Bassi C et al. (1994) Derivative surgical treatment. In: Pederzoli P, Cavallini G, Bassi C, Falconi M (eds) Facing pancreatic dilemma. Springer-Verlag, Berlin Heidelberg New York, pp 199–213

Prinz RA (1993) Surgical options in chronic pancreatitis. Int J Pancreatol 14:97–105

Prinz RA, Aranha GV, Greenleem HB (1985) Combined pancreatic duct and upper gastrointestinal and biliary tract drainage in chronic pancreatitis. Arch Surg 120:361–366

Procacci C, Graziani R, Zamboni G et al. (1997) Cystic dystrophy of the duodenal wall: radiological findings. Radiology 205:741–747

Puestow CB, Gillesby WJ (1958) Retrograde surgical drainage of pancreas for chronic pancreatitis. Arch Surg 76:898–906

Rosch T, Schusdziarra V, Born P et al. (2000) Modern imaging methods versus clinical assessment in the evaluation of hospital in-patients with suspected pancreatic disease. Am J Gastroenterol 95:2261–2270

Rothlin MA, Lopfe M, Schlumpf R, Largiader F (1998) Long-term results of hepaticojejunostomy for benign lesions of the bile ducts. Am J Surg 175:22–26

Russel C (1998) Indications for surgery. In: Beger HG, Warshaw AL, Buechler MW, et al (eds) The pancreas. Blackwell Science, London, pp 815–823

Sauerbruch T, Holl J, Sackmann M, Paumgartner G (1992) Extracorporeal lithotripsy of pancreatic stones in patients with chronic pancreatitis and pain: a prospective follow up study. Gut 33:969–972

Sarfeh IJ, Rypins EB, Jakpwaz JG, Juler GL (1988) A prospective, randomized clinical investigation of cholecystoenterostomy and choledochoenterostomy. Am J Surg 155:411–414

Sawyer R, Frey CF (1994) Is there still a role for distal pancreatectomy in surgery for chronic pancreatitis. Am J Surg 168:6–9

Seiler CA, Friess H, Buechler MW (1998) Thrombosis of the portal and splenic vein. In: Beger HG, Warshaw AL, Buechler MW, et al (eds) The pancreas. Blackwell Science, London, pp 761–765

Smith CD, Behrns KE, van Heerden JA, Sarr MG (1994) Radical pancreatoduodenectomy for misdiagnosed pancreatic mass. Br J Surg 81:585–589

Smits ME, Badiga SM, Rauws AJ et al. (1995) Long term results of pancreatic stents in chronic pancreatitis. Gastrointest Endosc 42:452–456

Stahl TJ, O'Connors AM, Ansel HJ, Venes JA (1998) Partial biliary obstruction caused by chronic pancreatitis. Ann Surg 207:26–32

Sugerman HJ, Barnhart GR, Newsome HH (1986) Selective drainage for pancreatic, biliary, and duodenal obstruction secondary to chronic fibrosing pancreatitis. Ann Surg 203:558–567

Talamini G, Bassi C, Falconi M et al. (1996) Pain relapses in the first 10 years of chronic pancreatitis. Am J Surg 171:565–569

Talamini G, Falconi M, Bassi C et al. (1999a) Incidence of cancer in the course of chronic pancreatitis. Am J Gastroenterol 94:1253–1260

Talamini G, Bassi C, Falconi M et al. (1999b) Early detection of pancreatic cancer following the diagnosis of chronic pancreatitis. Digestion 60:554–561

Taylor B (2003) Carcinoma of the head of the pancreas versus chronic pancreatitis: diagnostic dilemma with significant consequences. World J Surg 27:1249–1257

Thompson JS, Murayama KM, Edney JA, Rikkers LF (1994) Pancreaticoduodenectomy for suspected but unproven malignancy. Am J Surg 168:571–573

Traverso LW, Longmire WP (1978) Preservation of the pylorus in pancreatico-duodenectomy. Surg Gynecol Obstet 146:659–662

Warshaw AL (1988) Conservation of pancreatic tissue by combined gastric, biliary, and pancreatic duct drainage for pain for chronic pancreatitis. Am J Surg 149:563–569

Whipple AO, Pearson WB, Mullins CR (1935) Treatment of carcinoma of the ampulla of Vater. Ann Surg 102:763–769

Witz M, Shkolnik Z, Dinbar A (1989) Intraoperative pancreatic biopsy – a diagnostic dilemma. J Surg Oncol 42:117–119

Yeo CJ, Bastidas JA, Lynch-Nyhan A, Fishman EK, Zinner MJ, Cameron JL (1990) The natural history of pancreatic pseudocysts documented by computer tomography. Surg Gynecol Obstet 170:411–417

Subject Index

A

abdominal
- pain 15, 107, 130
- trauma 270
- ultrasound 20
abscess 63
acetaldehyde 118
- toxicity 6
acinar
- atrophy 195
- carcinoma 161, 286
- cell 9
- - atrophy 154
- - damage 10
- - necrosis 9
- filling 83, 192
acquired immunodeficiency syndrome (AIDS) 50
activator protein 1 (AP-1) 10, 236
acute necrotizing pancreatitis 386
acute pancreatitis 3, 62, 84
- acute bleeding 300
- alcohol-induced 5
- complications 66
- features 15
- hemorrhagic complications 71
- MRI severity index 87
- pathophysiology 3
- resolution 41
- staging 61
- vascular complications 71
acute respiratory distress syndrome (ARDS) 11
adenocarcinoma 330, 338
- of the papilla 150
adipose tissue infiltration 234
albumin 6
alcohol
- abuse 50, 85, 117
- dehydrogenase (ADH) 118
alcoholic pancreatitis 5, 17, 51, 59, 171, 192, 232
ampulla of Vater 4
ampullary adenocarcinoma 360
amylase 191
anaplastic carcinoma 285
annular pancreas 123, 132, 150
antinuclear antibody 121
APACHE II score 18, 62
apparent diffusion coefficient (ADC) 101, 202
arterial
- bleeding 297
- disruption 288, 295, 296
- pseudoaneursysm 319
- spin labeling (ASL) 101
ascariasis 4
ascites 324
atrophy of acinar and islet tissue 183
autoimmune pancreatitis 60, 97, 100, 121, 131, 134, 143, 145, 168, 183, 195, 203, 240, 338
- steroid treatment 203
autophagic vacuole 8

B

bacterial cholangitis 373
Balthazar-Ranson scoring system 20
bariatric surgery 211
bile duct
- carcinoma 242
- stenosis 241, 323
- stricture 58, 210
biliary
- calculi 4, 85
- cirrhosis 245, 25, 302, 323
- colic 53
- drainage 372
- duct stone 38
- enteric anastomosis 85
- lithiasis 120, 130
- microlithiasis 40, 156
- obstruction 213, 221, 265, 371, 372, 387
- sepsis 24
- sludge 19, 51
- sphincterotomy 222
- stenosis 373
- stones 38
- stricture 219, 252
- tract
- - congenital lesion 160
- - obstruction 306, 308
- tumor 131
Billroth II gastrectomy 211

bleeding 29, 295
- pancreatitis 299
- pseudocyst 288, 297
blunt abdominal trauma 270
bone window 168
breast cancer 102
breath-holding imaging 80
Brunner's gland 247, 249
brush cytology 218
bull's eye 168

C

calcific pancreatitis 373
calcitonin-gene related peptide 236
calcium 9
- crystals 119
- deposits 154
capsule-like rim 168, 171, 176, 344, 346
carbonic anhydrase 121, 241
cathepsin B 8
cationic
- trypsin 121
- trypsinogen 133
- - gene 120, 237
cellular debris 281
chain-of-lakes appearance 176
cholangiocarcinoma 245
cholangiography 210
cholangitis 16, 19, 252, 302
cholecystitis 53
cholecysto-jejunostomy 388
cholecystokinin (CCK) 4
cholecystolithiasis 51
choledochal cyst 123, 152
choledochocele 152
choledocho-enterostomy 387, 388
choledocholithiasis 19, 21, 38, 40, 85, 198
cholelithiasis 19, 39, 49, 50, 283
cholestasis 302
chronic inflammation of papilla 156
chronic pancreatitis 60, 117, 209
- Cambridge classification 218
- idiopathic 183
- malabsorption 265
- non-obstructive 145
- pathology 231
- pathophysiology 117
- TIGAR-O classification 231
- ultrasonographic diagnosis 143
chymotrypsin 238, 251
collagen vascular disease 99
colonoscopy 323
common bile duct (CBD) 4, 19, 149, 193, 196, 198, 199, 285, 302
- stones 51, 85
- stricture 264, 372
computed tomography (CT) 49
- chronic pancreatitis 149
- limitations in diagnosis 58
- severity index 65, 86
- staging 63
- - limitations and pitfalls 65
concomitant pancreatic cancer 254
C-reactive protein (CRP) 18
Crohn's disease 241, 245, 338
Cullen's sign 16, 17, 53, 61
cyst rupture 263
cyst-enterostomy 377
cyst-gastrostomy 22, 28
cystic
- duodenal dystrophy 346
- dystrophy 134, 145, 147, 196, 264
- - of duodenum 283
- - of the duodenal wall 120, 131, 247
- ectasia 164, 361, 365
- fibrosis 120, 176, 238, 365
- - gene mutation (CFTR) 168
- - transmembrane conductance regulator gene 122
- neoplasia 350, 379
- pancreatic tumor 69
- tumor 161
cystjejunostomy 22, 28
cystoenteric fistula 379
cytokine 10, 51, 61

D

diabetes 133, 237, 265
diagnostic ultrasound 33
diffuse autoimmune chronic pancreatitis 174
diffusion-weighted imaging (DWI) 101, 202
disseminated intravascular coagulopathy 262
double-duct sign 200, 346
duct
- fibrosis 252
- of Santorini 5, 120, 122, 154
- of Wirsung 37, 120, 122
- penetrating sign 338
ductal
- adenocarcinoma 131, 161, 163, 164, 198, 218, 285, 330, 339, 350
- carcinoma 265
- hypertension 210
- leak 213
- obstruction 118, 119, 221, 357
- stone 168
- - bull's eye type 168
duct-penetrating sign 200
duodenal
- cystic dystrophy 161, 162
- diverticulum 122

- duplication 152
- dystrophy 156
- obstruction 388
- stenosis 58, 253, 323
- wall cyst 247
- wall dystrophy 156
duodeno-cephalo-pancreatectomy 131, 134
duodenopancreatectomy 283
duodenum-preserving pancreatic head resection 386
dynamic contrast enhanced imaging 83

E

ecchymoses in the flanks 16
echogenicity of the parenchyma 141
echotexture of pancreas 34
ectasia 176
edematous pancreatitis 52, 86, 312
elastase 10
encapsulated hemorrhagic cyst 263
endocavity gas bubble 43
endocrine
- function failure 129
- insufficiency 117
endoductal protein plug 154
endoscopic
- cystenterostomy 379
- drainage 374, 377
- retrograde cholangiopancreatography (ERCP) 19, 20, 50, 152, 184, 209, 371
- - biopsy 218
- - complications 212
- - complications assessment 218
- - diagnostic 215
- - stent removal 224
- - technical principles 210
- - tissue sampling 218
- sphincterotomy 40
endoscopy 371
endotherapy 201, 221, 223, 224, 381
endotoxin 11
enzymatic peritonitis 263
esophagogastroduodenoscopy 378
ESWL, *see* extracorporal shock-wave lithotripsy
ethanol 118
exocytosis 118
external fistula 321
extracorporal shock-wave lithotripsy (ESWL) 201, 219
extraluminal duodenal diverticulum 150
extravasated pancreatic enzyme 96
extravasation of activated pancreatic enzyme 70

F

Fallopian tube 16
fat
- necrosis 66
- suppression 186
fatty acid ethyl ester (FAEE) 6, 118
fever 16
fibroblast 235, 251
- growth factor (FGF) 235
fibrocalculous pancreatic diabetes 252
fibrocystic gene mutation 133, 176
fibroinflammatory pseudotumor 243
fibrosis 118, 194, 249, 264, 347
- in the duodenal wall 353
- pseudo-capsule 274
- pseudotumor 246
fine needle aspiration (FNA) 24
fistula 198, 264, 317
fistulography 317, 318, 321
flank ecchymosis 16, 61
fluid collection 36, 56, 66, 311
- hemorrhage-like 93
focal
- autoimmune chronic pancreatitis 175
- chronic pancreatitis 329
- fibrosis 154
- inflammatory mass 198, 200
- pancreatitis 101
focused abdominal sonogram for trauma (FAST) 113
follicular hyperplasia 244

G

gadolinium 186
- chelate agent 84
gallbladder 51
- stones 51
gallstone 19, 38, 57
- acute pancreatitis 67
- pancreatitis 4, 85
gastric outlet obstruction 160, 263
gastrointestinal bleeding 29
gene mutation 121, 132
glandular
- atrophy 168, 231
- echotexture 141
- infection 41
Glasgow criteria 18, 62
glucose transporter 356
graduated bougienage 222
granulocyte 121
granulocytic epithelial lesion (GEL) 241
Grey-Turner's sign 16, 17, 53, 61
groove pancreatitis 58, 59, 120, 131, 232, 247, 283, 346, 353, 354, 371

H

haemosuccus pancreaticus 300, 316
half-Fourier acquisition single shot turbo spin echo (HASTE) sequence 82, 281, 315

harmonic imaging 144
Hashimoto's thyroiditis 338
hematocrit 17
hemodialysis 84
hemorrhage 29, 72, 90, 316
hemorrhagic
- fluid collection 92
- pancreatitis 92
- pseudocyst 280
hereditary pancreatitis 119, 232, 237, 238
hydrostatic balloon 377
- dilatation 222
hyperamylasemia 16, 53, 107, 108
hypercalcemia 6, 171
hypergammaglobulinemia 240
hyperlipoproteinemia 6
hyperparathyroidism 171, 252
hypertriglyceridemia 6
hypervascular pseudo-mass 160
hypoalbuminemia 262
hypocalcemia 262
hypoproteinemia 262
hypovolemic ischemia 11

I

idiopathic chronic pancreatitis 183, 237
idiopathic pancreatitis 40, 251
IgG4-related systemic disease 245
infected
- pancreatic necrosis 24, 68, 263
- pseudocyst 42, 263
inflammatory
- myofibroblastic tumor 246
- pancreatic disease 119
- pancreopathy 261
- pseudotumor 246
- stenosis of the papilla 159
interleukin (IL)
- IL-1 51
- IL-1b 11
internal
- fistula 318, 383
- pancreatic fistula 254
interstitial
- edema 34
- pancreatitis 21, 52
- stenosis 321
intraductal
- calculi 143
- mucin-producing tumor 131
- papillary mucinous tumor (IPMT) 145, 163, 253, 357, 386
- - of the collateral duct 285
- stone 130
- tumor 164, 347
- ultrasound 337
intralobular fibrosis 233, 234, 250
intraluminal
- duodenal diverticulum 152
- mucous plugging 238
intrapancreatic hematoma 111
intraparenchymal
- fluid collection 89
- hemorrhage 316
intraperitoneal pancreatic fluid 73
intrasplenic pseudocyst 325
isolated left-sided portal hypertension 71

J

juxtapapillary
- duodenal adenocarcinoma 160
- neoplasm 357

K

keratin 8 gene 120
K-ras mutation 218

L

lactoferrin 241
left-sided portal hypertension 265
leukocytosis 21, 22, 107
lipase 16, 191
lipoprotein 6
lithostathine 117, 118
lithotripsy 219, 385
liver
- fibrosis 102
- parenchyma 86
lung injury 11
- pancreatitis-induced 12
lymphadenopathy 60, 176, 246
lymphocyte 121
lymphoid follicles 244
lymphoplasmacellular pancreatitis 246
lymphoplasmacytic sclerosing pancreatitis 97, 241, 246
lymphoplasmatic cholecystitis 245

M

macrophage 9
magnetic resonance
- cholangiopancreatography (MRCP) 38, 79, 184
- - patient preparation 81
- - projective 187

- - protocol 81
- - secretin-MRCP (s-MRCP) 79, 80, 82, 184, 187, 318
- elastography 102
- imaging (MRI) 79
- spectroscopy 101
main pancreatic duct
- diffuse dilation 357
maldigestion 117
malnutrition 265
mass-forming pancreatitis 131, 145, 203, 245, 330
mastocyte 262
mature pseudocyst 276, 283
maximum intensity projection (MIP) 313
mesenchymal tumor 150
metabolic
- chronic pancreatitis 252
- entrapment process 356
methemalbumine 18, 61
microlithiasis 120, 130, 149
Mikulicz's disease 241, 245
minor papilla stenting 150
mucin deposit 363
mucinous cystic
- neoplasm 253
- pancreatic tumor 283
- tumor 281
mucoviscidosis 238
multifocal idiopathic fibrosclerosis 245
multiorgan failure 261, 311
multiplanar reformation (MPR) 313
multi-slice spiral computed tomography 337
myocardial depression 11
myofibroblast 246, 251

N

nasocystic drain 377
nasopancreatic catheter 212
necrosectomy 19, 24, 27
necrosis-fibrosis sequence 184, 236, 237
necrotic hemorrhagic pancreatitis 296
necrotizing
- pancreatitis 21–23, 52, 61, 88, 93, 133, 261
- vasculitis 52
needle-aspiration biopsy 286
- pseudocyst 286
needle-knife sphincterotomy 375
neoplasm 166, 167
neoplastic
- inflammatory myofibroblastic tumor 246
- obstruction 361
nephrogenic systemic fibrosis (NSF) 84
neuroendocrine tumor 150, 164, 286, 338
neutrophils 10
non-alcoholic duct-destructive chronic pancreatitis 97
non-bleeding pseudoaneurysm 297
non-breath-holding imaging 80
non-functioning pancreatic neuroendocrine tumor 160
non-Hodgkin lymphoma 176
non-obstructuve chronic pancreatitis 145, 164
nuclear factor κB (NF-κB) 10, 236
numerical detection system 62

O

obesity 17
obliterated phlebitis 195
obstructing neoplasm 145
obstruction of the gastro-intestinal tract 288
obstructive
- chronic pancreatitis 145, 152, 154, 155, 157, 250
- - CT diagnosis 156
- jaundice 288
- pancreatitis 118
occult microlithiasis 51
optical coherence tomography (OCT) 219
organ injury scale (OIS) 107
osteoclast-like giant cell tumor 286

P

p53 218
PAF 11, 12
pain
- associated with chain-of-lake dilatation of the Wirsung duct 385
- associated with segmental dilatation of the Wirsung duct 386
- associated with uniform dilatation of the Wirsung duct 385
- groove pancreatitis 386
- suspected tumor 386
pancreas
- adenocarcinoma 131
- cystic tumor 161
- divisum 5, 80, 83, 85, 97, 122, 132, 150, 160, 164, 165, 342
- - inversum 338, 345
- echotexture 34
- hypoechoic area 35
- size 34
- trauma 5
- traumatic injury 107
pancreatectomy 73, 113
pancreatic
- abscess 56, 68, 264, 287, 316
- adenocarcinoma 133, 145, 176, 195, 279
- amylase 53
- ascites 37, 39, 56, 73, 266, 324, 380, 383
- atrophy 140, 234
- calcification 141

pancreatic (*continued*)
- carcinoma 101
- collections 312
- digestive enzyme 7
- duct 199
- - adenocarcinoma 179
- - cannulation 210
- - changes 141, 144
- - dilatation 141
- - disruption 22, 27, 109, 111
- - fistula 302
- - imaging 186
- - leaks 380
- - obstruction 4, 238
- - stenting 223
- - stones 210, 219
- - stricture 221
- echotexture 40, 141
- edema 109, 110
- endocrine function 221
- enzyme 51
- exocrine function 188
- fibrosis 183, 252
- fistula 317, 374
- flow output 188, 189
- fluid collection 379
- fracture 109
- gland 52, 54, 56, 63, 133, 139, 154, 171
- - necrosis 66
- head fibrosis 323
- hematoma 112
- laceration 109
- lipase 51
- lymphoma 242
- malformation 132
- necrosis 27, 52, 61, 65, 68, 89, 262, 311, 313, 380
- - sterile 27
- neoplasm 4, 85, 101, 216, 371
- parenchyma 55, 64, 139, 144, 154, 184, 194, 248
- pseudocyst 22, 69, 213
- ribonuclease 18, 61
- secretory trypsin inhibitor (PSTI) 118, 120, 122, 133, 214
- sphincterotomy 134, 201, 220
- stellate cells (PSC) 118
- stenting 201
- - techniques 222
- trauma 107
- traumatic injury 107
- - clinical classification 107
- - imaging diagnosis 108
- tumor 123, 160, 163
- - slow-growing 131
- volume 140
pancreatic-abdominal fistula 73
pancreatic-enteric fistula 318
pancreatico-biliary fistula 306, 318
pancreatico-cutaneous fistula 321, 380
pancreatico-duodenectomy 386
pancreatico-jejunostomy 73, 224, 385, 387, 388
pancreatico-pleural fistula 320
pancreatico-venous fistula 319
pancreatitis
- acute, *see there*
- associated with gene mutation 121
- calcium-induced 6
- chronic, *see there*
- drug-induced 7
- ERCP-related 108
- following cardiac surgery 7
- gallstone-induced 4
- hemorrhage 297
- hypertriglyceridemia 6
- idiopathic 38
- infectious agent 7
- mass-forming 131, 145, 203, 241
- neoplasm-associated 4
- segmental 58
- splenic involvement 325
- tumor-forming 241
- ultrasound 139
pancreatitis-associated protein 18
pancreato-cutaneous fistula 264
pancreatography 210, 218
pancreatoscopy 209, 365
papilla of Vater 40, 51, 385
- stenosis 119
- tumor 123
papillary
- hyperplasia 252
- neoplasm 164
- stenosis 385
- tumor 160
paraampullary duodenal wall cyst 247
paraduodenal pancreatitis 195, 196, 232, 247, 248
parathyroid disease 171
parenchymal
- atrophy 164
- echotexture 144
- fibrosis 168, 183
- ischemia 66
- laceration 108
- necrosis 88
peptic ulcer 324
percutaneous transhepatic cholangiography (PTC) 295
perfusion imaging 100
periampullary diverticulum 122
periductal
- fibrosis 232, 242
- inflammation 117
- inflammatory cellular infiltrate 171
perilobular fibrosis 233, 237
peripancreatic
- edema 92

- exudate 186
- fat necrosis 88
- fluid collection 36, 63, 89, 93, 112, 262
- necrosis 27
peritonitis 325, 379
periumbilical ecchymosis 61
phased-array radiofrequency coil 80
phlebitis 246, 247
phospholipase 10
pig tail catheter 28
plasma cell granuloma 246
platelet-derived growth factor 235
pleural effusion 19, 292, 320, 383
plump myofibroblast 243
polyarthritis 254
polymorphonuclear cell 262
portal
- hypertension 286
- vein
- - fistula 302
- - thrombosis 29
positron-emitting tomography 354
post-ERCP pancreatitis 212
post-sphincterotomy bleeding 213
post-surgical fistula 321
post-traumatic fistula 321
prednisone 344
primary sclerosing
- cholangitis 99
- pancreatitis 97
primary chronic pancreatitis 152, 164, 169
procarboxypeptidase B 18
protein plug 233
pseudoaneurysm 29, 44, 71, 72, 197, 202, 218, 265, 288, 295
- hemorrhage 263
pseudocapsule 276, 281
pseudocyst 37, 42, 44, 56, 63, 68, 69, 70, 94, 133, 156, 193, 196, 210, 213, 219, 238, 253, 263, 311, 71, 383
- associated to pancreatic tumor 278
- CT imaging 276
- drainage 201
- endoscopic ultrasound imaging 282
- evolution 286
- fistula 289
- imaging 269
- infection 40, 288
- post-traumatic 271
- rupture 289
- transpapillary drainage 377
- ultrasound 276
pseudotumor 330, 344, 346
pseudotumoral mass 353
Puestow procedure 373
Purtscher's retinopathy 16
pyelophlebitis 305
pylorus-preserving pancreatico-duodenectomy 386

Q

quality of life 383

R

Ranson's criteria 18, 62
reactive oxygen species (ROS) 236
Recklinghausen's disease 150
relapsing pancreatitis 149, 153
retention cyst 193, 253, 266
retroperitoneal fibrosis 195, 246
rheumatoid arthritis 338

S

Santorinicele 80
sclero-odditis 264
sclerosing
- cholangitis 195, 245, 246, 338
- sialoadenitis 245
sclerotherapy 302
secretin 101, 187, 203
- administration 191
- stimulation 111
segmental pancreatitis 58
self-expanding metal stent (SEMS) 373
sensitivity encoding 80
serum protease inhibitor 7
- Kazal type 1 (SPINK1) 122, 172, 173
serous cystadenoma 161, 281, 283
serum
- alkaline phosphatase 372, 387
- amylase 16, 53, 108
- lipase level 35
severe acute pancreatitis (SAP) 156, 158, 270
sialoadenitis 195
signal-to-noise ratio (SNR) 80
simultaneous acquisition of spatial harmonics (SMASH) 80
single shot fast spin echo (SSFSE) sequence 82, 315
Sjögren's syndrome 99, 241, 246, 338
smooth muscle hyperplasia 249
solid duodenal dystrophy 164, 170
solid papillary tumor 285
sphincter of Oddi 188
- dysfunction 83, 120, 130, 212
- stenosis 131
sphincterotomy 130, 150, 210, 212, 224
- endoscopic 38
- wire-guided 220
SPINK1, *see* serine protease inhibitor Kazal type 1
spleen rupture 325
splenectomy 28, 302
splenic

- abscess 325
- artery aneurysm 99
- hemorrhage 325
- thrombosis 305
- venous thrombosis 29, 71, 96, 197, 254, 265, 302
splenomegaly 71, 96
steatorrhoea 117, 129, 133, 189, 232, 237, 265
stenosis of the papilla of Vater 119
stent
- dysfunction 223
- removal 223
sterile pancreatic necrosis 27
stone extraction balloon 220
stricturoplasty 222
substance P 236
supraampullary duodenum 248
systemic inflammatory response syndrome (SIRS) 262

T

T lymphocyte 241, 244
tachycardia 16
teardrop sign 338
telomerase activity 218
thrombophlebitis 288, 302
- of the spleno-portal venous axis 304
thrombosis of the pancreatic vein 288
thyroiditis 195
time-to-inflow deceleration 193
total excreted volume 189
total parenteral nutrition (TPN) 24
trans-abdominal ultrasound 361
transforming growth factor (TGF) 235
trans-hepatic portography 320
transpapillary drainage of pseudocyst 377
trauma to the pancreas 5
triglyceride 6
tri-nitro-benzene sulfonic acid (TNBS) 121
tropical pancreatitis 183, 252
true neoplasm 246
trypsin 7, 8, 122
trypsinogen 7
- activation peptide (TAP) 18, 62
tumor necrosis factor 51
- alpha (TNF-α) 11
turbo-spin echo imaging 111

U

ulcerative colitis 99, 240, 241, 245
ultrasound (US) 33
- chronic pancreatitis 139
- contrast-enhanced 145
- diagnostic 33
- needle aspiration 35
uncinate process 54, 285, 336
unilocular cystic mass 285

V

vasculitis 246
vasoactive peptide 61
venous thrombosis 28, 202, 286, 295, 302
volume rendering 313

W

Whipple resection 58
wirsungorrhage 300

Z

zymogen granules 262

List of Contributors

GIULIA ARMATURA, MD
Department of Surgery Sciences
Policlinico "GB Rossi"
University of Verona
Piazzale LA Scuro 10
37134 Verona
Italy

MARIA ANTONIETTA BALI, MD
Department of Radiology
MR Imaging Division
Cliniques Universitaires de Bruxelles
Hôpital Erasme
Université Libre de Bruxelles
Route de Lennik 808
1070 Brussels
Belgium

EMIL J. BALTHAZAR, MD
Professor, Department of Radiology
Bellevue Hospital
NYU-Langone Medical Center
Room 3W37
462 First Avenue
New York, NY 10016
USA

Email: *emiljmd@aol.com*
Balthe01@endeavor.med.nyu.edu

PETER A. BANKS, MD
Director, Center for Pancreatic Disease
Division of Gastroenterology
Brigham and Women's Hospital
Professor of Medicine
Harvard Medical School
75 Francis Street
Boston, MA 02115
USA

Email: pabanks@partners.org

DAFNA BAR-SAGI, PhD
Department of Biochemistry
NYU-Langone Medical Center
550 First Avenue
New York NY, 10016
USA

CLAUDIO BASSI, MD
Surgical and Gastroenterological Department
Hospital "GB Rossi"
University of Verona
Piazzale LA Scuro 10
37134 Verona
Italy

Email: claudio.bassi@univr.it

CARLO BIASIUTTI, MD
Department of Radiology
Policlinico "GB Rossi"
University of Verona
Piazzale LA Scuro 10
37134 Verona
Italy

Email: carlo.biasiutti@azosp.vr.it

LETIZIA BONINSEGNA, MD
Surgical and Gastroenterological Department
Hospital "GB Rossi"
University of Verona
Piazzale LA Scuro, 10
37134 Verona
Italy

COSTANZA BRUNO, MD
Department of Radiology
Policlinico "GB Rossi"
University of Verona
Piazzale LA Scuro 10
37134 Verona
Italy

Email: costanza.bruno@azosp.vr.it

GIOVANNI BUTTURINI, MD
Surgical and Gastroenterological Department
Hospital "GB Rossi"
University of Verona
Piazzale LA Scuro 10
37134 Verona
Italy

Chiara Calciolari, MD
Department of Radiology
Policlinico "GB Rossi"
University of Verona
Piazzale LA Scuro 10
37134 Verona
Italy

Paola Capelli, MD
Department of Pathology
University of Verona
Strada le Grazie 8
37134 Verona
Italy
Email: paola.capelli@azosp.vr.it

Giovanni Carbognin, MD
Department of Radiology
Policlinico "GB Rossi"
University of Verona
Piazzale LA Scuro 10
37134 Verona
Italy
Email: giovanni.carbognin@azosp.vr.it

Giorgio Cavallini, MD
Internal Medicine Section C
Department of Gastroenterology
Policlinico "GB Rossi"
University of Verona
Piazzale LA Scuro 10
37134 Verona
Italy

Daniela Cenzi, MD
Department of Radiology
Ospedale Borgo Trento
Piazzale Stefani 1
37126 Verona
Italy

Lorenzo Cereser, MD
Department of Radiology
MR Imaging Division
Cliniques Universitaires de Bruxelles
Hôpital Erasme
Université Libre de Bruxelles
Route de Lennik 808
1070 Brussels
Belgium

Daniela Coser, MD
Department of Radiology
Policlinico "GB Rossi"
University of Verona
Piazzale LA Scuro 10
37134 Verona
Italy

Myriam Delhaye, MD, PhD
Department of Gastroenterology
Hopital Erasme
Université Libre de Bruxelles
Route de Lennik 808
1070 Brussels
Belgium
Email: Myriam.Delhaye@erasme.ulb.ac.be

David L. Diehl, MD, FACP
Adjunct Associate Clinical Professor of Medicine
NYU-Langone School of Medicine
Geisinger Medical Center
Department of
Gastroenterology and Nutrition
100 North Academy Ave, 21-11
Danville, PA 17822
USA
Email: ddiehl@mol.net

Mirko D'Onofrio, MD
Department of Radiology
Policlinico "GB Rossi"
University of Verona
Piazzale LA Scuro 10
37134 Verona
Italy
Email: mirko.donofrio@univr.it

Niccolò Faccioli, MD
Department of Radiology
Policlinico "GB Rossi"
University of Verona
Piazzale LA Scuro 10
37134 Verona
Italy

Massimo Falconi, MD
Surgical and Gastroenterological Department
Hospital "GB Rossi"
University of Verona
Piazzale LA Scuro 10
37134 Verona
Italy
Email: massimo.falconi@univr.it

Giovanni Foti, MD
Department of Radiology
Policlinico "GB Rossi"
University of Verona
Piazzale LA Scuro 10
37134 Verona
Italy

Francesca Franzoso, MD
Department of Radiology
Policlinico "GB Rossi"
University of Verona
Piazzale LA Scuro 10
37134 Verona
Italy

Luca Frulloni, MD, PhD
Department of Gastroenteroloy
Policlinico "GB Rossi"
Piazzale LA Scuro 10
37134 Verona
Italy
Email: luca.frulloni@univr.it

Rossella Graziani, MD
Department of Radiology
Policlinico "GB Rossi"
University of Verona
Piazzale LA Scuro 10
37134 Verona
Italy
Email: rossella.graziani@azosp.vr.it

Alessandro Guarise, MD
Department of Radiology
San Bassiano Hospital
Via dei Lotti 41
36024 Bassano del Grappa (VI)
Italy

Elizabeth Hecht, MD
Department of Radiology
NYU-Langone Medical Center
560 First Avenue, Suite HW 202
New York, NY 10016
USA
Email: hechte01@med.nyu.edu
emh100@hotmail.com

Peter Kingman, MD
Department of Surgery
Memorial Sloan-Kettering Cancer Center
New York, NY 10021
USA

Günter Klöppel, MD
Professor and Head, Department of Pathology
University of Kiel
Michaelistrasse 11
24105 Kiel
Germany

Richard S. Kwon, MD
Center for Pancreatic Disease
Division of Gastroenterology
Brigham and Women's Hospital
Harvard Medical School
75 Francis Street
Boston, MA 02115
USA
Email: rkwon@partners.org

John Mallen-St. Clair, BA, MSc
Department of Biochemistry
NYU-Langone Medical Center
550 First Avenue
New York, NY 10016
USA

Giancarlo Mansueto, MD
Department of Radiology Institute
University of Verona
Piazzale LA Scuro 10
37134 Verona
Italy
Email:giancarlo.mansueto@univr.it

Celso Matos, MD
Department of Radiology
MR Imaging Division
Cliniques Universitaires de Bruxelles
Hôpital Erasme
Université Libre de Bruxelles
Route de Lennik 808
1070 Brussels
Belgium
Email: cmatos@ulb.ac.be

Alec J. Megibow, MD, MPH, FACR
Professor, Department of Radiology
NYU-Langone Medical Center
550 First Avenue
New York, NY 10016
USA
Email: Alec.Megibow@Med.Nyu.Edu

Salvatore Minniti, MD
Department of Radiology
Policlinico "GB Rossi"
University of Verona
Piazzale LA Scuro 10
37134 Verona
Italy

Giovanni Morana, MD
Department of Radiology
General Hospital Cà Foncello
Piazza Ospedale 1
31100 Treviso
Italy

Koenraad J. Mortele, MD
Center for Pancreatic Disease
Department of Radiology
Division of Abdominal Imaging and Intervention
Brigham and Women's Hospital
Harvard Medical School
75 Francis Street
Boston, MA 02115
USA

Email: kmortele@partners.org

Marinella Neri, MD
Department of Radiology
Policlinico "GB Rossi"
University of Verona
Piazzale LA Scuro 10
37134 Verona
Italy

Paolo Pederzoli, MD
Surgical and Gastroenterological Department
Hospital "GB Rossi"
University of Verona
Piazzale LA Scuro, 10
37134 Verona
Italy

Roberto Pozzi Mucelli, MD
Department of Radiology
Policlinico "GB Rossi"
University of Verona
Piazzale LA Scuro 10
37134 Verona
Italy

Email: roberto.pozzimucelli@univr.it

Ricardo Sante Murano, MD
Department of Radiology
Policlinico "GB Rossi"
University of Verona
Piazzale LA Scuro 10
37134 Verona
Italy

Nora Sartori, MD
Surgical and Gastroenterological Department
Hospital "GB Rossi"
University of Verona
Piazzale LA Scuro 10
37134 Verona
Italy

Giacomo Schenal, MD
Department of Radiology
Ospedale Borgo Trento
Piazzale Stefani 1
37126 Verona
Italy

Peter Shamamian, MD
Department of Surgery
Medical University of South Carolina
Charleston, SC 29425
USA

Email: shamamia@musc.edu

Alessia Tognolini, MD
Department of Radiology
Policlinico "GB Rossi"
University of Verona
Piazzale LA Scuro 10
37134 Verona
Italy

Giuseppe Zamboni, MD
Department of Pathology
University of Verona
Ospedale S. Cuore-Don Calabria
Via don Sempreboni, 5
37024 Negrar-Verona
Italy

Email: giuseppe.zamboni@sacrocuore.it

MEDICAL RADIOLOGY Diagnostic Imaging and Radiation Oncology

Titles in the series already published

DIAGNOSTIC IMAGING

Innovations in Diagnostic Imaging
Edited by J. H. Anderson

Radiology of the Upper Urinary Tract
Edited by E. K. Lang

The Thymus - Diagnostic Imaging, Functions, and Pathologic Anatomy
Edited by E. Walter, E. Willich, and W. R. Webb

Interventional Neuroradiology
Edited by A. Valavanis

Radiology of the Lower Urinary Tract
Edited by E. K. Lang

Contrast-Enhanced MRI of the Breast
S. Heywang-Köbrunner and R. Beck

Spiral CT of the Chest
Edited by M. Rémy-Jardin and J. Rémy

Radiological Diagnosis of Breast Diseases
Edited by M. Friedrich and E. A. Sickles

Radiology of Trauma
Edited by M. Heller and A. Fink

Biliary Tract Radiology
Edited by P. Rossi. Co-edited by M. Brezi

Radiological Imaging of Sports Injuries
Edited by C. Masciocchi

Modern Imaging of the Alimentary Tube
Edited by A. R. Margulis

Diagnosis and Therapy of Spinal Tumors
Edited by P. R. Algra, J. Valk and J. J. Heimans

Interventional Magnetic Resonance Imaging
Edited by J. F. Debatin and G. Adam

Abdominal and Pelvic MRI
Edited by A. Heuck and M. Reiser

Orthopedic Imaging
Techniques and Applications
Edited by A. M. Davies and H. Pettersson

Radiology of the Female Pelvic Organs
Edited by E. K. Lang

Magnetic Resonance of the Heart and Great Vessels
Clinical Applications
Edited by J. Bogaert, A. J. Duerinckx, and F. E. Rademakers

Modern Head and Neck Imaging
Edited by S. K. Mukherji and J. A. Castelijns

Radiological Imaging of Endocrine Diseases
Edited by J. N. Bruneton in collaboration with B. Padovani and M.-Y. Mourou

Radiology of the Pancreas
2nd Revised Edition
Edited by A. L. Baert. Co-edited by G. Delorme and L. Van Hoe

Trends in Contrast Media
Edited by H. S. Thomsen, R. N. Muller, and R. F. Mattrey

Functional MRI
Edited by C. T. W. Moonen and P. A. Bandettini

Emergency Pediatric Radiology
Edited by H. Carty

Liver Malignancies
Diagnostic and Interventional Radiology
Edited by C. Bartolozzi and R. Lencioni

Spiral CT of the Abdomen
Edited by F. Terrier, M. Grossholz, and C. D. Becker

Medical Imaging of the Spleen
Edited by A. M. De Schepper and F. Vanhoenacker

Radiology of Peripheral Vascular Diseases
Edited by E. Zeitler

Radiology of Blunt Trauma of the Chest
P. Schnyder and M. Wintermark

Portal Hypertension
Diagnostic Imaging and Imaging-Guided Therapy
Edited by P. Rossi. Co-edited by P. Ricci and L. Broglia

Virtual Endoscopy and Related 3D Techniques
Edited by P. Rogalla, J. Terwisscha van Scheltinga and B. Hamm

Recent Advances in Diagnostic Neuroradiology
Edited by Ph. Demaerel

Transfontanellar Doppler Imaging in Neonates
A. Couture, C. Veyrac

Radiology of AIDS
A Practical Approach
Edited by J. W. A. J. Reeders and P. C. Goodman

CT of the Peritoneum
A. Rossi, G. Rossi

Magnetic Resonance Angiography
2nd Revised Edition
Edited by I. P. Arlart, G. M. Bongartz, and G. Marchal

Applications of Sonography in Head and Neck Pathology
Edited by J. N. Bruneton in collaboration with C. Raffaelli, O. Dassonville

3D Image Processing
Techniques and Clinical Applications
Edited by D. Caramella and C. Bartolozzi

Imaging of the Larynx
Edited by R. Hermans

Pediatric ENT Radiology
Edited by S. J. King and A. E. Boothroyd

Imaging of Orbital and Visual Pathway Pathology
Edited by W. S. Müller-Forell

Radiological Imaging of the Small Intestine
Edited by N. C. Gourtsoyiannis

Imaging of the Knee
Techniques and Applications
Edited by A. M. Davies and V. N. Cassar-Pullicino

Perinatal Imaging
From Ultrasound to MR Imaging
Edited by F. E. Avni

Diagnostic and Interventional Radiology in Liver Transplantation
Edited by E. Bücheler, V. Nicolas, C. E. Broelsch, X. Rogiers and G. Krupski

Imaging of the Pancreas
Cystic and Rare Tumors
Edited by C. Procacci and A. J. Megibow

Imaging of the Foot & Ankle
Techniques and Applications
Edited by A. M. Davies, R. W. Whitehouse and J. P. R. Jenkins

Radiological Imaging of the Ureter
Edited by F. Joffre, Ph. Otal and M. Soulie

Radiology of the Petrous Bone
Edited by M. Lemmerling and S. S. Kollias

Imaging of the Shoulder
Techniques and Applications
Edited by A. M. Davies and J. Hodler

Interventional Radiology in Cancer
Edited by A. Adam, R. F. Dondelinger, and P. R. Mueller

Imaging and Intervention in Abdominal Trauma
Edited by R. F. Dondelinger

Radiology of the Pharynx and the Esophagus
Edited by O. Ekberg

Radiological Imaging in Hematological Malignancies
Edited by A. Guermazi

Functional Imaging of the Chest
Edited by H.-U. Kauczor

Duplex and Color Doppler Imaging of the Venous System
Edited by G. H. Mostbeck

Multidetector-Row CT of the Thorax
Edited by U. J. Schoepf

Radiology and Imaging of the Colon
Edited by A. H. Chapman

Multidetector-Row CT Angiography
Edited by C. Catalano and R. Passariello

Focal Liver Lesions
Detection, Characterization, Ablation
Edited by R. Lencioni, D. Cioni, and C. Bartolozzi

Imaging in Treatment Planning for Sinonasal Diseases
Edited by R. Maroldi and P. Nicolai

Clinical Cardiac MRI
With Interactive CD-ROM
Edited by J. Bogaert, S. Dymarkowski, and A. M. Taylor

Dynamic Contrast-Enhanced Magnetic Resonance Imaging in Oncology
Edited by A. Jackson, D. L. Buckley, and G. J. M. Parker

Contrast Media in Ultrasonography
Basic Principles and Clinical Applications
Edited by E. Quaia

Paediatric Musculoskeletal Disease
With an Emphasis on Ultrasound
Edited by D. Wilson

MR Imaging in White Matter Diseases of the Brain and Spinal Cord
Edited by M. Filippi, N. De Stefano, V. Dousset, and J. C. McGowan

Imaging of the Hip & Bony Pelvis
Techniques and Applications
Edited by A. M. Davies, K. Johnson, and R. W. Whitehouse

Imaging of Kidney Cancer
Edited by A. Guermazi

Magnetic Resonance Imaging in Ischemic Stroke
Edited by R. von Kummer and T. Back

Diagnostic Nuclear Medicine
2nd Revised Edition
Edited by C. Schiepers

Imaging of Occupational and Environmental Disorders of the Chest
Edited by P. A. Gevenois and P. De Vuyst

Virtual Colonoscopy
A Practical Guide
Edited by P. Lefere and S. Gryspeerdt

Contrast Media
Safety Issues and ESUR Guidelines
Edited by H. S. Thomsen

Head and Neck Cancer Imaging
Edited by R. Hermans

Vascular Embolotherapy
A Comprehensive Approach
Volume 1: *General Principles, Chest, Abdomen, and Great Vessels*
Edited by J. Golzarian. Co-edited by S. Sun and M. J. Sharafuddin

Vascular Embolotherapy
A Comprehensive Approach
Volume 2: *Oncology, Trauma, Gene Therapy, Vascular Malformations, and Neck*
Edited by J. Golzarian. Co-edited by S. Sun and M. J. Sharafuddin

Vascular Interventional Radiology
Current Evidence in Endovascular Surgery
Edited by M. G. Cowling

Ultrasound of the Gastrointestinal Tract
Edited by G. Maconi and G. Bianchi Porro

Parallel Imaging in Clinical MR Applications
Edited by S. O. Schoenberg, O. Dietrich, and M. F. Reiser

MRI and CT of the Female Pelvis
Edited by B. Hamm and R. Forstner

Imaging of Orthopedic Sports Injuries
Edited by F. M. Vanhoenacker, M. Maas and J. L. Gielen

Ultrasound of the Musculoskeletal System
S. Bianchi and C. Martinoli

Clinical Functional MRI
Presurgical Functional Neuroimaging
Edited by C. Stippich

Radiation Dose from Adult and Pediatric Multidetector Computed Tomography
Edited by D. Tack and P. A. Gevenois

Spinal Imaging
Diagnostic Imaging of the Spine and Spinal Cord
Edited by J. Van Goethem, L. van den Hauwe and P. M. Parizel

Computed Tomography of the Lung
A Pattern Approach
J. A. Verschakelen and W. De Wever

Imaging in Transplantation
Edited by A. Bankier

Radiological Imaging of the Neonatal Chest
2nd Revised Edition
Edited by V. Donoghue

Radiological Imaging of the Digestive Tract in Infants and Children
Edited by A. S. Devos and J. G. Blickman

Pediatric Chest Imaging
Chest Imaging in Infants and Children
2nd Revised Edition
Edited by J. Lucaya and J. L. Strife

Color Doppler US of the Penis
Edited by M. Bertolotto

Radiology of the Stomach and Duodenum
Edited by A. H. Freeman and E. Sala

Imaging in Pediatric Skeletal Trauma
Techniques and Applications
Edited by K. J. Johnson and E. Bache

Image Processing in Radiology
Current Applications
Edited by E. Neri, D. Caramella, C. Bartolozzi

Screening and Preventive Diagnosis with Radiological Imaging
Edited by M. F. Reiser, G. van Kaick, C. Fink, S. O. Schoenberg

Percutaneous Tumor Ablation in Medical Radiology
Edited by T. J. Vogl, T. K. Helmberger, M. G. Mack, M. F. Reiser

Liver Radioembolization with ^{90}Y Microspheres
Edited by J. I. Bilbao, M. F. Reiser

Pediatric Uroradiology
2nd Revised Edition
Edited by R. Fotter

Radiology of Osteoporosis
2nd Revised Edition
Edited by S. Grampp

Gastrointestinal Tract Sonography in Fetuses and Children
A. Couture, C. Baud, J. L. Ferran, M. Saguintaah and C. Veyrac

Intracranial Vascular Malformations and Aneurysms
2nd Revised Edition
Edited by M. Forsting and I. Wanke

High-Resolution Sonography of the Peripheral Nervous System
2nd Revised Edition
Edited by S. Peer and G. Bodner

Imaging Pelvic Floor Disorders
2nd Revised Edition
Edited by J. Stoker, S. A. Taylor, and J. O. L. DeLancey

Coronary Radiology
2nd Revised Edition
Edited by M. Oudkerk and M. F. Reiser

Integrated Cardiothoracic Imaging with MDCT
Edited by M. Rémy-Jardin and J. Rémy

Multislice CT
3rd Revised Edition
Edited by M. F. Reiser, C. R. Becker, K. Nikolaou, G. Glazer

MRI of the Lung
Edited by H.-U. Kauczor

Imaging in Percutaneous Musculoskeletal Interventions
Edited by A. Gangi, S. Guth, and A. Guermazi

Contrast Media
Safety Issues and ESUR Guidelines
2nd Revised Edition
Edited by H. S. Thomsen and J. W. A. Webb

Inflammatory Diseases of the Brain
Edited by S. Hähnel

Dural Cavernous Sinus Fistulas
Diagnostic and Endovascular Therapy
Goetz Benndorf

Imaging of the Pancreas
Acute and Chronic Pancreatitis
Edited by E. J. Balthazar, A. J. Megibow, and R. Pozzi Mucelli

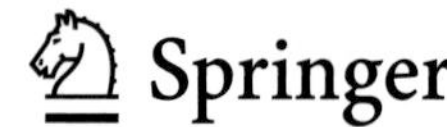

Medical Radiology Diagnostic Imaging and Radiation Oncology

Titles in the series already published

Radiation Oncology

Lung Cancer
Edited by C. W. Scarantino

Innovations in Radiation Oncology
Edited by H. R. Withers and L. J. Peters

Radiation Therapy of Head and Neck Cancer
Edited by G. E. Laramore

Gastrointestinal Cancer – Radiation Therapy
Edited by R. R. Dobelbower, Jr.

Radiation Exposure and Occupational Risks
Edited by E. Scherer, C. Streffer, and K.-R. Trott

Interventional Radiation
Therapy Techniques – Brachytherapy
Edited by R. Sauer

Radiopathology of Organs and Tissues
Edited by E. Scherer, C. Streffer, and K.-R. Trott

Concomitant Continuous Infusion
Chemotherapy and Radiation
Edited by M. Rotman and C. J. Rosenthal

Intraoperative Radiotherapy – Clinical Experiences and Results
Edited by F. A. Calvo, M. Santos, and L. W. Brady

Interstitial and Intracavitary Thermoradiotherapy
Edited by M. H. Seegenschmiedt and R. Sauer

Non-Disseminated Breast Cancer
Controversial Issues in Management
Edited by G. H. Fletcher and S. H. Levitt

Current Topics in Clinical Radiobiology of Tumors
Edited by H.-P. Beck-Bornholdt

Practical Approaches to Cancer Invasion and Metastases
A Compendium of Radiation Oncologists' Responses to 40 Histories
Edited by A. R. Kagan with the Assistance of R. J. Steckel

Radiation Therapy in Pediatric Oncology
Edited by J. R. Cassady

Radiation Therapy Physics
Edited by A. R. Smith

Late Sequelae in Oncology
Edited by J. Dunst, R. Sauer

Mediastinal Tumors. Update 1995
Edited by D. E. Wood, C. R. Thomas, Jr.

Thermoradiotherapy and Thermochemotherapy
Volume 1:
Biology, Physiology, and Physics
Volume 2:
Clinical Applications
Edited by M. H. Seegenschmiedt, P. Fessenden and C. C. Vernon

Carcinoma of the Prostate
Innovations in Management
Edited by Z. Petrovich, L. Baert, and L. W. Brady

Radiation Oncology of Gynecological Cancers
Edited by H. W. Vahrson

Carcinoma of the Bladder
Innovations in Management
Edited by Z. Petrovich, L. Baert, and L. W. Brady

Blood Perfusion and Microenvironment of Human Tumors
Implications for Clinical Radiooncology
Edited by M. Molls and P. Vaupel

Radiation Therapy of Benign Diseases
A Clinical Guide
2nd Revised Edition
S. E. Order and S. S. Donaldson

Carcinoma of the Kidney and Testis, and Rare Urologic Malignancies
Innovations in Management
Edited by Z. Petrovich, L. Baert, and L. W. Brady

Progress and Perspectives in the Treatment of Lung Cancer
Edited by P. Van Houtte, J. Klastersky, and P. Rocmans

Combined Modality Therapy of Central Nervous System Tumors
Edited by Z. Petrovich, L. W. Brady, M. L. Apuzzo, and M. Bamberg

Age-Related Macular Degeneration
Current Treatment Concepts
Edited by W. E. Alberti, G. Richard, and R. H. Sagerman

Radiotherapy of Intraocular and Orbital Tumors
2nd Revised Edition
Edited by R. H. Sagerman and W. E. Alberti

Modification of Radiation Response
Cytokines, Growth Factors, and Other Biolgical Targets
Edited by C. Nieder, L. Milas and K. K. Ang

Radiation Oncology for Cure and Palliation
R. G. Parker, N. A. Janjan and M. T. Selch

Clinical Target Volumes in Conformal and Intensity Modulated Radiation Therapy
A Clinical Guide to Cancer Treatment
Edited by V. Grégoire, P. Scalliet, and K. K. Ang

Advances in Radiation Oncology in Lung Cancer
Edited by B. Jeremić

New Technologies in Radiation Oncology
Edited by W. Schlegel, T. Bortfeld, and A.-L. Grosu

Multimodal Concepts for Integration of Cytotoxic Drugs and Radiation Therapy
Edited by J. M. Brown, M. P. Mehta, and C. Nieder

Technical Basis of Radiation Therapy
Practical Clinical Applications
4th Revised Edition
Edited by S. H. Levitt, J. A. Purdy, C. A. Perez, and S. Vijayakumar

CURED I • LENT
Late Effects of Cancer Treatment on Normal Tissues
Edited by P. Rubin, L. S. Constine, L. B. Marks, and P. Okunieff

Radiotherapy for Non-Malignant Disorders
Contemporary Concepts and Clinical Results
Edited by M. H. Seegenschmiedt, H.-B. Makoski, K.-R. Trott, and L. W. Brady

CURED II • LENT
Cancer Survivorship Research and Education
Late Effects on Normal Tissues
Edited by P. Rubin, L. S. Constine, L. B. Marks, and P. Okunieff

Radiation Oncology
An Evidence-Based Approach
Edited by J. J. Lu and L. W. Brady

Primary Optic Nerve Sheath Meningioma
Edited by B. Jeremić, and S. Pitz

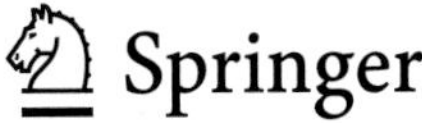

Printing and Binding: Stürtz GmbH, Würzburg